Pocket Companion of Critical Care: Immediate Concerns

ROBERT R. KIRBY, M.D.
Professor of Anesthesiology
University of Florida College of Medicine
Gainesville, Florida

ROBERT W. TAYLOR, M.D.
Assistant Professor of Medicine
Baylor College of Medicine
Director, Medical Intensive Care Unit
The Methodist Hospital
Houston, Texas

JOSEPH M. CIVETTA, M.D.
Professor of Surgery, Anesthesiology, Medicine, and Pathology
University of Miami School of Medicine
Director, Surgical Intensive Care Unit
University of Miami/Jackson Memorial Medical Center
Miami, Florida

Pocket Companion of Critical Care: Immediate Concerns

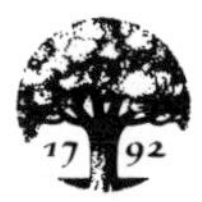

J. B. LIPPINCOTT COMPANY
Philadelphia
Grand Rapids
New York
St. Louis
San Francisco
London
Sydney
Tokyo

Acquisitions Editor: Nancy Mullins
Production Manager: Janet Greenwood
Production: Ruttle, Shaw & Wetherill
Compositor: Ruttle, Shaw & Wetherill
Printer/Binder: R. R. Donnelley & Sons

1 3 5 6 4 2

Library of Congress Cataloging-in-Publication Data

Pocket companion of critical care : immediate concerns / Robert R. Kirby, Robert W. Taylor, Joseph M. Civetta.
p. cm.
Consists primarily of information compiled from the larger comprehensive textbook, Critical care / [edited by] Joseph M. Civetta, Robert W. Taylor, Robert R. Kirby. c1988.
Includes bibliographical references.
ISBN 0-397-51030-6
1. Critical care medicine—Handbooks, manuals, etc. I. Kirby, Robert R. II. Taylor, Robert W. (Robert Wesley), 1949– . III. Civetta, Joseph M. IV. Critical care.
[DNLM: 1. Critical Care—handbooks. WX 39 P741]
RC86.8.P63 1990
616' .028—dc20
DNLM/DLC
for Library of Congress 89-13406
CIP

The authors and publisher have exerted every effort to ensure that drug selection and dosage set forth in this text are in accord with current recommendations and practice at the time of publication. However, in view of ongoing research, changes in government regulations, and the constant flow of information relating to drug therapy and drug reactions, the reader is urged to check the package insert for each drug for any change in indications and dosage and for added warnings and precautions. This is particularly important when the recommended agent is a new or infrequently employed drug.

Preface

One's first exposure to a busy intensive care unit (ICU) can be unsettling at best and panic-provoking at worst. Even seasoned ICU personnel can be frustrated by the seeming chaos associated with the diagnosis and treatment of critical illness. Frequent requirements for immediate decisions and implantation of complicated therapy make it essential that potentially life-saving issues be sorted out in some meaningful fashion. In this fashion, a reasoned approach with a realistic hope of success may be achieved. The corollary, of course, is that decisions concerning when to decrease or cease efforts in hopeless cases are equally important.

This book attempts to accomplish the aforementioned goals in a logical, systematic, and perhaps most importantly, concise fashion. Major organ system dysfunction in medical and surgical patients is discussed with primary emphasis focused on how and what to do in the first 24 to 48 hours of a patient's ICU admission. Most of the information has been compiled from the larger comprehensive textbook, *Critical Care*. For those individuals who desire a more in-depth presentation of a particular subject, the relevant chapter in the latter publication is listed.

As with *Critical Care,* we hope that *Pocket Companion of Critical Care: Immediate Concerns* will be both read and useful. For the neophyte it should prove valuable in formulating an approach to the bewildering number and variety of illnesses in the ICU population. For the experienced practitioner—physician, nurse, respiratory therapist, or other health care provider—it should prove to be a valuable resource that reinforces the knowledge base that is already present. In some instances, it may suggest a new approach or recall to mind one previously learned but subsequently forgotten.

The author/editors are first and foremost clinicians in medicine, surgery, and anesthesiology. We have all had research experience, but have never left the clinical arena. Our interests are widely divergent in some areas but convergent in others. Hopefully, this fact will be apparent and will result in both pleasurable and informative reading.

Robert R. Kirby, M.D.
Robert W. Taylor, M.D.
Joseph M. Civetta, M.D.

Contents

V RESPIRATORY DISORDERS 291

VI NEUROLOGIC/PSYCHIATRIC DISORDERS 401

XI HEMATOLOGIC/ONCOLOGIC DISORDERS 565

XII SKIN AND MUSCLE DISORDERS 597

XIII ICU INFECTIONS 615

XIV ENVIRONMENTAL HAZARDS 647

Pocket Companion of Critical Care: Immediate Concerns

I. Fundamental Considerations

1
Clinical Assessment in the ICU

Controversies surrounding the accuracy of currently available techniques make it imperative that careful clinical assessment be used to correlate with invasive measurements whenever possible. For example, the differences noted between invasive and noninvasive blood pressure measurements are well documented and have led to the perception that "at times, the reading, which is considered the more 'normal' of the two or more in keeping with the patient's clinical condition, is chosen to represent arterial pressure." Also, inaccuracies associated with the measurement of pulmonary artery pressures are reported that make clinical correlation and integration of data vitally important. The care and the setup of electronic equipment require time and precision if accurate and reproducible results are to be recorded. Of concern in modern intensive care units (ICUs) is the apparent lack of similar precision in the performance of a clinical examination. Proper lighting, patient position, equipment, and, perhaps most important, time are required to make appropriate judgments. The early morning rounds scarcely allow enough time to read the enormously detailed flow sheet and fail to provide for appropriate patient evaluation.

As described by Goldenheim and Kazemi, "Critically ill patients require frequent monitoring of their vital signs, which in addition to providing important data about cardiopulmonary function, brings a member of the health care team into close contact with the patient. This permits frequent observation of the patient's sensorium, skin temperature and color, and respiratory effort." Obviously, the intent is to integrate the objective with the subjective—the so-called "feel" of the experienced ICU nurse or clinician. It is the subjective information that, when appropriately used, provides the cornerstone on which all therapeutic decisions should be based.

RESPIRATORY ASSESSMENT

The patient who is seen to be breathing is in respiratory failure until proven otherwise. As an axiom, this statement is useful because it draws attention to the obvious, which is often overlooked. On or off a ventilator, use of accessory muscles of respiration and (in adult patients) rates greater than 30 per minute indicate respiratory insufficiency. The blood gases may appear adequate, and, in some cases, patients may tolerate the condition well. In the long term, however, the likelihood is that the patient will require some intervention.

Another observation that is misinterpreted often concerns the patient who is "fighting the ventilator," that is, the patient's breathing pattern is asynchronous with ventilator cycling, and the patient and care team are all uncomfortable. Normally, this observation should be interpreted that the patient is not receiving adequate ventilatory support rather than that the patient's efforts are inappropriate. A normal ventilatory pattern is one that is unobtrusive to the observer, that is, each inhalation is followed by passive exhalation, with a pause before a subsequent breath. Tachypnea in adults (rates above 30 breaths per minute) is usually an indication of respiratory distress. In fact, newer ventilatory support modes (mandatory minute ventilation, pressure support) are often adjusted in an attempt to control respiratory rate rather than in an attempt to provide either a specific tidal volume or inspiratory pressure. Another important feature of patients receiving mechanical ventilation is the appropriate auscultatory clinical examination. Too often, respiratory rate is counted by placing a hand on the abdomen and counting the number of times per minute that the abdominal effort is sensed. Unfortunately, although respiratory effort is initiated during this maneuver, gas passage into the lungs is often asynchronous and does not necessarily equal the abdominal effort. The appropriate way to count respirations in any ICU or recovery room setting is by placing a stethoscope over the lung fields and auscultating each breath.

An additional influence of clinical evaluation is seen in the often difficult decision of whether to intubate a patient. Certainly, arterial blood gases are a poor indicator, and all students are warned of the possibility that a normal P_{CO_2} may be a reflection of inadequacy rather than appropriate gas exchange. This is true in patients who initially hyperventilate but then tire and develop normocapnia which, if not treated, rapidly leads to decompensation. The clinician can often decide on intubation by observing the patient, noting the degree of respiratory effort, and counting breaths. In adults, rates greater than 30 are poorly tolerated and should signal caution. Also, the patient's ability to converse provides an indication of air hunger. The individual should be asked to breathe in and then count aloud on exhalation. Patients who cannot count beyond five or ten are at extreme risk and should be monitored closely in an environment in which intubation facilities are available instantly. Below five, prophylactic intubation is indicated, and in the gray zone of five to ten many would advocate mechanical support. Although not particularly scientific, these guidelines often help in a doubtful patient who demonstrates acceptable "numbers."

HEMODYNAMIC ASSESSMENT

Assessment of the circulatory system should not be left to cardiac output and blood gas evaluations. Again, simple clinical assessment often helps to determine the volume status of a patient, and, although clinical prediction of invasively obtained filling pressures may be low, it is unwise to hesitate in providing appropriate therapy while waiting for invasive monitoring to be established. Certainly, patients can indicate their volume status in answer to the simple question of "are you thirsty," which often helps to clarify an otherwise confusing situation. Patients who are truly thirsty, can differentiate the sensation of thirst from that of a dry mouth. Often a low intravascular volume and associated high serum osmolarity are reflected clinically as thirst. On the other hand, patients who are satisfied with a sponging of the mouth to alleviate dryness usually do not demonstrate signs or symptoms of a low intravascular volume. Unfortunately, urine output and concentrating ability do not always reflect accurately intravascular volume because of coincident hormonal abnormalities associated with anesthesia or stress.

Other indicators of hemodynamic stability are the rate of temperature restitution after surgery and the changes in blood pressure associated with rewarming. Certainly, patients who return to the recovery room or ICU at 34°C may exhibit hypertension and tachycardia. As they are rewarmed, it is not unusual to see marked decreases in blood pressure associated with continued tachycardia. This should not be surprising because of the increased intravascular space made available by peripheral vasodilation, and appropriate volume resuscitation should be anticipated during this period. On the other hand, these changes may be minimized by using vasodilating drugs such as nitroprusside during the operative stage, which may prevent vasoconstriction and enable adequate maintenance of intravascular volume. Clinically, the speed at which a patient rewarms and the degree of hemodynamic instability encountered are often indicative of the relative state of intravascular volume and hemodynamic compromise. Patients with low filling pressures and cardiac outputs tend to require a longer time for rewarming, associated with a metabolic acidosis and large swings in pressure as the temperature rises. In addition, the requirement for passive heaters is greater than that seen in patients with adequate preload and stable cardiac output.

IATROGENIC CONCERNS

Perhaps the most important aspect of clinical evaluation in critical care medicine—the prevention of iatrogenesis—is often overlooked or undervalued. A morning rounding challenge for all critical-care-based physicians should be to determine the number of mistakes and potential mistakes that are evident in the setup of the patient's monitoring equipment, ventilator, or associated items such as chest tubes and urinary catheters. In addition, charting errors and numbers of medications should be noted. In all instances, recorded data should be scrutinized and the patient's environment checked for hazards. For example, inappropriate ventilator settings may provoke respiratory paradox and a worsened patient condition. Problems may be as simple as an inappropriately set peak flow rate or inspiratory sensitivity, either of which can provoke an apparent paradox between patient and machine. In addition, calibration constants on cardiac output computers, location of flow-through temperature probes, attention to details of injectate volume, and zero reference points for transducers can all affect the perceived appropriateness of care.

All clinicians should become familiar with the noises of the ICU, and the sounds of a ventilator that works under stress should be distinguished from those of one that is working normally. In the former situation, give careful attention to the patient and make appropriate adjustments to the mechanical device. Usually the patient and his condition determine the ventilatory requirement, rather than *vice versa*. In addition, the amount of data recorded on most patients is extensive, and clinicians must not get overwhelmed by a regurgitation of normal data that obscure the critical points; rather, detailed appraisal of appropriate abnormalities should be routine for all rounding teams. In this way, the subtle areas of ICU practice may be exposed. For example, the suddenly abnormal blood gas may be due to inappropriate sampling, with excess heparin remaining in the sample syringe, rather than to sudden deterioration of the patient's condition. Appropriate critical and clinical appraisal of the patient may keep the clinician aware that although subtle changes may be reflected only by sophisticated monitoring techniques, major changes are unusual without some form of clinical manifestation. In many instances, the clinician works outside the conventions of normal numbers and purely within the boundaries of clinical intuition and careful physical examination. For these techniques to be valuable, repeated assessment is as important for clinical decision-making as it is for trend monitoring and interventional management techniques.

For further information, please see Chapter 25 in Civetta JM, Taylor RW, Kirby RR: Critical Care. *Philadelphia: J. B. Lippincott, 1988*

BIBLIOGRAPHY

Allardyce DB: Monitoring of the critically ill patient. *Can J Surg* 1978; 21:75

Chuyn DA: A comparison of intra-arterial and auscultatory blood pressure readings. *Heart Lung* 1985; 14:223

Connors AF, McCaffree DR, Gray BA: Evaluation of right heart catheterization in the critically ill patient without acute myocardial infarction. *N Engl J Med* 1983; 308:263

Del Guercio LRM, Cohn JD: Monitoring operating risk in the elderly. *JAMA* 1980; 243:1350

Drake JJ: Locating the external reference point for central venous pressure determination. *Nurs Res* 1974; 23:475

Eichorn JH, Cooper JB, Cullen DJ, et al: Standards for patient monitoring during anesthesia at Harvard Medical School. *JAMA* 1986; 256:1017

Goldenheim PD, Kazemi H: Cardiopulmonary monitoring of critically ill patients: I. *N Engl J Med* 1984; 311:717

Henning RJ, Wiener F, Valdes S, et al: Measurement of toe temperature for assessing the severity of acute circulatory failure. *Surg Gynecol Obstet* 1979; 149:1

Holder DA: Does hemodynamic monitoring complement conventional methods of assessment in the critically ill cardiac patient? *Can Med Assoc J* 1979; 121:895

Knaus WA, Draper EA, Wagner DP, et al: An evaluation of outcome from intensive care in major medical centers. *Ann Intern Med* 1986; 104:410

Maloney JV: The trouble with patient monitoring. *Ann Surg* 1968; 168:605

Miller L: Neurological assessment: A practical guide for the critical care nurse. *J Neurosurg Nurs* 1979; 11:2

Nadeau S, Noble WH: Misinterpretation of pressure measurements from the pulmonary artery catheter. *Can Anaesth Soc J* 1986; 33:352

Pollack MM, Urs ER, Getson PR, et al: Accurate prediction of the outcome of pediatric intensive care. *N Engl J Med* 1987; 316:134

Rao TLK, Jacobs KH, El-Etr AA: Reinfarction following anesthesia in patients with myocardial infarction. *Anesthesiology* 1983; 59:499

Schroeder SA: Outcome assessment 70 years later. Are we ready? *N Engl J Med* 1987; 316:160

Sibbald WJ, Cunningham DR, Chin DN: Noncardiac or cardiac pulmonary edema? A practical approach to clinical differentiation in critically ill patients. *Chest* 1983; 84:452

Venus B, Mathru M, Smith RA, et al: Direct versus indirect blood pressure measurements in critically ill patients. *Heart Lung* 1985; 14:228

Webster's New Collegiate Dictionary, Springfield, Massachusetts, G & C Merrian, 1977

2

Fluids and Electrolytes in the Critically Ill

FLUID COMPARTMENTS

Total body water makes up 60% of the body weight in an average male and approximately 50% in an average female. In thin males and females, the values are 65% and 55%, respectively, whereas in obese persons, they are 60% and 50%. In a 70-kg lean adult man, the intracellular compartment contains 66% (28 liters) of total body water and the extracellular compartment 34% (14 liters). The extracellular compartment is composed of intravascular and interstitial subcompartments. The former contains approximately 3.5 liters and the latter approximately 10.5 liters (Figs. 2-1 and 2-2).

If no solute is present, the added fluid distributes evenly through the total body water until the concentrations of solute in both compartments are equal. Clinically, this sequence only occurs when dextrose solutions are infused.

In the prototypical 70-kg man, 30 minutes after rapid infusion of 1 liter of 5% dextrose in water (D_5W), the compartments are enlarged to the following dimensions: total body water, 43 liters; intracellular water, 28.8 liters; extracellular water, 14.2 liters; interstitial water, 10.6 liters; and intravascular water, 3.6 liters (Fig. 2-3). After 30 minutes, only 100 ml additional volume is in the intravascular compartment. In contrast, 30 minutes after rapid infusion of 1 liter of Ringer's lactate solution, total body water is 43 liters; intracellular water, 28 liters; extracellular water, 15 liters; interstitial water, 11.2 liters; and intravascular water, 3.8 liters (Fig. 2-4). Here, we have enlarged the intravascular compartment by 300 ml, or 200 ml more than results from the same volume infusion of D_5W.

This line of reasoning becomes somewhat more complicated when colloid solutions are considered. The half-life of albumin is approximately 20 days in the body but about 16 hours in plasma. Ten percent of infused albumin leaves the vascular space within 2 hours, and 75% within 2 days. The membranes between the fluid compartments are semipermeable; thus albumin, like crystalloid solutions, crosses over, but at a slower rate. If we rapidly infuse 100 ml of 25% albumin into a healthy individual, 30 minutes later essentially all of the infused volume is within the intravascular compartment (Fig. 2-5). In our 70-kg man, the volume changes are as follows: total body water, 42.1

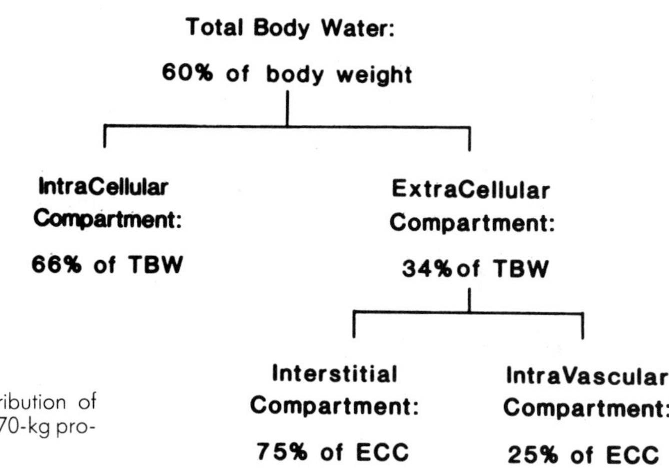

Figure 2-1 Distribution of body water in a 70-kg prototypical man.

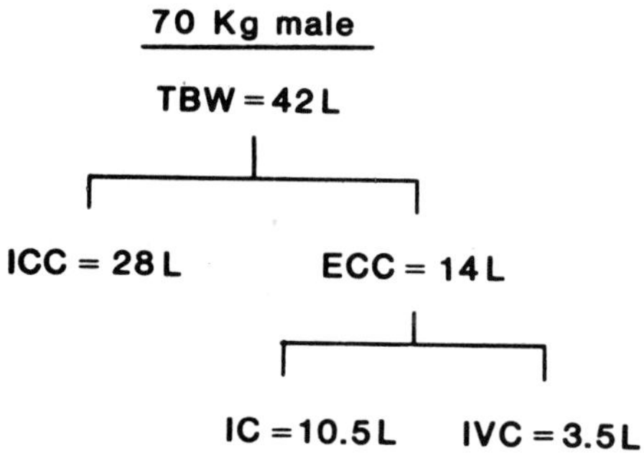

70 Kg male

TBW = 42 L

ICC = 28 L

ECC = 14 L

IC = 10.5 L

IVC = 3.5 L

Figure 2-2 Normal fluid volumes of the intracellular and extracellular compartments (*ICC, ECC*). TBW = total body water; IC = interstitial compartment; IVC = intravascular compartment.

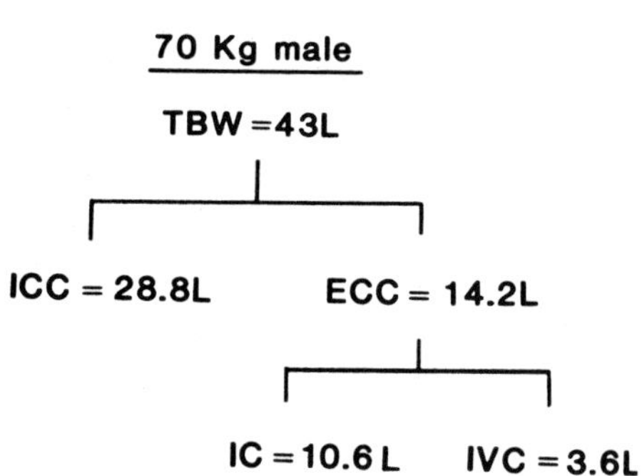

Figure 2-3 Effects of infusion of 1 liter of D_5W.

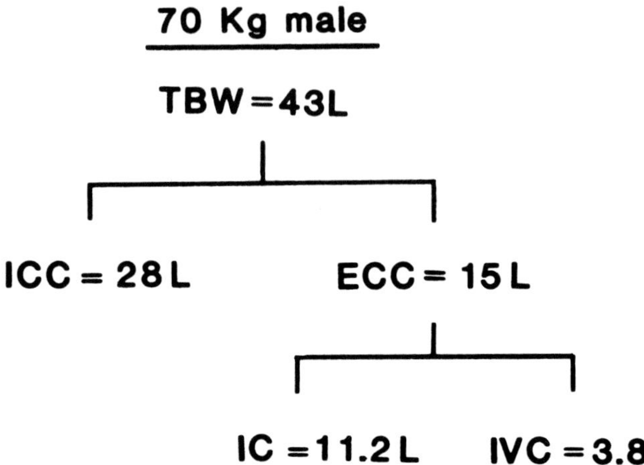

Figure 2-4 Effects of infusion of 1 liter of Ringer's lactate.

liters; intracellular water, 28 liters; extracellular water, 14.1 liters; interstitial water, 10.5 liters; and intravascular water, 3.6 liters. Thus, immediately after infusion, the intravascular compartment is increased by only 100 ml. However, each gram of intravascular albumin is thought to "bind" 18 ml of water because of its oncotic activity. Thus the 25 g in 100 ml of infused albumin theoretically draws another 450 ml of interstitial fluid into the intravascular space. After equilibration, the extracellular compartment still is composed of

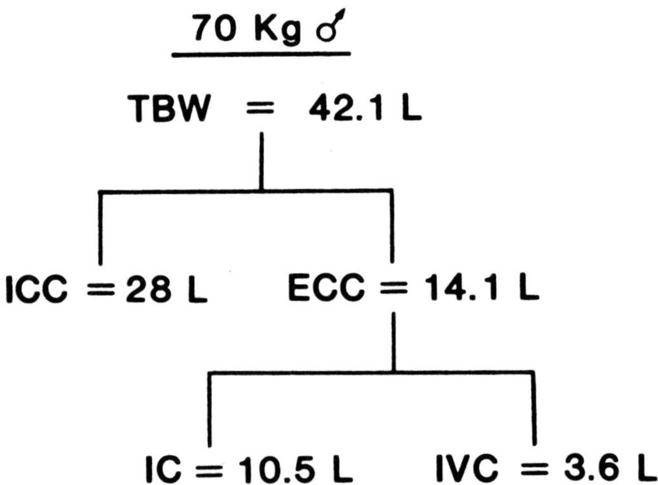

Figure 2-5 Distribution of 100 ml of 25% albumin 30 minutes after infusion.

14.1 liters; however, the interstitial compartment decreases to 10.05 liters, and the intravascular compartment increases to 4.05 liters.

DISORDERS OF SODIUM AND WATER METABOLISM

HYPONATREMIA

Isotonic

Isotonic hyponatremia (Table 2-1) is characterized by a low serum Na^+ but a normal measured plasma osmolality. Common causes include hyperproteinemic states (multiple myeloma, Waldenström's macroglobulinemia) and hyperlipidemic states (familial lipoprotein lipase deficiency and hyperlipoproteinemias secondary to diabetes mellitus, alcohol abuse, and use of oral contraceptives). Clinical laboratories report serum Na^+ results in meq/liter of *plasma,* rather than meq/liter of *plasma water.* Thus the reported concentration is artifactually low. This difference can be corrected by the formula in Table 2-2. Attempts to correct the pseudohyponatremia, especially if diuretics are used, can result in significant iatrogenic complications.

Hypertonic

Hypertonic hyponatremia (Table 2-3) is diagnosed by low serum Na^+ and plasma osmolality > 290 mOsm/kg H_2O. Management entails restoration of the free water deficit, volume deficit, and hyperglycemia to normal values. First correct the measured serum Na^+ to its normal euglycemic value:

$$Na^+_{euglycemic} = \text{measured } Na^+ + 0.028\,(\text{glucose} - 100)$$

Signs of hypovolemia can be addressed by infusion of isotonic saline solution.

Next anticipate correcting the underlying cause. In the diabetic patient, the presence of occult infection, myocardial ischemia, trauma, a cerebrovascular accident, or anesthetic/surgical stress should be assessed. Glycerol and mannitol are most often used to treat cerebral edema. If laboratory abnormalities become clinically relevant, these treatments should be considered.

Two major complications can result from the treatment of hypertonic hypernatremia related to either diabetic ketoacidosis or nonketotic hyperos-

TABLE 2-1 ISOTONIC HYPONATREMIA

Diagnosis:	↓ Na^+; normal osmolality
Causes:	Hyperproteinemic states Hyperlipidemic states
Management:	Work-up underlying cause Do not panic
Complications:	Related to underlying disease

TABLE 2-2 DECREASE IN SERUM SODIUM WITH HYPERLIPIDEMIA

HYPERLIPIDEMIA
Decrease (meq/liter) = Plasma lipid (mg/dl) × 0.002
HYPERPROTEINEMIA
Decrease (meq/liter) = Increment of total protein > 8 g/dl × 0.25

molar coma. Hypoglycemia, either relative or absolute, resulting from aggressive insulin therapy is avoidable. Clinically apparent cerebral edema is an uncommon complication of therapy for diabetic ketoacidosis. A recent paper documented six cases of subclinical brain swelling found on repetitive computed tomography scans of the head in boys aged 11 to 14 years with diabetic ketoacidosis. The mechanism of the alterations in brain volume is not entirely clear, but may be related to vigorous hydration, insulin therapy, or damage of cerebral capillary endothelium. Although no specific therapy prevents cerebral edema, mannitol may be useful in its treatment. We recommend slow correction of both glucose and water deficit in patients with diabetic ketoacidosis and nonketotic hyperosmolar coma as a possible means to reduce the occurrence of cerebral edema, although evidence on this point is lacking.

Hypotonic

Hypotonic (true) hyponatremia (Table 2-4) is characterized by a decrease in serum Na^+ and plasma osmolality. Certain laboratory data are valuable, particularly serum chloride (Cl^-), HCO_3^-, K^+, BUN, creatinine, glucose, and, of course, Na^+. Urinary measurements must include Na^+, K^+, Cl^-, and osmolality. An accurate determination of urine output also is essential. Numerous drugs can be associated with isovolemic true hyponatremia (Table 2-5).

TABLE 2-3 HYPERTONIC HYPONATREMIA

Diagnosis:	↓ Na^+, plasma osmolality > 290 mOsm/kg H_2O
Causes:	Hyperglycemia
	Mannitol
	Gylcerol
Management:	Correct volume deficit
	1. Insulin to slowly decrease glucose
	2. Hypotonic saline to correct free water deficit
	Correct underlying cause
	1. Why is patient hyperglycemic?
	2. Why is glycerol or mannitol in use?
Complications:	Hypoglycemia
	Cerebral edema

TABLE 2-4 HYPOTONIC HYPONATREMIA

Diagnosis:	↓ Na^+, plasma osmolality < 270 mOsm/kg H_2O Differentiate type by assessment of ECF volume
Causes:	Hypovolemic 1. Extrarenal: GI loss—vomiting, diarrhea Burns Third space (*e.g.*, pancreatitis) 2. Renal: Diuretics Adrenal failure Renal parenchymal disease Hypervolemic 1. Advanced renal disease: Acute renal failure Chronic renal insufficiency 2. Edematous states: Congestive heart failure Cirrhosis of the liver Nephrotic syndrome Severe hypoproteinemia 2° nutritional/GI disease Isovolemic 1. Stress 2. Adrenal insufficiency 3. Hypothyroidism 4. Drugs 5. K^+ depletion/diuretic use 6. Psychogenic polydipsia 7. SIADH
Management:	Hypovolemic—isotonic saline Hypervolemic/isovolemic—restrict free H_2O Manage underlying disorders
Complications:	CNS—seizures, coma, death, residual effects Decompensation of underlying disorders

TABLE 2-5 DRUGS ASSOCIATED WITH ISOVOLEMIC TRUE HYPONATREMIA

Agent	**Mechanism***
Morphine	1
Chlorpropamide	1,2
Nonsteroidal anti-inflammatory agents (*e.g.*, aspirin)	2
Vincristine	1
Cyclophosphamide	?
Clofibrate	1
Carbamazepine	1
?Antipsychotics	?
?Antidepressants	?
Oxytocin	Stimulates ADH

*1 = stimulates central release of ADH; 2 = potentiates peripheral action of ADH.

HYPERNATREMIA

Water Loss

Pure water loss (Table 2-6) occurs with increased insensible loss of water through the skin and in thyrotoxicosis. The most important step in diagnosis and management is clinical evaluation of the ECF volume and calculation of the approximate water deficit. Whenever possible, water replacement should be done slowly with oral fluids. Replacement should be rapid only if severe symptoms and hypertonicity are present. In this case, enough free water (D_5W) should be given to replace half of the calculated deficit, with the remainder infused over the subsequent 24 to 48 hours.

The major complications of pure water loss hypernatremia are isotonic water intoxication and cerebral edema resulting from too rapid correction of hypertonicity.

Diabetes Insipidus. Diabetes insipidus (DI) is central or nephrogenic. Central DI can be idiopathic or associated with head trauma, neurosurgical procedures, brain tumors, CNS granulomatous disease (tuberculosis and sarcoidosis), intracranial aneurysms, meningitis, encephalitis, and Guillain-Barré syndrome. It may be complete or partial.

Nephrogenic DI can be congenital or acquired, with the latter more common and less severe than the former. Several disease processes are associ-

TABLE 2-6 HYPERNATREMIA: PURE WATER LOSS

Diagnosis:	↑ Na^+, urine osmolality ≥2 × plasma osmolality (except in diabetes insipidus), moderate azotemia, ↓ urine volume, appropriate clinical picture
Causes:	↑ Insensible loss from skin, lungs 1. ↑ Environmental temperature 2. Fever 3. Thyrotoxicosis 4. Burn injury 5. Inadequately humidified ventilator 6. Diabetes insipidus
Management:	Calculate water deficit: $0.6 \times \text{body wt (kg)} \times \frac{PNa^+}{140} - 1$ Correct underlying cause if possible Replace water deficit
Complications:	Isotonic water intoxication

ated with nephrogenic DI, including sickle cell nephropathy, chronic pyelonephritis, and multiple myeloma. Hypercalcemia, hypokalemia secondary to diminished medullary hypertonicity, and drugs such as lithium, demeclocycline, amphotericin B, and methoxyflurane also cause nephrogenic DI.

The hallmark of DI is polydipsia and polyuria, with urinary output ranging from 3 to 15 liters/day. The diagnosis of central DI is made by stimulating ADH release. ADH causes urine osmolality to increase above 800 mOsm/kg H_2O. No additional increase occurs with exogenous ADH injection. Therapy for complete central DI includes a synthetic nasal spray, 1-desamino-8-D-arginine vasopressin (DDAVP), which is more potent and has a longer half-life than the parent hormone and controls urine output for 12 to 24 hours after a single dose. Also available are vasopressin tannate in oil, 2 to 5 units IM every 24 to 48 hours; and lysine vasopressin, administered as a nasal spray every 4 to 6 hours. Nephrogenic DI is somewhat more difficult to treat in that it is not responsive to ADH or to agents that enhance the renal response to this hormone. Acquired nephrogenic DI is initially treated by correcting the underlying cause (*e.g.*, hyperkalemia or hypercalcemia); drugs such as lithium or demeclocycline should be terminated. Thiazide diuretics or salt and protein restriction enhance proximal fluid reabsorption by decreasing distal fluid delivery. In congenital nephrogenic DI, urine output may be decreased by as much as 50% through the use of thiazide diuretics.

Hypotonic Fluid Loss

CAUSES. Hypotonic fluid loss is the most common form of hypernatremia (Table 2-7). Management involves replacement of the ECF loss with normal saline, followed by correction of the free water deficit with hypotonic solutions (Table 2-8). Complications include vascular collapse and isotonic water intoxication with overly rapid correction. Peritoneal dialysis or hemodialysis may be used.

TABLE 2-7 HYPOTONIC FLUID LOSS

Diagnosis:	↑ Na^+, signs and symptoms ECF depletion, oliguria (unless due to use of osmotic agents), U_{Na^+} variable
Causes:	Gastroenteritis
	Osmotic diuresis
	(1) Urea secondary to high-protein tube feeding
	(2) Glucose
	(3) Mannitol or glycerol
	Peritoneal dialysis
Management:	Replace ECF loss with physiologic saline or colloid
	Then use hypotonic solutions to slowly correct free water deficit
Complications:	Vascular collapse
	Isotonic water intoxication and cerebral edema

TABLE 2-8 CALCULATING NA^+ AND WATER ABNORMALITIES IN WATER LOSS HYPERNATREMIA

$$Na^+ \text{ excess (meq)} = 0.6 \times \text{body weight (kg)} \times (\text{current } P_{Na^+} - 140)$$

$$\text{Water deficit (liters)} = 0.6 \times \text{body weight (kg)} \times \frac{\text{current } P_{Na^+}}{140} - 1$$

POTASSIUM DISORDERS

HYPOKALEMIA

Hypokalemia is defined arbitrarily as a serum K^+ level ≤ 3.5 meq/liter. Essential to the evaluation of this disorder are spot urinary K^+ and Cl^- levels, arterial *p*H and HCO_3^-, a careful history and physical examination, and perusal of the patient's list of medications. Causes are listed in Table 2-9. Problems in the ICU commonly are drug-induced through increased $Na^+ - K^+$ exchange, increased Na^+ delivery to the distal tubule, and cellular shifts (Table 2-10).

A spot urine K^+ may be obtained to differentiate hypokalemia due to gastrointestinal losses from that due to renal losses. In the former, urinary K^+ should be less than 20 meq/liter, whereas in the latter, the value is greater than 20 meq/liter. A better index is the fractional excretion of K^+, which is equal to urine K^+/plasma K^+ divided by urine creatinine/plasma creatinine $\times$ 100. A fractional excretion less than 6% is compatible with appropriate K^+ conservation.

Clinical features of hypokalemia include impaired neuromuscular function (weakness, paralysis, myonecrosis), paralytic ileus, cardiac abnormalities (conduction defects, dysrhythmias, altered sensitivity to digitalis, and, possibly, myocardial cell necrosis), renal abnormalities, and neuropsychiatric disturbances (depression, faulty memory, confusion). In an emergency situation (e.g., myonecrosis or significant dysrhythmias), K^+ should be replaced intravenously by a solution containing 40 to 60 meq/liter, infused at a rate ≤ 40 meq/hour.

If oral intake is not possible, K^+ can be administered intravenously at a concentration of 40 meq/liter, given at a rate of approximately 10 meq/hour. Magnesium deficit, if present, must be corrected in order to correct the hypokalemia.

HYPERKALEMIA

Hyperkalemia (Table 2-11) is defined arbitrarily as a K^+ value above 5.5 meq/liter. It generally is treated if there is an abrupt rise from normal to ≥ 6.5 meq/liter, or if *any* level is associated with electrocardiographic (EKG) changes. Drugs, some of which are listed in Table 2-12, can cause hyperkalemia.

TABLE 2-9 HYPOKALEMIA

Definition:	$K^+ \leq 3.5$ meq/liter
Diagnosis:	K^+, spot U_{K^+}, history, medication list, U_{Cl^-}, arterial pH, P_{CO_2}, HCO_3^-
Causes:	Factitious (1) WBC count (> 100,000 at room temperature) Intracellular shift (1) Alkalemia (2) Insulin therapy (3) β-adrenergic stimulation (4) Anabolism Gastrointestinal loss (1) Diarrhea (2) Vomiting (3) Enteric or biliary fistula Renal loss (1) Increased urinary flow (2) Hypomagnesemia (3) Increased mineralocorticoid activity Drugs
Management:	Correct K^+ abnormality (1) Emergency: IV (peripheral vein)—≤ 40 meq/hr in a concentration of 40 to 60 meq/liter (2) Nonemergency Oral—wax matrix KCl 40 to 120 meq/day Intravenous—10 meq/hr in a concentration of 40 meq/liter Correct Mg^{++} abnormality if present Work-up cause
Complications:	Hyperkalemia with rapid/excessive correction Due to hypokalemia (see text)

Clinical features of hyperkalemia primarily involve neuromuscular abnormalities. Weakness, paresthesias, descending paralysis, and flaccid quadriplegia are seen. Cardiac abnormalities are the most feared sequelae of hyperkalemia and include conduction defects as well as dysrhythmias. Hyponatremia and acidosis potentiate the adverse effects of hyperkalemia on the heart. With a serum K^+ of 5.5 to 6.5 meq/liter, one sees peaking or "tenting" of the T-waves. An elevation > 6.5 meq/liter produces flattening of the P-wave, prolongation of the PR interval, and a widening or slurring of the QRS complex. At levels > 8 meq/liter, a sine wave pattern and ventricular fibrillation or cardiac arrest ensue.

Emergency management of hyperkalemia involves several interventions. First, 10 ml to 30 ml of a 10% solution of calcium gluconate is injected intravenously over 3 to 5 minutes, with continuous EKG monitoring. The onset

TABLE 2-10 DRUGS ASSOCIATED WITH HYPOKALEMIA

Agent	Mechanism
Laxatives Hypertonic enemas	↑ Gastrointestinal loss
Amphotericin B Polymyxin B Outdated tetracycline Gentamicin-cephalexin combination PGF_2 Neomycin	Direct toxic effect on renal tubule
Steroids (IV, oral, nasal) Carbenoxalone L-dopa Gentamicin	Enhanced $Na^+ - K^+$ exchange
Thiazides Furosemide Ethacrynic acid Bumetanide	Increased distal tubular Na^+ delivery
Penicillin Ampicillin Carbenicillin Nacillin Ticarcillin	Presence of nonreabsorbable anions in the distal tubule
Barium Lithium β-Agonists	Cellular K^+ shifts

(Modified from Nanji AA: Drug-induced electrolyte disorders. *Drug Intell Clin Pharm* 1983; 17:175)

of action is within several circulation times, but the duration is only 30 to 60 minutes, thus a second dose may be required.

If hypovolemia and hyponatremia are present, a bolus of normal saline may be given intravenously. More commonly, $NaHCO_3$, 50 ml to 100 ml of a 7.5% solution, is used. Both Na^+ and $NaHCO_3$ enhance intracellular movement of K^+, and the onset of action is within 15 to 30 minutes. A glucose-insulin infusion can be useful: 500 ml of a 10% dextrose solution plus 10 units of regular insulin should be infused intravenously over 1 hour; the onset of action is within 15 to 30 minutes.

Loop diuretics such as furosemide, ethacrynic acid, or bumetanide facilitate distal tubular Na^+ delivery and thus increase K^+ excretion. Oral or rectal sodium or calcium polystyrene sulfonate, in combination with a sorbitol solution, will exchange Na^+ or CA^{++} for K^+ in the gastrointestinal tract. The enema is effective at approximately 60 minutes, whereas the oral form takes 120 minutes. If these measures are ineffective or if renal failure is present, peritoneal dialysis or hemodialysis can be initiated. A transvenous pacemaker

TABLE 2-11 HYPERKALEMIA

Diagnosis:	$K^+ \geq 5.5$ meq/liter
Causes:	Factitious
	1. Thrombocytosis
	2. Leukocytosis
	3. Hemolysis
	4. Infectious mononucleosis
	Increased intake
	1. Banked blood (> 5 days old)
	2. Rapid IV infusion of K^+
	Abnormal distribution
	1. Acidemia (some forms)
	2. Catabolism
	3. Extracellular hypertonicity
	4. Insulin deficiency
	5. β-Blockers
	Decreased renal K^+ secretion
	1. Acute renal failure
	2. Decreased mineralocorticoid activity
	3. Decreased urinary Na^+
	Drugs
Management:	Emergency
	1. 10–30 ml 10% calcium gluconate
	2. Saline solution or sodium bicarbonate (50–100 ml 7.5% solution)
	3. Glucose insulin (500 ml 10% dextrose plus 10 units regular insulin IV infusion over 1 hr)
	4. Loop diuretics
	5. Sodium or calcium polystyrene sulfonate + sorbitol, given orally (25 g/dose) or by retention enema (50 g/dose)
	6. Dialysis
	7. Transvenous pacemaker
	Nonemergency
	1. K^+ restriction (40–60) meq/day)
	2. Correct acidosis or hypovolemia if present
	3. Treat underlying disease
Complications:	Hypokalemia
	Due to hyperkalemia (see text)

is indicated when atrioventricular block or severe bradycardia is not reversed within minutes following calcium gluconate or $NaHCO_3$ infusion.

CALCIUM DISORDERS

HYPOCALCEMIA

Hypocalcemia is reflected by Ca^{++} levels < 2.0 meq/liter or total serum CA < 8.5 mg/dl (Table 2-13).

Parathyroid insufficiency is seen most commonly in an acquired form after neck surgery. It may also occur following trauma to the neck and from tumor, sarcoid, and amyloid infiltration. Parathyroid suppression also results from hypomagnesemia and hypermagnesemia, burns, sepsis, and pancreatitis.

Vitamin-D-related hypocalcemia is associated with impaired vitamin D activation, as in renal failure, and vitamin D deficiency when this vitamin is not added to intravenous parenteral nutrition solutions. Rhabdomyolysis causes hypocalcemia by inhibiting renal synthesis of $1{,}25(OH)_2D$ and by causing Ca precipitation in the injured muscle. Finally, many drugs can induce hypocalcemia (Table 2-14).

Clinical features include weakness, fatigue, and neuromuscular irritability that ranges from muscle spasms to seizures. Chvostek's sign is demonstrated by tapping over the facial nerve where it passes through the parotid gland; ipsilateral contraction of the facial muscles suggests hypocalcemic-induced irritability. Trousseau's sign is evoked when a blood pressure cuff on the upper arm is inflated to 20 mm Hg above systolic pressure and held at that level for 3 minutes; myotonic carpal spasm of the wrist muscles is seen.

TABLE 2-12 DRUGS ASSOCIATED WITH HYPERKALEMIA

Agent	Mechanism
KCl Oral electrolyte solution K-Penicillin Soup Oxprenolol + K^+	Increased intake (exogenous load)
Barbiturates Heroin Phencyclidine Amphetamines Other narcotics and sedatives	Abnormal distribution—drug-induced rhabdomyolysis
Succinylcholine	Abnormal distribution—leakage
Digoxin	Abnormal distribution—inhibition of Na^+-K^+-ATPase
Arginine	Abnormal distribution—displacement from cells
Amiloride/hydrochlorothiazide	Abnormal distribution—mechanism unknown
Triamterene Amiloride Spironolactone Indomethacin Captopril Heparin	Decreased urinary excretion

(Nanji AA: Drug-induced electrolyte disorders. *Drug Intell Clin Pharm* 1983; 17:175)

Cardiovascular abnormalities include dysrhythmias, digitalis insensitivity, prolongation of the QT and ST segments of the EKG, and terminal T-wave inversion.

Management of severe and symptomatic hypocalcemia includes calcium gluconate, 10 ml of a 10% solution, injected intravenously over 10 minutes; or $CaCl_2$, 10 ml of a 10% solution in 500 ml of D_5W, infused over 30 minutes. If symptoms persist, supplemental Ca may be infused at a rate of 1 to 2 mg/kg body weight/hour. When hyperphosphatemia or K^+ deficits exist, they also must be corrected.

TABLE 2-13 HYPOCALCEMIA

Diagnosis:	$Ca^{++} < 2.0$ meq/liter (4.0 mg/dl), or serum Ca < 4.3 meq/liter (8.5 mg/dl)
Causes:	Parathormone related 1. Parathyroid insufficiency 2. Parathyroid suppression Vitamin D related 1. Impaired vitamin D activation 2. Increased loss of vitamin D Miscellaneous 1. Hyperphosphatemia 2. Drugs 3. Hypoalbuminemia 4. Fat embolism
Management:	Severe, symptomatic 1. Calcium gluconate (10 ml 10% solution over 10 min), or calcium chloride (10 ml 10% solution in 50 ml D_5W over 30 min) 2. If symptoms persist: 1–2 mg/kg/hr of elemental calcium 3. Correct magnesium and potassium deficits, if present 4. Treat hyperphosphatemia if present 5. Monitor symptoms and serum total or ionized calcium levels Asymptomatic 1. Calcium gluconate or calcium lactate (2–4 g/day, divided doses every 6 h) 2. If needed, add a vitamin D preparation[16] Work-up cause
Complications:	Inadequate therapy 1. Seizures 2. Laryngospasm/respiratory arrest 3. Congestive heart failure 4. Dysrhythmias Excessive therapy 1. Hypercalcemia 2. If hyperphosphatemia present, soft tissue calcification when calcium-phosphate product > 40–60

TABLE 2-14 DRUGS ASSOCIATED WITH HYPOCALCEMIA

Agent	Mechanism
Heparin	Pseudohypocalcemia
Phosphate	↑ Phosphate load
Magnesium sulfate Colchicine Furosemide Calcitonin Mithramycin Propylthiouracil Cimetidine	↓ Parathormone secretion/action
Phenytoin	↓ Active vitamin D production/action
Phenobarbital Aspirin Estrogens Glutethimide	
Gentamicin Tobramycin Capreomycin Neomycin Carbenicillin Cisplatin Amphotericin B Polymyxin B Digitalis Diuretics Purgatives/laxatives	Hypomagnesemia
Citrate EDTA	Chelating agents

(Nanji AA: Drug-induced electrolyte disorders. *Drug Intell Clin Pharm* 1983; 17:175)

HYPERCALCEMIA

Hypercalcemia is defined by $Ca^{++} > 2.6$ meq/liter or total serum Ca > 10.5 mg/dl (Table 2-15). Causes are listed in Table 2-16. Several drugs can also significantly increase calcium levels (Table 2-17).

Cardiovascular effects include an increase in peripheral vascular resistance, hypertension, and potentiation of the cardiac effects of digoxin. Electrocardiographic changes include prolongation of the PR interval, widening of the QRS interval, shortening of the ST segment, and a slight flattening of T-waves. Biphasic T-waves and QRS voltage increase also are reported. Hypercalcemic crisis involves intravascular volume depletion, renal insuffi-

TABLE 2-15 HYPERCALCEMIA

Diagnosis:	Ca^{++} > 2.6 meq/liter (5.0 mg/dl) Serum Ca > 5.4 meq/liter (10.5 mg/dl)
Causes:	Impaired homeostatic control 1. ↑ PTH production 2. ↑ 1,25-$(OH)_2$ vitamin D Overwhelmed homeostatic control 1. Skeletal mobilization of calcium 2. ↓ Renal excretion of calcium Reduced bone formation Drugs
Mangement:	Emergency treatment 1. Normal saline (2–3 liters over 3–6 hr) 2. Furosemide (40–100 mg IV every 2–4 hr) 3. Mithramycin (25 μg/kg IV every 3–4 days) 4. Calcitonin (4 MRC units/kg SC every 12 hr) 5. Steroids Hydrocortisone (3mg/kg/day in divided doses every 6 hr) Prednisone (40–80 mg/day) 6. Hemodialysis or peritoneal dialysis Nonemergency treatment 1. Adequate fluid intake 2. Withdrawal of drugs causing hypercalcemia 3. Restriction of oral calcium 4. Mobilization, if possible
Complications:	Inadequate therapy 1. Severe dehydration 2. Renal failure 3. Coma and death Excessive therapy 1. Related to agents used (see text) 2. Hypocalcemia

ciency, and coma. Therapy includes intravenous infusion of normal saline, 2 to 3 liters over 3 to 6 hours, and furosemide, 40 mg to 100 mg IV every 2 to 4 hours.

When this therapy is ineffective or contraindicated, administration of mithramycin, 25 μg/kg body weight IV every 3 to 4 days, or calcitonin, 4 MRC units per kg body weight SC every 12 hours, may be initiated. The Ca-lowering effect with mithramycin is seen within 12 to 24 hours. Significant toxicity, including nephrotoxicity, thrombocytopenia, hepatocellular necrosis, nausea, vomiting, Na^+ retention, and hypokalemia can occur with this agent.

Calcitonin usually results in a decrease in Ca 1 to 2 hours after initiation of therapy. Side-effects are less serious than those of mithramycin and include nausea, facial flushing, and diarrhea. In patients with renal failure or congestive heart failure, hemodialysis or peritoneal dialysis occasionally is used to decrease serum calcium rapidly.

TABLE 2-16 DIFFERENTIAL DIAGNOSIS OF HYPERCALCEMIA

MOST COMMON
Malignancy
- PTH-like material
  - Lung, hypernephroma, lymphoma, multiple myeloma
- Osteoclast activating factor
  - Lymphoma, multiple myeloma
  - Prostaglandins
  - Solid tumors (lungs, breast, kidney)

Endocrine
- Parathyroid hormone
  - Primary hyperparathyroidism

LESS COMMON
Endocrine
- Hyperthyroidism
- Pheochromocytoma
- Adrenal insufficiency
- Acromegaly

Drug use or intoxication
- Hypervitaminosis (A and D)
- Thiazide diuretics
- Lithium
- Hormonal treatment of cancer
- Milk-alkali syndrome

Granulomatous diseases
- Berylliosis
- Coccidiodomycosis
- Histoplasmosis
- Sarcoid
- Tuberculosis

Immobilization
- Especially with underlying bone disease and/or high bone turnover

Miscellaneous
- Critically ill patients
- Paget's disease
- After renal transplant
- Recovery from acute renal failure
- Phosphate depletion syndrome
- Familial hypocalciuric hypercalcemia

PHOSPHORUS DISORDERS

HYPOPHOSPHATEMIA

The strict definition of hypophosphatemia includes a serum $PO_4 < 3$ mg/dl while the patient is in the fasting state (Table 2-18). When the serum PO_4 level is less than 2 mg/dl, the urine should contain less than 100 mg of phosphate per day. Amounts in excess of this value suggest hyperparathyroidism or a primary renal dysfunction. Five major categories of causes are

TABLE 2-17 DRUGS ASSOCIATED WITH HYPERCALCEMIA

Agent	Mechanism
Intravenous lipid emulsion	Pseudohypercalcemia (when fluorometric technique used to measure calcium)
Self-administered calcium and vitamin D	Factitious
Vitamins D and A	Increased bone reabsorption
Low-dose furosemide (oral)	Decreased urinary calcium excretion
Thiazides	Multifactorial
Chlorthalidone	
Lithium	
Tamoxifen	Unknown
Estrogens	
β-Adrenergic agents	Increased PTH release

(Nanji AA: Drug-induced electrolyte disorders. *Drug Intell Clin Pharm* 1983; 17:175)

intracellular anabolic shifts (*i.e.*, recovery from malnutrition and burns), gram-negative bacteremia, alcoholism, alkalosis (respiratory and metabolic), and diabetic ketoacidosis or salicylate poisoning. Clinical manifestations include acute skeletal myopathy with profound weakness and, occasionally, respiratory muscle paralysis; cardiomyopathy; neurologic dysfunction; hematologic disorders with decreased platelet adhesiveness, phagocytic impairment, and hemolysis of red cells; and, in chronic deficiency states, skeletal dysfunction with increased bone turnover and decreased mineralization.

Management of profound depletion (serum PO_4 < 1 mg/dl) includes

TABLE 2-18 HYPOPHOSPHATEMIA

Diagnosis:	Serum PO_4 < 1 meq/liter (3 mg/dl) in fasting state
Causes:	Intracellular shift
	Renal loss
	Gastrointestinal
	Iatrogenic
	Drugs
Management:	Profound depletion (< 1mg/dl)
	(1) Potassium phosphate or sodium phosphate (2.5–5.0 mg/kg/6 hr)
	(2) Follow serum phosphate, calcium, magnesium, potassium levels every 12 hr
	(3) When phosphate ≥ 2 mg/dl, switch to oral agents
	Depletion (≤ 2 mg/dl)
	(1) Whole cow's milk (1 mg phosphate/ml; 1500–2000 ml/day)
	(2) NEUTRA-PHOS (250 mg/tablet; 2 tablets every 8–12 hr)
	(3) Phospho-soda (129 mg/ml; give 5 ml every 8–12 hr)
Complications:	Metastatic calcifications
	Hyperphosphatemia

TABLE 2-19 HYPERPHOSPHATEMIA

Diagnosis:	Serum PO_4 > 1.5 meq/liter (4.5 mg/dl) in fasting state
Causes:	Decreased renal excretion
	Increased intracellular to extracelluar shift
	Increased phosphate ingestion
Management:	Restrict PO_4 intake (< 200 mg/day)
	Saline infusion
	Acetazolamide
	Oral phosphate binders
	Correct hypocalcemia
	Peritoneal dialysis or hemodialysis
Complications:	Hypophosphatemia
	Hypocalcemia
	Metastatic calcification

intravenous potassium phosphate or sodium phosphate in a dose of 2.5 to 5 mg/kg every 6 hours. Serum PO_4, Ca^{++}, Mg^{++}, and K^+ levels must be measured every 12 hours. Intravenous PO_4 must not be given to patients with hypercalcemia; the hypercalcemia must be corrected first to prevent metastatic calcifications.

HYPERPHOSPHATEMIA

CAUSES. Hyperphosphatemia is defined by a fasting serum PO_4 > 4.5 mg/dl (Table 2-19). Common causes include decreased renal PO_4 excretion, renal failure, hyperthyroidism, growth hormone excess, and use of diphosphonates. Another cause is increased intracellular-to-extracellular PO_4 shifts (seen in rhabdomyolysis, sepsis, severe hypothermia, malignant hyperthermia, sepsis, and tumor chemotherapy). Urinary excretion of PO_4 is enhanced by saline infusion and acetazolamide, 500 mg every 6 hours. If hypocalcemia is present, it should be corrected. In renal failure, PO_4 may be eliminated through peritoneal dialysis or hemodialysis.

For further information, please see Chapter 41 in Civetta JM, Taylor RW, Kirby RR: Critical Care. *Philadelphia: J. B. Lippincott, 1988*

BIBLIOGRAPHY

Arieff AI: Hyponatremia, convulsions, respiratory arrest and permanent brain damage after elective surgery in healthy women. *N Engl J Med* 1986; 314:1529

Ayus JC, Krothapalli RK, Arieff AI: Changing concepts in treatment of severe symptomatic hyponatremia. *Am J Med* 1985; 78:897

Cox M: Potassium homeostasis. In Beck LK (ed): Body fluid and electrolyte disorders. *Med Clin North Am* 1981; 65:363

Forster J, Querusio L, Burchard KW, et al: Hypercalcemia in critically ill surgical patients. *Ann Surg* 1985; 202:512

Krane EJ, Rockoff MA, Wallman JK, et al: Subclinical brain swelling in children during treatment of diabetic ketoacidosis. *N Engl J Med* 1985; 312:1147

Lau K: Phosphate disorders. In Kokko JP, Tannen RL (eds): *Fluids and Electrolytes,* p. 398. Philadelphia, WB Saunders, 1986

Metildi LA, Shackford SR, Virgilio RW, et al: Crystalloid versus colloid in fluid resuscitation of patients with severe pulmonary insufficiency. *Surg Gynecol Obstet* 1984; 158:207

Pak CYC: Calcium disorders—Hypercalcemia and hypocalcemia. In Kokko JP, Tannen RL (eds): *Fluids and Electrolytes,* p. 472. Philadelphia, WB Saunders, 1986

Rackow EC, Falk JL, Fein IA: Fluid resuscitation in circulatory shock. *Crit Care Med* 1983; 11:839

3
Hyperosmolar States

EVALUATION OF HYPEROSMOLAR STATES

The initial evaluation of the hyperosmolar state is depicted in Figure 3-1.

HYPONATREMIA

A discrepancy between measured and calculated plasma osmolality of greater than 10 mOsm/kg H_2O suggests the presence of a nonsodium solute. In the absence of a change in body water, the plasma sodium concentration decreases approximately 1.6 meq/liter for each 100 mg/dl rise in the plasma glucose concentration.

HYPERNATREMIA

Volume Depletion

Clinically, one sees poor skin turgor, dryness of skin and mucous membranes, postural changes in pulse and blood pressure, hypotension, azotemia, and oliguria.

Volume Overload

Clinical signs of interstitial (e.g., peripheral edema) and intravascular volume overload (e.g., pulmonary edema) may be present. This syndrome may result from the administration of sodium bicarbonate, hypertonic saline, or salt tablets. Exogenous use of fludrocortisone, primary aldosteronism, Cushing's syndrome, and congenital adrenal hyperplasia are also causes.

Normal Volume

These patients usually present with signs and symptoms of intracellular fluid loss, including thirst, weakness, and neurologic features.

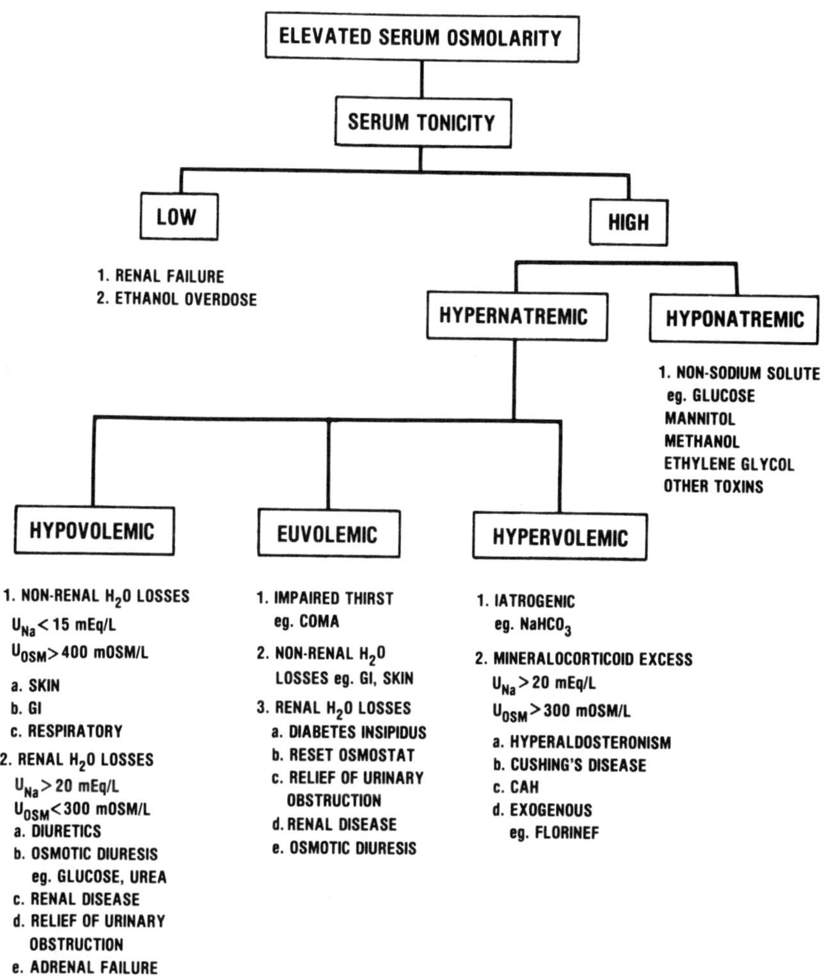

Figure 3-1 Evaluation of hypertonic states.

CLINICAL FEATURES (TABLE 3-1)

Hypotension is uncommon until 20% to 30% of intravascular fluid is lost, which would require about 12 liters of total body water loss. The brain is most susceptible to volume shifts (*e.g.*, cellular dehydration) because it is in a closed container (the skull). Most symptomatic patients have a plasma osmolality greater than 350 mOsm/kg H_2O.

Loss of CNS cellular volume puts mechanical traction on the delicate

TABLE 3-1 Clinical Features in Patients with Hypertonic Syndromes

General	Cardiovascular
Dehydration (poor skin turgor)	Volume depletion
Thirst, polydipsia	Hypotension, shock
Neurologic	Renal
	Oliguria or polyuria, nocturia
Weakness, lethargy, mental dullness, coma	Bladder distension
Iritability	
Hyperactive reflexes	Hydronephrosis
Spasticity, nystagmus, ataxia, or muscle twitching	Renal insufficiency
Seizures	
Focal Abnormalities	
Cerebral hemorrhage	
Subarachnoid hemorrhage	
Venous thrombosis	

cerebral vessels and may cause vascular damage, including subcortical parenchymal hemorrhage, subarachnoid hemorrhage, and venous thrombosis. Massive polyuria may lead to cardiovascular compromise with hypotension and shock.

TREATMENT

Treatment of hypertonicity is aimed at replacing water deficits, matching intercurrent losses, and decreasing ongoing losses, if possible (Fig. 3-2).

HYPERTONICITY WITH HYPONATREMIA

Treatment of hypertonic syndromes associated with hyponatremia rests with reducing the elevated concentration of the nonsodium solute (e.g., glucose, mannitol, toxin). Insulin alone, however, should not be administered to a hyperglycemic patient with relative hypertonicity since an acute insulin-induced shift of glucose into the ICF may acutely reduce intravascular volume and precipitate hypotension and shock.

HYPERTONICITY WITH HYPERNATREMIA

The water deficit can be calculated from the plasma osmolality or plasma sodium concentration as follows: Deficit = (0.6)(weight in kg)(1 – 140/actual Na^+). If the patient shows initial neurologic improvement and later deteriorates, cerebral edema should be suspected. If fundoscopic examination or lumbar puncture reveals clinical features that suggest cerebral edema, administration of fluid should be stopped and osmotherapy with hypertonic saline or mannitol begun.

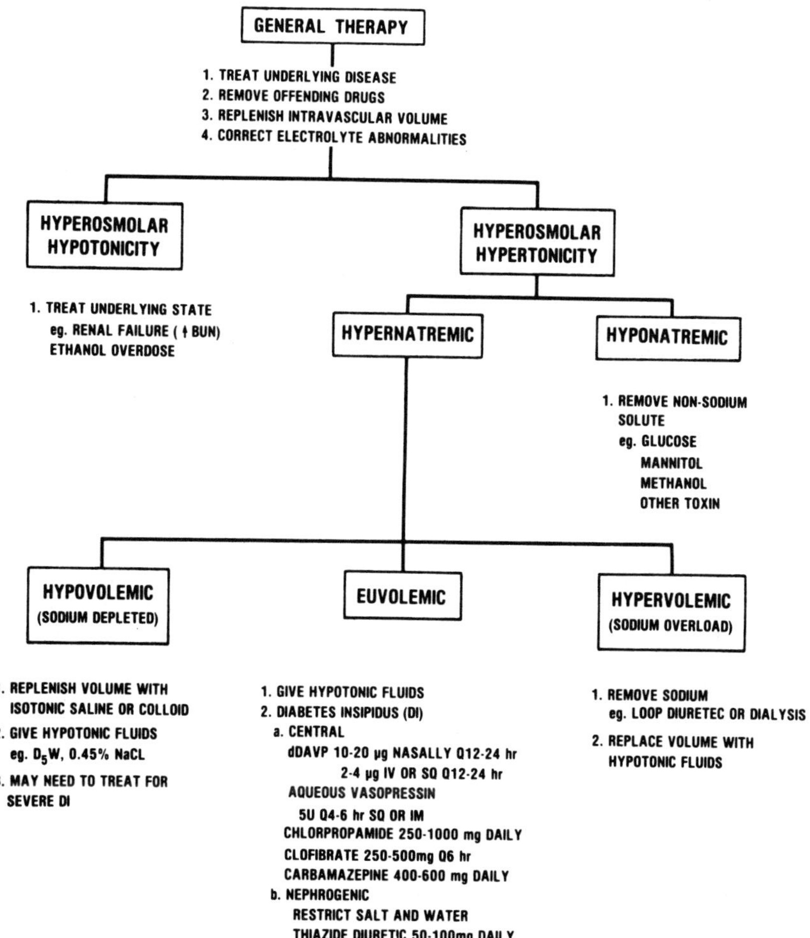

Figure 3-2 Treatment of hypertonic states.

HYPERNATREMIA SECONDARY TO WATER LOSS

If the patient is hypovolemic, intravascular volume must be replaced first, usually with balanced electrolyte solutions. Once intravascular volume is corrected, water deficits can be replaced enterally or intravenously, depending on the patient's clinical status. If 5% glucose solution is used to replenish body water, the infusion rate must be adjusted to avoid glycosuria. Otherwise, the resulting osmotic diuresis may exacerbate the hyperosmolar state.

SODIUM OVERLOAD

In sodium overload states, sodium can be removed from the body with loop diuretics or dialysis and volume replaced with hypotonic fluids. Acute ECF volume overload may cause pulmonary edema and congestive heart failure. Acute cerebral dehydration may cause seizures; intravenous furosemide should be given immediately and hypotonic fluid infusion begun to replace water deficits. In patients who are oliguric despite diuretics, phlebotomy and 5% dextrose infusion can buy time until dialysis can be started. Electrolyte status must be monitored to avoid hypokalemia and hypomagnesemia.

For further information, please see Chapter 42 in Civetta JM, Taylor RW, Kirby RR: Critical Care. *Philadelphia: J. B. Lippincott, 1988*

BIBLIOGRAPHY

Balestrieri F, Chernow B, Rainey T: Post-craniotomy diabetes insipidus—Who's at risk. *Crit Care Med* 1982; 10:108

Chernow B, Willey S, Zaloga GP: Critical care endocrinology. In Shoemaker WC (ed): *Textbook of Critical Care*. Philadelphia, WB Saunders, 2nd ed, pp 736–766, 1988

Cobb WE, Spare S, Reichlin S: Neurogenic diabetes insipidus—Management with dDAVP. *Ann Intern Med* 1978; 88:183

Culpepper RM, Hebert SC, Andreoli TE: The posterior pituitary and water metabolism. In Wilson JD, Foster DW (eds): *Williams Textbook of Endocrinology*, 7th ed, pp 633–642. Philadelphia, WB Saunders, 1985

Feig PU, McCurdy DK: The hypertonic state. *N Engl J Med* 1977; 297–1444

Gennari EJ: Serum osmolality. *N Engl J Med* 1984; 310:102

Humes HD, Narins RG, Brenner BM: Disorders of water balance. *Hosp Pract* 1979; March:133

Kleeman CR: CNS manifestations of disordered salt and water balance. *Hosp Pract* 1979; May:59

Miller M, Kalkos T, Moses AM, et al: Recognition of partial defects in anti-diuretic hormone secretion. *Ann Intern Med* 1970; 73:721

Moses AM, Notman DD: Diabetes insipidus and syndrome of inappropriate anti-diuretic hormone secretion (SIADH). *Adv Intern Med* 1982; 27:73

Narins RG, Jones ER, Stom MC, et al: Diagnostic strategies in disorders of fluid, electrolyte and acid-base homeostasis. *Am J Med* 1982; 72:496

Singer I, Forrest JN: Drug-induced states of nephrogenic diabetes insipidus. *Kidney Int* 1976; 10:82

Zaloga GP, Chernow B: Insulin, glucagon and growth hormone. In Chernow B (ed): *The Pharmacologic Approach to the Critically Ill Patient*, pp 562–585. Baltimore, Williams & Wilkins, 1983

Zaloga GP, Chernow B: Life threatening electrolyte and metabolic abnormalities. In Parillo JE (ed): *Current Therapy in Critical Care Medicine* pp 245–257. Toronto, BC Decker, 1987

4
Acid–Base Problem Solving

Systemic diseases are often accompanied by alterations in acid–base regulation. Occasionlly, the abnormalities that result may become life-threatening, and the clinician must be able to differentiate and treat them. Failure to do so may result in morbidity or mortality that is preventable by the application of a few basic principles. This chapter does not discuss the various pathophysiological mechanisms by which alterations of acid–base occur, but rather focuses on simple, effective methods of diagnosis and treatment.

Historically, the subject of acid–base regulation has been made unnecessarily difficult by the use of terms such as "CO_2 combining power," "base excess," "buffer base," "standard bicarbonate," and "alkali reserve"—none of which has any readily apparent clinical meaning. When additional modifiers are added—for example, a "negative base excess"—these terms become almost incomprehensible. Regardless of the terminology used, however, acid–base disturbances involve one simple fact: the normal concentration or, more specifically, the activity, of the hydrogen ion (H^+) has been altered. We define acids as substances which, when in solution, dissociate to form H^+ and an anion (e.g., Cl^-, SO_4^{2-}, HPO_4^{2-}). Conversely, bases are substances which, when in solution, combine with (remove) H^+. The general reaction describing this relationship is

$$HA \leftrightarrows H^+ + A^-, \qquad (1)$$

where HA represents an acid (H^+ donor) and A^- its conjugate base.

RESPIRATORY DERANGEMENTS

Carbon dioxide alters H^+ according to the following reversible reaction:

$$CO_2 + H_2O \leftrightarrows H_2CO_3 \leftrightarrows H^+ + HCO_3^-. \qquad (2)$$

Respiratory derangements, by virtue of their effect on the partial pressure of arterial carbon dioxide (Pa_{CO_2}), may cause major changes in H^+ concentration within the body. For each acute 10 mm Hg deviation of Pa_{CO_2} above or below 40 mm Hg, the *p*H changes by approximately 0.07 units. In actuality, this change is not entirely linear, but with small acute changes in Pa_{CO_2}, the accuracy of the arterial blood gas values can be checked by knowing the approximate magnitude of change in *p*H that *should* occur for a given change in Pa_{CO_2}.

Since there is a straightforward relationship between Pa_{CO_2} and alveolar ventilation, correction of the respiratory component in acid–base derangements is easy (at least in theory). If the *p*H is decreased and the Pa_{CO_2} levels are increased, an increase in alveolar ventilation will lower Pa_{CO_2} and return *p*H to normal. The opposite is also true. Remember that if *alveolar* ventilation is halved, Pa_{CO_2} is approximately doubled. Similary, if *alveolar* ventilation is doubled, Pa_{CO_2} decreases by half. Respiratory disturbances and H^+ concentration can be easily assessed and corrected if the following relationship is appreciated:

$$\uparrow \dot{V}_A \rightarrow \downarrow CO_2 \rightarrow \uparrow pH. \quad (3)$$

METABOLIC DISTURBANCES

Hydrogen ion concentration also is affected by nonrespiratory ("metabolic") processes. Syndromes of metabolic acidosis fall into two patterns that can be separated by calculating the anion gap.

$$\text{Anion Gap} = Na^+ - (Cl^- + HCO_3^-). \quad (4)$$

This "gap" represents unmeasured anions, most of which are offset by H^+. Thus an increased anion gap often implies the presence of a metabolic acidosis. Alternatively, Cl^- may increase as H^+ concentration rises (Table 4-1). Causes of metabolic alkalosis can be categorized according to a

TABLE 4-1 TYPES OF METABOLIC ACIDOSIS

Anion Gap
Renal failure
Diabetic ketoacidosis
Salicylism
Lactic acidosis (and starvation)
Toxins
Methanol
Paraldehyde
Ethylene glycol
Hyperchloremic
Renal tubular acidosis
Acetazolamide therapy
Diarrhea
Ureteral diversions
Addition of HCl (NH_4Cl, HCl, arginine, lysine)
Early renal failure

pattern of anion (Cl^-) depletion into Cl^- responsive or Cl^- resistant types (Table 4-2).

Just as the change in Pa_{CO_2} from a normal value of 40 mm Hg is the prime indicator of respiratory acid–base disturbance, a change in bicarbonate (HCO_3^-) concentration generally reflects disturbances that are metabolic in origin.

The normal value for plasma HCO_3^- is 24 mmol/liter. Bicarbonate is a "buffer." In the simplest terms, buffers, within their operational range, react with H^+ ions when these ions are present in excessive quantities, removing them from solution and thereby minimizing the increase in acidity that would otherwise occur. Conversely, if the milieu becomes too alkaline, the buffers release H^+ and, in so doing, tend to return the *p*H toward normal. Quantitatively, HCO_3^- is the most important ECF buffer, representing 75% to 80% of the total ECF against metabolically produced or exogenously administered acids. The other important buffers are hemoglobin, protein, and phosphates.

PROBLEM SOLVING

Determination of arterial *p*H by itself does not allow categorization of the H^+ excess or deficit. Arterial P_{CO_2} also must be known. For example, if a patient has an arterial *p*H of 7.0 and a Pa_{CO_2} of 40 mm Hg, metabolic acidosis is present, since ventilation, by definition, is normal. The H^+ measured by the *p*H electrode is only a miniscule part of the patient's total H^+ load. As an example, if the arterial *p*H is reduced from 7.44 (H^+ = 36 nmol/liter) to 7.14 (H^+ = 72 nmol/liter) by an infusion of 0.1 M hydrochloric acid, approximately 14×10^6 nmol of H^+/liter ECF is added. Of this total, only 36 nmol/liter are responsible for the decrease of *p*H. The rest is buffered and thus rendered "harmless." If we can determine the change in body buffers, we can quantitate the H^+ that was added to or lost from the system. Since HCO_3^- is the major buffer, any change in its concentration can be interpreted as reflecting changes in H^+, with which it combines.

Extracellular fluid in a normal adult is composed of the interstitial fluid and

TABLE 4-2 TYPES OF METABOLIC ALKALOSIS

Cl^- Responsive	Cl^- Resistant
Vomiting or nasogastric suction	Adrenal disorders
Diuretic therapy	Hyperaldosteronism
Cl^- wasting diarrhea	Cushing's disease
Posthypercapnic alkalosis	Exogenous steroids
Carbenicillin or penicillin therapy	Bartter's syndrome
	Refeeding alkalosis
	Severe potassium depletion
	HCO_3^- therapy

plasma, and is equal to 20% of the body weight. If you know the amount of HCO_3^- change per liter from normal, and calculate the number of liters of ECF, a quantitative estimate of the HCO_3^- deficit (or excess) can be made. Consider the following example of a patient with a slight metabolic acidosis:

$$
\begin{aligned}
\text{Normal } HCO_3^- &= 24 \text{ mmol/liter} \\
\text{Actual } HCO_3^- &= 20 \text{ mmol/liter} \\
\text{Difference (normal} - \text{actual)} &= 4 \text{ mmol/liter} \\
\text{Body weight} &= 70 \text{ kg} \\
\text{ECF (20\% body weight)} &= 14 \text{ kg (14 liter).} \\
HCO_3^- \text{ deficit} &= \text{Body weight} \times \text{\%ECF} \\
&\quad \times HCO_3^- \text{ deficit/liter} \\
&= 70 \text{ kg} \times 0.2 \times 4 \text{ mmol/liter} \\
&= 56 \text{ mmol.}
\end{aligned} \tag{5}
$$

If changes in HCO_3^- always indicated only metabolic (non-respiratory) acidosis or alkalosis, the presence and degree of the abnormality would be easily ascertained, as in the preceding example. However, this is not the case. Any process that changes Pa_{CO_2} (hyperventilation or hypoventilation, increased or decreased carbon dioxide production) also results in a change in HCO_3^- (see Equation 2).

The amount by which HCO_3^- is altered by different levels of Pa_{CO_2} depends on whether the change is acute or chronic. If you wish to determine how much of a decrease in HCO_3^- resulted from the buffering of acid, you must first determine whether Pa_{CO_2} is normal. If it is, you can assume that the change noted is nonrespiratory. If Pa_{CO_2} is increased or decreased from a normal value of 40 mm Hg, however, you must first determine how much this change altered HCO_3^-. Only then can any additional change in HCO_3^-, over and above that resulting from Pa_{CO_2} change, be considered nonrespiratory in origin.

During acute and chronic hypocapnia and hypercapnia, changes in HCO_3^- are almost linear over the range of Pa_{CO_2} (20–100 mm Hg) encountered in altered pathologic states. Thus, you can predict what HCO_3^- "should be" for any Pa_{CO_2}. This observation leads to certain rules of thumb to characterize various acid–base abnormalities. These are as follow:

1 During acute hypercapnia, HCO_3^- increases 1 mmol/liter for each 10 mm Hg increase in Pa_{CO_2} above 40 mm Hg.

2 During chronic hypercapnia, HCO_3^- increases 4 mmol/liter for each 10 mm Hg increase in Pa_{CO_2} above 40 mm Hg.

3 During acute hypocapnia, HCO_3^- decreases 2 mmol/liter for every 10 mm Hg decrease in Pa_{CO_2} below 40 mm Hg.

4 During chronic hypocapnia, HCO_3^- decreases 5 to 7 mmol/liter for every 10 mm Hg decrease in Pa_{CO_2} below 40 mm Hg.

The rules of thumb make the delineation of acid–base disordes relatively simple, as demonstrated by two clinical examples.

> *Case 1:* An otherwise healthy, 35-year-old, 70-kg man sustains acute airway obstruction. Repeated attempts at tracheal intubation are unsuccessful and he regurgitates and aspirates liquid gastric contents. Finally, an endotracheal tube is inserted. An arterial blood sample is sent to the blood gas laboratory and the following values are reported: Pa_{CO_2} = 70 mm Hg; arterial *p*H = 7.10; HCO_3^- = 21 mmol/liter.

To determine what type of acid–base disturbance this patient has, a stepwise analysis might proceed in the following manner. By convention, arterial *p*H below 7.36 represents acidemia (above 7.44 is alkalemia). Thus, the patient is acidemic and, because the Pa_{CO_2} is 70 mm Hg, at least a portion of the acidemia is respiratory. Is there also a component of nonrespiratory or metabolic acidosis? Application of rule of thumb 1 suggests that HCO_3^- should be at least 3 mmol above the normal values of 24 mmol/liter if only Pa_{CO_2} is changed. The predicted HCO_3^- is 27 mmol/liter; hence a deficit of 6 mmol/liter exists. A combined respiratory acidemia and metabolic acidosis are present.

> *Case 2:* A 56-year-old, 70-kg man with chronic obstructive pulmonary disease and a resting Pa_{CO_2} of 70 mm Hg sustains an acute perioperative myocardial infarction. The blood pressure is 80/50 mm Hg, and he is diaphoretic, cool, and clammy. Arterial blood gas analysis shows the following:
>
> Pa_{CO_2} = 70 mm Hg; arterial *p*H = 7.10; HCO_3^- = 21 mmol/liter.

Here, the laboratory values are identical to those in case 1, but the clinical setting is considerably different. The arterial *p*H of 7.10 confirms acidemia and the Pa_{CO_2} of 70 mm Hg reveals that respiratory factors are present. However, in this instance, one is dealing with chronic hypercapnia, and the application of rule of thumb 3 predicts an HCO_3^- of 36 mmol/liter. Actual HCO_3^- is only 21 mmol/liter, a deficit of 15 mmol/liter. The metabolic, or nonrespiratory, component of acidosis is much greater than in Case 1.

Major revisions in thought concerning the role of HCO_3^- therapy are taking place. The American Heart Association now urges restraint in the use of sodium bicarbonate during cardiopulmonary resuscitation (as opposed to their previous rather cavalier approach). Experimentally, HCO_3^- administered to correct severe hypoxic lactic acidosis actually increases lactate production. Part of the difficulty may be related to the fact that carbon dioxide elaborated by the reaction of H^+ and HCO_3^- (Equation 2) rapidly diffuses across cell membranes, creating intracellular acidosis even while the extracellular acidosis is decreased.

For further information, please see Chapter 32 in Civetta JM, Taylor RW, Kirby RR: Critical Care. *Philadelphia: J. B. Lippincott, 1988*

BIBLIOGRAPHY

American Heart Association: Standards and guidelines for cardiopulmonary resuscitation and emergency cardiac care: Part III. Adult advanced cardiac life support *JAMA* 1986; 255:2933

Bernards WC: *Interpretation of Clinical Acid–Base Data. Regional Refresher Courses in Anesthesiology,* pp 17–28. Philadelphia, JB Lippincott, 1973

Brackett NC Jr, Cohen JJ, Schwartz WB: Carbon dioxide titration curve of normal man. *N Engl J Med* 1965; 272:6

Brackett NC Jr, Wingo CF, Muren O, et al: Acid–base response to chronic hypercapnia in man. *N Engl J Med* 1969; 280:124

Cohen JJ, Brackett NC Jr, Schwartz WB: The nature of carbon dioxide titration curve in the normal dog. *J Clin Invest* 1964; 43:777

Graf H, Leach W, Arieff AI: Evidence for a detrimental effect of bicarbonate therapy in hypoxic lactic acidosis. *Science* 1986; 227:754

Robinson JR: *Fundamentals of Acid–Base Regulation,* 5th ed. Philadelphia, Blackwell Scientific Publications. 1975

Schwartz WB, Brackett NC Jr, Cohen JJ: The response of extra-cellular hydrogen ion concentration to graded degrees of chronic hypercapnia: The physiologic limits of the defense of pH. *J Clin Invest* 1965; 44:291

Schwartz WB, Relman AS: A critique of the parameters used in the evaluation of acid–base disorders. *N Engl J Med* 1963; 268:1382

5 Nutritional Requirements

Table 5-1 describes nutritional assessment measures used in the critical care setting.

ASSESSMENT OF PROTEIN REQUIREMENTS

A normal, unstressed person ingesting adequate nonprotein calories requires approximately 1 g/kg/day of high biologic value protein to maintain nitrogen equilibrium (Table 5-2).

Compared with normal persons, highly catabolic patients burn a larger proportion of infused amino acids as fuel, even with high caloric intakes. On the basis of nitrogen balance data, most experts recommend infusion of 1.5 to 2.0 g/kg/day of conventional high biologic value amino acids to counteract this phenomenon.

FUEL METABOLISM DURING CRITICAL ILLNESS

ASSESSING THE QUANTITY OF FUEL REQUIRED

Measurements may be made in the clinical setting using a "metabolic cart"; generation of heat (referred to as "metabolic rate") is proportional to the rate of oxygen consumption and carbon dioxide production. Similar information may be obtained using a Douglas bag and flow-meter for collecting inspired and expired air. For patients with pulmonary artery balloon flotation catheters, the Fick method may be used to calculate oxygen consumption from cardiac output, hemoglobin concentration, and arterial and mixed venous oxygen saturations. Metabolic rate in kilocalories per 24 hours is roughly equal to 7.25 times the calculated oxygen consumption (Table 5-3).

TABLE 5-1 NUTRITIONAL ASSESSMENT MEASURES USED IN THE CRITICAL CARE SETTING

Measure	Comment
Delayed cutaneous hypersensitivity	Correlates well with survival in the critical care setting and appears related to nutritional status but is affected by many non-nutrition-dependent factors
Lymphocyte count	Large overlap between well-nourished and malnourished populations; unclear relationship to survival
Serum complement, fibronectin levels	Appear related to nutritional status and to likelihood of survival of critical illness but are affected by many non-nutrition related influences
Serum albumin levels	Do not decline significantly during noncatabolic states except during severe emaciation; decline rapidly during acutely catabolic states regardless of nutritional status
Other hepatic-derived serum protein levels	Levels may be influenced more by biologic expediency during acute insults than by "nutritional status" *per se*
Mid-arm muscle circumference	Possible relationship to diaphragmatic and cardiac muscle mass
Fasting urea nitrogen excretion rate	Assesses rate of endogenous protein catabolism; urinary urea excretion rate represents approximately 85% of total nitrogen excreted in the urine
Nitrogen balance	Useful for assessing the efficacy of a nutritional regimen: nitrogen balance = (amino acid/protein infused/24 hours)/(6.25) − (UUN excreted in 24 hours)/(.85) − 4; should be performed weekly

TABLE 5-2 RECOMMENDED AMINO ACID/PROTEIN ADMINISTRATION RATES FOR SPECIFIC POPULATIONS WITH ADEQUATE NONPROTEIN CALORIC INTAKE

Population	Rate (g/kg/day)
Normal individuals, unstressed	1.0
Postoperative patients	2.1–2.6[110]
Septic patients	1.5[70]
Multiply traumatized patients	1.8[71]
Burned patients	1.5–3.0[69]

Determine nitrogen balance at weekly intervals to assess adequacy of amino acid/protein administration.
In the most highly catabolic patients, insulin administered to maintain serum glucose at 100 to 150 g/dl markedly enhances nitrogen retention, possibly due to its effect on skeletal muscle.

TABLE 5-3 METHODS FOR ESTIMATING THE RATE OF CALORIC INFUSION

Metabolic cart or Douglas bag and spirometer

Metabolic rate, kcal/day (approximate) = (3.94)($\dot{V}_{O_2}$, liters/day) + 1.11 ($\dot{V}_{CO_2}$, liters/day)

Reverse Fick method

$\dot{V}_{O_2}$, ml/min = (1.34)(CO)(H6)($Sa_{O_2} - S\bar{v}_{O_2}$) + 0.0031(CO)($Pa_{O_2} - P\bar{v}_{O_2}$)
$\dot{V}_{O_2}$, liters/day = ($\dot{V}_{O_2}$, ml/min)(1.44)
Assume $\dot{V}_{O_2} \ll \dot{V}_{CO_2}$
Metabolic rate, kcal/day (approximate) = (5.05)(1.44)($\dot{V}_{O_2}$, ml/min)
= (7.27) $\dot{V}_{O_2}$, ml/min)

kcal/kg/day method (stress factors)*

Normal resting metabolic rate	25 kcal/kg/day
Septic patients	30–40 kcal/kg/day
Multiply traumatized patients	25–35 kcal/kg/day
Burned patients	25–50 kcal/kg/day

*Large variability in caloric expenditure is due to the multifactorial etiology of increased metabolic rate; no single value for a stress factor can adequately represent all patients in a given disease category (see text). Patients in any disease category who are undergoing hemodynamic resuscitation may have lower than normal metabolic rates; nutritional supplementation should be reduced appropriately or withheld.

TABLE 5-4 RELATIVE ADVANTAGES AND DISADVANTAGES OF SOME COMMERCIALLY AVAILABLE CALORIC SUBSTRATES

Fuel	Advantages	Disadvantages
Glucose	1. Possibly more likely to promote nitrogen retention in the most highly catabolic patients (data inconclusive) 2. Less expensive	1. Stimulates increased oxygen consumption (may be undesirable for patients with impaired oxygen transport) 2. Stimulates markedly increased CO_2 production (may be undesirable for patients with respiratory compromise or those being weaned from mechanical ventilation) 3. Hyperglycemia
Long-chain triglyceride	1. Less likely than glucose to increase CO_2 production 2. Possibly less likely than glucose to promote increased oxygen consumption (data inconclusive) 3. Contains arachidonic acid precursors which prevent development of essential fatty acid deficiency	1. May cause arterial oxygen desaturation (usually not a problem clinically) 2. Preliminary animal data suggest possible immune depression 3. May not be metabolized in certain patients; serum turbidity should be checked 24 hours after infusion 4. Does not appear to promote nitrogen retention in the absence of carbohydrate
Medium-chain triglyceride	1. Does not require enzymatic digestion for GI absorption 2. May not require carnitine for entry into mitochondria 3. Has not been reported to cause arterial oxygen desaturation	1. Does not contain essential fatty acids 2. Does not appear to promote nitrogen retention in the absence of carbohydrate

ASSESSING THE TYPE OF FUEL TO BE INFUSED

The introduction of intravenous nonglucose fuels has increased therapeutic options while somewhat confusing the treatment of ICU patients. Three types of commercially available caloric substrates are described in Table 5-4.

For further information, please see Chapter 44 in Civetta JM, Taylor RW, Kirby RR: Critical Care. *Philadelphia: J. B. Lippincott, 1988*

BIBLIOGRAPHY

Askanazi J, Nordenstrom J, Rosenbaum SH, et al: Nutrition for the patient with respiratory failure: Glucose vs. fat. *Anesthesiology* 1981; 54:373

Askanazi J, Rosenbaum SH, Hyman AK, et al: Respiratory changes induced by the large glucose loads of total parenteral nutrition. *JAMA* 1980; 243:1444

Bozzetti F: Parenteral nutrition in surgical patients. *Surg Gynecol Obstet* 1976; 142:16

Brennan MF, Cerra R, Daly JM, et al: Report of a research workshop: Branched-chain amino acids in stress and injury. *JPEN* 1986; 10:446–452

Elwyn DH, Kinney JM, Malayappa J, et al: Influence of increasing carbohydrate intake on glucose kinetics in injured patients. *Ann Surg* 1979; 190:117

Greene HL: Response of the bowel to injury and the transition from parenteral to enteral feedings. *Acta Chir Scand* (Suppl) 1983; 517:21

Gump FE, Long C, Killian P, Kinney JM: Studies of glucose intolerance in septic patients. *J Trauma* 1974; 14:378

Iapichino G, Radrizzani D, Solca M, et al: The main determinants of nitrogen balance during total parenteral nutrition in critically ill injured patients. *Intensive Care Med* 1984; 10:251

Kresowik TK, Dechert RE, Mault JR, et al: Does nutritional support affect survival in critically ill patients? *Surg Forum* 1985; Vol. 36

Nordenstrom J, Carpentier YA, Askanazi J, et al: Free fatty acid mobilization and oxidation during total parenteral nutrition in trauma and infection. *Ann Surg* 1983; 198:725

Nuwer N, Cerra FB, Shronts EP, et al: Does modified amino acid total parenteral nutrition alter immune response in high level surgical stress? *JPEN* 1983; 7:521

O'Donnell TF, Clowes GHA, Blackburn GL, et al: Proteolysis associated with a deficit of peripheral energy fuel substrates in septic man. *Surgery* 1976; 80:192

Quebbeman EJ, Ausman RK, Schneider TC: A re-evaluation of energy expenditure during parenteral nutrition. *Ann Surg* 1982; 152:282

Soroff HS, Pearson E, Artz CP: An estimation of the nitrogen requirements for equilibrium in burned patients. *Surg Gynecol Obstet* 1961; 63:159

6
Enteral and Parenteral Nutrition

SELECTION OF PATIENTS AND INDICATIONS FOR NUTRITIONAL SUPPORT

TARGET POSSIBLY ACHIEVABLE

Patients are prime candidates for nasogastric or nasointestinal feeding if the gastrointestinal tract is normal, as in severe systemic illness, anorexia, (usually secondary to disease and malnutrition), neurologic impairment preventing oral feeding, substantially increased requirements with relative anorexia, (*e.g.*, in burn cases), or chronic obstructive lung disease with severe dyspnea. However, in disease of the pharynx, esophagus, or stomach, or surgery of the esophagus, stomach, or pancreas, patients usually require intubation of the stomach or intestine by percutaneous gastrostomy or operative jejunostomy.

If there is an abnormality of the intestinal tract, such as short bowel with more than 60 cm of small intestine available, inflammatory bowel disease, or chronic partial bowel obstruction, diets must be delivered carefully with the aid of a pump to avoid surges and consequent distention of the bowel.

Patients in the ICU who cannot receive an oral diet or enteral feeding need parenteral nutrition (PN) if they are already starved, have been on hypocaloric solutions (*e.g.*, 5% dextrose in water) for a week or more, or are malnourished and unlikely to start eating within a week. Patients with massive bowel resection, (*i.e.*, leaving less than 60 cm), chronic bowel obstruction, extensive bowel disease, radiation enteritis, and end-jejunostomy, where oral feeding results in uncontrolled fluid and electrolyte losses, also need PN, as do those who, because of drug or other treatment, are constantly nauseated and unable to eat, (*e.g.*, those undergoing radiotherapy or chemotherapy for prolonged periods).

In several GI disorders, symptoms become worse if the patients are fed orally. For example, patients with pancreatitis will develop pain and elevated serum amylase. In patients with a high intestinal fistula, the output will increase and the fistula will open if oral feeding is undertaken.

NUTRIENT REQUIREMENTS FOR ENTERAL AND PARENTERAL FEEDING

PROTEIN REQUIREMENTS

Give 1.0 to 1.5 g/kg ideal body weight/day of a balanced amino acid mixture and monitor the response of plasma proteins and urea nitrogen excretion.

ENERGY REQUIREMENTS

Needs can be predicted with reasonable accuracy by the Harris–Benedict equation for normal man.

$$\text{Men: kcal/day} = 66 + (13.8 \times W) + (5.0 \times H) - (6.8 \times A)$$
$$\text{Women: kcal/day} = 655 + (9.6 \times W) + (1.8 \times H) - (4.7 \times A),$$

where W = body weight in kilograms, H = height in centimeters, and A = age in years.

To the basal energy expenditure (BEE) must be added the thermogenic effect of food (10%) to give resting energy expenditure (REE) in the bedridden patient. Injury, sepsis, and burns were once thought to increase energy requirements by roughly 30%, 60%, and 100%, respectively, but the degree of hypermetabolism in injured and or septic patients has come into question recently. It should be recognized that an increase in metabolic rate of even 60%, when referred to the BEE (which is about 25 kcal/kg/day), works out to a requirement of only 40 kcal/kg/day, or 2800 kcal in the 70-kg man.

The optimal caloric intake in the majority of patients is between 32 and 35 kcal/kg/day, with a maximum of 40 kcal/kg/day.

ELECTROLYTE REQUIREMENTS

Sodium

RECOMMENDATION. In the average patient, about 100 to 120 mmol/day of sodium can be given, with supplemental sodium to cover any abnormal losses through the GI tract. In severely malnourished patients and those with cardiopulmonary disease, the sodium intake should be restricted to 50 to 60 mmol/day and the amount infused increased gradually as the patient tolerates the fluid load.

Potassium

RECOMMENDATION. To determine potassium requirement during PN, three facts need to be considered. First, glucose infusions increase the need for potassium. Second, about 3 meq of K^+ is retained with each gram of nitrogen. Third, total deficit of potassium may amount to between 800 and 900 mmol in the 50 to 70 kg adult. The infusion of about 80 to 120 meq/day will aid in replenishing stores and meeting daily needs.

Magnesium

RECOMMENDATION. Magnesium should always be included in PN regimens. At least 12 to 15 mmol/day should be given and extra should be added to cover losses in GI secretions.

Phosphorus

RECOMMENDATION. The total needs for phosphorus amount to about 14 to 16 mmol/day when a glucose-lipid source of nonprotein energy is given. These requirements are increased when glucose is given as the sole caloric source.

MICRONUTRIENT REQUIREMENTS

Trace Elements

Iron. A dilute solution of iron–dextran can be used to provide 1 mg of iron per day to meet physiologic losses. This should be increased to 2 mg/day in females. Additional needs related to abnormal losses should be met by infusing a calculated amount of iron–dextran.

Zinc. Adults should ingest 15 mg/day of zinc. Increased catabolism and GI losses increased requirements by 12 mg/liter of small-intestinal fluid lost and 17 mg/liter of stool, measured in the NPO state.

Copper. Requirements are 0.3 mg/day in patients without diarrhea, rising to 0.5 mg/day in those with diarrhea, and falling to 0.1 mg/day in patients with abnormal liver function.

Vitamins

Vitamin A. The recommended daily dose of vitamin A by the parenteral route is 2500 IV.

Vitamin C. About 300 to 500 mg/day will maintain normal to high blood levels of vitamin C in patients receiving TPN.

Vitamin D. Intravenous vitamin D is not recommended.

Vitamin K. Administering 10 mg per week of Synkayvite, a water-soluble analogue, maintains normal coagulation parameters over several months in patients receiving long-term TPN.

Thiamine. Five mg/day should be sufficient for most patients receiving TPN.

Riboflavin. In patients receiving TPN, 5 mg/day is recommended as a safe amount for avoiding deficiency.

Niacin. Observations of circulating levels of niacin in long-term TPN indicate that about 50 mg/day is a safe intake that avoids deficiency.

Pantothenate. Studies of blood levels of pantothenic acid suggest that 15 mg/day is a suitable intake in TPN.

Pyridoxine. An intake of 5 mg/day is sufficient to maintain normal blood levels of pyridoxine in long-term TPN.

Folic Acid and Vitamin B_{12}. The recommended daily intake in PN is 600 μg of folic acid and 12 μg of vitamin B_{12}.

Biotin. The American Medical Association has recommended administration of 60 μg/day for patients receiving TPN.

TECHNIQUES OF ADMINISTRATION

ENTERAL NUTRITION

The principle of administering nutrients through nasogastric or nasoenteral tubes is to infuse the nutrient at a rate at which it can be absorbed so that diarrhea and gastrointestinal discomfort do not occur. Gastric emptying is normally controlled so as to release about 2.6 kcal/min or 150 kcal/hr. The osmolarity (or osmolar concentration) is not of as much concern as the rate at which calories (osmoles) are infused. If gastric emptying is erratic, thus releasing gushes of high-osmolarity fluid into the intestine, diarrhea will occur.

Technical Details of Entry to GI Tract

Tubes vary in size from 5 to 8 Fr. Gastric tubes are 80 cm to 90 cm long and enteral tubes are 108 cm to 110 cm. The stylet and tubes are lubricated with PAM, a lecithin spray. This makes the withdrawal easy, even when the tube is curled. The patient should lie on the left side or be seated if possible. The tube is inserted through a nostril and advanced through the pharynx and esophagus to about 50 cm. Then 50 ml of air is injected and the tube advanced along the greater curvature of the stomach until it is as close to the pylorus as possible. For all critically ill patients, use longer tubes, placed under fluoroscopic control into the distal duodenum or preferably beyond the duodenojejunal flexure.

In patients with delayed gastric emptying, pass the tube into the duodenum with the aid of a gastroscope. The tube with the stylet inserted is laid alongside the gastroscope and the tip secured with a polypectomy snare passed through the channel. The scope is then advanced with the tube into the duodenum and the snare freed. The tube is advanced with the stylet and the gastroscope is withdrawn.

Operative Insertion of Feeding Tube

CERVICAL PHARYNGOSTOMY. This procedure has limited usefulness, but the tube can be inserted during a neck dissection when it is anticipated that oral feeding will be delayed. The tube is comfortable and can be kept in place for long periods.

GASTROSTOMY. Percutaneously inserted tubes should be used. In brief, a gastroscope is passed and, after transilluminating the stomach, a 16-gauge Medicut catheter is inserted transabdominally through an area anesthetized with 2% lidocaine. A #2 silk suture is passed through the Medicut catheter and grasped with forceps passed through the gastroscope. The silk suture is pulled through the mouth by withdrawing the scope. Then a 16-F Malecot catheter is trimmed to remove the flare at the end opposite the mushroom, and the end is tied with a #2 silk suture and forced into another Medicut catheter. The suture is pulled out of the tip of the Medicut catheter and tied to the other suture protruding through the mouth. Then the Malecot catheter is pulled in a retrograde direction and out of the skin opening.

JEJUNOSTOMY. The simplest technique, least likely to cause sepsis from leaks, is the needle catheter jejunostomy. This technique is useful after surgery such as Whipple's procedure, where it is anticipated that the patient may not be able to eat for a prolonged period.

Selection of Feeding Mixtures

The feeding mixtures used enterally can be classified into the categories listed below. (Detailed compositions are given in Table 6-1.)

Types of Mixtures

POLYMERIC DIETS. These include: (1) blenderized formulas, which are composed of whole foods, (2) lactose-containing milk-based diets, which are palatable and can be taken orally and (3) lactose-free formulas, which are palatable and can be given to lactose-intolerant patients.

DEFINED FORMULA OR ELEMENTAL DIETS. These formulas are not palatable and must be given nasoenterally. Because they are predigested, they can be easily absorbed and are thus ideal for patients with pancreatic insufficiency or short bowel.

MODULAR DIETS. These diets are composed of separate modules of protein, fat, carbohydrate, electrolytes and trace elements. Because they can be combined in different ratios, they are valuable for feeding patients with specific needs.

SODIUM CONTENT OF ENTERAL DIETS. The sodium concentration of most enteral formulas is 20 to 30 mM. Because absorption of glucose released by digestion of saccharides in the diet requires Na^+ for transport, the low sodium content of the diet hinders carbohydrate absorption and promotes diarrhea. Add sodium to a final concentration of 100 mM to decrease diarrhea.

Delivery of Nutrients

Starter Regimens. Start with full-strength feeding, given slowly to be sure that there is no gastric retention. If there is no evidence of obstruction or retention over the first 8 hours, the rate is increased from 50 to 125 ml/hr over the first 3 days.

Use of Pumps. Constancy of nutrient inflow to avoid diarrhea is best achieved with a pump.

Contamination. Nutritional solutions become contaminated and grow bacteria easily. They should be prepared in a sterile manner or obtained in prepackaged sterile bags and infused so that the bag does not hang longer than 8 hours.

PARENTERAL NUTRITION

Nutrition Prescription

There is an increasing tendency to provide all nutrients, including lipid, in a 3-liter plastic bag. The mixture is stable for 24 hours. Instability may be due to excessive quantities of divalent cations (Ca^{2+}, Mg^{2+}, and Zn^{2+}).

Catheter Care and Tubing Change

The dressing on the catheter exit site should be changed at least once a week. It should also be changed if it becomes infected.

COMPLICATIONS

ENTERAL NUTRITION

Misplaced Tube. Problems related to misplaced tubes can be avoided by taking radiographic films before infusion in all cases.

Gastric Retention and Aspiration. Use of nasoenteral, rather than nasogastric, feeding for critically ill patients avoids gastric retention and aspiration. If gastric feeding is used, the residual volume is checked and, if it exceeds 150 ml, infusion is resumed at half the rate and the residual is determined every 4 hours. To minimize aspiration, the patient can be fed with the head raised to 30°.

Diarrhea and GI Discomfort. Factors that can cause diarrhea and gastrointestinal discomfort during EN, and measures to correct them, are as follows:

1 Lack of sodium in the formula—add sodium.

2 Uncontrolled flow into the intestine—use pump to regulate flow.

(Text continued on page 53)

TABLE 6-1 APPROXIMATE COMPOSITION OF REPRESENTATIVE NUTRITIONAL SUPPLEMENTS

Name of Supplement	Standard Serving Size	Calories per 100 ml	Carbohydrate		Protein		Fats		Sodium	Osmolarity mOsm/liter	Recommended Daily Volume	Flavors Available	Properties
			Source	g/100 ml	Source	g/100 ml	Source	g/100 ml	mg/100 ml				
Vivonex (Norwich Eaton)	300 ml	100	Glucose Oligosaccharides	22.6	L-Amino acids	2.0	Safflower oil	0.07	86	550	1800 ml	Unflavored Flavoring packages availables: chocolate, beef broth, orange, grape, strawberry, vanilla, tomato	Elemental diet Minimal residue Lactose-free
Vivonex HN (Norwich Eaton)	300 ml	100	Glucose Oligosaccharides	20.2	L-Amino acids	4.6	Safflower oil	0.09	77	810	3000 ml	Same as Vivonex	High protein Elemental
Flexical (Mead-Johnson)	250 ml	100	Sucrose Dextrins	15.5	Casein protein hydrolysate L-amino acids	2.68	Soy oil MCT oil* Lecithin	3.4	35	805	2000 ml	—	Minimal residue Low residue Lactose-free
Isocal (Mead-Johnson	250 ml	100	Corn syrup solids	2.15	Calcium & sodium caseinates Soy protein isolate	3.25	Soy oil MCT oil Lecithin	4.2	50	350	2000 ml	—	Lactose-free
Precision LR (Doyle)	300 ml	106	Maltodextrin Sucrose	23.7	Egg white solids	2.5	Vegetable oil	0.07	67	525	1710 ml	Cherry, lemon, lime, orange	Low residue Lactose-free
Precision isotonic (Doyle)	250 ml	100	Glucose Oligosaccharides Sucrose	15.0	Egg white solids	3.0	Vegetable oil	3.1	80	300	1560	Vanilla	Isotonic Low residue Lactose-free
Precision HN (Doyle)	300 ml	100	Maltodextrin Sucrose	20.7	Egg white solids	4.2	Vegetable oil	0.04	93	580	3000 ml	Citrus fruit	High protein Low residue Lactose-free

Vital (Ross)	300 ml	100	Glucose Oligosaccharides Polysaccharides	18.9	Soy, whey Meat (hydrolyzed)	4.1	Sunflower oil	1.0	38	450	1500 + ml	Banana	Complete hydrolyzed diet
Nutri-1000 (Cutter)	10 oz 32 ox	100	Corn syrup solids Milk Sucrose	10.0	Skim milk Sodium caseinate	3.25	Soy oil (hydrogenated) Coconut oil	5.2	50	400	2000 ml	Vanilla, chocolate	Medium residue 5 g lactose/ 100 ml (also a lactose-free product)
Citrotein (Doyle)	190 ml	66	Sucrose Maltodextrin	12.3	Egg white solids	4.0	Vegetable oil	0.17	68	503	1152 ml	Orange	Lactose-free
Ensure (Ross)	250 ml	106	Corn syrup solids Sucrose	14.4	Calcium caseinate Soy protein isolate	3.7	Corn oil	3.7	74	460	1900 ml	Vanilla, black walnut Flavor packages available: vanilla, orange, cherry, lemon, pecan, strawberry	Medium residue Lactose-free
Portagen (Mead-Johnson)	250 ml	100	Corn syrup solids Sucrose	10.4	Sodium caseinate	3.4	MCT oil Corn oil Lecithin	5.0	62	354	1200 ml	—	Lactose-free
Sustacal (Mead-Johnson)	360 ml	100	Sucrose Corn syrup solids	13.7	Conc. skim milk Sodium & calcium caseinate Soy protein isolates	5.1	Soy oil	2.3	92	625	1080 ml	Vanilla, chocolate	Medium residue
Meritene (Dolye)	300 ml	100	Corn syrup solids Sucrose	12.0	Conc. skim milk Sodium & calcium caseinate	6.0	Vegetable oil	3.0	90	560	1040 ml	Vanilla, eggnog, chocolate	Milk base ~ 57g lactose/1000 kcal

(continued on page 52)

TABLE 6-1 *(continued from page 51)*

Name of Supple-ment	Standard Serving Size	Calories per 100 ml	Carbohydrate		Protein		Fats		Sodium				
			Source	g/100 ml	Source	g/100 ml	Source	g/100 ml	mg/100 ml	Osmo-larity mOsm/liter	Recom-mended Daily Volume	Flavors Available	Properties
Lolactene (Doyle)	Similar to Meritene with < 4.0 g lactose/1000 kcal												
Cutter II (Cutter)	200 ml	100	Sucrose Orange juice Farina Conc. of green beans & carrots	12.1	NFDM† Beef Egg yolk	3.75	Corn oil Egg yolk	4.0	63	435–510	2000 ml	—	Moderate residue ~ 37 g lac-tose/1000 kcal
Compleat-B (Doyle)	400 ml	100	Maltodextrin NFDM Sucrose Green bean puree Pea puree Orange juice Peach puree	12.0	Beef puree NFDM	4.0	Corn oil	4.0	140	490	1600 ml	—	Moderate residue ~ 24 g lac-tose/1000 kcal
Sustagen (Mead-John-son)	240 ml	160	Corn syrup solids Dextrose	27.2	NFDM Powdered whole milk Calcium cas-einate	9.6	Milk fat	1.4	108	1620	1750 ml	Vanilla, chocolate	High calorie High protein Lactose con-taining
Amin-Aid (McGaw)	340 ml	200	Maltodextrin Sucrose	32.4	Essential amino acids Histidine	1.9	Soy oil	7.0	13	1125	—	—	Elemental diet Supplement Low electro-lyte Lactose-free

(Kirshner JB, Shorter RG: Inflammatory Bowel Disease, 2nd ed. Philadelphia, Lea & Febiger, 1980. Published with permission.)
*MCT = medium-chain triglyceride.
†NFDM = nonfat dry milk.

3 Bacterial contamination—change bags and sets every 24 hours; reduce hang times to 8 hours; use aseptic preparation of solutions.

4 Infusing ice cold solutions—warm to room temperature before feeding.

5 Use of broad-spectrum antibiotics—review use of antibiotics; culture stools for *Clostridium difficile* and test for its toxin.

6 Intercurrent GI problem—examine patient for GI disease.

Electrolyte Disturbance. Osmotic diarrhea can cause hypernatremia, hyperchloremia, and dehydration. Intravenous infusion of free water will control the problem. The cause—inadequate nutrient absorption—should be evaluated and the rate of infusion adjusted.

Technical Complications

Complications of Catheter Insertion. INJURY TO LUNG AND PLEURA. Pneumothorax is the most common complication of catheter insertion. If a patient manifests dyspnea, chest pain, or cyanosis after catheter insertion, tension pneumothorax, or other pleural complication should be suspected. Insertion of a large-bore needle or a thoracostomy tube is performed if the patient is unstable.

INJURY TO THE ARTERY AND VEIN. Injury to the subclavian artery or vein can be treated by removing the needle or catheter and applying direct pressure. The radial and ulnar pulses on the injured side should be checked frequently. If the tip of the catheter lacerates the vein and terminates in the pleural space, infusion of fluid will quickly produce chest pain, dyspnea, and, possibly, shock. A chest radiograph and aspiration of the chest will confirm this diagnosis. This complication can be avoided if the infusion is maintained at a "keep open" rate until the position of the catheter is confirmed radiographically. Treatment should include immediate discontinuation of the infusion, catheter removal, and evacuation of the pleural space by a thoracostomy tube.

INJURY TO BRACHIAL PLEXUS. If there is nerve damage, reflected by radial, ulnar, or median nerve signs, remove the catheter.

INJURY TO THORACIC DUCT. Injury to the thoracic duct from a left subclavian catheter will be obvious when clear lymph drains from the insertion site. Treatment involves removal of the catheter.

INJURY TO MEDIASTINUM. Insertion of a temporary catheter may occasionally cause a mediastinal hematoma. Rarely, a large hematoma could cause compression of the superior vena cava. Surgery would be required to evacuate the hematoma and relieve the obstruction.

EMBOLUS. Air embolism can occur at the time of catheter insertion when the syringe is removed prior to threading of the catheter. It can be avoided by having the patient perform a Valsalva maneuver, during this step in the technique. Embolism of the catheter can occur, if it has been inserted through a needle, upon pulling back on the catheter and adjusting its position while the needle is still in the vein. Intravenous removal with a guide-wire snare technique can be performed with image intensification in the cardiac catheterization unit.

MALPOSITION OF THE CATHETER. On occasion, during insertion the catheter will enter the ipsilateal internal jugular vein or cross over to the contralateral innominate vein. If malposition occurs, it should be corrected by repositioning under fluoroscopic control. If this is not possible, the catheter should be removed and a new catheter inserted.

CARDIAC COMPLICATIONS. Cardiac dysrhythmias may occur if the catheter is positioned within the right atrium or ventricle. This complication can be avoided by correct positioning of the catheter within the SVC.

Septic Complications

If a fever develops during the administration of PN, a close examination for focal sources must be carried out. In particular, injection abscesses, phlebitis, chest infection, urinary tract infection, and abdominal sepsis should be considered. Certain patients are at greater risk for catheter sepsis than others, including anergic patients, those receiving steroids, and those with acute pancreatitis and severe inflammatory bowel disease. If the blood cultures are positive or if the fever continues, the temporary subclavian catheter should be removed. Even after catheter removal, fever and positive blood cultures will persist in certain circumstances. Antibiotics are used.

Metabolic Complications

The blood glucose levels should be measured regularly, and exogenous insulin may be infused by a constant infusion. If the patient is acutely ill and has low blood pressure or poor peripheral circulation, intravenous infusion (in contrast to subcutaneous administration) is the only way to ensure that injected insulin is available to the body. The intravenous route allows careful control of blood glucose in the unstable patient, and the needs for insulin with a constant infusion are low compared with the amounts required using intermittent dosing.

Hypoglycemia. Symptoms include weakness, trembling, diaphoresis, headache, chills, rapid pulse, and decreased consciousness. If the volume infused falls behind schedule, the rate should not be increased to "catch up."

Electrolyte Imbalances. The most common imbalances are related to potassium, phosphorus, and magnesium ions. During active protein synthesis and anabolism, the level of these ions in the plasma may fall. These should be corrected immediately, usually through a change in the PN prescription.

Hyperlipoproteinemia. An elevation of blood lipids may occur as a result of overproduction of lipids from endogenous sources, overinfusion of exogenous lipids, reduced utilization, or from infusing carbohydrates in excess of needs.

Hypercholesterolemia. Hypercholesterolemia may be seen when lipid emulsions are infused at high rates (*i.e.*, in excess of 2 g/kg/day). The elevation returns to normal within a few days of discontinuing the infusion.

Abnormalities of Liver Function. Fatty liver results from the infusion of carbohydrate in excess of caloric needs or from a deficiency of essential fatty acids. The patient presents with a large tender liver and an elevation of serum glutamic-oxaloacetic transaminase (SGOT) or serum aspartate transaminase (AST).

For further information, please see Chapter 45 in Civetta JM, Taylor RW, Kirby RR: Critical Care. *Philadelphia: J. B. Lippincott, 1988*

BIBLIOGRAPHY

Anderson GH, Patel DG, Jeejeebhoy KN: Design and evaluation by nitrogen balance and blood aminograms of an amino acid mixture for total parenteral nutrition of adults with gastrointestinal disease. *J Clin Invest* 1974; 53:904

Dickenson RJ, Ashton MG, Axon ATR, et al: Controlled trial of intravenous hyperalimentation and total bowel rest as an adjunct to routine therapy of acute colitis. *Gastroenterology* 1980; 79:1199

Finch CA, Huebers H: Perspectives in iron metabolism. *N Engl J Med* 1982; 306:1520

Greenberg GR, Fleming CR, Jeejeebhoy KN, et al: Controlled trial of bowel rest and nutritional support in the management of Crohn's disease (abstr). *Gastroenterology* 1985; 88:1405

Halperin ML, Wolman SL, Greenberg GR: Paracellular recirculation of sodium is essential to support nutrient absorption in the gastrointestinal tract: An hypothesis. *Clin Invest Med* 1986; 9:209

Hill GL, King RFGJ, Smith RC, et al: Multi-element analysis of the living body by neutron activation analysis—Application to critically ill patients receiving intravenous nutrition. *Br J Surg* 1979; 66:868

Keohane PP, Attrill H, Love M, et al: Relation between osmolality of diet and gastrointestinal side effects in enteral nutrition. *Br Med J* 1984; 288:678

Koretz RL: What supports nutritional support? *Dig Dis Sci* 1984; 29:577

O'Morain C, Segal AW, Levi AJ: Elemental diets as primary therapy of acute Crohn's disease: A controlled trial. *Br Med J* 1984; 288:1859

Saverymuttu S, Hodgson HJF, Chadwick VS: Controlled trial comparing prednisolone with an elemental diet plus non-absorbable antibiotics in active Crohn's disease. *Gut* 1985; 26:994

Wolman SL, Anderson GH, Marliss EB, et al: Zinc in total parenteral nutrition: Requirements and metabolic effects. *Gastroenterology* 1979; 76:458

Young GA, Collins JP, HIll GL: Plasma proteins in patients receiving intravenous amino acids or intravenous hyperalimentation after major surgery. *Am J Clin Nutr* 1979; 32:1192

II.
The Surgical Patient

7

Preoperative Evaluation of High-Risk Elective Surgical Patients

Preoperative evaluation of a critically ill patient may vary from rapid diagnosis and resuscitation for a life-threatening emergency to a detailed analysis of the suitability of a physiologically compromised patient to undergo major operation. In the first case, preoperative evaluation includes therapy, and that evaluation is necessarily brief and narrowly focused. This chapter presents the decision process involved in evaluating high-risk patients for operation or patients undergoing high-risk procedures. In order to begin this analysis, an understanding of perioperative risks is essential.

OVERALL PERIOPERATIVE RISK

Physicians caring for patients in the perioperative period know that morbidity and mortality occur but often underestimate the risk by tenfold to 100-fold. Ten percent of surgical patients experience a complication. This morbidity is difficult to quantify, and a consensus view on its clinical importance is not available. Mortality, on the other hand, is a more easily defined end-point, and more information is available for analysis.

Perioperative mortality for elective surgical procedures ranges from 0.5% to 1.9% and is dependent upon numerous modifying factors, including patient age and concurrent diseases; surgical procedure; institution; and postoperative care. In a series of more than 100,000 patients, the perioperative mortality was 0.5% if no concurrent preoperative medical condition was present; it increased to 2.1% with obesity, 7% with ischemic heart disease, and 15.8% with cardiac failure. Mortality was further increased twofold to fivefold for each of these conditions if the operation was emergent rather than elective. The reported mortality for patients older than 65 years of age is 4.9%. Although the data are not clear-cut, age appears to identify patients at increased risk for perioperative death. The important factor may not be age *per se*, but rather that older patients have more concurrent diseases, placing them at risk in the perioperative period. The American Society of Anesthesiologists' (ASA) physical status classification system (Table 7–1), although not intended to be a measure of risk, nevertheless correlates with increasing perioperative mortality (Table 7–2) and identifies an increasingly ill patient population.

The impact of the proposed surgical procedure on a high-risk patient also needs to be understood if appropriate perioperative management is to be attained. Goldman outlined a cardiac risk stratification system for patients undergoing a variety of noncardiac surgical procedures, which is widely used as an estimate of cardiac risk. However, Jeffrey evaluated Goldman's index in a select group, patients undergoing aortic surgery, and documented that cardiac risk was under-estimated from threefold to sevenfold, depending on the Goldman class. This work indicates that the physiologic trespass imposed by different procedures needs to be considered when one determines the appropriateness of preoperative evaluation in high-risk patients.

Qualifications of the physicians caring for the patient also need to be ascertained. Slogoff reported that perioperative morbidity and perioperative myocardial infarction varied sevenfold between anesthesiologists practicing in the same institution. Thus, although they seldom are considered formally in risk stratification, physicians caring for a patient perioperatively—anesthesiologists, internists, and surgeons alike—are an important determinant of the type and extent of preoperative evaluation that is appropriate for an individual high-risk patient.

WHO SHOULD BE EVALUATED?

When one considers patients at higher risk, are there any general guidelines to direct the preoperative evaluation? Two important variables, age and the urgency of the operation, cannot be altered. Therefore, you should direct your evaluation to variables in which improvement is possible: concurrent disease, the anesthetic, and the operative procedure. The increased risk associated with aging may indicate that a more detailed evaluation is desirable. Infections in high-risk patients are not covered in any detail in this chapter. Nevertheless, they are involved in a large percentage of delayed

TABLE 7–1. DEFINITIONS OF AMERICAN SOCIETY OF ANESTHESIOLOGISTS (ASA) PHYSICAL STATUS CLASSIFICATION

Physical Status	Definition
1	Healthy patient
2	Mild systemic disease; no functional limitation
3	Severe systemic disease; definite functional limitation
4	Severe systemic disease that is constant threat to life
5	Moribund patient; unlikely to survive 24 hours, with or without operation

TABLE 7–2. PERIOPERATIVE MORTALITY IN PATIENTS STRATIFIED ACCORDING TO ASA CLASSIFICATION

Physical Status	Anesthetics	Deaths	Mortality (%)	Mortality Factor*
1	50,703	43	0.08	NA
2	12,601	34	0.27	3.4
3	3,626	66	1.8	22.5
4	850	66	7.8	97.5
5	608	57	9.4	117.5

(Modified from Vacanti)
*The factor mortality was increased over that in ASA I patients.

perioperative deaths. Every effort should be made to prevent them if they have not occurred, and to treat them if they have.

Concurrent diseases associated with the most significant perioperative complications or the highest mortality are those involving the cardiovasular, pulmonary, and neurologic systems. When organ-system dysfunction is examined in each of these areas, some unifying signs and symptoms appear to be useful as indicators of increased risk or the need for a more detailed preoperative evaluation (Table 7–3). Additionally, some high-risk operations

TABLE 7–3. INDICATORS OF INCREASED PERIOPERATIVE RISK AND NEED FOR MORE DETAILED PREOPERATIVE EVALUATION IN HIGH-RISK PATIENTS

Cardiovascular
- S_3 Gallop
- Jugular venous distention
- Myocardial infarction within 6 months
- Dysrhythmias*
- Age > 70 years
- Emergency operation
- Important AS
- Poor general health

Pulmonary
- Chronic lung disease
- $FEV_1 < 2.0$ liters
- Obesity
- Hypercarbia at rest
- Age > 70 years
- Site of operation
- Smoking history

Neurologic
- CNS injury
- Carotoid bruit†

(Modified from Goldman, Tisi, and Wolf)
*Other than sinus or PACs, or PVCs > 5/min.
†As a marker for ischemic heart disease.

demand a more detailed evaluation either preoperatively or intraoperatively, even in healthy asymptomatic patients.

HOW TO PROCEED

CARDIOVASCULAR DISEASE

Cardiovascular complications contribute to a significant percentage of perioperative mortality because of their prevalence within the surgical population and their immediate life-threatening nature. If we are to limit the impact of cardiovascular complications on perioperative morbidity and mortality, we must recognize that cardiovascular disease is present.

The physical examination *may* be helpful if signs point toward a diagnosis of congestive heart failure but often is of limited value if one attempts to rely on it to predict other cardiovascular functions. Some data suggest that correct predictions of cardiac index and pulmonary artery occulsion pressure are possible, based on physical findings alone, in patients with acute myocardial infarctions. Yet, in critically ill patients, the predictive value of the physical examination appears limited. Conners evaluated such individuals without myocardial damage. Physical examination was associated with a correct prediction of cardiac index and pulmonary artery occlusion pressure only in 44% and 42% of patients, respectively. The number of correct predictions did not correlate with observer experience; residents and attending staff were equally (in)effective. Thus, the concept that physician experience enables more accurate prediction of cardiovascular function is open to question.

Goldman has suggested that in patients receiving general anesthetics, and undergoing elective operation, hypertension does not result in an increased risk provided that [1] the diastolic blood pressure is stable and not more than 110 mm Hg and [2] intraoperative and recovery room blood pressures are closely monitored and are treated so that changes more than 50% above or more than 33% below the preoperative value do not occur for more than 10 minutes.

The nature of the patient's symptoms and physical findings should dictate the extent of the preoperative laboratory assessment. Because congestive heart failure, recent myocardial infarction, and aortic stenosis all carry a significantly increased risk at operation, they should be searched for and defined by the available laboratory testing.

PULMONARY DISEASE

The nearly universal impairment of pulmonary function in the perioperative period makes pulmonary risk assessment central to a complete preoperative evaluation. Perioperative pulmonary complications range from 2% to 70%, depending on the criteria used to identify them. Despite this wide variation, high-risk patients can be identified and management altered to lessen the risk of pulmonary problems. The evaluation of suitability for operation in patients with compromised pulmonary function has a long history.

A careful history often directs the preoperative evaluation of the high-risk surgical patient. Limited exercise tolerance, increased sputum production, and a history of wheezing demand a more thorough examination before surgery. Obesity, age, smoking history, and the site of operation are additional risk factors identifiable before laboratory testing. The physical examination will reinforce the history yet, as is the case with certain cardiovascular measurements, may not allow prediction of cardiopulmonary function in patients with chronic obstructive pulmonary disease.

Through the years, one pulmonary function test has been sought that allows assessment of the suitability for operation in the compromised pulmonary patient. At present, however, the most practical approach is to combine a number of examinations. Arterial blood gas and pH measurements assess oxygenation and ventilatory adequacy. Hypoxemia is not as predictive of high perioperative risk as is hypercarbia. In patients with hypercarbia, perioperative pulmonary complications are higher than in those who can maintain normal alveolar ventilation.

Pulmonary spirometry commonly is performed on patients undergoing routine operation. A forced expiratory volume at 1 second (FEV_1) less than 2 liters suggests the strong possibilty of postoperative pulmonary dysfunction. Because thoracic and upper abdominal surgery impose approximately the same decrement on post-operative pulmonary function, at least during the immediate postoperative period, use of this general guide seems appropriate. Additional information may be obtained if maximal voluntary ventilation (MVV) is measured.

In general, a reduction of forced vital capacity (FVC) is associated with a restrictive physiologic defect, whereas a reduction of FEV_1 suggests airway obstruction. A better definition of pulmonary reserve involves calculation of the FEV_1/FVC ratio, which normally is 0.85 or greater. Should this value improve after the administration of a bronchodilator, aggressive preoperative therapy (when time allows) may lessen perioperative risk. The importance of such evaluation and treatment is obvious when the immediate postoperative changes in pulmonary function are considered. Recall that in upper abdominal surgery, a significant reduction of FVC and FRC occurs. The reduction of lung volumes is related not only to pain, but also to apparent diaphragmatic dysfunction.

When a high-risk patient is scheduled to undergo pulmonary resection, more specialized pulmonary function testing may be indicated. In addition to the older split lung function technique of bronchospirometry, radioisotope lung scanning techniques (ventilation and perfusion scans) can be used. Further, right heart catheterization, allowing measurement of pulmonary artery pressures and cardiac function, helps to stratify patients with serious pulmonary impairment. Such tests should be performed when routine pulmonary function testing shows FVC to be less than 50% predicted (or less than 15 ml/kg); FEV_1 less than 50% predicted (or less than 2 liters); MVV less than 50% predicted (or less than 50 liters/min).

NEUROLOGIC DISEASE

Exacerbation of major neurologic disease in the perioperative period is not as common, and often not as immediately life-threatening, as are major cardiovascular and pulmonary complications, Nonetheless, significant time is spent screening patients preoperatively for cerebrovascular disease. This effort may be related to the deeply ingrained concept that perioperative strokes are caused by intraoperative hypotension coupled with carotid arterial disease. Most physicians now recognize that cerebral infarctions related to carotid arterial disease usually are caused by artery-to-artery thromboembolism.

The history and physical examination must be used to screen patients for neurologic disease because routine laboratory testing of central nervous system function is not available. Above the age of 55 years, up to one in six patients has a carotid bruit or neurologic symptoms suggestive of carotid arterial disease. When the patient is asymptomatic but has a carotid bruit, no further investigation appears necessary if Ropper's data (Table 7–4) can be extrapolated to all high-risk surgical patients. Should symptoms of extracranial carotid vascular disease be present, further diagnostic work-up may be required.

Methods of assessing the extracranial carotid circulation involve estimates of flow (ophthalmodynamometry, ultrasonic carotid artery doppler studies) and anatomy (ultrasonic B-mode imaging, carotid arteriography). Noninvasive measures generally are considered adequate unless more than 70% luminal narrowing of one carotid, more than 50% narrowing of both carotids, or significant ulceration (> 0.5 cm in diameter) is noted. If these features are present, arteriography is indicated. Perhaps more important is the recognition that carotid bruits are often a marker for more life-threatening ischemic heart

TABLE 7–4. INCIDENCE OF CAROTID BRUIT AND STROKE IN ELECTIVE SURGICAL PATIENTS

	Stroke	
Auscultation of Neck	**Number**	**%**
Carotid bruit (n = 104)	1	0.96
No carotid bruit (n = 631)	4	0.63
Total (n = 735)	5*	0.68

(Modified from Ropper)
*Strokes occurred only in patients undergoing coronary artery bypass grafting.

disease. Myocardial infarction occurs 2.5 times more commonly in patients with asymptomatic bruits than in age-matched controls without bruits.

For further information, please see Chapter 15 in Civetta JM, Taylor RW, Kirby RR: Critical Care. *Philadelphia: J. B. Lippincott, 1988*

BIBLIOGRAPHY

Boushy SF, Billeq DM, North LB, et al: Clinical course related to preoperative and postoperative pulmonary function in patients with bronchogenic carcinoma. *Chest* 1971; 59:383

Cohen MM, Duncan PG, Pope WDB, et al: A survey of 112,000 anaesthetics at one teaching hospital (1975–83). *Can Anaesth Soc J* 1986; 33:22

Conners AF, McCaffree DR, Gray BA: Evaluation of right-heart catheterization in the critically ill patient without myocardial infarction. *N Engl J Med* 1983; 308:263

Didolkar MS, Moore RH, Takita H: Evaluation of the risk in pulmonary resection for bronchogenic carcinoma. *Am J Surg* 1974; 127:700

Dureuil B, Desmonts JM, Mankikian B, et al: Effects of aminophylline on diaphragmatic dysfunction after upper abdominal surgery. *Anesthesiology* 1985; 62:242

Farrow SC, Fowkes FGR, Lunn JN, et al: Epidemiology in anaesthesia: II. Factors affecting mortality in the hospital. *Br J Anaesth* 1982; 54:811

Farrow SC, Fowkes FGR, Lunn JN, et al: Epidemiology in anaesthesia: III. Mortality risk in patients with co-existing disease. *Br J Anaesth* 1982; 54:819

Forrester JS, Diamond GA, Swan HJC: Correlative classification of clinical and hemodynamic function after acute myocardial infarction. *Am J Cardiol* 1977; 39:137

Goldman L, Caldera DL: Risks of general anesthesia and elective operation in the hypertensive patient. *Anesthesiology* 1979; 50:285

Goldman L, Caldera DL, Nussbaum SR, et al: Multifactorial index of cardiac risk in non-cardiac surgical procedures. *N Engl J Med* 1977; 297:845

Hospital Mortality: PHS Hospitals, United States, 1974–1975, p. 190. Ann Arbor, Commission on Professional and Hospital Activities, 1977

Jeffrey CC, Kunsman J, Cullen DJ, et al: A prospective evaluation of cardiac risk index. *Anesthesiology* 1983; 58:462

Kronlund SF, Phillips WR: Physician knowledge or risks of surgical and invasive diagnostic procedures. *West J Med* 1985; 142:565

Ropper AH, Wechsler LR, Wilson LS: Carotid bruit and the risk of stroke in elective surgery. *N Engl J Med* 1982; 307:1388

Simmoneau G, Vivien A, Sartene, et al: Diaphragm dysfunction induced by upper abdominal surgery. Role of postoperative pain. *Am Rev Respir Dis* 1983; 128:899

Slogoff S, Keats AS: Does perioperative myocardial ischemia lead to postoperative myocardial infarction? *Anesthesiology* 1985; 62:107

Tisi GM: Preoperative evaluation of pulmonary function: Validity, indications and benefits. *Am Rev Respir Dis* 1979; 119:293

Tisi GM: *Pulmonary Physiology in Clinical Medicine,* p. 109. Baltimore, Williams & Wilkins, 1980

Toole JF: Editorial: Surgery for patients with carotid-artery murmurs. *N Engl J Med* 1982; 307:1401

Unger K, Shaw D, Karlinger JS, et al: Evaluation of left ventricular function in patients with chronic obstructive lung disease. *Chest* 1975; 68:135

Vacanti CJ, VanHouten RJ, Hill RC: A statistical analysis of the relationship of physical status to postoperative mortality in 68,388 cases. *Anesth Analg* 1970; 49:564

Wolf PA, Kannel WB, Sorlie P, et al: A symptomatic carotid bruit and risk of stroke. The Framingham study. *JAMA* 1981; 245:1442

8

Trauma: Secondary Triage in the ICU

INITIAL ICU EVALUATION

OXYGENATION AND VENTILATION

Arterial blood gas values are the best indicators of oxygenation and ventilation. However, the Pa_{O_2} must be correlated with the FI_{O_2} and the appearance of the chest radiograph to fully appreciate the severity of the patient's problem. Initially, hypoxemia must be corrected by ruling out simple causes (e.g., pneumothorax), increasing the FI_{O_2} or increasing PEEP.

Ventilation is a separate function intimately related to oxygenation. In the unintubated conscious patient, increased respiratory and pulse rates, sweating, and flaring of the alae nasae may all be signs of hypercapnia. Alternatively, these signs may be absent with central nervous system depression from drug overdose, anesthetics, or massive head injury. Physical findings of upper airway obstruction include inspiratory stridor, suprasternal and intercostal retractions, and paradoxical motion of the chest wall. If clearing of the upper airway does not resolve the obstruction, tracheal intubation or cricothyroidotomy may be indicated.

PERFUSION

Blood pressure, the color, warmth, and speed of capillary refill of the extremities, and urine output are sensitive parameters which can be assessed quickly. A sinusoidal arterial pulse tracing in the mechanically ventilated patient may be a sign of hypovolemia. The arterial blood presssure consistently diminishes during the inspiratory cycle of positive-pressure ventilation due to diminished venous return.

Most trauma victims will already have a central venous pressure (CVP) catheter in position. A low CVP associated with poor perfusion is helpful. However, a normal or high CVP may not indicate normovolemia. The possibility of cardiac tamponade (causing equalization of the arterial, pulmonary artery, and central venous pressures) must always be considered in any trauma patient or one who has had central venous catheterization.

RENAL FUNCTION

Separate assessment of renal function is important because development of acute renal failure (ARF) doubles the mortality rate in the ICU. Hourly monitoring of urine output is essential. Differentiation between acute tubular necrosis (ATN) and prerenal azotemia may be difficult. Measurement of serum and urine sodium, creatinine, urea, and water may help (Table 8–1). In patients with rhabdomyolysis (compartment syndrome, crush injury, compression necrosis of skeletal muscle), osmotic diuresis with mannitol and alkalinization of the urine with sodium bicarbonate are indicated. Obstructive uropathy is an uncommon cause of renal failure in the trauma patient and can be ruled out by renal ultrasound.

Restoration of intravascular volume and the judicious use of low-dose

TABLE 8-1 DIFFERENTIATING PRERENAL AZOTEMIA AND ACUTE TUBULAR NECROSIS

Index	Prerenal (Functional ARF)	ATN (Parnechymal ARF)
(Indices of tubular reabsorption of sodium)		
RFI	<1	>1
FE(Na)	<1	>1
U(Na)	<20 meq/liter	>40 meq/liter
(Indices of tubular reabsorption of water)		
C(H_2O)	<0	>0
U(osm)/S(osm)	>2	<1.1
U(Cr)/S(Cr)	>40	<20
U(urea)/S(urea)	>20	<10
Urine SG	>1.020	<1.010
U(osm)	>500 mOsm/liter	350 mOsm/liter
S(urea)/S(Cr)	>10:1	ca 10

RFI (renal failure index) = U(Na)/U(Cr)/S(Cr);
FE(Na) = U(Na)/S(Na)/U(Cr)/S(Cr) × 100;
U(Na) = Urine sodium concentration;
S(Na) = Serum sodium concentration;
U(Cr) = Urine creatinine concentration;
S(Cr) = Serum creatinine concentration;
C(H_2O) (Free water clearance) = S(osm)/U(osm) × U(vol) × U(vol);
U(osm) = Urine osmolality;
S(osm) = Serum osmolality;
U(vol) = Urine volume;
SG = specific gravity;
ca = approximately.

dopamine (2–5 μg/kg/min) to optimize renal blood flow may help maintain urine output. Loop diuretics, however, should rarely if ever be used in the first 24 hours in the treatment of the multiple trauma victim.

NEUROLOGIC FUNCTION

The Glasgow Coma Scale (GCS) provides an objective assessment of the patient's neurologic status.

DIAGNOSTIC PROCEDURES

Patients with blunt chest trauma need a careful review of the chest radiograph and EKG as well as the arterial blood gases. Acute life-threatening problems such as hemothorax or pneumothorax, cardiac tamponade, and ruptured diaphragm should have been diagnosed by now. Look for pneumomediastinum and atelectasis that may indicate a bronchial tear or an esophageal injury. Consider the possibility of an aortic arch injury. The presence of a left apical cap, widened mediastinum, blurring of the aortic knob, downward shift of the left main stem bronchus, or fractured left first or second ribs are all radiologic indications for arch aortography.

Double contrast CT scans of the abdomen and peritoneal lavage are methods of searching for intraperitoneal injury short of laparotomy.

After the chest and abdomen have been examined, a search for missed, but function-threatening, injuries should be made. Radiographs of the axial skeleton should be reviewed and correlated with the physical examination. Missed fractures should be identified and treated. Is a spine fracture present? If so, is it stable or unstable? Should special radiographic views or a CT scan be taken at this time to help decide on treatment? How much can the patient be moved?

Where and how were the intravenous catheters placed? As a general rule, all vascular access lines placed in trauma patients in the emergency department should be removed within 24 hours. They often have been placed swiftly without strict attention to aseptic technique. Failure to change them sets the stage for septic thrombophlebitis and generalized sepsis several days later.

ONGOING ICU EVALUATION

NEUROLOGIC

What is the patient's GCS? Has it changed? Are pupillary reactions to light symmetric? Is the patient moving all extremities? Is an intracranial pressure (ICP) monitor in place? If so, what is the ICP, and has it been easy to control?

CARDIOVASCULAR

What is the patient's heart rate and rhythm? Is he requiring drugs to augment inotropy or control dysrhythmias? Does the patient have a new heart murmur? Is a new S_3 or S_4 present? What is the CVP, PAOP, cardiac output, blood pressure, and urine output?

RESPIRATORY

Is the patient intubated? If not, can he generate a good cough? What is the amount and character of the tracheal aspirate? What is the F_{IO_2}, Pa_{O_2} and pH? What is the V_T, respiratory rate, peak inspiratory pressure, and PEEP? Are there any changes on today's radiograph?

GASTROINTESTINAL

Is the abdomen soft or firm, scaphoid or distended? What is the nasogastric output? Is the patient receiving antacids? Can tube feedings begin? If not, should hyperalimentation be started? Is there any evidence of intra-abdominal hemorrhage or pus? Is the patient jaundiced?

WOUNDS

Are the wounds clean or dirty, open or closed? Are they granulating? Do they need debridement? Are antibiotics indicated?

INPUT AND OUTPUT

What is the exact input and output? Is the balance positive or negative? What about the electrolytes, BUN, creatinine, and blood sugar? What changes are required in the fluid orders?

HEMATOLOGIC STATUS

Are the hemoglobin and hematocrit stable? Should we measure the prothrombin time, partial thromboplastin time, and platelet count? What about the possibility of disseminated intravascular coagulation?

SEPSIS

Is the patient receiving antibiotics? What organisms have been cultured from where? What are the sensitivities of the organisms? Is the patient's creatinine rising? If so, should the dose of aminoglycoside be altered? Where is the source of sepsis, and what is being done about it? The intravenous catheters should be changed, blood, sputum, urine, and wound cultures obtained, antibiotics started, and occult (intrathoracic, intracranial, and intra-abdominal) sources of sepsis identified.

For further information, please see Chapter 46 in Civetta JM, Taylor RW, Kirby RR: Critical Care. *Philadelphia: J. B. Lippincott, 1988*

BIBLIOGRAPHY

Advanced Trauma Life Support Manual, Committee on Trauma, American College of Surgeons, p. 57, 1984

Anderson RJ, Linas SL, Berns AS, et al: Nonoliguric acute renal failure. *N Engl J Med* 1977; 296:1134

Blaisdell WF, Trunkey DD: *Trauma Management: Vol 1. Abdominal Trauma.* Thieme-Stratton, Georg Thiem Verlag, 1982

Lee WC, Uddo JF Jr, Nance FC: Surgical judgment in the management of abdominal stab wounds. Utilizing clinical criteria from a 10-year experience. *Ann Surg* 1984; 199:549

McLellan BA, Hanna SS, Montoya DR, et al: Analysis of peritoneal lavage parameters in blunt abdominal trauma. *J Trauma* 1985; 25:393

Petty TL, Ashbaugh DG: The adult respiratory distress syndrome—Clinical features and factors influencing prognosis and principles of management. *Chest* 1971; 70:233

Trunkey DD, Lewis FR: Current Therapy of Trauma, 1984–1985. In *Abdominal Trauma.* Philadelphia, BC Decker, 1984

Valeri RC, Feingold H, Cassidy G, et al: Hypothermia-induced reversible platelet dysfunction. *Ann Surg* 1987; 205:175

Werwath DL, Schwab CW, Scholton JR, Robinett W: Microwave ovens: A safe method of warming crystalloids *Am Surg* 1984; 50:656

9 Evaluation of Bleeding

Abnormal bleeding during or following a surgical procedure, or after traumatic injury, is due either to a failure of local hemostasis (termed "surgical bleeding") or to a defect in the coagulation mechanism. Although catastrophic hemorrhage is readily evident, bleeding after admission to the intensive care unit (ICU) may, at other times, be occult. Signs of hypovolemia may be mistaken for inadequate fluid replacement or vasodilatation, and a slowly falling hematocrit may be erroneously attributed to "hemodilution." Abnormal bleeding in the surgical or trauma patient requires immediate acquisition of information about previous bleeding tendencies or the administration of drugs that interfere with the coagulation mechanism. Careful examination will usually (but not always) disclose if bleeding is localized surgical bleeding, or if it is secondary to a generalized coagulopathy. To complete the evaluation of abnormal bleeding, use a sequence of laboratory determinations outlined by the algorithm in Figure 9–1. While this approach can be very useful, it is equally important to recall that bleeding postoperatively is commonly due to technical errors (surgical bleeding), anticoagulation therapy, or sepsis.

SURGICAL BLEEDING

The most common cause for postoperative bleeding is imperfect or incomplete attention to hemostasis during the procedure. Severe postoperative hemorrhage may present as profound hypotension or shock, or be recognized as blood exiting through tubes or drainage tracts. Blood in tubes and drains may clot, however, and there can be significant bleeding without outward manifestations. The rate and magnitude of blood loss is quantitated by measuring external losses, or it can be related to the number of units of blood used for replacement. Since surgical bleeding is dependent on technical aspects, discussion with members of the operative team may reveal intraoperative problems which increase its likelihood. This suspicion will be further heightened if the usual tests of coagulation are normal. Prompt reoperation is mandatory in the presence of massive bleeding because unabated blood loss is associated with profound systemic effects. In the absence of these factors, the decision to reoperate depends on less quantifiable factors such as the potential benefits of removing an extravascular collection of blood versus the stresses of a second operation.

NONSURGICAL BLEEDING

Defects in primary hemostasis (local vasoconstriction and formation of platelet plugs) or in secondary hemostasis (transformation of fibrinogen to cross-linked fibrin) are either congenital or acquired. Disorders of primary hemostasis are differentiated from those of secondary hemostasis by the platelet count and template bleeding time (Fig. 9–1).

DISORDERS OF PRIMARY HEMOSTASIS

A decrease in the number of circulating platelets or an alteration in platelet function results in disorders of primary hemostasis. Thrombocytopenia may be due to dilution following multiple transfusions, decreased production secondary to suppression of bone marrow megakaryocytes, sequestration in the spleen, or increased destruction such as occurs during sepsis. Not uncommonly, more than one process occurs, causing a severe defect in primary hemostasis.

A prolonged bleeding time associated with a normal platelet count indicates a defect in platelet function. Ingestion of aspirin is probably the most common cause of defective platelet function. The defect (blocking formation of thromboxane) is permanent for the life of the platelet, usually 8 to 10 days, and administration of platelets is necessary to correct the abnormal bleeding time. A single 325-mg dose of aspirin will prolong the bleeding time longer than 6 minutes in 50% to 60% of patients. This emphasizes the importance of determining the medications that have been given to the patient with abnormal hemostasis. Platelet function is reversibly affected by hypothermia, a frequent complication in trauma patients and in surgical patients undergoing extensive procedures. Thus, the treatment of hypothermia should be a major priority in the postoperative bleeding patient.

DISORDERS OF SECONDARY HEMOSTASIS

If the platelet count and bleeding time are normal, the patient most likely has a disorder of secondary hemostasis. A prolonged partial thromboplastin time (PTT) with a normal prothrombin time (PT) suggests an inherited defect in coagulation. The major inherited bleeding disorders are factor VIII deficiency (hemophilia A), factor IX deficiency (hemophilia B), and von Willebrand's disease. Hemophilia A and B account for approximately 75% and 20%, respectively, of all inherited factor deficiencies. Patients with large wounds or patients who are about to undergo major surgery should have complete

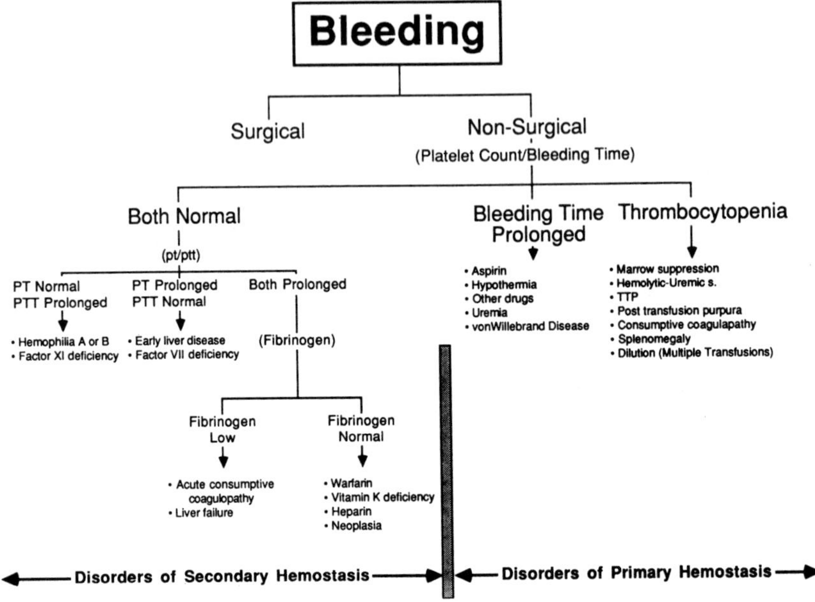

Figure 9-1 Causes of abnormal bleeding in a surgical patient. Bleeding must first be differentiated as either a failure of local hemostasis ("surgical bleeding") or a defect in the coagulation mechanism. Coagulation disorders are further segregated into disorders of primary hemostasis encompassing qualitative or quantitative platelet defects and disorders of secondary hemostasis involving coagulation factor deficiencies. Virtually all disorders of coagulation encountered in the surgical patient are acquired defects and are identified by routine laboratory tests.

replacement of the deficient factor in consultation with a hematologist. Liver disease and factor VII deficiency produce a prolonged PT in association with a normal PTT.

Prolongation of both the PT and PTT are indicative of acquired disorders of coagulation. Included in this group are bleeding associated with warfarin administration or heparin infusion, vitamin K deficiency, consumptive coagulopathy, liver failure, and neoplasia. Patients receiving warfarin in the therapeutic range seldom develop spontaneous hemorrhage. However, they may demonstrate abnormal bleeding after surgery. Administration of fresh frozen plasma will be necessary to correct this defect. Anticoagulation with heparin during peripheral vascular or cardiovascular procedures may extend into the postoperative period, impairing hemostasis. Vitamin K deficiency may be present in the chronically ill or malnourished patient. The administration of vitamin K, although specific, will not quickly correct the defect induced by vitamin K deficiency in a bleeding patient. Administration of fresh frozen plasma is, therefore, necessary.

The other causes of an acquired coagulopathy are further differentiated by determining the fibrinogen level. A diminished fibrinogen level suggests the diagnosis of an acute consumptive coagulopathy, which is supported by other evidence that indicates on-going intravascular coagulation. This process also involves consumption of platelets, lowering the platelet count. When consumptive coagulopathy induced by sepsis is present, the most immediate goal is identification and treatment of the septic focus before attention is directed entirely to correcting the coagulopathy. If the initiating event is not diagnosed and successfully treated, therapy will ultimately fail. Neoplasia is associated with a consumptive coagulopathy, but it usually occurs in a chronic, less fulminant form. Abnormalities in coagulation parameters, including the fibrinogen level may not always be present.

For further information, please see Chapter 58 in Civetta JM, Taylor RW, Kirby RR: Critical Care. *Philadelphia: J. B. Lippincott, 1988*

BIBLIOGRAPHY

Bick RL: Alterations of hemostasis associated with surgery, cardiopulmonary bypass surgery, and prosthetic devices. In Ratnoff OD, Forbes CD (eds.): *Disorders of Hemostasis,* p. 379. Orlando, Grune & Stratton, 1984

Bick RL: Disseminated intravascular coagulation and related syndromes: Etiology, pathophysiology, diagnosis, and management. *Am J Hematol* 1978; 5:265

Kane KK: Fibrinolysis—A review. *Ann Clin Lab Sci* 1984; 14(6):443

Prentice CRM: Acquired coagulation disorders. *Clin Haematol* 1985; 14(2):413

Risbery B, Medegard A, Heideman M, et al: Early activation of humoral proteolytic systems in patients with multiple trauma. *Crit Care Med* 1986; 14(11):917

Sirridge M: Laboratory evaluation of the bleeding patient. *Clin Lab Med* 1984; 4(2):285

Subcommittee on ATLS of the American College of Surgeons. Shock. In: *Advanced Trauma and Life Support. Course Manual,* p 47. American College of Surgeons, 1984.

10
Abdominal Trauma

In abdominal trauma, significant injuries may not yet have been diagnosed due to subtle presentation or incomplete initial evaluation. Specific details concerning the anatomic injuries and their surgical repair are crucial so that the initial intensive care unit (ICU) plan may provide for the after effects of the injury, its physiologic consequences, and reparative measures.

GENERAL CONSIDERATIONS

ANATOMY

In addition to the more obvious landmarks, intra-abdominal contents can rise to the level of the fourth intercostal space during expiration. Penetrating injuries to the lower chest may cause intra-abdominal injuries.

MECHANISM OF INJURY

In general, there is an ascending order of severity starting with knife or other types of stab wounds, low-velocity gunshot wounds, high-velocity gunshot wounds, and blunt trauma.

DIAGNOSTIC EVALUATION AND MANAGEMENT

Gunshot wounds to the abdomen cause internal injuries in over 90% of cases. Most patients will undergo laparotomy immediately after resuscitation. If the wound is deemed tangential and superficial, frequent reevaluation will be necessary to determine if intra-abdominal or retroperitoneal injuries are present.

Because stab wounds cause internal injuries in only 30% to 40% of cases, patients may be subjected to selective management. Laparotomy is usually performed if the patient presents with hypotension, signs of peritoneal irritation, evisceration through the stab wound, blood in the nasogastric tube, hematuria, blood in the rectum, or pneumoperitoneum.

Diagnostic peritoneal lavage (DPL) is often used to identify intra-abdominal injuries. In penetrating trauma, lavage may be considered positive if the red blood cell (RBC) count is greater than 20,000 mm^3, white blood count (WBC) greater than 500, amylase greater than 175 units, or bile, bacteria, or intestinal contents are identified in the lavage fluid. An open technique for DPL should be used if the patient has a pelvic fracture, is pregnant, is in the pediatric age group, or has had previous surgery. If the red cell count is greater than 100,000/mm^3, DPL is considered positive after blunt trauma. The other criteria are the same. Abdominal computed tomography (CT) scans are currently used to evaluate blunt abdominal trauma. It would seem to be particularly useful to evaluate retroperitoneal structures, the spleen, and the liver.

MORTALITY AND MORBIDITY

The overall mortality rate for stab wounds is approximately 2% to 3%, for gunshot wounds, 10% to 12%, and for blunt trauma, 25%. If intraoperative deaths are excluded, the causes of death include bleeding, associated head injury, pneumonia, respiratory failure, sepsis, and multisystem organ failure (MSOF). The mortality rate also increases with an increased number of abdominal organ injuries. Early deaths are usually due to shock and hemorrhage, whereas late deaths result from sepsis and MSOF.

The most common complications include atelectasis, coagulopathies, acidosis and cardiovascular collapse, adult respiratory distress syndrome (ARDS), pneumonitis, acute renal failure, phlebitis, small bowel obstruction, intra-abdominal abscess, and postoperative abdominal hemorrhage. Patients with major injuries have corresponding major physiologic abnormalities soon after operation. Most are related to cardiorespiratory and oxygen transport functions initially. Nonoperated trauma patients who remain unstable or become unstable during their initial ICU stay should be considered for intra-abdominal hemorrhage or injury to solid or hollow viscus.

SPECIFIC ORGAN INJURIES

LIVER

Injuries are divided into five classes from capsular tear to bilobar destruction or hepatic vein injury. Approximately 75% will be capsular tears (Class I) or nonbleeding parenchymal wounds (Class II). Bleeding parenchymal wounds (Class III) and major fracture or unilobar destruction account for about 10% each. Class I and II injuries have few if any sequelae. In Class III injuries, postoperative bleeding and hepatic dysfunction are more common. Class IV patients have major injury and, therefore, are usually physiologically quite unstable. Packing and the military antishock trousers (MAST) may be used to control bleeding postoperatively. In addition to coagulopathy, hypothermia, acidosis, and bleeding, these patients often have marked respiratory insufficiency. Patients with Class V injuries have a very high intra-operative mortality rate; survivors can be predicted to be extremely unstable.

SPLEEN

The majority of injuries include major lacerations or severe fractures. Splenic salvage is usually attempted if the patients are stable and do not have a shattered spleen. Approximately 50% of splenic injuries can be salvaged; however, operating time and blood loss may be increased. Postoperative complications include atelectasis, pneumonia, and pleural effusion. Pancreatitis and wound infections are also common. Thrombocytosis and intra-abdominal abscesses are late complications of note.

PANCREAS

Pancreatic injuries often occur in association with major vessel injuries, and early deaths usually reflect hemorrhage or profound shock. Specific complications related to pancreatic injuries include fistulas, recurrent abdominal abscesses, and pulmonary complications. Fistulas, pseudocysts, and abscesses can be expected in approximately 25% to 30% of patients with significant pancreatic injury.

DUODENUM

Significant duodenal injuries have approximately 30% mortality and require major extirpative and reconstructive procedures. Postoperative complications include anastomotic leakage and intra-abdominal abscesses, as well as the complications common to all abdominal surgery. Tube gastrostomy, duodenostomy, and jejunostomy are often used to decompress the injured and repaired duodenal segment. Proper functioning of these tubes is necessary to permit the injured duodenum to heal. Fixation is essential, initially, and both tape and sutures must be checked and changed at regular intervals to prevent displacement.

BILIARY TRACT

Although uncommon, these injuries may be difficult to repair technically because of the small size of the ducts encountered; T tubes or other drains may be used in an attempt to stent a repair. Complications following biliary tract injuries include obstructive jaundice, pancreatitis, fistula, cholangitis, and hemobilia.

ESOPHAGUS

Esophageal injuries may escape initial diagnosis. Early severe sepsis and mediastinal air may be present. A gastrostomy and/or cervical esophagostomy may be used for decompression and diversion during the initial postoperative period.

STOMACH AND SMALL BOWEL

Relatively frequently injured in penetrating and blunt trauma, surgical repair is usually straightforward. Anastomotic leaks, fistula, and intra-abdominal abscesses are potential complications but rare because these organs heal well.

COLON AND RECTUM

Resection of the involved segment with proximal diverting colostomy is usually performed in complicated cases. Specific details and a diagram of the procedure performed should be entered into the patient's record since many variations and combinations of surgical procedures can be performed. Intra-abdominal abscess and fecal fistula may occur.

DIAPHRAGM

Penetrating chest injuries often damage the diaphragm as well. Diagnostic peritoneal lavage may be positive, or fluid may exit through a thoracostomy tube. Whenever discovered, diaphragmatic injuries should be repaired because of the possibility of incarceration of abdominal viscera with subsequent strangulation.

FINAL CAVEATS

The patient admitted following laparotomy for significant intra-abdominal injuries can be expected to have an unstable initial course. The degree of injury and initial instability also set the stage for late organ dysfunction and sepsis.

In the nonoperative patient, one must maintain a high index of suspicion to detect intra-abdominal injuries. Because the rate of successful treatment diminishes the longer diagnosis is delayed, the ICU team has a special responsibility to perform repeated evaluations of the patient who may have suffered as yet undiagnosed intra-abdominal injuries.

For further information, please see Chapter 50 in Civetta JM, Taylor RW, Kirby RR: Critical Care. *Philadelphia: J. B. Lippincott, 1988*

BIBLIOGRAPHY

Baker ME, Blinder RA, Rice RP: Diagnostic imaging of abdominal fluid collections and abscesses. *CRC Crit Rev Diag Imag* 1986; 25:233

Berne CJ, Donovan AJ, Hagen WE: Combined duodenal pancreatic trauma: The role of end-to-side gastrojejunostomy. *Arch Surg* 1986; 96:713

Brown GL, Richardson JD: Traumatic diaphragmatic hernia: A continuing challenge. *Ann Thoracic Surg* 1985; 39:170

Busuttil RW, Kitahama A, Cerise E, et al: Management of blunt and penetrating injuries to the porta hepatis. *Ann Surg* 1980; 191:641

Cogbill TH, Moore EE, Kashuk, JL: Changing trends in the management of pancreatic trauma. *Arch Surg* 1982; 117:722

Committee on Trauma Research, National Research Council: *Injury in America*. National Academy Press, Washington, DC, 1985

Cook A, Levine BA, Rusing R: Traditional treatment of colon injuries. *Arch Surg* 1984; 119:591

Federle MP, Goldberg HI, Kaiser JA, et al: Evaluation of abdominal trauma by computed tomography. *Radiology* 1981; 138:637

Fuller WD, Hunt J, Altemeirer WA: Prophylactic antibiotics in penetrating wounds of the abdomen. *J Trauma* 1972; 12:282

Miller L, Bennett EV, Root HD, et al: Management of penetrating and blunt diaphragmatic injury. *J Trauma* 1984; 24:403

Nichols RL, Smith JW, Klein PB, et al: Risk of infection after penetrating injuries of the abdomen. *N Engl J Med* 1984; 311:1065

Orloff MJ, Charters AC: Injuries of the small bowel and mesentery and retroperitoneal hematoma. *Surg Clin North Am* 1972; 52:729

Sherman R: Perspectives in management of trauma to the spleen: 1979 presidential address, American Association for the Surgery of Trauma. *J Trauma* 1980; 20:1

Soderstrom CA, Maekawan K, DuPreist RW Jr, et al: Gallbladder injuries resulting from blunt abdominal trauma. *Ann Surg* 1981; 193:60

Symbas PN, Hatcher CR Jr, Vlasis SE: Esophageal gunshot wounds. *Ann Surg* 1980; 191:703

Trunkey DD, Shires GT, McClelland R: Management of liver trauma in 811 consecutive patients. *Ann Surg* 1974; 170:722

11 The Acute Abdomen

ACUTE ABDOMEN ON ADMISSION

A patient entering an intensive care unit (ICU) with abdominal pain or signs of peritoneal irritation has an acute abdominal problem until alternate explanations are found. Fever of unknown origin, jaundice, hematemesis, and hematochezia also should lead to a careful examination for an acute abdominal source of symptoms. When an acute problem is recognized through physical examination and history, the physician then can use a series of diagnostic tests to determine a specific diagnosis. The major decision then is whether to treat the problem with or without surgery.

Ruptured appendix, perforated viscus, gangrenous cholecystitis, pancreatic or intraperitoneal abscess, cholangitis, uncontrollable bleeding, strangulated bowel, and peritonitis all require surgical intervention. Stress ulcer without perforation, hepatitis, pancreatitis, sickle cell crises, and nonthrombotic mesenteric ischemia are best treated medically.

The differentiation of pathologic conditions is dependent on the location and presentation of the symptoms. Laboratory tests are adjunctive, whereas radiographic techniques can often be diagnostic. A complete blood count (CBC), including differential, is useful in differentiating an infectious process, but a white blood cell (WBC) count can also be elevated in stress states. The serum amylase level is usually elevated in pancreatitis; liver functions are abnormal in biliary disease. Bilirubin can be elevated in sepsis, hemolysis, and hepatitis as well as in biliary obstructive disease. Testing stools and nasogastric aspirates for blood is helpful in differentiating a source of bleeding.

An upright or right lateral decubitus abdominal film should be obtained to look for free air, air-fluid levels, and soft-tissue densities. Contrast studies are rarely helpful and are difficult to perform. Ultrasound is a useful bedside adjunct in the differentiation of biliary and pancreatic from hepatic cellular diseases. Ultrasound can delineate pelvic abscesses but is limited in midabdominal processes. Computed tomography (CT) scans are useful in diagnosing abdominal masses and pathology, although they require a labor-intensive transport to the radiology suite. Less efficacious are gallium and indium scans.

Peritoneal lavage has been an accurate tool in the diagnosis of abdominal trauma. It has also been used in the diagnosis of pancreatitis and mesenteric thrombosis with ischemic gut. The presence of red blood cells (RBC), more than 500 WBC, increased amylase, or bacteria on Gram stain are all indicative of an acute abdominal process.

The most important therapeutic decision is whether or not surgery is necessary. Although well-defined abscesses can be drained under CT guidance, other surgical problems require abdominal exploration to control the process.

Unless contraindicated, a nasogastric tube should be placed for decompression and antacid administered for stress prophylaxis in all patients with acute abdominal problems. Vigorous resuscitation with isotonic fluids is frequently necessary secondary to third space losses and bleeding. Broad-spectrum antibiotics with gram-negative and anaerobic coverage may be helpful and should be used.

The most important aspects are early recognition of the problem and early initiation of the appropriate therapy before shock, sepsis, and multiple organ system failure (MOSF) supervene.

ACUTE ABDOMEN DEVELOPING IN THE PATIENT IN THE ICU

Critically ill patients are especially prone to develop abdominal catastrophies that are frequently insidious in onset. Although appendicitis, calculous cholecystitis, diverticulitis, and other common causes of acute abdominal problems exist in critically ill patients, the incidence is not significantly higher than in the general population. Instead, patients in the ICU are subject to a different set of disease processes. All patients in ICUs who are not improving as they should when the primary disorder has been adequately treated must be examined for possible abdominal catastrophy.

Patients on ventilators for respiratory failure are at a high risk for gastrointestinal bleeding and paralytic ileus. Aggressive antacid therapy should be followed by early endoscopy if the bleeding persists.

Prolonged intravenous hyperalimentation associated with septicemia and discontinuation of enteral feedings increases the risk of acalculus cholecystitis. Fever of unknown origin associated with right upper quadrant symptoms and signs of hepatic dysfunction must be aggressively pursued with ultrasound and DISIDA scans, if warranted, to determine the presence of acute biliary disease. Early surgical intervention is indicated if the diagnosis is biliary sepsis or obstruction.

Low flow states associated with cardiac difficulties or prolonged hypotension in elderly patients increase the risk of nonocclusive mesenteric thrombosis. Patients with abdominal pain out of proportion to physical findings, nausea, vomiting, hematochezia, leukocytosis, and low-grade fever should be aggressively studied. Sigmoidoscopy followed by angiography and the instillation of vasodilating agents have been helpful in the diagnosis and treatment of this disorder. A similar syndrome may develop following aortic aneurysm resection, especially when the inferior mesenteric arterial supply is disrupted at surgery.

A diabetic whose ketoacidosis has not improved despite fluids and insulin should be examined closely for the presence of intra-abdominal infection or strangulated bowel. Persistence of severe acidosis in any patient may be a sign of ischemic gut. Recurrent fever and leukocytosis in patients following abdominal surgery indicates abdominal infection until proven otherwise.

For further information, please see Chapter 49 in Civetta JM, Taylor RW, Kirby RR: Critical Care. *Philadelphia: J. B. Lippincott, 1988*

BIBLIOGRAPHY

Aranha GV, Goldberg NB: Surgical problems in patients on ventilators. *Crit Care Med* 1981; 478

Brewer RJ, Golden GT, Hitch DD, et al: Abdominal pain: An analysis of 1,000 consecutive cases in a university hospital emergency room. *Am J Surg* 1976; 131:219

DiPiro JT, Mansberger JA, David JA: Current concepts in clinical therapeutics: Intra-abdominal infections. *Clin Pharmacol* 1986; 5:34

Hinsdale JG, Jaffe BM: Re-operation for intra-abdominal sepsis. Indications and results in modern critical care setting. *An Surg* 1984; 199:31

Norwood SH, Civetta JM: Abdominal CT scanning in critically ill surgical patients. *Ann Surg* 1985; 202:166

12
The Complicated Postoperative Abdomen

Evaluating the abdomen for complications after elective abdominal operations is a difficult diagnostic problem. Postoperative pain, ileus, and ventilatory and hemodynamic support can often mask the usual findings that herald an acute abdomen.

Patients having abdominal surgery frequently require ICU observation because of the complexity of the operation or other nonabdominal risk factors, such as poor cardiac or respiratory function. If a potentially life-threatening complication has a reasonable chance of developing postoperatively, then ICU observation is required after major elective abdominal surgery. The sympathetic response to pain (sinus tachycardia, hypertension) can adversely affect patients with poor cardiac function. These side-effects, combined with rapid changes in volume status, may be all that is necessary to produce a perioperative myocardial infarction. Even in the absence of extra-abdominal risk factors, many patients who require intra-abdominal procedures need ICU observation postoperatively to prevent the occasional complication which, if unrecognized, could be catastrophic to the patient's outcome. Following prolonged abdominal operations, patients usually require aggressive hour-to-hour volume replacement. ''Stents'' and drains placed at surgery must be carefully protected because dislodgement will often require reoperation for replacement. Significant hypothermia postoperatively can predispose to life-threatening cardiac dysrhythmias which must be recognized and treated rapidly.

Although there are many complications specific to certain abdominal operations (discussed later), postoperative intra-abdominal hemorrhage can complicate any elective or emergency laparotomy. The diagnosis is not difficult if hypotension and tachycardia and the rapid development of abdominal distention are present. In the ICU patient the findings are often more subtle, especially if hourly attention to urine output and preload has maintained relatively normal intravascular volume. A persistent sinus tachycardia above 120 to 130 beats per minute (unresponsive to pain medication) should raise the question of intra-abdominal bleeding, despite the absence of hypotension. A decreasing hematocrit value is often attributed to ''dilutional effects,'' but should certainly suggest continued blood loss. If the rate of bleeding is slow, several hours may elapse before the diagnosis can be confirmed. A painful abdominal incision and the patient's altered mental status (from anesthesia or postoperative analgesics) will often hinder accurate physical examination; significant abdominal distention may not develop until 1 to 3 liters of blood accumulate within the peritoneal cavity.

Most bleeding complications from technical surgical errors become apparent within the first 24 to 48 hours postoperatively. Hemorrhage following aortic reconstruction or pancreatic surgery may occur at any time during the postoperative recovery period. Because of the lack of objective findings on physical examination, the diagnosis of intra-abdominal hemorrhage in the postoperative ICU patient may be delayed unless there is a constant, high index of suspicion. Persistent tachycardia and the need for 1 or 2 units of blood to maintain a stable hemoglobin level over 12 to 24 hours may be the only clues. Abdominal radiographs may demonstrate a general haziness with nonvisualization of the psoas margins. Bowel gas patterns may show separation of the intestines from the lateral abdominal wall, indicating that the bowels are floating ventrally on the pooled intraperitoneal blood. Absence of these radiographic findings does not rule out the diagnosis, and bleeding is often not confirmed until the abdomen is reexplored.

In addition to bleeding complications, certain abdominal operations require ICU management because of problems that are specific to the particular operation. Although usually easily managed, hypoglycemia, hypoalbuminemia, and hypophosphatemia are common complications following major hepatic resections. Hemobilia, though rare, can develop after elective hepatic resections and may be unrecognized as the cause for postoperative blood loss. Pyogenic liver abscess can be a lethal complication and should be suspected if fever and jaundice reappear. Complete hepatic failure may develop from septic complications or from lack of enough functional hepatic tissue following resection. This lethal problem does not usually occur if 20% of normal liver remains and no postoperative problems develop that reduce oxygen delivery to the remaining liver.

Acute pancreatitis, ductal or anastomotic disruptions, and external pancreatic fistulas can develop following elective pancreatic procedures. Pancreatic pseudocysts and abscesses can occur later as a result of these early postoperative complications. Subtotal or total pancreatectomy can also cause specific metabolic problems such as brittle diabetes and pancreatic exocrine insufficiency.

Patients undergoing major abdominal vascular reconstruction frequently have significant cardiac and respiratory risk factors. Early graft thrombosis and infection can be life-threatening complications postoperatively.

Most problems arising from complicated gastrointestinal or biliary tract procedures result from bile or intestinal contents leaking into the peritoneal cavity, from infectious complications, or from biliary or alimentary tract obstruction.

Proper evaluation of the abdomen postoperatively requires understanding of the physiologic changes that occur after laparotomy. The abdominal incision should be free of significant edema, erythema, or fluid drainage. The skin edges should be completely apposed. Serosanguinous drainage is often the first sign of wound dehiscence and, if suspected, surgical consultation should be obtained as soon as possible. Immediate treatment is confined to covering the incision with a dry, sterile dressing.

Paralytic ileus develops following any abdominal operation and may cause minimal abdominal distention due to the inability to move intestinal secretions and gas. Bowel sounds generally return by 24 to 72 hours, primarily because of the early return of small bowl function. Oral intake cannot be resumed, however, until the stomach (which regains peristalsis at 24 to 48 hours) and large bowel (which may not return to normal function for 5 days) are functioning properly.

Sepsis continues to be the most common cause of death in critically ill surgical patients. Following elective surgery, a persistent sinus tachycardia (>120 beats/min), respiratory dysfunction, and hyperglycemia combined with a continued positive fluid balance and paralytic ileus after the seventh postoperative day should raise the suspicion of intra-abdominal sepsis.

The evaluation for sepsis requires a thorough knowledge of the patient's history, clinical condition, type of surgery performed, and elapsed time since laparotomy, plus an appropriately directed physical examination followed by tests to confirm clinical suspicions. Life-threatening complications must be considered, but the evaluation should be clinically relevant so that tests which are of little benefit are excluded. Intra-abdominal sepsis is rarely clinically apparent within the first 48 hours following operation. From 48 hours to 7 days postoperatively, warning signs begin to develop, but diagnostic tests, such as computed tomography (CT) scan, are often unreliable for confirming the diagnosis. After 1 week, diagnostic testing usually becomes more helpful but such tests should be done only if the results would alter therapy. A critical assessment of the overall prognosis in terms of underlying disease and degree of organ system dysfunction should precede continued aggressive support and repeated diagnostic tests which may be of little benefit.

It is important to become familiar with the various anatomic complications that may develop in the immediate postoperative period. Various internal and external fistulas can develop postoperatively, causing significant metabolic derangements if the lost fluid and electrolytes are not properly replaced. The volume of fluid lost must be accurately recorded and replaced. Although electrolyte content can be estimated, it is good practice to measure the electrolytes to guide proper replacement.

Most abdominal wound infections become clinically apparent within the first 7 to 10 days postoperatively. The incubation period for staphylococcal wound infection is generally 4 to 6 days, whereas gram-negative organisms require 7 to 14 days. Early wound infections (within 48 hours postoperatively) should raise the suspicion of group A streptococcal or clostridial infection, especially if severe incisional pain accompanies the clinical findings. Although rare, these are lethal infections if not rapidly recognized and treated.

The proper utilization of "surgical hardware" and a knowledge of "tube technology" are important in determining a successful outcome. Various tubes and drains are placed for decompression, feeding, or drainage. No tube should ever be removed from a patient without prior consultation with the operating surgeon. Also, attempts should never be made to replace a tube or drain that has been accidently dislodged without prior discussion with the operating surgeon.

EVALUATING THE ELECTIVE POSTOPERATIVE PATIENT

REASONS FOR ICU CARE

Surgical patients frequently require care in the ICU after elective abdominal operations. The requirement for intensive care may be merely a need for "close observation," but is more often due to a combination of the potential complications that can occur from the complexity of the operation and the relative risk factors of the patient.

Patients with poor cardiac or respiratory function often require monitoring and careful observation after intra-abdominal operations because of the physiologic stress that develops. Pain can significantly restrict respiratory function after abdominal procedures and careful attention to vigorous pulmonary toilet and pain relief, without respiratory depression, will help prevent postoperative pulmonary complications. Patients with marginal cardiac function also need careful attention to prevent the adverse effects of sinus tachycardia and other dysrhythmias that may develop from pain. Elevated heart rates and minor hypovolemic changes from fluid losses may be just enough to precipitate a perioperative myocardial infarction.

Preoperative physiologic assessment may certainly benefit high-risk patients and enhance intraoperative and postoperative management (see Chapter 7). Continuous epidural analgesia in the postoperative period may also benefit those patients with marginal pulmonary function. Pulmonary artery catheterization for monitoring the high-risk patient requires ICU facilities, because nursing expertise and monitoring capabilities are rarely found outside a critical care unit.

Even in the absence of patient risk factors, many intra-abdominal procedures require ICU observation for a certain time postoperatively to prevent the occasional complication that if unrecognized could be catastrophic to the patient's outcome. Other intra-abdominal procedures often create a "labor-intensive" patient whose postoperative care literally requires one or even two full-time nurses to fulfill the patient's needs.

Many prolonged abdominal operations, such as aortic reconstruction or pancreatic surgery, will often require aggressive hour-to-hour fluid replacement to prevent hypotension from "third space" losses. It is not unusual for patients with postoperative peripheral vascular problems to require 6 to 12 liters of intravenous fluid in the first 24 hours to maintain adequate arterial pressure and renal perfusion. Various drains and anastomotic "stents" are frequently placed which, if inadvertently removed by the sedated or disoriented patient, would necessitate reoperation for replacement. Such careful observation and continuous monitoring usually cannot be guaranteed on a general surgical ward.

Morbidly obese patients are both high risk and labor intensive. Abdominal operations are more difficult in obese patients and the probability of postoperative pulmonary, cardiac, and infectious complications is considered much higher. Indeed, merely turning such massive endomorphs requires several people. Prevention of pneumonia requires hourly respiratory care.

It is important to understand that from the operating surgeon's viewpoint, there is usually a "critical observation period" for most patients following major abdominal operations. If the complication is potentially life-threatening, with a reasonable chance of developing, then ICU observation is required. It is important that the ICU staff understand thse complications and their clinical presentations. Continuous communication with the operating surgeon is mandatory for effective postoperative care.

Prolonged elective abdominal operations often require close postoperative observation, especially if significant hypothermia develops intraoperatively. Rewarming can lead to rapid changes in acid–base balance, occasionally producing cardiac dysrhythmias from electrolyte changes (particularly potassium and ionized calcium). Rewarming and shivering also cause major increases in oxygen consumption which can be detrimental to the patient with marginal cardiac or respiratory function who is unable to increase oxygen delivery to meet these needs (without hemodynamic support).

COMMON ABDOMINAL PROCEDURES REQUIRING ICU MANAGEMENT

Liver Resections

Patients can develop a myriad of metabolic derangements following hepatic resections for primary or metastatic carcinoma. Hypoglycemia, hypoalbuminemia, and hypophosphatemia are common in the immediate postoperative period but are generally easily managed with continuous infusions of 10% to 20% dextrose solutions supplemented with potassium phosphate. Albumin levels are customarily maintained within the normal range with supplemental infusions.

Major hepatic resections can cause significant catabolism and negative nitrogen balance. It is generally believed that these abnormalities may be associated with significant increases in operative morbidity and mortality; therefore, parenteral or enteral protein and calorie supplementation is recommended.

The degree of abnormality observed in biochemical liver function parameters following liver resection depends on the amount and the quality of remaining liver tissue. No specific abnormal liver function patterns are observed. Liver function tests may be abnormal for several days or weeks following major resections. Lactic dehydrogenase (LDH), serum glutamic-oxaloacetic transaminase (SGOT), and serum glutamic-pyruvic transaminase (SGPT) levels generally return to normal after about 1 week if there are no postoperative complications, but this is not a specific trend. Alkaline phosphatase levels tend to remain elevated up to several months postoperatively; hyperbilirubinemia develops within 72 hours and persists for 3 to 4 weeks.

Despite decreases in prothrombin, factors V, VII, IX, X, and plasminogen levels, hemorrhagic diathesis is uncommon. Platelet counts are depressed for 1 to 2 weeks. Fibrinogen levels may decrease, along with intermittent increases in fibrin split products. These findings in the presence of a decreasing hematocrit value postoperatively may indicate a coagulopathy. If intra-abdominal hemorrhage is suspected, abnormalities in clotting factors should not delay abdominal reexploration, because the cause is most likely from a correctable source at the surgical site, and continued intra-abdominal bleeding may indeed lead to a consumptive or fibrinolytic coagulopathy.

Hemobilia can occur in the immediate postoperative period from a communication between a parenchymal branch of the hepatic arterial system and the biliary tree. Hemobilia is diagnosed easily if a T tube has been placed in the common bile duct at the time of surgery. Otherwise, the diagnosis may go unrecognized. The classical presentation of right upper quadrant pain, jaundice, and gastrointestinal bleeding may all be obscured in the postoperative period unless bleeding is massive. Generally hemobilia presents as intermittent gastrointestinal bleeding because clotting occurs within the biliary ducts until a critical level of bile (which lyses blood clots) accumulates and causes rebleeding. Unless blood refluxes into the stomach, appearing in the nasogastric tube, this rare complication may go unrecognized until the patient passes a bloody or melenic stool. The diagnosis is confirmed by duodenoscopy demonstrating blood flowing from the sphincter of Oddi. The preferred treatment is hepatic arteriography with selective embolization of the bleeding site. Hepatic infarction can occur with embolization; therefore, reexploration may be a safer maneuver for hepatic preservation in the immediate postoperative period, depending on the extent of the hepatic resection.

Pyogenic liver abscess following resection is often a lethal complication with mortality rates reported to be 50% or greater despite aggressive therapy. The mortality rate for undrained liver abscesses approaches 100%. Liver abscesses do not usually develop until after the 10th postoperative day and making the diagnosis in the postoperative patient can be very difficult. Jaundice associated with pyogenic liver abscess is an ominous sign. There are generally no discriminating levels, because all patients who undergo liver resection develop some degree of jaundice in the postoperative period. If jaundice has resolved postoperatively but reappears, especially if associated with fever, then pyogenic hepatic abscess must be ruled out.

Physical examination is often unreliable in the postoperative period, although right upper quadrant pain to palpation may be helpful if the patient has recovered from the discomfort of abdominal surgery.

Atelectasis of the right lung base, elevation of the right hemidiaphragm, or a right pleural effusion on chest radiograph may suggest the diagnosis. Ultrasonography or CT may confirm the diagnosis, depending on the amount of liver remaining and the elapsed time since surgery. Early diagnosis and percutaneous or operative drainage is the only hope for survival. Antibiotics are required for 4 to 6 weeks in conjunction with drainage.

Transient episodes of hypovolemia, prolonged dysrhythmias, or other factors reducing cardiac output and hepatic blood flow may be enough to reduce oxygen delivery to the remaining hepatocytes and cause irreversible injury at a time when there is no hepatic reserve. Bilirubin levels exceeding 20 mg/dl in the absence of major hematomas or large numbers of blood transfusions usually signify irreversible hepatic failure and further supportive efforts are usually unsuccessful unless a reversible septic focus can be identified and treated.

Pancreatic Operations

The pancreas lies retroperitoneally, in close association with the duodenum, common bile duct, aorta, and splenic, superior mesenteric, and portal veins, and the inferior vena cava. This location, combined with the abundant pancreatic blood supply and its exocrine and endocrine secretions, make pancreatic surgery an often treacherous undertaking.

Hemorrhage is the most common complication and generally presents as any other form of intra-abdominal bleeding. Significant fluid losses can occur following major retroperitoneal dissections for total or subtotal pancreatectomy and hypovolemic shock can develop without bleeding unless aggressive volume replacement is given postoperatively.

Acute pancreatitis can develop following any operation on the pancreas or biliary tract. It is usually caused by disruption of the pancreatic ducts with leakage of pancreatic secretions into the retroperitoneum. This can develop from a major anastomotic leak or merely from an intraoperative pancreatic needle biopsy. Postoperative pancreatitis can develop immediately or may not occur until several days to weeks postoperatively. In ICU patients, the diagnosis should be suspected if ileus and positive fluid balance persist past the usual postoperative period for resolution. Physical findings are not specific in the immediate postoperative period, but the diagnosis can be confirmed by documenting hyperamylasemia or elevated urine amylase levels. Postoperative pancreatitis carries a significant risk for major hemorrhage because of the pancreas' retroperitoneal juxtaposition to many major blood vessels and its own rich vascular supply. Bleeding may develop as early as 3 or 4 days or as late as 3 weeks postoperatively, usually secondary to erosion of major blood vessels by pancreatic secretions. The mortality rate from postoperative hemorrhagic pancreatitis is extremely high. Immediate surgery and radical pancreatic debridement are necessary for patient survival.

Ductal or anastomotic disruptions can cause pancreatic ascites if the secretions are not confined to the retroperitoneum. Abdominal distention may develop rapidly since normal pancreatic secretions range from 700 to 1500 ml/day. Hyperamylasemia is usually present, but ascitic fluid levels are often at least ten times higher. Operative closure of the internal leak is usually necessary.

External pancreatic fistulas can develop after pancreatic procedures. Clear, colorless fluid may be seen on the wound dressing. The diagnosis is confirmed by a high amylase content in the clear fluid. Eighty percent of external pancreatic fistulas will close unless they are exposed to biliary or intestinal contents. High-volume fistulas (>500 ml) or fistulas persisting for longer than 6 weeks usually require operative closure.

Pancreatic pseudocysts can develop following acute pancreatitis from ductal disruption with leakage of pancreatic fluid. Pseudocysts may not be clinically apparent postoperatively, but can be late manifestations of acute pancreatitis or complications from anastomotic leaks. Massive hemorrhage into a pseudocyst can be a life-threatening complication. Hyperamylasemia, a palpable abdominal epigastric mass, and a prior history of pancreatitis suggest the diagnosis.

Pancreatic abscess is a late complication of pancreatic surgery. Abscesses develop in approximately 5% of patients with acute pancreatitis. Immediate pancreatic exploration and drainage is necessary if the diagnosis is clinically suspected and confirmed by CT scan or ultrasound. Abscesses can erode into major retroperitoneal blood vessels and adjacent organs. The mortality rate for this complication is reported to be as high as 35%.

All of these complications can occur after any pancreatic operation, but certain procedures tend to be more frequently accompanied by complications. Several operations are performed for patients with chronic pancreatitis. These include distal pancreatectomy with pancreatojejunostomy (Duval procedure), longitudinal pancreatojejunostomy (Puestow procedure), and subtotal and total pancreatectomy. The most common problem following the Duval and Puestow procedures is anastomotic leak. Bleeding, acute pancreatitis, and infectious complications are uncommon following these procedures because extensive retroperitoneal dissection is not required. Patients rarely need ICU care following these drainage procedures unless they have other medical problems.

Subtotal and total pancreatectomy for chronic pancreatitis predispose to all of the problems previously described as well as some specific metabolic problems. It is reported that only 20% of normal pancreatic tissue is required to prevent diabetes. Mild diabetes is a common problem in patients with chronic pancreatitis. All patients will require insulin replacement following subtotal or total pancreatectomy. Careful monitoring of the serum glucose level in the postoperative period is required. Due to the lack of glucagon production from the alpha cells (which have also been removed) only very small amounts of insulin (5–20 U/day) are required. Careful titration of glucose and insulin is necessary to prevent profound changes that can occur with only small amounts of glucose or insulin. Pancreatic exocrine insufficiency also develops, but this is not usually a problem in the critical care setting since patients are not taking food orally.

Pancreatoduodenectomy (Whipple procedure) and total pancreatectomy are performed for resectable pancreatic or duodenal malignancies. The above-described complications develop more often in malignant disease than in benign disease. Hemorrhage and anastomotic leaking are the most common postoperative complications. Mortality rates reported for these operations range from 5% to 35%.

Major Abdominal Vascular Procedures

Patients undergoing aortic reconstruction for occlusive disease or abdominal aortic aneurysm require careful postoperative ICU management. Most patients with symptomatic peripheral vascular disease also have significant cardiac and respiratory risk factors. The most common cause of death in these patients is myocardial infarction, and intraoperative and postoperative hemodynamic monitoring are often beneficial. Hemorrhage may develop postoperatively, but abdominal distention may not develop if the bleeding is confined to the retroperitoneum. Careful fluid management results in maintenance of arterial blood pressure and several hours may pass before bleeding is apparent. Significant hemorrhage requires immediate return to the operating room. The most common cause is technical error, but occasionally no specific bleeding site is found, and hemorrhage may be attributed to prolonged heparin activity or coagulopathy.

Early graft thrombosis can also occur; this should be considered if a drop in the segmental doppler pressures of one or both extremities develops. Immediate heparinization and reexploration are needed if graft thrombosis develops.

Early graft infections are first recognized when a wound infection develops in one of the groin incisions. Drainage of the localized abscess may reveal involvement of the distal limb of the graft. Occasionally bleeding from the groin incision, usually occurring a week to 10 days postoperatively, will be the first sign of a graft infection. Either presentation mandates immediate removal of the infected graft. Vascular surgery procedures and complications are described in greater detail in Chapter 15.

Complicated Gastrointestinal and Biliary Procedures

The most common complications occurring after major gastrointestinal or biliary operations result from bile or intestinal leakage into the peritoneal cavity, infection, or obstruction of the biliary system or a portion of the alimentary tract. After these types of procedures, ICU care is required generally only if the operation is extensively prolonged or if the patient had other significant risk factors or intraoperative complications.

Other than bleeding, few immediate intra-abdominal problems develop. Occasionally a major bile leak can develop and if not properly drained, severe bile peritonitis and hypotension can develop rapidly. The patient presents with generalized, severe abdominal pain and distention. Bowel necrosis can present in a similar fashion and should be suspected following bowel operations that require transection of one or more bowel loops and mesentery for creation of various anastomoses. Occasionally the blood supply can be compromised from the procedures and necrosis will occur.

Most anastomotic leaks are not apparent until 4 to 7 days postoperatively when the patient develops a persistent fever, ileus, or other diversion from the normal postoperative course.

For further information, please see Chapter 52 in Civetta JM, Taylor RW, Kirby RR: Critical Care. *Philadelphia: J. B. Lippincott, 1988*

BIBLIOGRAPHY

Balasegaram M: Management of hepatic abscess. *Curr Prob surg* 1981; 18:285

Bradley EL, Clement JL, Gonzales AC: The natural history of pancreatic pseudocysts: A unified concept of management. *Am J Surg* 1979; 137:135

Cameron JL, Kieffer RS, Anderson WJ, Zuidema GD: Internal pancreatic fistulas: Pancreatic ascites and pleural effusions. *Ann Surg* 1976; 184:587

Flint LM: Liver failure. *Surg Clin North Am* 1982; 62:157

Frey CF: Hemorrhagic pancreatitis. *Am J Surg* 1979; 137:616.

Frey CF, Child CG, Fry W: Pancreatectomy for chronic pancreatitis. *Ann Surg* 1976; 184:403

Lorentzen J, Nielson OM, Arendrup H, et al: Vascular graft infections. *Surgery* 1985; 98:81

McClave S: Pancreatic abscess: 10 year experience at the University of South Florida. *Am J Gastroenterol* 1986; 81:180

McDonald AP, Howard RJ: Pyogenic liver abscesses. *World J Surg* 1980; 4:369

Nielsen ML, Mygind T: Selective arterial embolization in traumatic hemobilia. *World J Surg* 1980; 4:357

Pinkerton JA, Sawyers JL, Foster JH: A study of the postoperative course after hepatic lobectomy. *Ann Surg* 1971; 173:800

Ranson JHC: Acute pancreatitis: Where are we? *Surg Clin North Am* 1981; 61:55

Rout WR, Zuidema GD: Complications in hepatic surgery and trauma. In Greenfield LJ (ed): *Complications in Surgery and Trauma,* p 547. Philadelphia, JB Lippincott, 1984

Stone HH, Long WD, Smith RB, Haynes CD: Physiologic considerations in major hepatic resections. *Am J Surg* 1969; 117:78

Trapnell JE: Pathophysiology of acute pancreatitis. *World J Surg* 1981; 5:319

Trojanowski JQ, Harrist TJ, Athanosoulis CA, Greenfield AJ: Hepatic and splenic infarction: Complications of therapeutic transcatheter embolization. *Am J Surg* 1980; 139:272

Warshaw A, Rattner DW: Timing of surgical drainage for pancreatic pseudocyst. *Ann Surg* 1986; 202:720

Whittemore AD, Clowes AW, Couch NP, Mannick JA: Secondary femoropopliteal construction. *Ann Surg* 1981; 193:35

13 Thoracic Surgery

Admission of a thoracic surgical patient to the intensive care unit (ICU) should initiate a series of immediate actions designed to stabilize the patient and to anticipate problems. Routine orders common to all patients are essential (*e.g.*, fluid or blood orders, medications, and laboratory tests). Ventilator orders are immediately transcribed and changed as dictated by blood gas determinations. If the patient has come directly from surgery, the $F_{I_{O_2}}$, rate and tidal volume (V_T) may need to be changed. Patients under anesthesia are usually maintained on 100% oxygen which is unnecessary and undesirable in most ICU patients. The average patient will do well with an inspired oxygen fraction ($F_{I_{O_2}}$) of 0.40, V_T of 15 ml/kg and an intermittent mandatory ventilation (IMV) rate of 8. We have found it helpful in most patients, initially, to add 4 to 5 cm of positive end-expiratory pressure (PEEP) to maintian a normal functional residual volume. This low level of PEEP reduces atelectasis, maintains lung expansion, and may actually aid in decreasing air leak through the chest tubes because a fully expanded lung in apposition to the chest wall is essential in sealing off the alveolar and bronchiolar air leaks that always occur after pulmonary surgery.

It is important to obtain an upright chest film as soon as possible. Films taken in the supine position may not give an accurate estimation of the degree of pneumothorax or fluid which may be present. Most nurses and radiology technicians will obtain a supine film unless specifically ordered to get an upright film. It is not difficult to elevate the head of the bed and support the patient while obtaining a film in the 75° to 90° position. The film should be carefully evaluated for the following:

1 Position of endotracheal tube

2 Position of chest tubes

3 Position of monitoring catheters

4 Presence of pneumothorax

5 Amount of fluid or blood in the thorax

6 Presence of atelectasis or pulmonary infiltrate

7 Degree of mediastinal shift

8 Width of the mediastinum in trauma patients.

Pain control is very important in thoracic surgical patients. Unless they have had intercostal blocks, thoracic patients awake with excruciating pain; this leads them to thrash about in bed, to pull on intravenous and monitoring lines, and to fight the ventilator. If they are not using the ventilator, they tend to take shallow, irregular respirations which lead to poor ventilation and carbon dioxide retention. As discussed later in detail, intravenous pain control is best.

It is essential that chest tubes function properly. All connections should be checked, secured, and wrapped with tape to prevent leaks. Suction is usually set at 20 cm H_2O negative pressure, and the fluid level in the bottles should be noted on an hourly basis to record the amount of blood loss. The apical chest tube should be removing air from the thorax as evidenced by bubbling in the water seal bottle, and the posterior tube should be draining blood; a few clots are inevitable, but if the tube becomes filled with clot, it must be opened. The early occurrence of large quantities of clot may indicate excessive blood loss, since rapid bleeding usually leads to clotting while slow bleeding usually results in defibrination and liquid blood, which is easily removed by the tube.

Finally, the ICU physician and nurse should have a clear idea as to the expected medical course of the patient and the possible complications. The most common problem that we have observed in the ICU, particularly in private hospitals, is the "too many doctors syndrome" in which a phalanx of super specialists, in succession, together with their fellows and residents, daily assault the nursing staff with multiple, complex, sometimes contradictory, orders and fill the chart with endless illegible notes. Since each specialist is often narrowly focused on his or her own interests, sometimes the most fundamental problems (e.g., the patient's nutrition) may be overlooked. It is imperative for the ICU physician to maintain a broad overview of the patient as a whole. One person or team needs to coordinate and integrate care to prevent unnecessary confusion.

BLUNT TRAUMA

RIB FRACTURES

Usually ribs four through ten are the ones fractured, since the scapula and shoulder girdle effectively protect the upper ribs, and the 11th and 12 ribs are so short and flexible that they are uncommonly fractured. One or two rib fractures are usually no cause for alarm and can be treated on an outpatient basis with analgesics and splinting one side of the chest without danger to the patient. However, three or more fractures are better managed by hospitalization and further observation of the patient. One or two rib fractures in an elderly patient, in the patient with COPD, or in the patient with other significant trauma may become important because the decrease in VC and decreased ability to clear secretions, which occur with such fractures, may assume a significance out of proportion to the apparent injury. If the VC exceeds 15 ml/kg, the patient will probably do well with analgesics or intercostal nerve blocks and continued observation. In the ICU, nerve blocks with 0.25% bupivocaine with epinephrine 1:200,000 are extremely useful in helping the patient to cough, to breath deeply with an incentive spirometer, and to move around in bed or into a bedside chair. A comfortable patient whose pain is controlled will feel better, will do better, and will be able to cooperate much better than a patient sedated with morphine who continues to have intermittent pain.

FLAIL CHEST

A flail chest occurs when instability of the chest wall produces paradoxical motion with inspiration. This dramatically reduces VC and efforts by the patient to increase depth of respiration and to increase minute ventilation are inefficient; they increase paradox and increase oxygen consumption due to the increased work of breathing. Fractures or fracture–dislocations in two areas are usually necessary to produce significant flail chest. A combination of radiographs and palpation of the chest is necessary to evaluate the injury; it is common for patients to have dislocations of the costochondral junctions, which are not visible on film, associated with posterior rib fractures. If one detects motion or fractures in two locations in three or more ribs, the patient is at high risk for the development of significant impairment of ventilation. Lewis has emphasized that patients with rib fractures or flail chest should be evaluated by measuring the VC. Normal VC is 60 to 70 ml/kg; a minimally adequate VC is 15 ml/kg. A decrease in the VC to this level is an indication for intubation and ventilatory support.

A flail chest which was minimal or unnoticed in the emergency room may not become significant or obvious until 8 to 24 hours later when the splinting afforded by the voluntary and involuntary contractions of chest wall muscles is lost. At this time the patient may decompensate rapidly. Patients with multiple rib fractures or minimal flail chest should be followed closely in the ICU with serial blood gas determinations. Deterioration in blood gases may be an indication for intubation even though the VC may appear to be adequate. If one waits for the VC to reach minimal levels, the first indication of serious trouble may be a respiratory or cardiac arrest.

Treatment

Conservative Management. Patients with a mild to moderate flail chest can often be managed without ventilatory assistance if there is no underlying pulmonary contusion or other significant injury. The patient should be given supplemental oxygen to maintain the Pa_{O_2} at approximately 80, and the pain should be controlled with intercostal blocks and minimal narcotic analgesia. Careful pulmonary toilet with coughing, nasotracheal suction, and chest physiotherapy will usually be adequate to clear pulmonary secretions. If chest physiotherapy is used, the patient should have adequate analgesia with nerve blocks, or the pain may be intolerable. Pneumothorax is a common complication of intercostal blocks. If one occurs in a patient whose ventilation is already compromised, the patient's condition may deteriorate rapidly.

Internal Stabilization with Ventilator Support. The use of this technique is the standard by which other methods must be measured. In 1982, James and Moore reviewed the results of treatment of flail chest prior to and after 1970 when the use of long-term ventilator support became generalized. In six series reported before 1970, the average mortality rate was 33%; in six series reported after 1970, the average mortality rate was 18%. Specific ventilator management must be individualized; however, the use of IMV with approximately 5 cm of PEEP has proven to be an excellent method to maintain the patient's oxygenation, to maintain adequate residual volume, and to allow maximum comfort for the patient. Initially, it is advisable to intubate the patient transnasally or transorally. After the patient is stabilized, usually a matter of 48 to 72 hours, a tracheotomy may be advisable. Most patients will require ventilation for 10 to 21 days. They are much easier to manage and are more comfortable with a tracheotomy. A few patients with moderate flail chest will improve rapidly after intubation and will not require long-term ventilation; in these cases endotracheal intubation for approximately 7 days will be sufficient to wean them from the ventilator and tracheotomy may not be required.

PULMONARY CONTUSION

Pulmonary contusions are extremely common after blunt trauma to the chest. They are usually easy to diagnose in a patient with rib fractures or flail chest where they are seen as localized infiltrates or opacities on an early chest film. Subsequent chest films show increasing opacification of the areas for 24 to 48 hours and then gradual resolution over the next 7 days. From the standpoint of the ICU physician, it is important to understand that severe bilateral pulmonary contusions may occur in the absence of rib fractures or flail chest. The admitting chest film may appear normal, and the first sign of pulmonary contusion may be progressive hypoxemia. Serial chest films will reveal the contusion. One should be particularly alert to the possibility of pulmonary contusion in a patient who has chest wall bruises and contusions in the absence of rib fractures. These patients may require intubation and ventilatory support if they develop progressive hypoxia. In the absence of other indications for mechanical ventilation, they can usually be managed with supplemental oxygen.

Although most pulmonary contusions result in localized hematomas which are absorbed and which lead to minimal morbidity, massive trauma may lead to severe generalized pulmonary injury which may be bilateral and which may lead to or coexist with ARDS. Management of these patients remains controversial. The usual admonition is "to keep the patients dry" to decrease or prevent the accumulation of pulmonary water, to use diuretics to remove excess water, and to use plasma, blood, or albumin to maintain the plasma oncotic pressure in order to decrease the capillary leak which occurs in severely damaged lungs. This protocol seems logical but is ineffective. The capillary leak occurs whether or not colloids are given, and if important extracellular fluid deficits are not adequately replenished, the morbidity and mortality may increase. Adult respiratory distress syndrome is the sum total of a complicated series of antecedent physiologic events, and whether incident to pulmonary contusion, or other causes, attention should be directed toward management of the whole patient. It has been demonstrated, and subsequent studies have confirmed, that significant extracellular fluid volume losses occur in surgical patients. The management of these patients requires the judicious replenishment of these losses with a balanced salt solution as well as replenishment of blood. This may initially require large volumes of crystalloids. The best managed patient is one whose CVP, blood pressure, urine output, and pulmonary artery occlusion pressure (PAOP) are normal; under these conditions the patient is less apt to have significant pulmonary failure; if pulmonary failure occurs, it is easier to manage if the cardiovascular function is as near normal as possible.

It is certainly wise not to give the patient more fluid than is necessary to maintain a normal cardiovascular and renal function, but the *milieu interieur* described by Claude Bernard includes the entire body, and it is not probable that the lung can be isolated from the *milieu* and made selectively "dry."

CARDIAC CONTUSION

Although it can result from any direct trauma to the anterior chest wall, cardiac contusion usually occurs when the driver of a vehicle hits the steering wheel with his chest. Bruises or abrasions of the anterior chest or presternal area are usually present, but the patient may complain of nothing more than soreness over the anterior chest. The diagnosis should be suspected in any patient who gives a history of an injury to the anterior chest in a vehicle accident. Fortunately most cardiac contusions are not serious and require nothing more than supportive treatment. In patient who have significant injury, the most common findings are cardiac dysrhythmias, heart block, and tachycardia. Right bundle branch block is common. The diagnosis is established when the MB band of the creatine kinase (CK), expressed as a percentage of the total CK, is elevated. The cardiospecific enzyme, CK–MB, is released from necrotic myocardium, and an elevation of the CK–MB to 5% or more indicates significant damage to the myocardium. Since the right ventricle is anterior and is the most commonly injured portion of the heart, the amount of muscle involved may not be enough to cause an elevation in the CK. Technetium scans have been disappointing in the diagnosis of myocardial injury except in the unusual instance of transmural ventricular damage. The presence of murmurs may indicate septal, valvular, or papillary muscle injury, and in these cases two-dimensional echocardiography may be helpful. Electrocardiographic-gated blood-pool radionuclide angiography has been reported to be an accurate method to evaluate myocardial injury.

Serial EKGs are the best screening method for evaluation of patients with myocardial contusion. Usually the ST elevation, dysrhythmias, and heart block will subside in several days, occasionally in several weeks, and the patient will have no sequelae. The treatment of myocardial contusion consists of close monitoring and the use of those measures normally used in the management of myocardial infarction. A complete cardiology work-up will be necessary for patients who have complications.

AORTIC RUPTURE

These injuries occur from sudden deceleration, usually from automobile accidents, but occasionally from falls from height. They almost always occur at the aortic isthmus just distal to the subclavian artery. Eighty percent of the patients will die within a few minutes after injury; of those who survive to reach a hospital 80% will die within 24 hours if the rupture is not surgically repaired. Almost all of the remainder will be dead within a few weeks though an occasional patient will develop a chronic aneurysm. It is important for those working in an ICU to have a high degree of suspicion for aortic rupture because it may not be diagnosed in the early evaluation of severely traumatized patients. Many of the patients, perhaps 35% to 40%, will have little external evidence of chest trauma. The majority will have multiple extrathoracic injuries which demand immediate attention. The most suggestive physical findings are the presence of a systolic murmur, especially over the back, and a pressure differential between the upper and lower extremities which causes a relative hypotension in the lower extremities; these signs are not consistent; however, and their absence does not rule out the injury.

These patients survive to reach the hospital only because the aortic tear is incomplete, the intima and media are torn, leaving the adventitia to contain the blood flow; this results in an expanding adventitial hematoma. Early chest films, especially the hurried anteroposterior films taken in most emergency rooms, may not suggest the diagnosis. The characteristic findings are widening of the superior mediastinum, blurring or obliteration of the aortic knob, displacement of the trachea to the left, pleural cap, and downward displacement of the left main stem bronchus. Any patient admitted to the ICU with a history of deceleration injury should be carefully followed with serial chest films; if there is any question as to the possibility of aortic rupture, an aortogram should be performed, and, if positive, the patient should be taken to surgery for definitive repair. Incomplete tears of the subclavian, innominate, and carotid vessels also occasionally occur; they produce similar radiographic findings, and an aortogram is diagnostic.

PENETRATING TRAUMA

Although penetrating wounds to the chest are a surgical problem, and most patients will have definite treatment before they are admitted to the ICU, it is necessary to monitor them carefully for secondary problems or additional hidden wounds.

PULMONARY WOUNDS

When the penetrating wound has damaged only the lung, the patient will usually have a hemopneumothorax. In most instances, inserting chest tubes will be sufficient treatment. When the lung is expanded by evacuation of the pneumothorax, it will usually provide sufficient tamponade to stop the bleeding in the low-pressure pulmonary vessels. The tube will also evacuate the blood to allow complete expansion of the lung and will provide measurement of the amount of continued bleeding. Although many trauma centers successfully use one posterolateral chest tube, the use of two chest tubes, one placed posterolaterally to remove blood and one placed posterolaterally or anteriorly to the apex of the chest to remove air is preferable. The apical tube will not remove a significant amount of blood, but it is much more efficient in removing air. In the presence of significant continued bleeding, it is possible for the posterior tube to become plugged with clot; in this event the air will not be adequately evacuated and a tension pneumothorax may occur. Most low-velocity gunshot wounds and stab wounds to the pulmonary parenchyma can be managed with chest tubes, and no surgery is necessary. Bleeding may be brisk initially, but usually drops below 100 ml/hr within several hours; if the bleeding continues at 200 ml/hr for more than 4 to 6 hours, or if the initial evacuation of blood was 1500 ml or more, then thoracotomy is almost always indicated. Such a large hemorrhage usually indicates that a systemic chest wall artery or a major pulmonary vessel is injured.

High-velocity missile wounds present a different set of problems. The cavitation effect produced by absorption of the enormous kinetic energy of the missile may destroy a large amount of lung, may injure larger bronchi, or may produce such large pulmonary hematomas that surgery is indicated early in the management of the injury. Many high-velocity combat injuries can be managed initially with chest tubes alone. However, a large percentage of these patients will later require thoracotomy for pulmonary resection, decortication, and evacuation of empyema and infected clot. In the civilian setting the best results are obtained by early thoracotomy, evacuation of blood and clots, and the resection of severely damaged lung to prevent continued air leak, hemorrhage, and empyema.

Patients with high-velocity penetration wounds are also more apt to have air embolism than patients with blunt or low-velocity trauma, though it may occur in any patient who has disruption of the pulmonary parenchyma. Air embolism is more common than was formerly appreciated. It occurs when air from ruptured bronchi is forced into pulmonary veins from which it enters the systemic circulation through the left atrium. It may enter the coronary arteries and cause sudden severe dysrhythmias and ventricular fibrillation; or it may enter the cerebral circulation where it causes severe neurologic symptoms. If the air embolus is large enough, it may appear that the patient has had a sudden massive cerebrovascular accident. With smaller emboli, the patient may develop a variety of focal neurologic signs and symptoms. The presence of air embolism is often not appreciated until the patient is intubated and placed on positive-pressure ventilation, which increases the pressure gradient between the open bronchus and the open pulmonary vein. It is commonly associated with significant continued hemoptysis, which diagnostic feature is not always helpful without other signs because of the frequency with which hemoptysis is seen in pulmonary injury. Nevertheless, any patient who has penetrating chest trauma or a lung laceration from a fractured rib, and who develops unexplained neurologic and cardiac symptoms, should be carefully evaluated for air embolism. Air in the retinal arteries if present, is diagnostic, but this is not always seen, and in the case of massive embolism, there may be no time to look. If air embolism occurs, positive-pressure ventilation should be stopped and the patient taken immediately to surgery. Massive air embolism may require immediate thoracotomy in the emergency room or in the ICU in which event the pulmonary hilum should be clamped to prevent further entrance of air into the atrium; positive-pressure ventilation can then be reestablished and the patient taken to the operating room for definitive surgery.

TRACHEOBRONCHIAL INJURIES

Tracheobronchial injury incident to penetrating trauma is usually associated with damage to major blood vessels, and the indications for surgery are clear. When tracheobronchial injuries are caused by blunt trauma and deceleration, the diagnosis may not be immediately obvious. Such injury to the trachea usually causes a vertical tear of the membranous portion within a few centimeters of the carina. The major bronchi are usually torn transversely near the take off of the upper lobe bronchi. It is these that are sometimes missed.

These injuries should be suspected in a patient who has severe mediastinal emphysema, a large continuing air leak, and continued pneumothorax despite adequate chest tube suction. Massive subcutaneous emphysema may occur over the entire body leading to a grotesque, bloated appearance of the patient, closure of the eyelids, and a characteristic crackling feeling when the skin is indented with the examining finger. The subcutaneous emphysema is not, of itself, dangerous, but it incites great anxiety on the part of the patient and family. If the diagnosis is suspected, bronchoscopy should be performed as soon as the patient is stabilized and, if the diagnosis is confirmed, early surgery is indicated. If the diagnosis is missed, bronchial stenosis invariably occurs, and late repairs are often unsuccessful.

For further information, please see Chapter 47 in Civetta JM, Taylor RW, Kirby RR: Critical Care. *Philadelphia: J. B. Lippincott, 1988*

BIBLIOGRAPHY

Bitto T, et al: Pneumothorax during positive-pressure mechanical ventilation. *J Thoracic Cardiovasc Surg* 1985; 89:585

Branthwaite MA: Monitoring respiratory function in the critically ill. *Intensive Care Med* 1982; 8(3):111–113

Hasembos M, et al: Postoperative analgesia by epidural versus intramuscular nicomorphine after thoracotomy. Part II. *Acta Anaesthesiol Scand* 1985; 29:5787

Hurst JM, DeHaven CB, Branson RD: Use of CPAP mask as the sole mode of ventilatory support in trauma patients with mild to moderate respiratory insufficiency. *J Trauma* 1985; 25 (11):1065–1068

Lewis FR: *Current Therapy of Trauma,* pp. 235–236. Philadelphia, BC Decker, 1986

Mangano DT: Monitoring pulmonary arterial pressure in coronary artery disease. *Anesthesiology* 1980; 53:364–370

Mitchell RR, et al: Oxygen wash-in method for monitoring functional residual capacity. *Crit Care Med* 1982; 10(8):529–533

Newell JD, Underwood GH, Kelley MJ: The ICU chest film: Cardiac versus pulmonary disease. *Cardiol Clin* 1983; 1(4):729–743

Nyhus LM: Presidential address: Academic surgery—points of view. *Surgery* 1985; 98(4):619–624

Rithalia SV, Ng Y, Tinker J: Measurement of transcutaneous PCO_2 in critically ill patients. *Resuscitation* 1982; 10:13–18

Taylor GA, et al: Symposium on trauma: 1. Controversies in the management of pulmonary contusion. *Can J Surg* 1982; 25(2):167–170

Watt I, Ledingham IM: Mortality amongst multiple trauma patients admitted to an intensive therapy unit. *Anesthesia* 1984; 39:973

Waxman K, Shoemaker WC: Management of postoperative and posttraumatic respiratory failure in the intensive care unit. *Surg Clin North Am* 1980; 60(6):1413–1428

14

Postoperative Management of the Cardiac Surgery Patient

DYSRHYTHMIAS

Cardiac dysrhythmias occur in nearly 50% of patients. As a general rule, the urgency of therapy corresponds to the hemodynamic effect of the dysrhythmia. The exception is ventricular ectopic activity where treatment may be indicated despite lack of significant hemodynamic alteration. Continuous electrocardiographic (EKG) monitoring is indicated for the first 48 hours, although telemetered monitoring for a longer interval may be desirable. Table 14-1 summarizes the common dysrhythmias and their appropriate treatment.

With ventricular fibrillation (VF) if a defibrillator is immediately at hand, defibrillation with 300 J is the initial treatment; otherwise, external cardiac compression, ventilation with 100% oxygen, and mobilization of the "arrest" team are used, followed by defibrillation as soon as the instrument is available. After successful defibrillation, a lidocaine infusion is begun. If defibrillation is not immediately successful, cardiac massage is reinstituted and treatment continues, most commonly by the witnessed arrest protocol of the American Heart Association. In cases of refractory VF, procainamide, 15 to 20 mg/kg or 1 g, is often useful. Bretylium tosylate may also be used; however, significant hypotension is often problematic with this drug in the postoperative patient.

After effective rhythm is restored, consideration should be given to antidysrhythmic therapy. The medications and uses are classified in Table 14-2.

BLEEDING

Excessive postoperative bleeding occurs in approximately 4% of cardiac surgical patients (Table 14-3). Such bleeding usually is easily quantitated in chest drainage containers. At times bleeding can be occult; collection in the pleural cavity may be associated with unexplained hypotension and hypovolemia. If bleeding is extensive, decreased breath sounds are detected, and

TABLE 14-1 COMMON DYSRHYTHMIAS IN POSTOPERATIVE CARDIAC SURGICAL PATIENTS

Dysrhythmia	Treatment
Ectopic rhythms	
Atrial premature contractions	1. Usually none required but may indicate hypokalemia
Ventrical premature contractions	1. None if < 5–6 min, if unifocal, and if not close to T wave 2. Lidocaine 1.5 mg/kg bolus, plus infusion 1–4 mg/min 3. Overdrive pacing 4. Check electrolytes for hypokalemia
Tachydysrhythmias	
Paroxysmal atrial tachycardia	1. Rapid atrial pacing 2. Propranolol 3. Vagal tone (carotid massage, hypertension, anticholinesterases) 4. Cardioversion 5. Digoxin (dysrhythmia may be precipitated by digitalis toxicity)
Atrial flutter	1. Rapid atrial pacing 2. β-blockade 3. Verapamil 4. Cardioversion 5. Digoxin
Atrial fibrillation	1. Digoxin 2. Cardioversion
Ventricular tachycardia	1. Lidocaine if stable 2. Cardioversion
Ventricular fibrillation	1. Defibrillation 2. Cardiac arrest protocol 3. If refractory, then procainamide or bretylium
Bradydysrhythmias	
Sinus or nodal bradycardia	1. Atrial pacing when available 2. Atropine 3. Isoproterenol (rarely needed) 4. Electrical pacing (rarely needed)
Atrioventricular dissociation with slow ventricular response	1. Ventricular pacing (preferably AV sequential) 2. Atropine—rarely successful 3. Isoproterenol 4. Temporary pacing (transvenous, esophageal, transcutaneous, transthoracic)

dullness to percussion over the involved chest cavity is present. A chest radiograph aids the diagnosis.

Blood in the pericardial sac leads to pericardial tamponade. Rapid buildup can produce sudden cardiovascular collapse, while slower accumulation results in a condition which is difficult to diagnose. Diastolic filling is impeded, resulting in decreased blood pressure and cardiac output. Muffled heart tones, a low voltage EKG, jugular venous distention, and pulsus paradoxus are nonspecific findings which may be confusing after cardiac surgery.

TABLE 14-2 CLASSIFICATION AND USE OF ANTIDYSRHYTHMIC DRUGS

I Membrane Stabilizers A	B	C	II Beta-Receptor Blockers	III Drugs Prolonging Repolarization	IV Calcium Channel Blockers
Electrophysiologic effects					
QRS duration ↑ ERP ↑, APD ↑ QRS duration ↑ phase 0 ↓ Depolarization prolonged Conduction velocity decreased	APD ↓, ERP/APD ↓ QRS duration ±	Marked ↓ phase 0 Marked ↓ conduction velocity, marked ↑ QRS duration	↓ Vmax ↑ APD ↑ DRP ↑ ERP/APD	↑ APD, ERP, and ERP/APD	Prolonged depolarization and ↑ APD duration
Pharmacologic effects					
Interference with fast-channel (sodium) conductivity			Blockage of β-adrenergic receptor	Possibly interference with sodium and calcium exchange	Interference with slow-channel (calcium) conductivity
Prototype drugs					
Quinidine Procainamide Disopyramide Diphenylhydantoin	Lidocaine Mexiletine Tocainide	Lorcainide Encainide Flecainide	Propranolol Metoprolol Esmolol	Bretylium	Verapamil Nifedipine Diltiazem Lidoflazine
Antidysrhythmic use					
Supraventricular and ventricular dysrhythmias	Ventricular ectopy	Supraventricular and ventricular dysrhythmias	Tachydysrhythmias	Refractory ventricular fibrillation	Primarily atrial flutter, slows rate in atrial fibrillation

ERP = effective refractory period; APD = action potential duration.

TABLE 14-3 ETIOLOGY OF EXCESSIVE BLEEDING

Lack of Surgical Hemostasis
Normal coagulation studies
Needs reexploration
Coagulopathy
Preoperative medication, especially aspirin
Preoperative coagulopathy
Inadequate heparin reversal
Heparin rebound
Large overdose of protamine
Massive transfusion with dilution of platelets and factors V, VIII
Transfusion reaction
Disseminated intravascular coagulation
Primary fibrinolysis (very rare)

VENTILATION/OXYGENATION

Ventilator settings should be employed according to Table 14-4.

After a 20-minute stabilization period, check arterial blood gas partial pressures and pH, and adjust the ventilator settings accordingly. Minor adjustments in ventilator rate often are necessary. Positive end-expiratory airway

TABLE 14-4 MECHANICAL VENTILATORY SUPPORT

Mode	IMV, CMV, assist/control are the same if the patient is paralyzed. IMV or A/C allow the patient to increase ventilation as he awakens, and paralysis is reversed.
F_{IO_2}	Frequently, FRC is decreased during transport. It is safest to place the patient on 0.8 to 1.0 initially.
V_T	12–15 ml/kg for peak inspiratory pressure (PIP) 35 cm H_2O or less. Large V_Ts help open atelectatic alveoli. Excessive V_Ts may disrupt internal mammary artery anastomosis. The emphasis is on a cooperative interaction among all involved in the patient's care.
Rate	Adjust to give minute ventilation of 120 ml/kg at 37°C with decrease of 10 ml/kg/°C.
PEEP/CPAP	5 cm H_2O should be added. Contraindications: low blood pressure and cardiac output; hyperinflated lungs with air trapping (bronchospasm or severe emphysema); endobronchial intubation; pneumothorax.
Flow rate	Slower flow rates decrease airways resistance due to turbulent flow; may improve distribution of inspired gases. 30–40 liters/min is a reasonable starting point.
I:E Ratio	Should be 1:2 or less. Longer expiratory times allow complete exhalation, preventing air trapping; interferes less with venous return.
Inflation hold	Can be set at 0.5 sec or greater to help open alveoli.
Alarms	Peak airway pressure alarm set 15–20 cm above usual PIP. Low inspiratory pressure alarm ("disconnect") set 10 cm H_2O below usual PIP. Low exhaled volume alarm set 30% below mechanical tidal volume until patient begins spontaneous breathing.

pressure (PEEP) between 5 and 10 cm H_2O usually allows weaning of the fraction of inspired oxygen (FI_{O_2}) to 0.4 or less while the Pa_{O_2} remains between 70 and 90 mm Hg.

When weaning is initiated (Table 14-5) it can be done in a single step to spontaneous breathing with continuous positive airway pressure (CPAP), or more gradually by decreasing the ventilator rate in 2 breaths/min decrements using intermittent mandatory ventilation (IMV) as long as arterial blood pH is above 7.35.

The patient is ready for tracheal extubation when the criteria in Table 14-6 are satisfied. Hemodynamic instability and excessive bleeding are important contraindications to extubation, even if pulmonary function is normal.

MONITORING

BLOOD PRESSURE

A confounding difficulty with peripheral arterial pressure measurement is that intense vasoconstriction resulting from shock, hypothermia, and cardiopulmonary bypass causes peripheral underestimation of the central aortic pressure. This phenomenon is sufficiently predictable following hypothermic bypass, even after warming and the use of vasodilators, that treatment of hypotension in that setting should not be undertaken before the pressure is verified with an independent measurement, preferably directly from the aorta.

TABLE 14-5 WEANING FROM VENTILATORY SUPPORT

Wean inspired oxygen concentration
- Decrease FI_{O_2} to 0.35
- Maintain Pa_{O_2} at least 70 mm Hg
- Add PEEP if necessary
- Consider cardiac effects of PEEP

Wean ventilation rate: IMV wean
- Reduce IMV rate 2 breaths/min decrements
- Continue if pH 7.35 or above
- At lower rates consider work of breathing

Wean ventilation rate: T-piece wean
- Ventilate fully on assist-control
- T-piece trial when strong and stable
- Consider CPAP instead of T piece to maintain FRC

Wean CPAP last
- CPAP improves FRC, FI_{O_2} does not
- Reduce CPAP in 2.5-cm H_2O decrements until 5.0 cm H_2O
- If CPAP requirements prolonged, consider increasing rate to decrease work of breathing

Extubate
- Measure muscle strength (FVC, PNP)
- Assess CNS status (awake, alert, narcotics)
- Remove endotracheal tube

TABLE 14-6 EXTUBATION CRITERIA

Oxygenation
Pa_{O_2} 70–90 mm Hg on 5 cm CPAP and Fi_{O_2} 0.4 or less
Ventilation
pH at least 7.35 on CPAP 30 min
Rate 24/min or less
$V_D/V_T \leq 0.6$
Muscle strength
Head lift 5 sec
FVC at least 15 ml/kg
PNP at least −25 cm H_2O
Airway protection
Gag and swallow reflexes intact
Hemodynamics
Cardiac output and blood pressure adequate
Inotropic support minimal
Intra-aortic balloon pump removed
No excessive bleeding
No need for reexploration
CNS status
Awake, alert, cooperative, eager to be extubated

PULMONARY ARTERY PRESSURE

Selective rather than routine use of pulmonary artery (PA) catheters is the appropriate choice in cardiac surgical patients. However, PA catheterization should be used unhesitatingly if the patient's hemodynamic status deviates significantly from that which is expected.

ELECTROCARDIOGRAPH

A variety of lead systems can be used to detect rhythm disturbances; the principle is to select one for each patient which provides readily visible atrial and ventricular EKG waveforms. Since most postoperative cardiac surgical patients have temporary atrial and ventricular pacing leads, the atrial electrogram is easily obtained to determine the relationship between the P wave and the QRS complex. The atrial pacing wire is connected to the precordial lead of a suitably isolated EKG system which is then monitored. Alternatively, the atrial wire and the left arm electrode are connected while standard limb lead I is monitored (the atrial pacing wire becomes the positive electrode).

FLUIDS THERAPY

Oxygen delivery must be considered during volume replacement. It can be improved by the infusion of red blood cells (RBC) until hemoglobin is 12 g/dl. Improvement also results from increasing cardiac output, a first step of which is to optimize preload.

Coagulation defects usually are corrected with fresh frozen plasma or platelets. Fresh frozen plasma carries the risk of transfusion-induced hepatitis and acquired immune deficiency syndrome (AIDS), and should not be used for volume expansion in the absence of specific coagulation defects.

If the hemoglobin concentration is optimal, and coagulation is adequate, but the patient needs preload augmentation, the choice is between crystalloid and colloid. Isotonic crystalloids such as Ringer's lactate or normal saline are effective and inexpensive. Colloids such as hydroxyethylstarch or albumin are two to four times more effective for intravascular volume expansion, but are more expensive. Because of the capillary leak induced by cardiopulmonary bypass, significant portions of administered colloid will leak into the pulmonary interstitium and may be more difficult than crystalloid to mobilize.

How much fluid to give is determined in part by "construction" of ventricular function curves. No single, optimal filling pressure applies to all patients; furthermore, the optimal filling pressure for an individual patient changes with time as ventricular compliance is altered. Measure CVP or PAOP and cardiac output, administer a rapid fluid bolus, and repeat the measurements. If little change in either measurement occurs, repeat the rapid bolus until the filling pressures rise. If a rise in filling pressure is associated with an increase in cardiac output, repeat the procedure, looking for further increases or maintenance of filling pressures at a constant level. When PAOP rises above 15 mm Hg, give smaller fluid boluses. If it reaches 18 to 20 mm Hg without a corresponding increase in cardiac output, consider another approach such as afterload reduction or inotropic support.

COMPLICATIONS

ATELECTASIS

Atelectasis occurs in 60% to 84% of patients after cardiopulmonary bypass. Treatment involves opening alveoli with high peak inflation pressure and inflation hold, and maintaining them open with PEEP or CPAP.

ENDOTRACHEAL TUBE MALPOSITION

This complication is most likely to occur during transport from the OR to the ICU. Changes in head position can cause inadvertent bronchial intubation or tracheal extubation. Accidental extubation can be minimized by the use of hand restraints, secure taping of the endotracheal tube, proper positioning of ventilator hoses, and care in moving the intubated patient.

PNEUMOTHORAX

Pneumothorax is commonly produced by opening the pleural cavity during sternotomy or internal mammary artery dissection. It can occur in any mechanically ventilated patient. Proper lung expansion depends on a functioning thoracostomy tube. The tube should be connected to a water seal drainage system during transport to the ICU. Proper lung inflation should be checked on the postoperative chest radiograph.

BRONCHOSPASM

Bronchospasm can develop after cardiopulmonary bypass. Possible etiologies include preexistent bronchospastic diseases, protamine reaction, or noncardiogenic pulmonary edema. Treatment includes nebulized beta-adrenergic agents, aminophylline infusion, steroids, and possibly antihistamines.

PULMONARY EDEMA

Permeability

This type of pulmonary edema (noncardiogenic) results from anaphylactic reactions to drugs such as protamine, from transfusion reactions, or from postperfusion syndrome ("pump lung") which occurs rarely and unpredictably after cardiopulmonary bypass times greater than 2 hours. Treatment includes epinephrine, 0.01 to 0.1 μg/kg/min, careful fluid administration, and PEEP to support oxygenation.

Hydrostatic

Hydrostatic (cardiogenic) pulmonary edema results from increased interstitial lung water due to the increased pulmonary artery pressure associated with left-sided heart failure. Treatment includes ventilatory support, while therapeutic efforts are directed to improve cardiac function.

PULMONARY EMBOLUS

Pulmonary embolus is rare after cardiac surgery unless prolonged immobilization, low cardiac output, or dysrhythmias are prevalent. Differentiating pulmonary embolus from perioperative myocardial infarction or cardiac tamponade is difficult.

PNEUMONIA

Pneumonia is rare in the acute postoperative period unless infection existed preoperatively or aspiration occurred perioperatively. Temperature elevations above 38°C are common during rewarming and during the first postoperative day. The white blood cell count is frequently elevated. Cultures should not be obtained unless these changes persist into the second postoperative day.

PHRENIC NERVE PARALYSIS

Phrenic nerve paralysis occurs after cardiac surgery in about 1.5% of patients. If bilateral, ventilatory mechanics are inadequate to clear secretions and perhaps even to provide adequate ventilation. Bilateral paralysis should be suspected in a ventilator-dependent patient if paradoxical abdominal wall movement and postural orthopnea occur when the ventilator rate is decreased. The diagnosis is confirmed by observing diaphragmatic movement under fluoroscopy.

Neurologic Dysfunction

A recent large series reported a 16% incidence of cerebral dysfunction on the first postoperative day. Neurologic function was normal in all but 6.4% by the 10th postoperative day. New motor deficits were reported in 3% of patients after cardiopulmonary bypass.

Damage to the central nervous system (CNS) includes cerebral vascular accident (CVA), postoperative psychosis or delirium, and minimal brain dysfunction. Ischemia due to poor perfusion is responsible for some CVAs, but the importance of flow rate and perfusion pressure during cardiopulmonary bypass is controversial. Mean arterial pressure below 50 mm Hg results in electroencephalographic changes indicative of ischemia. Nevertheless, many investigators believe that as long as flow rates are adequate, perfusion pressure is relatively unimportant. Evidence has been presented that perfusion with both low pressures (50–60 mm Hg) and low flow (30–50 ml/kg) does not increase the incidence of neurologic complications.

Emboli are believed to be responsible for most CVAs associated with cardiac surgery. Air remaining in the heart and pulmonary veins, despite careful attempts at removal, and atheromatous plaques broken off during manipulation of the aorta can still reach the brain.

Delirium or psychosis after bypass occurs in as many as 28% of patients. Severe illness, sleep deprivation, and sensory isolation in the ICU are possible etiologies. Treatment includes haloperidol, along with reorientation and reassurance by the staff and family.

RENAL INSUFFICIENCY

Moderate to severe acute renal failure after cardiac surgery occurs in up to 7% of patients and has an associated mortality rate of 65% to 88%. Predictors of acute renal failure include preoperative renal dysfunction, old age, left ventricular dysfunction, prolonged hypotension, prolonged surgery and bypass time, and excessive hemolysis.

For further information, please see Chapter 48 in Civetta JM, Taylor RW, Kirby RR: Critical Care. *Philadelphia, J. B. Lippincott, 1988*

BIBLIOGRAPHY

Abel RM, Buckley MJ, Austen WG, et al: Etiology, incidence, and prognosis of renal failure following cardiac operations. Results of a prospective analysis of 500 consecutive patients. *J Thorac Cardiovasc Surg* 1976; 71:323

Angelini P, Feldman MI, Lufschanowski R, et al: Cardiac arrhythmias during and after heart surgery: Diagnosis and management. *Prog Cardiovasc Dis* 1974; 16:469

Bachmann F, McKenna R, Cole ER, et al: The hemostatic mechanism after open-heart surgery. I. Studies on plasma coagulation factors and fibrinolysis in 512 patients after extracorporeal circulation. *J Thorac Cardiovasc Surg* 1975; 70:76

Conrardy PA, Goodman LR, Lainge F, et al: Alteration of endotracheal tube position. Flexion and extension of the neck. *Crit Care Med* 1976; 4:8

Culliford AT, Thomas S, Spencer FC: Fulminating noncardiogenic pulmonary edema. A newly recognized hazard during cardiac operations. *J Thorac Cardiovasc Surg* 1980; 80:868

Hilberman M, Kamm B, Lamy M, et al: An analysis of potential physiological predictors of respiratory adequacy following cardiac surgery. *J Thorac Cardiovasc Surg* 1976; 71:711

Hilberman M, Myers BD, Carrie BJ, et al: Acute renal failure following cardiac surgery. *J Thorac Cardiovasc Surg* 1979; 77:880

Markland ON, Moorthy SS, Mahomed Y, et al: Postoperative phrenic nerve palsy in patients with open-heart surgery. *Ann Thorac Surg* 1985; 39:68

Slogoff S, Girgis KZ, Keats AS: Etiologic factors in neuropsychiatric complications associated with cardiopulmonary bypass. *Anesth Analg* 1982; 61:903

15
Vascular Surgery and Trauma

BASIC PRINCIPLES

CIRCULATION

Baseline examination of the extremities distal to the reconstruction should be obtained when the patient arrives in the ICU. Initially, following aortic or extra-anatomic reconstructions, neither distal pulses nor doppler signals may be present because of vasoconstriction from hypothermia. In nearly all of these patients, a doppler signal will be audible in the feet once the patient becomes normothermic (usually within 6 to 8 hr). If it is not, the surgeon should be notified.

Hypertension

The most convenient way of managing hypertensive crises is the infusion of drugs which have a rapid onset of action and a short half-life. Sodium nitroprusside can be used as a continuous infusion and titrated to the desired physiologic effect. Patients with ischemic coronary artery disease may have the potential for a "coronary steal" phenomenon when given nitroprusside. Therefore, the drug of choice in such patients may be intravenous nitroglycerine. Labetalol, is a combined, nonselective antagonist of both alpha- and beta-adrenergic receptors. Initial doses should begin with the administration of 20 mg infused intravenously over 2 minutes. Repeat injections of 40 to 80 mg may be given every 10 minutes until a maximum dose of 300 mg has been given.

RESPIRATORY MANAGEMENT

The vast majority of patients can be extubated in the early postoperative period. In general, a mode·of ventilatory support which provides decreased inspiratory and expiratory work of breathing as well as the lowest mean airway pressure possible should be provided for these patients.

PAIN

Since these patients may tolerate poorly the alpha-blockade effects of potent long-acting narcotics such as morphine, short-acting drugs (*i.e.*, fentanyl), which have fewer alpha-blockade side-effects than morphine, should be used.

PROBLEMS COMMON TO ALL VASCULAR RECONSTRUCTIONS

BLEEDING

Etiology. Common causes for postoperative bleeding, regardless of the operative location, include over-anticoagulation, improperly ligated venous or arterial branches, and leakage from the arterial suture line.

Diagnosis. Often, the first manifestation of wound bleeding is a blood-soaked dressing. This should be removed and the wound inspected. If skin edges are the source, there is usually minimal swelling of the wound and the bleeding site can be visualized. If the source is from the deep tissues, there is usually a moderate-to-massive degree of swelling. Large neck wound hematomas may produce respiratory distress requiring intubation.

Intra-abdominal bleeding is suggested by the presence of tachycardia, hypotension, and low pulmonary artery occlusion pressures which fail to improve after fluid boluses. A measurable increase in abdominal girth is a later finding, detectable only after 2 to 3 liters of blood have accumulated. Generally, if a patient receives 2 units of packed cells over a 2- to 3-hour period and fails to stabilize, significant bleeding is suggested. A coagulation profile should be obtained to rule out over-anticoagulation as a cause. The surgeon should be notified immediately about any bleeding complication.

Therapy. Skin edge bleeding may be controlled by compression, cautery with a silver nitrate stick, or with nylon sutures. Small wound hematomas may be observed. Large hematomas should be evacuated in the operating room. For intra-abdominal bleeding, fluids and blood should be administered to correct hypotension. If profound hypotension and rapid tachycardia develop, and there is no evidence for a cardiac cause or hypocoagulability, immediate reexploration is indicated. Over-anticoagulation should be treated with protamine sulfate (0.5–1 mg protamine/100 units of heparin given intraoperatively) and fresh frozen plasma.

GRAFT THROMBOSIS

Etiology. Common causes of early graft thrombosis are anastomotic stenosis, intimal flap, and twisting or kinking of the graft. Other causes include stenosis or occlusion of distal outflow vessels, low cardiac output, graft compression, and a small-diameter vein graft (infrainguinal reconstructions).

Diagnosis. Disappearance of a distal pulse palpable when the patient first arrives in the ICU suggests graft thrombosis. Disappearance of a previously audible doppler signal or a change from a biphasic to a monophasic signal also implies graft thrombosis. Clinical signs, such as the presence of pallor, mottled skin, and coolness of the extremity, are unreliable in the initial post-operative period.

Therapy. Once the diagnosis of graft occlusion is made, 5000 units of heparin should be given after the surgeon is consulted. Thrombectomy and correction of any technical error should then be performed.

WOUND INFECTION

Etiology. For neck wounds, intraoperative contamination is the most likely cause. For groin infections, possible causes are the presence of *Staphylococcus* in the creases, close proximity of the perineum, and contaminated inguinal lymphatics due to infected foot lesions.

Diagnosis. The first sign of infection is expanding erythema around the incision. If untreated the wound will become warm, tender, fluctuant, and purulent which suggests deep infection that may lead to graft infection. The surgeon should be informed when signs of wound infection appear.

Therapy. Once wound erythema appears, treatment should be initiated with intravenous antibiotics effective against *Staphylococcus.* If a foot infection is present, antibiotic coverage should include agents which are effective against the organisms present in the foot. Failure to treat wound infections aggressively may result in graft infection which often causes major amputation or death.

GRAFT INFECTION

Etiology. Graft contamination generally occurs at the time of implantation. Other factors contributing to graft infection are infected groin lymphatics, wound infection, and hematogenous seeding from a distant infected source, (*i.e.*, bladder, soft-tissue abscess).

Diagnosis. In most cases of infected aortofemoral grafts, clinical findings of infection first appear in the groin. The groin incision may be erythematous, swollen, and tender to palpation; purulent drainage may appear. If infection is confined to the abdomen, clinical signs are often subtle. The patient may present with malaise, low-grade fever, abdominal or back pain, anorexia, weight loss, and diaphoresis. Systemic sepsis, graft occlusion, and septic emboli are less common. If a draining sinus is present in a groin incision, contrast sinography is diagnostic for graft infection if the contrast outlines the graft. A computed tomography (CT) scan of the abdomen and pelvis is the most helpful test in diagnosing graft infection. Findings consistent with graft infection include perigraft fluid collections, loss of tissue planes, and perigraft air. Arteriography should be performed in all patients with graft infections to plan further operative therapy. It is not useful diagnostically.

Therapy. Proper operative therapy generally consists of removing the entire infected graft and extra-anatomic bypass to revascularize the extremities.

MANAGEMENT OF SPECIFIC RECONSTRUCTIONS

CAROTID/SUBCLAVIAN RECONSTRUCTIONS

Basic Considerations

Blood Pressure. After carotid endarterectomy, systolic blood pressure should be maintained between 110 and 160 mm Hg.

Neurologic. The patient must have a detailed baseline neurologic examination in the ICU.

Pain. Usually acetaminophen will suffice for pain. If this is not adequate, then codeine (30 mg PO or IM) may be administered.

Antiplatelet Therapy. Since endarterectomy creates a rough, thrombogenic surface within the artery, many surgeons prescribe aspirin, dyprimadole, or low-molecular-weight dextran.

Chest Radiograph. After subclavian artery reconstruction, a chest radiograph should be obtained to rule out a pneumothorax. An elevated hemidiaphragm caused by phrenic nerve injury should be noted.

Problems to be Anticipated

Postoperative Stroke/Transient Ischemic Attack (TIA). Any change in the patient's neurologic status must be immediately brought to the surgeon's attention. An ocular pneumoplethysmograph (OPG) may be used to determine patency of the carotid artery. If dense hemiplegia or aphasia develops, a heparin bolus should be given intravenously (5000 U). If the OPG reveals a patent artery and arteriography demonstrates a technical error, revision is required. If the arteriogram is normal, the patient should be returned to the ICU for evaluation of other possible causes for a TIA. If OPG and arteriography are not readily available, the safest course is to reexplore the patient and, if necessary, obtain an intraoperative arteriogram.

Headache. If the patient complains of a progressive increase in the severity of the headache or develops visual changes, vomiting, or an altered mental state, the physician should consider the possibility of an intracerebral hemorrhage. Patients with severe headaches should undergo a head CT scan immediately.

Nerve Injuries. Recurrent laryngeal nerve injuries present as prolonged postoperative hoarseness. Visualization of a paralyzed vocal cord during indirect laryngoscopy is diagnostic. Injury of both recurrent nerves following bilateral carotid endarterectomies may result in upper airway obstruction requiring tracheostomy.

Thoracic Duct Injury. Clear, light yellow fluid will persistently drain from the neck incision. If the amount of drainage is small, observation is indicated. A large volume of wound drainage requires reexploration for ligation of the thoracic duct.

MESENTERIC AND RENAL RECONSTRUCTIONS

Basic Considerations

Fluid Management. Patients undergoing renal artery revascularizations (especially bilateral reconstructions) often have a large volume deficit and may develop high urinary outputs (> 300 ml/hr) in the initial postoperative period. These patients can easily become dehydrated. Patients undergoing mesentereic revascularizations are also at risk for developing dehydration because of large third space losses which can occur when ischemic bowel is revascularized.

Hypertension. After renal revascularization, labile blood pressure in the immediate postoperative period is common. For hypertension over 180 mm Hg systolic, titrate the blood pressure to between 120 and 160 mm Hg systolic with a nitroprusside drip.

Problems to be Anticipated

Renal Artery Graft Stenosis/Thrombosis. Signs of graft stenosis or thrombosis are hypertension, renal failure, or flank pain due to renal infarction. If anuria occurs in the presence of adequate hydration after bilateral renal revascularization, the surgeon should be notified immediately. A decision must be made regarding the need for arteriography or reoperation for suspected graft occlusion.

Intestinal Infarction After Revascularization. Because of sequestration, a marked increase in fluid requirement may be one of the earliest signs of bowel infarction. Other findings include tachycardia, hypotension, marked leukocytosis (>20,000 WBC/mm^3), and unexplained metabolic acidosis. Once the diagnosis of graft thrombosis with intestinal infarction is suspected, the surgeon should be notified immediately. Arteriography should be performed urgently. If graft thrombosis is confirmed by arteriography, urgent reoperation for thrombectomy and revision of the mesenteric arterial graft is indicated. Bowel resection may also be required. If any bowel appears marginally viable, a second reexploration should be performed 24 hours later to examine the intestine.

DIRECT AORTIC RECONSTRUCTIONS

Problems to be Anticipated

Distal Embolization

If a large thrombus occludes a major vessel such as the femoral artery, this will produce findings similar to an acute graft limb occlusion. Microembolization will produce mottling and cyanosis of the toes and skin of the lower legs and feet leading to painful gangrene ("trash foot" syndrome).

If a major vessel becomes occluded, a 5000-unit bolus of heparin should be given and the patient returned to the operating room for a thrombectomy. Once microembolization has occurred, no effective medical or surgical therapy exists.

Patients at greatest risk for developing bowel ischemia are those who undergo repair of a ruptured abdominal aortic aneurysm, have a previously patent inferior mesenteric artery which was ligated intraoperatively, and have no mesenteric doppler signals present after the aortic reconstruction.

Any patient who develops bloody diarrhea or persistent nonbloody diarrhea should undergo flexible colonoscopic examination. Adequate examination should include visualization of the splenic flexure (40–50 cm from the anus). If superficial mucosal lesions are discovered on the initial examination, repeat examination should be performed every 24 or 48 hours to be certain that they are not progressing. Once ischemic lesions are identified on endoscopic examination, a decision must be made regarding observation or operation. If the lesions appear superficial and involve only the mucosa, it is safe to observe the patient with repeat endoscopic examination. If mucosal ischemia progresses, a colectomy should be performed. If the mucosa appears friable, necrotic, and hemorrhagic, then urgent colectomy, Hartmann's pouch, and end colostomy are required.

Acute Pancreatitis/Cholecystitis

Postoperative pancreatitis should be suspected in any patient who develops prolonged ileus (> 5 days) or exacerbation of abdominal pain with nausea and vomiting after oral feedings begin. Once this diagnosis is made, oral intake should be stopped and parenteral nutrition administered. A nasogastric tube is not required if the patient is not vomiting and otherwise has mild symptoms. Once the serum amylase level is normal, oral feedings can be resumed slowly.

Patients who develop unexplained right upper quadrant pain, fever, and leukocytosis should undergo an ultrasound examination of the gallbladder. Once the diagnosis of cholecystitis is made, appropriate antibiotics should be started. If there is no improvement within 24 hours, cholecystectomy or cholecystostomy, with the patient under local anesthesia if critically ill, should be performed.

EXTRA-ANATOMIC RECONSTRUCTIONS (FEMOROFEMORAL, AXILLOFEMORAL BYPASS)

Basic Considerations

Graft Tunnels

After the patient arrives in the ICU, the course of the subcutaneous graft tunnels should be inspected. A palpable pulse should usually be present over the graft except in obese patients and in those in whom a ringed graft was used. Swelling along the course of the tunnel may be a sign of bleeding.

Positioning

Since these grafts are superficial, the patient should not be allowed to lie on the side where an axillofemoral graft is located. Compressive devices, such as abdominal binders, should not be used.

Problems to be Anticipated

Brachial Plexus Injury

The most obvious finding is a neurologic deficit in the upper extremity which is noted when the patient awakens from anesthesia. Electromyography will define precisely which nerve roots have been injured.

INFRAINGUINAL RECONSTRUCTIONS

Basic Considerations

Leg Elevation

Since most patients develop leg swelling after an infrainguinal reconstruction, the extremities should be elevated above the level of the heart for 3 days. Bed rest is recommended during this time.

Problems to be Anticipated

Infection

In patients with foot infections, a prolonged course of antibiotics (7–10 days) is recommended, based on culture and sensitivity data. Patients without infections are given prophylactic antibiotics for 24 hours. Antibiotic coverage is especially important when a prosthetic graft is used in the presence of active infection. Whenever a leg becomes swollen after infrainguinal bypass, correct diagnosis is important. Other important causes of leg swelling after revascularization are deep venous thrombosis (DVT), compartment syndrome, and wound hematoma. With post-revascularization edema, the swelling is confined mainly to the calf and is often markedly improved with leg elevation. There is usually no calf tenderness except near the incision. Deep venous thrombosis is clinically difficult to differentiate from lymphedema. Since clinical findings are unreliable, the best tests to diagnose DVT are impedance plethysmography (IPG), venous ultrasound imaging, or venography. Swelling due to a wound hematoma is usually apparent on clinical examination. The swelling is mainly confined to the incision and discoloration and oozing may be present.

The best therapy for post-revascularization edema is bed rest and leg elevation. Patients with postoperative DVT should be started on continuous intravenous heparin at a rate which elevates the partial thromboplastin time to two times control. After 7 to 10 days, warfarin should be started and continued for 6 months. Large wound hematomas should be evacuated in the operating room; small hematomas may be observed.

THROMBOLYTIC THERAPY

INDICATIONS AND CONTRAINDICATIONS

Major indications and contraindications for the use of thrombolytic agents are listed in Table 15-1. Arterial thrombosis is most commonly treated by intra-arterial low-dose therapy. An important contraindication to thrombolytic therapy is acute arterial or graft thrombosis with limb-threatening ischemia.

TABLE 15-1 INDICATIONS AND CONTRAINDICATIONS FOR THROMBOLYTIC THERAPY

Indications
Acute deep venous thrombosis, < 3 days old
Pulmonary embolism–massive
Acute arterial occlusion
Acute arterial graft occlusion
Contraindications
Surgery–within 10 days
Organ biopsy–within 10 days
Arterial puncture–within 10 days
Parturition–within 10 days
GI bleeding–within 6 mo
Stroke–within 2 mo
Recent trauma
Uncontrolled hypertension
Cardiac thrombus
Coagulopathy
Severe hepatic or renal failure
Pregnancy
Childhood
Hemorrhagic retinopathy
Vascular graft implanted–within 6 mo
Active duodenal ulcer

Since thrombolytic agents usually require a minimum of 24 to 48 hours to restore perfusion, threatened limbs may become nonviable. Such patients should undergo urgent operative thrombectomy or arterial reconstruction.

ADMINISTRATION

Systemic Therapy (High Dose)

Streptokinase therapy is initiated with an intravenous loading dose of 250,000 units over 30 minutes then continued at 100,000 U/h for 24 hours for pulmonary embolism and for up to 72 hours for DVT. Urokinase therapy is initiated with an intravenous loading dose of 4400 U/kg body weight over 10 minutes then continued at a rate of 4400 U/kg/hr for 24 hours for pulmonary embolism.

Intra-arterial Therapy (Low Dose)

Under fluoroscopic guidance, an intra-arterial catheter is inserted and its tip is embedded into the thrombus. Streptokinase (5000 U/hr) or urokinase (440 U/kg/hr) infusion is begun. Start the patient on 600 to 800 units of intravenous heparin per hour to prevent pericatheter thrombus formation because this may produce an arterial occlusion when the catheter is withdrawn.

THERAPEUTIC MONITORING

High-Dose Therapy

Before therapy is begun, a baseline thrombin time, prothrombin time, partial thromboplastin time, platelet count, fibrinogen level, and hematocrit level should be obtained. Laboratory values should be obtained to document the existence of lytic state. A continued drop in hematocrit value may indicate occult bleeding (*i.e.*, retroperitoneal). Any evidence of bleeding is an absolute indication to discontinue therapy.

Low-Dose Intra-arterial Therapy

The same baseline laboratory tests are obtained prior to initiating infusion. A lytic state is evidenced by a thrombin time greater than 1.5 times the control value and a greater than 50% decrease in fibrinogen level. Bleeding is the main indication to terminate therapy. To follow the progress of thrombolysis, angiograms are obtained daily. The catheter tip is also further advanced so it can directly bathe the thrombus with the thrombolytic agent.

COMPLICATIONS

Hemorrhage

Many bleeding complications are relatively minor, but serious life-threatening complications, such as intracranial, gastrointestinal, or retroperitoneal bleeding, may also occur. When bleeding occurs, fibrinolytic therapy should be discontinued unless it occurs around a catheter site which is easily controlled by compression. Fresh frozen plasma should be given to replace deficient coagulation factors. If severe bleeding fails to respond to these measures, then epsilon-aminocaproic acid, a fibrinolysis inhibitor, should be administered as an intravenous 5-g loading dose followed by 1g/hr for 2 to 4 hours.

Allergic Reaction

Symptoms range from a skin rash to anaphylaxis. Mild allergic reactions are treated with antihistamines and steroids. More severe allergic reactions mandate cessation of SK infusion and treatment with large doses of steroids.

Distal Embolization

The limb will develop signs of severe ischemia, such as cyanosis, increasing foot pain, coolness, diminished sensation, and impaired motor function. Once these clinical signs appear, the surgeon should be notified and the thrombolytic therapy discontinued.

VASCULAR TRAUMA

COMMON PROBLEMS OF ALL RECONSTRUCTIONS DUE TO TRAUMA

In general, the same complications which occur after elective vascular reconstructions may also occur after reconstruction for traumatic injuries. The major difference between elective vascular reconstructions and posttraumatic reconstructions is that there are often several associated nonvascular injuries in the trauma victim which may have a more profound effect on the overall prognosis. Therefore, the ICU physician must be aware of potential complications that may arise from injured tissues in proximity to a repaired vascular injury.

MANAGEMENT OF SPECIFIC VASCULAR INJURIES

Aorta and Major Branches

Great Vessels. Injuries to the brachiocephalic vessels are often associated with injuries to other vital structures such as the trachea and esophagus. The ICU team should watch for signs of mediastinitis, subcutaneous emphysema, and pneumothorax in the postoperative period following repair of a great vessel injury.

Thoracic Aorta. Injuries to the thoracic aorta usually result in massive blood loss. Postoperative bleeding should be anticipated and is usually diagnosed by increased bloody drainage from the chest tubes.

Abdominal Aorta and Branches. Trauma to the abdominal aorta and any of its major intra-abdominal branches usually results in massive blood loss. The patient is often taken to the operating room *in extremis.* One of the most significant problems is bacterial contamination from concomitant injuries to the gastrointestinal tract. In general, most surgeons avoid placing prosthetic vascular grafts in patients with abdominal vascular injuries and bowel contamination because of the risk of infection.

Extremity Injuries

Arteriovenous Fistulae (AVF) and False Aneurysms. Clinical findings are the presence of a bruit or thrill over the injured area. A pulsatile mass may also be present. When these problems are suspected, the best test to confirm the diagnosis is arteriography. Generally, false aneurysms and AVFs should be repaired surgically, provided the patient is stable enough to undergo operation.

Fractures and Arterial Injuries. When the patient with an arterial injury associated with a fracture is admitted to the ICU, great care must be taken to keep the limb immobilized. Any forceful movement of the extremity may disrupt both the bone alignment and the vascular repair resulting in arterial thrombosis or possibly severe hemorrhage.

Venous Injuries. Careful observation for signs of a compartment syndrome is mandatory if a major deep vein is ligated. If the vein has been repaired, thrombosis may still occur. Development of marked calf tenderness and swelling are the first signs of this complication. To enhance venous blood flow, the legs should be elevated. Application of pneumatic compression boots over the extremity will also facilitate venous return. If the patient has no other serious injuries, start heparin as soon as possible after all major venous injuries.

Compartment Syndrome. Elevated compartment pressure above 30 mm Hg will result in nerve and muscle damage. If this pressure is not relieved, nerve damage will occur within minutes and will become permanent within 8 to 12 hours. Muscle death will begin within 4 hours and become maximal at 12 hours. Early signs of a developing compartment syndrome are fullness over an extremity with pain on palpation, paresthesia, weakness of the involved muscles, and diminished pulses. Paralysis, loss of sensation, and absent pulses are late findings which occur coincident with irreversible muscle necrosis. Patients who show signs of a compartment syndrome should undergo compartment pressure measurements. This involves inserting a catheter into the involved muscle compartment which is connected to a pressure transducer. If the compartment pressure is over 40 mm Hg, a fasciotomy should be performed. If the pressure remains between 30 to 40 mm Hg for over 4 hours, a fasciotomy should be performed. Fasciotomy should also be considered in patients with pressures less than 30 mm Hg who have clinical signs of compartment syndrome since no absolute critical pressure exists for every patient.

For further information, please see Chapter 53 in Civetta JM, Taylor RW, Kirby RR: Critical Care. *Philadelphia: J. B. Lippincott, 1988*

BIBLIOGRAPHY

Allen TW, Reul GJ, Morton JR, et al: Surgical management of aortic trauma. *J Trauma* 1972; 12:862

Bandyk DF: Vascular graft infection: Epidemiology, bacteriology, and pathogenesis. In Bernhard VM, Towne JB (eds): *Complications in Vascular Surgery,* 2nd ed, pp 471–485. Orlando, Grune & Stratton, 1985.

Bernhard VM, Towne JB: Complications in vascular surgery. In Moore WS (ed): *Vascular Surgery: A Comprehensive Review,* pp 737–776. New York, Grune & Stratton, 1983

Downs AR: Complications of abdominal aortic surgery. In Bernhard VM, Towne JB (eds): *Complications in Vascular Surgery,* 2nd ed pp 25–36. Orlando, Grune & Stratton, 1985

Hertzer, NR: Postoperative management and complications of extracranial carotid reconstruction. In Rutherford RB (ed): *Vascular Surgery,* 2nd ed, pp 1300–1316. Philadelphia, WB Saunders, 1984

Lim RC Jr, Trunkey DD, Blaisdell FW: Acute abdominal aortic injury: An analysis of operative and postoperative management. *Arch Surg* 1974; 109:706

Moore WS: Complications of vertebral and subclavian repair. In Bernhard VM, Towne JB (eds): *Complications in Vascular Surgery,* 2nd ed, pp 753–761. Orlando, Grune & Stratton, 1985

O'Hara PJ, Hertzer NR, Beven EG, et al: Surgical management of infected abdominal aortic grafts: Review of a 25-year experience. *J Vasc Surg* 1986; 3:725

Perdue GD Jr, Smith RB: Intra-abdominal vascular injury. *Surgery* 1968; 64:562

Reilly LM, Goldstone J: The infected aortic graft. In Bergan JJ, Yao JST (eds): *Reoperative Arterial Surgery,* pp 231–253. Orlando, Grune & Stratton, 1986

Warshaw AL, O'Hara PJ: Susceptibility of the pancreas to ischemic injury in shock. *Ann Surg* 1978; 188:197

Watkins L Jr, Gott VL: Blunt and penetrating trauma to the great vessels. In Glenn WL (ed): *Thoracic and Cardiovascular Surgery,* 4th ed, pp 1489–1497. Norwalk, Appleton-Century-Crofts, 1983

16

Relevant Surgical Aspects of Hepatobiliary Disease

FLUID MANAGEMENT IN CIRRHOTIC PATIENTS

Although postoperative cirrhotic patients may have the same diminished-functional extracellular volume requiring adequate replacement as do other patients, efforts must be taken to minimize ascites formation. Ascites formation is less of a clinical problem with central shunts than with selective shunts. Distal splenorenal shunt requires extensive retroperationeal dissection without portal and liver decompression and may be considered a model for ascites formation. It is much simpler to avoid than to treat tense ascites. If the patient is hypovolemic and hypotensive, appropriate resuscitation is indicated. Postoperative mild oliguria, however, is likely to be transient and unlikely to be a precursor of acute renal failure given adequate intraoperative fluid replacement. Judicious diuresis or administration of colloid usually achieves the desired outcome, reversal of oliguria without disproportionate ascites formation. The administration of sufficient crystalloid to increase urinary output, on the other hand, will usually create ascites. Diuresis may be ineffective if the urine sodium becomes scant or undetectable, and persistence will often produce azotemia. At this juncture a peritoneovenous shunt must be considered. Invasive monitoring may be necessary in the elderly patient with postnecrotic cirrhosis who may also have coronary artery disease.

CONTINUED BLEEDING

After emergency variceal decompression, the patient may return to the intensive care unit (ICU) with a Sengstaken–Blakemore tube still in place and with a Pitressin infusion. Both can usually be discontinued in less than 24 hours. If gastrointestinal bleeding persists, a technical problem with the shunt or an alternative bleeding site must be considered. Arteriography can identify a clotted or twisted anastomosis, and endoscopy may pinpoint the bleeding site. Hematologic parameters should be normalized with fresh frozen plasma and platelets.

ENCEPHALOPATHY

It is crucial to detect and correct precipitating cofactors such as sepsis, drugs, electrolyte and pH disturbances, gastrointestinal bleeding, hypoxia, hypercapnia, and azotemia. Coma in the early postoperative period is rarely due to the shunt itself, and thus requires an investigation of other etiologies.

LEAKING ASCITES

The incision must be carefully inspected for dehiscence, which must be treated operatively. A slow leak is more common and may be corrected by a running skin stitch and a layer of collodian. The ascites should be treated to allow the wound to seal. Paracentesis may be necessary to relieve severe abdominal distention. If tense, leaking ascites reaccumulates, a peritoneal catheter may be placed to drain sufficient fluid to decompress the wound. A peritoneovenous shunt may be necessary if this therapy is unsuccessful after 2 or 3 days.

INFECTED ASCITES

Signs of peritonitis, fever, and systemic sepsis may be absent in the postoperative cirrhotic patient. If a solitary organism is identified, it probably represents contamination during operation and usually responds to intravenous antibiotics or peritoneal lavage.

SURGICAL MANAGEMENT OF ASCITES

Refractory ascites can be managed by a central shunt, commonly a side-to-side portacaval or peritoneovenous shunt, often useful for patients with postoperative hepatorenal failure. Preoperative cultures of the ascites should be taken and a short course of prophylactic antibiotics administered in an effort to avoid shunt infection. The postoperative coagulopathy can be minimized with heparin, 5000 units subcutaneously twice daily. Flow through the shunt is maintained with an abdominal binder and incentive spirometry. Autoinfusion of ascites should be minimized if a coagulopathy occurs. If the coagulopathy cannot be reversed, the shunt may need to be removed. Early shunt infection may be accompanied by encephalopathy, systemic sepsis, and a bleeding diathesis. If antibiotics do not clear the infection, the shunt will have to be removed. Shunt failure may result from technical factors such as kinking at the clavicle, whereas late failures are almost always due to proteinaceous debris in the valve. In such cases, replacement will be effective.

MAJOR HEPATIC RESECTIONS

Peripheral edema and some ascites are common after major resections (greater than 50% of the liver). Routine administration of albumin rarely corrects the hypoalbuminemia and is expensive; its benefit has been difficult to prove prospectively. Postoperative hypoglycemia tends to be a more theoretical than practical problem, because it is readily controllable with a 5% or 10% glucose infusion. Hyperglycemia is more commonly observed. Persistent, marked prolongation of the prothrombin time and partial thromboplastin time should raise concern about the adequacy and viability of the liver remnant. However, a coagulopathy should not be considered as the primary etiology of bleeding until all mechanical causes have been corrected.

Hyperbilirubinemia accompanies major resections, especially when there is an increased pigment load from transfusions and impaired hepatocellular function from hypotension, medications, or infection. If the bilirubin level continues to rise after 14 days, bile duct injury must be considered. Evaluation may include radionuclide scanning if the hepatic dysfunction is not too abnormal. Ultrasonography and computed tomography (CT) scanning may be diagnostic. Percutaneous transhepatic cholangiography may define the proximal anatomy and allow percutaneous decompression if the patient is deemed too ill for surgery. Drains are routinely placed after liver surgery to evacuate bile. The persistent biliary fistula usually emanates from a major duct which may be defined by percutaneous transhepatic cholangiography. The large defect in the liver often fills in with an accumulation of hematoma, bile, and necrotic debris. If the patient becomes febrile, this locus must be evaluated for abscess formation by ultrasound or CT. Percutaneous placement of a sump drain is often therapeutic. Open drainage may be necessary.

HEMOBILIA

The classic triad is right upper quadrant pain, jaundice, and upper gastrointestinal bleeding. Although bleeding tamponades the source temporarily, after the clot dissolves, the bleeding resumes so that intermittent hemorrhage is common. Hemobilia most commonly follows trauma but may be a complication of liver biopsy or percutaneous transhepatic instrumentation. Angiography may be considered the mainstay of diagnosis and therapy since most hemobilia is arterial in origin, and hepatic arteriography with selective embolization usually controls the bleeding.

POSTOPERATIVE CHOLECYSTITIS

The classic presentation of right upper quadrant pain and a palpable mass is unusual in the ICU. A slow recovery, sepsis, or mild icterus should stimulate investigation. Radionuclide scan may show cystic duct obstruction, although visualization of the gallbladder does not exclude cholecystitis. Ultrasound or CT scans may demonstrate a thickened, inflamed gallbladder. Cholecystectomy or cholecystostomy may be performed, although percutaneous cholecystostomy may be useful in critically ill patients.

CHOLANGITIS

Most patients rapidly respond to fluids and broad-spectrum antibiotics. If the patient remains toxic, suppurative cholangitis must be considered, and immediate decompression of the biliary tree is necessary. Until recently, this meant emergency surgical placement of a T-tube in the common duct. Other options currently include endoscopic papillotomy or transhepatic biliary decompression.

BILIARY FISTULA AFTER CHOLECYSTECTOMY

Significant drainage after 2 or 3 days mandates investigation to rule out a bile duct injury. Endoscopic retrograde choledochopancreatography (ERCP) or transheptic cholangiography should be performed. If the leakage occurs from a cystic duct stump, it may spontaneously seal; a hepatic or common bile duct injury requires surgical repair. If the T-tube becomes partially dislodged in the early postoperative period, a water-soluble contrast study should be obtained. The interventional radiologist may be able to replace it. Otherwise, operation will be necessary to replace the T-tube, unless no distal obstruction occurred.

For further information, please see Chapter 51 in Civetta JM, Taylor RW, Kirby RR: Critical Care. *Philadelphia: J. B. Lippincott, 1988*

BIBLIOGRAPHY

Akovbiantz A, Schmid M, Schmid E: Postoperative syndromes after liver surgery. *Clin Gastroenterol* 1979; 8:471
Boey JH, Way LW: Acute cholangitis. *An Surg* 1980; 191:264
Cameron JL, Herlong HF, Sanfey H, et al: The Budd–Chiari syndrome. Treatment by mesenteric–systemic venous shunts. *Ann Surg* 1983; 198:335
Eckhauser FE, Pomerantz RA, Knol JA, et al: Early variceal rebleeding after successful distal splenorenal shunt. *Arch Surg* 1986; 121:547
Fulenwider TJ, Smith RB, Redd SC, et al: Peritoneovenous shunts. Lessons learned from an eight-year experience with 70 patients. *Arch Surg* 1984; 119:1133
Howard RJ: Acute acalculous cholecystitis. *Am J Surg* 1981; 141:194
Hutson DG, Livingstone A, Levi JU, Zeppa R: Early hepatic failure or upper gastroin-

testinal bleeding following a distal splenorenal shunt. *Surg Gynecol Obstet* 1982; 155:46

LaMont JT, Isselbacher KJ: Postoperative jaundice. *N Engl J Med* 1973; 288:305

Millikan WJ, Henderson JM, Sewell CW, et al: Approach to the spectrum of Budd–Chiari syndrome. Which patients require portal decompression? *Am J Surg* 1985; 149:167

Mirvis SE, Vainright JR, Nelson AW, et al: The diagnosis of acute acalculous cholecystitis. A comparison of sonography, scintigraphy, and CT. *Am J Radiol* 1986; 147:1171

17 Neurologic Injury

HEAD INJURY

Automobile accidents are the most common cause of head injury, followed by motorcycle and vehicle-pedestrian accidents, falls, assaults, gunshot and stab wounds, and recreational accidents. Head injury has been reported to occur in up to 71% of vehicular accidents, with 64% of the deaths attributed primarily to cerebral trauma. A majority of these victims are under the age of 30. It has been estimated that nearly 1 of every 25 people in the United States will suffer head trauma each year. In 75% of head injuries, avoidable potentiating factors are present, including cerebral or obstructive hypoxia resulting from airway or air space factors, hypotension secondary to hypovolemia or overzealous sedation, inadequate initial treatment, or delay in transfer. These factors contribute to death in 54% of head injury fatalities. Consequently, the potential for saving lives is great, and the ICU can play an important role in this process.

PATHOPHYSIOLOGY

Consciousness, the awareness of one's self and environment, is reflected in one's ability to be aroused, to perceive environmental stimuli, and to react appropriately on a cognitive and motor level. Arousability depends on the integrity of the reticular activating system of the brain stem, whereas cognitive ability depends on cerebral cortex integrity. The levels between consciousness and coma are determined by the distribution and extent of the pathologic process or insult. In concussions, generally no demonstrable gross lesions are present. Momentary loss of consciousness and amnesia are usually the only symptoms, although a focal deficit can occur if the insult is localized (e.g., cortical blindness resulting from a blow to the occipital lobe). Complete neurologic recovery occurs within 6 to 12 hours. If recovery does not occur, anoxic and metabolic causes have been ruled out, and no abnormalities have been demonstrated using computed tomography (CT), significant shearing forces were present and produced a "diffuse white matter injury."

Half of patients with prolonged unconsciousness have suffered intracranial hemorrhage, which may result in long-term or permanent dysfunction. The term "contusion" is used if abnormality is demonstrated on CT and implies a hemorrhagic event. Contusions may be associated with various states of awareness and, depending on their location, with focal deficits. They are caused by movement of the brain relative to its bony dural coverings, with areas of direct and indirect (contrecoup) impacts, resulting from brain mass acceleration–deceleration. These forces may also produce lacerations of the brain, causing intracerebral hemorrhages and intracerebral clots. Delayed intracerebral hematomas can be detected on follow-up CTs in cases that deteriorate or progress poorly. About 5% of intracranial hematomas result from injury to the meningeal arteries that supply the dura, causing an epidural hematoma. These arteries lie in grooves of the inner table of bones and are usually associated with fractures. Approximately 50% of patients with epidural hematoma will give a history of brief loss of consciousness followed by a lucid interval of up to several hours. Prognosis is generally good if surgical intervention precedes extreme neurologic decompensation. Subdural hematomas are the most frequent of the hematomas. They are classified as acute, subacute, or chronic, depending on the rate of progression of symptoms and the appearance of the clot at surgery. The bleeding is venous in origin, secondary to the avulsion of veins that bridge the dura and the cortical surface. Patients with subdural hematomas and alterations in consciousness are true surgical emergencies; operation within 6 hours of injury greatly enhances meaningful survivability. Patients with intracranial hematomas have a poorer outcome, particularly if they are above the age of 40.

Focal deficits can be immediate or delayed. Whereas immediate deficits may result from a specific injured area, delayed deficits represent an ongoing dynamic process, such as an expanding hematoma or worsening edema. Of greatest significance, late focal signs may herald impending brain herniation. In subfalcial herniation, the cortex is displaced across the midline, resulting in monoplegia of a leg. If herniation is extensive, hemiplegia can develop. Both types of paralysis develop on the side contralateral to the lesion. In uncal herniation through the tentorium, ipsilateral pupillary size dilatation will occur in addition to ipsilateral hemiparesis. A definitive assessment, such as a CT scan, or a shift of a calcified pineal is necessary to identify the actual side of the lesion for definitive surgery. Finally, there is cerebellar tonsillar herniation down through the foramen magnum. Here the eyes may be unilaterally or bilaterally diverging, with abnormalities in respiration and cardiovascular function, dysrhythmias, and hypotension.

IMMEDIATE DIAGNOSTIC PROCEDURES

Lateral skull films can document the presence of skull fractures or reveal air–fluid levels in sinuses or pneumoencephalus. If the pineal is calcified on an anteroposterior film, its position can indicate a shift away from the lesion. Films of the cervical spine should be examined for the commonly associated fractures. The CT scan is thought to be the most sensitive tool, missing virtually no underlying pathology except minor bony disruptions. In addition to reducing the need for other, more invasive, tests, CT scanning has decreased surgical explorations in cases of contusion or edema clincially mistaken for hematomas. Scans can also be used in serial fashion to assess outcome.

GUIDELINES FOR INTENSIVE CARE

With the exception of comatose patients and those with multiple injuries, some general guidelines are necessary to select head injury patients for ICU admission. Patients in the following categories should receive intensive care:

1 All acutely injured nonoperated patients with isolated head trauma who have demonstrable intracranial pathology, regardless of their Glasgow Coma Scale (GCS) score. This group includes very small subdural, epidural, and intraparenchymal hematomas or contusions.

2 In the absence of demonstrable intracranial pathology, patients with a GCS score of less than 13, which reflects a significant insult and possible pathologic lesion.

3 All postcraniotomy patients, with the exception of those who have undergone craniotomy for elevation of a depressed skull fracture without dural or cortical surface involvement.

4 Patients with focal signs, regardless of GCS score, demonstrable lesions by CT, or operation.

5 The multiple-injury trauma patient with some degree of neurologic involvement and hemodynamic or respiratory instability (e.g., a hypoxemic patient with rib fractures and underlying pulmonary contusion who has a high but abnormal GCS score).

6 Probable brain death patients during confirmation or preparation for organ procurement.

TREATMENT

The management of head injury is based on fundamental physiological principles. Brain extracellular fluid is only 20% to 30% of the amount found in other tissues. With injury, the normal blood–brain barrier is disrupted, resulting in fluid extravasation into an already minimal compartment. Also, cerebral arterial vessels lose their autoregulatory capacity (the ability to maintain a constant perfusion pressure over a wide range of systemic blood pressures; see Fig. 17-1): this can be local, regional, or global depending on the extent of injury. Perfusion of the injured area then becomes passive. The goal of therapy then is to limit extravasation of fluid while maintaining the intracranial blood volume.

The patient's head should be kept in a midline position and elevated to 30°. This enhances venous drainage and prevents kinking of the jugular venous system. The head-down position for cannulation of central veins

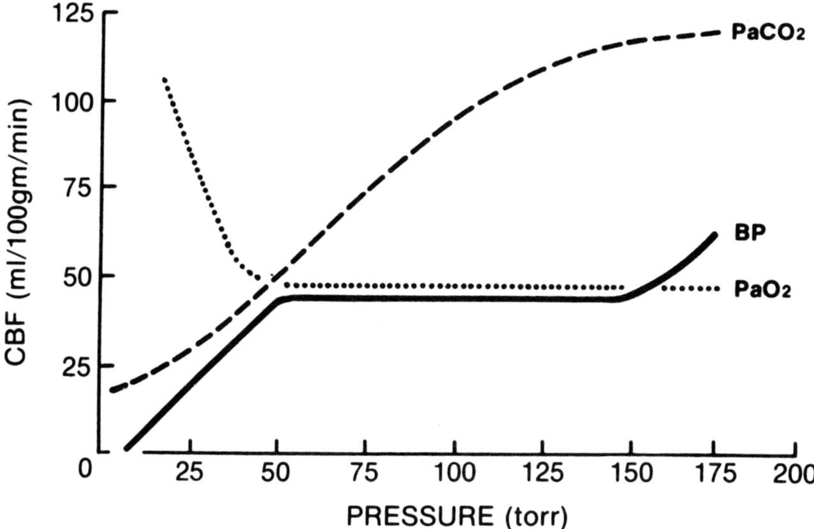

Figure 17-1 The effect of blood pressure *(BP)*, Pa_{O2}, and Pa_{CO2} on CBF in normal brain. (Shapiro HM: Intracranial hypertension: Therapeutic and anesthetic considerations. *Anesthesiology* 1975; 43:447)

should be avoided because this position leads to greatly increased intracranial blood volume and ICP. The procedure should be performed in a more upright position, but the operator must be careful to avoid air embolism.

Agitated behavior, coughing, straining, or anything that may increase intra-abdominal or intrathoracic pressure should be prevented because these pressures may increase ICP. The use of sedatives (barbiturates), analgesics (codeine), or muscle relaxants may be necessary to control muscle activity. Lidocaine, 25 mg to 50 mg, before endotracheal suctioning, may limit the cough reflex.

Blood Pressure

Arterial hypertension is a common finding in head-injured patients. It is probably secondary to the Cushing reflex, which is a normal physiological response to maintain perfusion to ischemic brain tissue. This may result in increased intracranial blood volume because of increased flow through non-autoregulated vessels, with resulting increased edema accumulation. Again, the brain-injured patient does not tolerate hypotension as readily as the non-head-injured patient; infarction is a real possibility. The mean arterial pressure, then, should be maintained in the normal range. If ICP is not monitored, the CPP (mean arterial pressure minus ICP) should be maintained above the critical level of 60 mm Hg to 100 mm Hg. (The assumes normal ICP; if abnormal ICP is suspected, it should be monitored.) In hypertension, vasodilators (trimethaphan), intravenous antihypertensives (α-methyldopa, verapamil, or β-blockers, if there are no medical contraindications), or sedation should be used. Nitroglycerine and sodium nitroprusside should be avoided because they increase venous capacitance and consequently increase intracranial blood volume.

Airway

Airway protection and ventilatory support are also of utmost importance. Pa_{O2} should be maintained near 100 mm Hg. If hypoxia develops (see Fig. 17-1), cerebral blood flow and intracranial blood volume will increase. Supplemental oxygen by mask may be used if airway protection is not necessary. If adequate oxygenation cannot be obtained, intubation and use of positive end-expiratory pressure (PEEP) is indicated. Although PEEP may raise intrathoracic pressure, obstruct venous inflow and, ultimately, increase ICP in a normal patient, in head-injured patients with respiratory failure, when pulmonary compliance is decreased, PEEP may not be transmitted and ICP may not be affected. The actual effect of PEEP on ICP can be measured if there is any concern. Respiratory failure is common in patients with head injuries. Hypercapnia should also be avoided because cerebral blood flow and volume are linearly increased with carbon dioxide tension. Because normal reflexes are lost in patients with depressed sensoria, airway control may be compromised. Oral airways or nasal trumpets may work temporarily but do not provide security for maintaining the airway or protection from aspiration of oral and gastric secretions. Consequently, intubation should be performed whenever doubt arises.

Seizure activity often accompanies head injury. Because seizure activity greatly increases cerebral metabolic activity and cerebral blood flow, anticonvulsant medications should be used for prophylaxis. Also, because each degree Celsius of temperature elevation will increase cerebral metabolic activity by approximately 6%, fevers should be controlled.

Other monitoring methods may aid management. Arterial catheterization can provide continual measurement for estimation of CPP and a route for blood sampling. When patients are given diuretics for the control of ICP, the pulmonary artery catheter is helpful in discriminating cardiac from respiratory abnormalities and assessing the response to treatment. I also use the pulmonary artery catheter to guide therapy with high-dose barbiturates because of their depressant effects upon the cardiovascular system.

Intracranial Pressure

The principle of treatment is that control of ICP to less than 20 mm Hg improves survival. The specific goals are (1) to limit formation of edema, maintain intracranial blood volume, and maintain blood pressure in the normal range to decrease blood flow through non-autoregulated areas; (2) to create an osmotic gradient toward the intravascular compartment; and (3) to eliminate obstruction to normal CSF movements or to prevent acute hydrocephalus. If intracranial hypertension (greater than 20 mm Hg) is present because of a lesion, other intracranial contents (the brain, blood, or CSF volume) must be decreased, individually or in combination, in an attempt to reduce the intracranial pressure to less than 20 mm Hg.

Hyperventilation has an almost immediate effect in decreasing intracranial blood volume. It can also be used on a long-term basis to maintain the lowered cranial blood volume by reducing Pa_{CO_2} to between 25 and 30 mm Hg. A Pa_{CO_2} of less than 22 mm Hg may create cerebral ischemia, which may cause cerebral vasodilatation (see Fig. 17-1) and, ultimately, increase intracranial blood volume. Although hyperventilation does reduce intracranial pressure, it is unclear how long this effect is maintained. After about 30 hours, the *p*H of CSF returns toward normal; hyperventilation may not have any effect. However, if the Pa_{CO_2} of blood is allowed to rise, CSF *p*H may fall and result in cerebral vasodilatation. Consequently, because prolonged hyperventilation does not seem to be detrimental as long as the systemic *p*H does not rise above 7.55, it can be used on a long-term basis or tapered gradually after 30 hours.

If hyperventilation fails to decrease the ICP to less than 20 mm Hg, mannitol, an osmotic diuretic, is given in an initial dose of 1.5 g/kg while monitoring ICP or level of consciousness. If this dose is infused in less than 15 minutes, the maximal effect will take place in approximately 20 minutes, with an average duration of action of about 3.5 hours. The extent and duration of response to mannitol vary; as a rule, the higher the initial intracranial pressure, the shorter is the response. Mannitol is then repeated in a dose of approximately 0.25 g/kg every 4 hours. Initially, serum osmolarity is measured every 4 hours. The dose of mannitol should then be adjusted to maintain the serum osmolarity at approximately 10 mOsm above normal, or about 290 to 300 mOsm. Maximal response of the ICP to mannitol is achieved at this level; higher levels do not increase the response. Rebound swelling (when the osmotically active particles move from the intravascular compartment to brain tissue, thus increasing interstitial fluid) is rarer with mannitol than with other hypertonic solutions. Furosemide (40–80 mg) can decrease intracranial pressure acutely by reducing intravascular volume. Furosemide, by unknown mechanisms, and acetazolamide, through carbonic anhydrase inhibition that limits ion exchange across the choroid plexus, have been reported to decrease the production of CSF.

If ICP is still greater than 20 mm Hg, venting of CSF can be performed if a ventricular cannula is present. The collecting bag for the CSF must not be placed lower than the level of the ventricles. If the ventricles are decompressed too rapidly and collapse, the brain may draw away from the dura, which may tear bridging veins between the dura and cortex and create a subdural hematoma. Sufficient CSF is slowly removed to lower ICP to 15 to 20 mm Hg. The frequency of venting is recorded because it varies and is an estimate of the severity of intracranial hypertension.

In summary, an elevation of ICP above 20 mm Hg is usually treated initially by hyperventilation because this approach can be effective in seconds. Even if the Pa_{CO_2} has been controlled for approximately 30 hours and there is an acute rise in ICP, hyperventilation can be tried again or CSF can be vented (if a ventriculostomy is present). If these abrupt rises in ICP appear to be periodic and are controlled by CSF venting, venting can be continued. If rises in pressure are more frequent and are not associated with periods of agitation (which should respond to sedation), mannitol could be used. Mannitol is necessary if ICP is measured by a bolt or an indwelling electronic device because CSF cannot be vented. Frequently, all three methods are used concomitantly to lower ICP.

Intracranial hypertension may not be controllable with these measures, and virtually all patients whose ICP cannot be controlled die. Barbiturates have been used to treat uncontrollable intracranial hypertension. Therapy has been used in many forms, ranging from seizure prophylaxis to dosages to reduce ICP to normal levels to high doses that induce an isoelectric electroencephalogram (EEG). Barbiturates reduce ICP either by reducing the cerebral metabolic rate or by lowering cerebral blood flow through peripheral venodilatation and depression of cardiac output. When used to control ICP, pentobarbital, 1 to 3 mg/kg, is given each hour until a maximum serum level of 30 to 50 mg/liter is obtained. This is also equivalent to the level associated with suppression of EEG activity. ICP is often controlled with lesser amounts, but greater doses have not been effective if ICP remains elevated. High-dose barbiturates were reported to increase the percentage of patients with useful recovery. However, in a subsequent controlled trial, the prophylactic use of pentobarbital did not improve outcome. Hypotension, sepsis, and hypothermia may occur with high-dose barbiturates. The pulmonary artery catheter should be used to monitor and maintain optimum cardiac function. Initiating a barbiturate coma is a major undertaking, requiring total management and care by experienced personnel. It might be viewed as a "last-ditch" effort to prevent death from uncontrolled intracranial hypertension.

Steroids are not currently used to treat cerebral edema or intracranial hypertension because they have not improved outcome in head trauma patients. They may, in fact, create glucose intolerance, cause immunosuppression, and suppress febrile responses suggestive of an undiagnosed infectious process.

A recent series reported no difference in outcome between the approach outlined here compared to little more than nursing care. The outcome is often so poor that it is difficult to demonstrate an effect of available therapeutic efforts. Perhaps further studies can delineate the important elements; at present, interventions are based on the pathophysiology described and do affect the intermediate parameters that are related to clinical outcome.

SPINAL CORD INJURY

Acute spinal cord injury occurs most commonly in young, active adults as a result of trauma. Injury to the vertebrae and connecting ligaments can occur without neurologic deficit; similarly, an injury to the spinal cord with resulting neurologic deficit can occur without evidence of injury to the spinal column.

Spinal cord injuries are devastating to the patient and family, and it may be considered even more devastating that spinal cord injury can occur during treatment of patients with injuries of the vertebral column. Because the potential for spinal cord injury may not have been fully recognized during initial evaluation prior to ICU admission, the intensivist must recognize situations with the potential for such injuries and institute preventive measures. Spinal trauma and potential spinal cord injury should be considered in all patients with head trauma, especially if the frontal and facial regions have been involved; in patients who have received penetrating injuries in proximity to or with a potential trajectory near the spinal column, especially in the cervical region; in patients who have suffered crush injuries or injuries due to falls; in patients with major multiple trauma; and in patients who have sustained accelerating–decelerating forces during accidents. These patients must be considered likely candidates for traumatic injuries to the vertebral column and potential spinal cord injury until definitive diagnostic studies have been obtained. Immobilization of the head and neck must be maintained until this diagnostic process has been completed. Cardiovascular and respiratory embarrassment may be present, as in other trauma patients, although special considerations apply to patients with spinal cord injury.

CERVICAL IMMOBILIZATION

Immobilization of the victim is usually performed by paramedics in the field. The intensivist must make an independent assessment of the need for and adequacy of such immobilization, whether the patient is first encountered in the emergency room, radiology department, or the ICU. Adequate immobilization must be maintained during the initial transportation of the patient. Current practices in intensive care often necessitate transport of the patient from the ICU to other areas of the hospital for diagnostic and therapeutic interventions, and adequate cervical immobilization during these periods shoud be considered the responsibility of the intensive care team.

Immobilization using a cervical collar should be considered precautionary and serves as a reminder that a potential cervical injury may exist. It should not be viewed as complete protection until a definitive diagnosis has been made. Patients are usually positioned on a spinal board, preferably at the scene of the accident, and this position is maintained throughout the diagnostic work-up. The head and cervical spine should be maintained in the sagittal plane. Sandbags are placed on either side of the head to prevent rotation. Adhesive strapping should be placed in continuous fashion from the spinal board, across the sandbags, and forehead, and back to the spinal board. This is an effective restraint and also reminds the patient to remain immobile. The conscious and cooperative patient should be instructed to remain supine and not to turn his head. If turning is necessary, it must be performed maintaining the alignment of the head and body ("log-rolling") while traction is maintained on the head.

Immobilization should be continued until the possibility of spinal injury has been eliminated or, in the case of existing injury, a more definitive form of cervical immobilization can be instituted.

For further information, please see Chatper 54 in Civetta JM, Taylor RW, Kirby RR: Critical Care. *Philadelphia: J. B. Lippincott, 1988*

BIBLIOGRAPHY

Berman IR, Ducker TB: Pulmonary, somatic and splanchnic circulatory responses to increased intracranial pressure. *Ann Surg* 1969; 169:210

Bowers SA, Marshall LF: Outcome in 200 consecutive cases of severe head injury treated in San Diego county: A prospective analysis. *Neurosurgery* 1980; 6:237

Brown FK: Cardiovascular effects of acutely raised intracranial pressure. *Am J Physiol* 1956; 185:510

Clifton GL, Grossman RG, Makela ME, et al: Neurological course and correlated computerized tomography findings after severe closed head injury. *J Neurosurg* 1980; 52:611

Cottrell JE, Bhagwandas G, Rappaport H, et al: Intracranial pressure during nitroglycerin-induced hypotension. *J Neurosurg* 1980; 53:309

Cottrell JE, Patel K, Turndorf H, et al: Intracranial pressure changes induced by sodium nitroprusside in patients with intracranial mass lesions. *J Neurosurg* 1978; 48:329

Diaz GF, Yock DH, Larson D, et al: Early diagnosis of delayed traumatic intracerebral hematoma. *J Neurosurg* 1979; 50:217

Gelpke GJ, Braakman R, Hakkema DF, et al: Comparison of outcome in two series of patients with severe head injuries. *J Neurosurg* 1983; 59:745

Jennett B, Bond M: Assessment of outcome after severe brain damage. *Lancet* 1975; 1:480

Jennett B, Teasdale G, Braakman R, et al: Prognosis of patients with severe head injury. *Neurosurgery* 1979; 4:282

Jennett B, Teasdale G, Galbraith S et al: Severe head injuries in three countries. *J Neurol Neurosurg Psychiatry* 1977; 40:291

Lanier WL, Stangland KJ, Scheithauer BW, et al: Effects of intravenous dextrose infusion and head position on neurologic outcome after complete cerebral ischemia. *Anes* 1985; 63:A110

Marshall LF, Shapiro HM: Examination by computerized axial tomography. *Int Anesthesia Clin* 1979; 17:391

Marshall LF, Smith RW, Rauscher LA, et al: Mannitol dose requirements in brain injured patients. *J Neurosurg* 1978; 48:169

Marshall LF, Smith RW, Shapiro HM: The outcome with aggressive treatment in severe head injury. *J Neurosurg* 1979; 50:26

Miller JD, Butterworth JF, Guderman SK, et al: Further experiences in the management of severe head injury. *J Neurosurg* 1981; 54:289

Nuelk DF, Gikas PW: Causes of death in automobile accidents. *JAMA* 1968; 203:98

Peerless SJ, Newcastle NB: Shear injuries to the brain. *Can Med Assoc J* 1967; 98:577

Roberts JR: Pathophysiology, diagnosis and treatment of head trauma *Topics Emerg Med* 1979; 1:41

Rose J, Valtonen S, Jennett B: Avoidable factors contributing to death after head injury. *Br Med J* 1977; 2:615

Severinghaus JW: Role of cerebrospinal fluid pH in normalization of cerebral blood flow in chronic hypocapnia. *Acta Neurol Scan* 1965; 14:116

Ward JD, Becker DP, Miller JD, et al: Failure of prophylactic barbiturate coma in the treatment of severe head injury. *J Neurosurg* 1985; 62:383

18
Multiple Fractures

When a physician encounters a patient with musculoskeletal injuries in the intensive care setting, often there is some bewilderment as to the proper medical and nursing management of the injured extremities, spine, and pelvis. This problem is greater if the patient has some type of traction device in place or one of the many external fixation frames applied to the extremities or pelvis. Questions may also arise as to how the patient can be moved in bed or transported from the intensive care unit (ICU) for additional diagnostic or therapeutic procedures.

This chapter is directed at the physician or nurse who is responsible for the care of patients with musculoskeletal injuries. An essential checklist is provided so that the patient can be assessed rapidly with regard to such points as neurovascular status of the extremities, proper alignment of traction and evaluation for injuries perhaps missed initially. The remainder of the chapter expands on the checklist and discusses in practical terms various orthopaedic techniques, some specific injuries, and possible complications and their prevention.

CHECKLIST FOR PATIENTS WITH MUSCULOSKELETAL INJURY

MENTAL STATUS

Patients with alterations in mental status may not be able to respond appropriately to the questions necessary to perform a thorough examination of the extremities and evaluation of the neurovascular system. This factor must be considered in the validity of the physical examination.

NEUROVASCULAR STATUS

The most common complication of a fracture or dislocation is a neurologic or vascular injury. Therefore, a comprehensive examination of sensory and motor function must be carried out and documented. Sensation is best evaluated by determining light touch, and motor function by observing active voluntary or involuntary motion. Any abnormalities should be reported to the responsible clinician.

Upper Extremity

Median nerve

Sensory–volar distal index finger tip

Motor–thumb abduction (movement away from the palm in the horizontal plane)

Ulnar nerve

Sensory–volar distal small finger tip

Motor–index finger abduction (movement toward the thumb in the plane of the palm)

Radial nerve

Sensory–dorsal first web space between the thumb and index

Motor–thumb extension at the distal joint

Lower Extremity

Superficial peroneal nerve

Sensory–dorsal foot between second and fourth toes

Motor–ankle eversion (movement toward outside of the leg)

Deep peroneal nerve

Sensory–dorsal first web space between great and second toes

Motor–ankle dorsiflexion, great toe extension

Posterior tibial nerve

Sensory–plantar surface of toes and foot

Motor–toe flexion

Vascular status should be determined by either palpation or doppler examination of the peripheral pulses at the wrist and ankle.

EXTREMITIES IMMOBILIZED IN CASTS OR SPLINTS

1. Check neurovascular status.
2. Check for swelling of exposed parts (should be able to place at least one finger's width between the case edge and skin).
3. Keep extremity elevated unless ordered otherwise.
4. Circumferential casts should not be applied acutely to patients with significant alterations in mental status.

PATIENTS IN TRACTION

1 Check neurovascular status.

2 Traction weights should be free of obstructions and not be resting on the floor or bed.

3 Skeletal traction pin should be connected to traction weight by a traction bow and rope. This system should not impinge against the traction splint. The interface between the traction pin and the skin should be without tension and allow access for pin care and dressings.

4 Avoid pressure points from the apparatus at the groin, knee (especially at the fibular head, laterally), heel area, foot, and toes.

5 In most cases the overall alignment of the extremity should be reasonably straight and not angulated.

6 The patient should be comfortable in traction and centered in the bed with the traction apparatus not touching the foot of the bed.

PATIENTS IN EXTERNAL FIXATION DEVICES

1 Pin sites should be clean without skin tension.

2 The device should not be touching the skin at any area.

3 The device should be rigid with all nuts and components tightened.

EXTREMITIES, PELVIS, AND SPINE—MISSED INJURIES

1 All extremities should be put through a full range of motion of nonimmobilized joints. Any joint pain, swelling or effusion must be regarded as a significant injury and requires complete radiographic examination.

2 Local swelling, ecchymosis, point tenderness, crepitus, and false motion are indicative of possible fracture and necessitate radiographs in two planes of the entire suspected bone and the adjacent joints.

3 Examine the pelvis by compressing the iliac crests together toward each other and applying anterior-posterior compression to each iliac crest. Any pain elicited by these maneuvers requires radiographic study.

4 Any neck or back pain should be investigated by examination of perineal sensation, rectal sphincter and bladder function, and radiographs in two planes of the entire spine. Until a diagnosis is made, the patient should be kept supine, with the neck immobilized.

COMPLICATIONS

SWELLING

All musculoskeletal injuries are accompanied by a variable amount of swelling. The degree of swelling is related to the type and magnitude of injury, with the greatest amount seen in displaced fractures and crush injuries. Swelling is secondary to hemorrhage from fractured bones and tissue edema is a response to injury. It is believed that maximal swelling occurs approximately 24 to 48 hours after injury.

Although some swelling is inevitable, excessive swelling should be avoided. If not, there will be increased local pain and the skin may form "fracture blisters" from rupture of the outer layers of the epidermis. The worst complication is the compartment syndrome, resulting in possible loss of the limb.

All injured extremities, both upper and lower, should be elevated above the heart level. Elevation assists in venous return by gravity drainage. Even marked amounts of swelling can be reduced if the limb is properly elevated. The only contraindications to elevation are reimplantations and suspected compartment syndromes, because elevation may decrease arterial flow in these conditions.

Extremities may be constricted by circumferential casts, dressings, elastic bandages, or braces. These can contribute to swelling by interfering with venous return and acting as tourniquets. The solution is to relieve the constriction by releasing tight dressings or bivalving the cast.

NEUROVASCULAR COMPROMISE

The most common complication of fractures or dislocations is a neurologic or vascular deficit. This deficit may occur at the time of the original trauma and be due to blunt or penetrating force. This type is not preventable. Nerve or vessel injury after the initial trauma is largely preventable. The functional outcome of the extremity, in most cases, is directly related to the integrity of the neurovascular systems.

Acute neural injury can be caused by contusion, stretching, or laceration. Most of the time there will be partial motor and sensory deficits in the injured nerve distribution. Rarely, there will be a complete absence of neural function. The recommended treatment is observation for these injuries since most are not lacerations and will recover function. If a nerve laceration is suspected, surgical exploration is indicated with possible repair.

Late neural injury has a variety of etiologies. One cause is direct pressure on a superficial nerve such as the common peroneal at the level of the fibular head, lateral to the knee. This pressure can be secondary to a poorly padded or tight cast or from improper positioning on a traction splint. In operated extremities in which a tourniquet has been used for hemostasis, a nerve palsy can result from prolonged tourniquet time or inappropriate pressure. The extremity will have a circumferential nerve deficit distal to the tourniquet site. Recovery is usually complete within a few days to weeks.

The cause of most vascular injuries associated with fractures or dislocations is the original trauma. Vessels may have partial or complete lacerations or intimal damage. An unusual cause is laceration by fracture fragments. The diagnosis of these lesions is typically made at the time of presentation to the hospital and treatment is begun promptly. Musculoskeletal injuries that have a fairly common association with vascular injuries are knee dislocations, supracondylar humeral fractures, and severe crush or open fractures of the tibia or forearm.

COMPARTMENT SYNDROME

One of the most devastating complications of fractures is the compartment syndrome. The pathophysiology of this condition begins with swelling within the deep fascial compartments of the extremities. The swelling may be secondary to fractures, crushing, vascular injury, constricting dressings, or several other causes. The deep fascial tissue is very dense and unyielding. If swelling continues unabated, the contents of the fascial compartments (nerves, blood vessels, muscles) will be compressed due to the lack of accommodation of the fascia to the increasing pressure. Microscopically, the initial event is arteriolar constriction which produces ischemia. The tissue response to this ischemia is an increase in capillary permeability and extravascular edema. This tissue edema leads to further increases in tissue pressure and compartment swelling with more ischemia. Thus, a vicious cycle is begun with progressive ischemia producing more swelling. If the pressure is not relieved within hours, irreversible tissue necrosis and permanent neural damage ensues.

Recognition is the key to preventing compartment syndromes. Subjectively, the patient will complain of progressive pain in the extremity which is out of proportion to that expected for the type of injury. Also, the pain usually is not relieved by otherwise adequate doses of analgesics. The patient may also complain of numbness and paresthesias in the distal extremity. In patients with altered mental status these subjective findings may be absent.

The earliest objective finding is decreased sensation to light touch in the distal extremity. Passive motion of the digits will refer pain to the involved compartment. This phenomenon is believed to be caused by stretching of ischemic muscles. The involved compartments will develop increasing tenseness to palpation. As the syndrome progresses, there will be muscle weakness and anesthesia of the distal skin, followed by total loss of muscle function. A very late sign is diminished or absent distal pulses.

The first step in a suspected compartment syndrome is to relieve all constriction around the extremity. Dressings should be released by cutting longitudinally. Circumferential casts must be bivalved, that is, opened along both long axes, through the cast material, with the underlying padding cut completely to the skin. If the pain is not immediately eased, the surgeon must be notified.

Methods have been devised to measure the compartment pressures in an extremity. A simple one that has been found to be effective and reasonably accurate is to set up the usual equipment to monitor an arterial line. An 18-gauge needle is attached to the tubing and flushed with heparinized saline. The arterial transducer should be at the level of the extremity to be tested and calibrated to zero. A small amount of local anesthesia may be used to infiltrate the skin and subcutaneous tissue only. The needle should then be inserted percutaneously and through the deep fascia into the compartment. A reading is taken to confirm proper placement of the needle. The pressure should fluctuate with active or passive motion of the muscles within the compartment tested. All compartments of the suspected part of the extremity should be measured and the pressures documented.

Pressures up to 30 mm Hg can be normal. Higher values may indicate a compartment syndrome. However, do not rely solely on the pressure measurements because the subjective complaints and physical examination are more definitive. Pressure measurements have been most helpful in equivocal cases or in patients with unreliable examinations such as those with closed-head trauma.

The definitive treatment for compartment syndrome is fasciotomy. The earlier the fasciotomy is done, the better are the chances for complete functional recovery. This condition is a true surgical emergency and there must be no delay once the diagnosis is made. At operation all compartments of the involved extremity are released through extensive incisions. The skin incisions are left open.

INFECTION

Sepsis in the musculoskeletal system is a dreaded complication, frequently necessitating multiple surgical procedures and prolonged antibiotic therapy with a poor functional outcome. Clearly, prevention of infection or its prompt treatment assumes paramount importance.

Infection rates differ depending on the type of injury and type of fracture treatment. Infection of a closed fracture is almost unheard of, whereas open fractures have had rates as high as 44%. Penetrating wounds to the knee joint carry approximately a 2% sepsis rate. It is axiomatic that the greater the damage to the bone and soft tissue, the greater the likelihood of infection.

Prevention of bone and joint sepsis is crucial in the severely injured patient with multiple fractures. The role of antibiotics in treating open fractures is now clearly established. All open fractures have bacterial contamination to a variable degree, depending mostly on the magnitude of injury. Therefore, the administration of antibiotics is therapeutic and not prophylactic. It is recommended that antibiotics be given immediately on hospital admission and continued for 2 to 3 days. Additionally, any further operative procedures on the open fracture should have 24 to 48 hours of perioperative antibiotic coverage. Essentially the same points should be considered for open joint wounds. Wound management for open fractures is controversial and many different protocols exist.

The diagnosis of an infected open fracture is not always straightforward. Subjectively, the patient may complain of increasing local pain at the fracture, especially with dressing changes or any manipulation of the limb. Objectively, there may be no local wound changes in early cases. Later, there will be increasing tenderness and erythema with some change in the character of the wound drainage. If some signs of inflammation are present, but if the wound drainage appears normal, exploration of the wound is indicated. Pockets of purulent material may be found deep in the extremity, particularly on the dependent side. At this stage, the patient may be febrile with leukocytosis and an elevated sedimentation rate. Deep wound cultures should be obtained and an intravenous cephalosporin antibiotic begun. In the more severe injuries (type III), there is a high incidence of gram-negative wound infections and an aminoglycoside should be added to the antibiotic regimen.

Any infected open fracture requires thorough surgical debridement. In a certain percentage of cases, retained foreign material is found or obviously necrotic bone or soft tissue. Serial debridements are indicated if the infection is resistant to treatment.

Septic joints can arise from direct penetrating injury and hematogenous seeding. Patients will complain of pain and inability to move the joint. Examination will reveal a hot, swollen, and tender joint with definite loss of motion. The joint effusion should be aspirated for Gram's stain, culture, and synovial analysis. *Staphylococcus aureus* is most common, but in a critically ill patient, gram-negative sepsis should be suspected.

In the traumatized patient the most effective treatment for a septic joint is drainage by surgical arthrotomy, with the appropriate intravenous antibiotic. In our hands, treatment by repeated aspiration has had a low rate of success, often requiring surgical drainage secondarily. A good functional result can be expected if the septic joint is treated promptly and aggressively.

For further information, please see Chapter 55 in Civetta JM, Taylor RW, Kirby RR: Critical Care. *Philadelphia: J. B. Lippincott, 1988*

BIBLIOGRAPHY

Brooker AF, Schmeisser G: *Orthopaedic Traction Manual,* p 81. Baltimore, Williams & Wilkins, 1980

Gustilo RB: *Management of Open Fractures and Their Complications,* p 133. Philadelphia, WB Saunders, 1982

Gustilo RB, Anderson JT: Prevention of infection in the treatment of 1,025 open fractures of long bones. *J Bone Joint Surg [AM]* 1976; 58:453

Johnson KD, Cadambi A, Siebert GB: Incidence of adult respiratory distress syndrome in patients with multiple musculoskeletal injuries: Effect of early operative stabilization of fractures. *J Trauma* 1985; 25:375

Mears, DC: *External Skeletal Fixation,* p 1. Baltimore, Williams & Wilkins, 1983

Mooney V, Claudi BF: Fractures of the shaft of the femur. In Rockwood CA, Green DP (eds): *Fractures in Adults,* vol 2, 2nd ed, p 1367. Philadelphia, JB Lippincott, 1984

Mubarak SJ, Hargen AR: Recognition and treatment of compartment syndromes. In Meyers MH (ed): *The Multiply Injured Patient with Complex Fractures,* p 71. Philadelphia, Lea & Febiger, 1984

Patazkis M, Harvey JP, Ivler D: Role of antibiotics in the management of open fractures. *J Bone Joint Surg [AM]* 1974; 56:532
Saucedo T, Matta J: The treatment of unstable pelvic ring injuries (abstr). In *Abstracts of the 53rd Annual Meeting of the American Academy of Orthopaedic Surgeons,* New Orleans, p 40, February 1986
Tile M: *Fractures of Pelvis and Acetabulum,* p 4. Baltimore, Williams & Wilkins, 1984
Walling AK, Housang S, Spiegel PG: Injuries to the knee ligaments with fractures of the femur. *J Bone Joint Surg [AM]* 1982; 64:1324
Whitesides TE, Haney TC, Morimoto K, et al: Tissue pressure measurements as a determinant for the need of fasciotomy. *Clin Orthop* 1975; 113:43
Wild JJ, Hanson GW, Tullos HS: Unstable fractures of the pelvis treated by external fixation. *J Bone Joint Surg [AM]* 1983; 64:1010

19
Urologic Surgery and Trauma

OPERATIVE PROCEDURES

Major urologic surgery can be conveniently categorized into upper abdominal (and thorax), lower abdominal, and pelvic procedures. Understanding these procedures and their indications can create awareness of their potential complications.

Upper abdominal operations include adrenalectomy for benign and frequently hormonally active tumors, radical adrenonephrectomy for adrenal and renal carcinomas, and retroperitoneal lymphadenectomy for testicular carcinoma and retroperitoneal tumors. In the immediate postoperative period the most common problems are respiratory and cardiovascular. Causes of early respiratory problems include postextubation hypoxemia, malfunction of the thoracostomy drainage system, or unsuspected pneumothorax. Respiratory problems usually appear as agitation, unresponsiveness, or severely abnormal blood gas results. If the patient's chest examination is not symmetric, pneumothorax must be presumed, and the chest tube must be examined for position and proper function and suction. Pulmonary embolism is rare in the immediate postoperative period; hypoxemia is usually caused by inadequate ventilation. For testicular cancer patients undergoing postchemotherapy (bleomycin) surgery, supplemental oxygen greater than 30% is contraindicated because it is associated with adult respiratory distress syndrome (ARDS), which is invariably fatal in these cases. Cardiovascular problems usually appear as patient unresponsiveness or hypotension. Causes for early cardiovascular instability are unrecognized postoperative hemorrhage, inadequate or excessive fluid replacement, myocardial infarction (MI), and adrenal medullary or cortical insufficiency. Hemorrhage, fluid replacement, and myocardial damage require focused attention on the patient's medical history, operative procedure, and physical examination; analysis of hemodynamic monitoring and urine output help to identify and treat the underlying problem. The possibility of acute adrenal insufficiency (catecholamine or glucocorticoid) as a cause of cardiovascular instability needs consideration.

Lower abdominal and pelvic procedures include radical cystectomy, total pelvic exenteration, and radical prostatectomy. In addition to cardiopulmonary problems, early postoperative complications include urinary drainage obstruction. In exenterative procedures where the bladder is removed or in radical prostatectomies where it is preserved, oliguria is one of the earlier abnormalities identified in cardiovascular instability or obstruction of urine egress. If urine output decreases, catheter obstruction must be ruled out by a physician. Only after mechanical malfunction is excluded can urine output be presumed to reflect a systemic problem.

TRAUMA

Urogenital trauma occurs from either blunt or penetrating injury. Electrical and thermal injuries are sufficiently rare to warrant exclusion from discussion. This classification system is important because the two types of injuries are often managed differently. Proximity injuries warrant evaluation since hematuria is not a sensitive predictor of the presence of severity of urologic injury. For example, a stab wound to the flank in a patient with a clear urinalysis should mandate an intravenous urogram because of the possibility of renal or ureteral injury. There is far less risk in evaluating a doubtful injury than there is in missing an injury by neglecting to do appropriate diagnostic tests. The most important principle in urogenital trauma is the *accurate preoperative delineation of the injury.* With modern radiographic techniques, including high-dose intravenous urography with nephrotomography, angiography, cystography, urethrography, and computed tomography scan, the urinary tract can be outlined in exquisite detail without the need for less precise and often meddlesome "exploration."

Blunt renal trauma, after appropriate evaluation radiographically, is usually managed nonoperatively, because these injuries invariably heal with minimal parenchymal loss. With penetrating renal injuries and an abnormal intravenous pyelogram, angiography is the next step. When knife wounds result in arteriovenous fistulae or arterial bleeding, the angiographer can embolize the appropriate vessel. However, surgery is necessary for gunshot wounds because of blast effect and resultant devitalized tissue. Ureteral injuries, usually asymptomatic and often without hematuria, are well defined by intravenous urography with extravasation of contrast; these injuries need to be surgically repaired.

Bladder injuries caused by blunt trauma are treated according to the anatomic site of extravasation. If there is intraperitoneal leakage, surgical repair is required. If leakage is confined to the retroperitoneum, urethral catheter drainage and antibiotics usually suffice. Penetrating bladder injuries need to be surgically repaired, and urethral injuries are treated with suprapubic cystostomy tubes to divert the urine. If the tear extends only part of the way through the urethra, healing will probably obviate an open surgical procedure. With urethral transection, urinary diversion with a suprapubic tube allows resolution of hematoma and facilitates later surgical repair.

Significant genital injuries usually require surgical correction. Injury to the erectile bodies of the penis, whether caused by blunt or penetrating trauma, requires an operation. Similarly, scrotal trauma, when there is bleeding or suspected testicular injury, requires surgical intervention.

For further information, please see Chapter 56 in Civetta JM, Taylor RW, Kirby RR: Critical Care. *Philadelphia: J. B. Lippincott, 1988*

BIBLIOGRAPHY

Brown DL, Kirby RR: Operative and perioperative critical care in the surgical patient. In Stamey TA (ed): *Monographs in Urology,* 1985; 6(6):1

Cass AS: Immediate radiologic evaluation and early surgical management of genital urinary injuries from external trauma. *J Urol* 1979; 122:772

Cass AS, Luxemberg M: Conservative or immediate surgical management of blunt renal trauma. *J Urol* 1983; 130:11

Donohue JP, Rowland RG: Complications of retroperitoneal lymph node dissection. *J Urol* 1981; 125:338

Fallon B, Wendt JC, Hawtey CE: Urological injury and assessment of patients with fractured pelvis. *J Urol* 1984; 131:712

Gibson GR: Urologic management and complications of fractured pelvis and ruptured urethra. *J Urol* 1974: 111:353

Goldman L: Cardiac risk and complications of non-cardiac surgery. *Ann Surg* 1983; 198:780

Hayes EE, Sandler CM, Corriere JN Jr: Management of the ruptured bladder secondary to blunt abdominal trauma. *J Urol* 1983; 129:946

Huleert JC, Grossman JE, Cummings KB: Risk factors of anesthesia and surgery in bleomycin treated patients. *J Urol* 1983; 130:163

Libertino JA, Eyre RC: Plan for management of complications after ileal conduit diversion. AUA Update Series 1984; vol 3(7)

Lieskovsky G, Pritchett TR, Skinner DG: Surgical management of renal cell carcinoma. In Stamey TA (ed): *Monographs in Urology,* 1984; 5(4):1

McAninch JR, Federle MP: Evaluation of renal injuries with computerized tomography. *J Urol* 1982; 128:456

Mendez R: Renal trauma. *J Urol* 1977; 118:698

Nicolaisen GS, McAninch JR, Marshall GA, et al: Renal trauma: Re-evaluation of the indications for radiographic assessment. *J Urol* 1985; 133:183

Ritchie JP, Skinner DG: Complications of urinary conduit diversion. In Smith RB, Skinner DG (eds): *Complications of Urologic Surgery: Prevention and Management,* p 209. Philadelphia, WB Saunders, 1976

Stewart BH: Adrenal surgery—Current state of the art. *J Urol* 1983; 129:1

Uflacker R, Paolini RM, Lima S: Management of traumatic hematuria by selective renal artery embolization. *J Urol* 1984; 132:662

20 The Gynecologic Patient

The gynecologic patient rarely presents to the ICU and postoperative hospitalization is usually short. In a review of women undergoing hysterectomy, the average postoperative stay was less than 1 week, and the incidence of life-threatening events was less than 0.2%.

Patients who present to the ICU, do so when (1) the extent of surgery is limited, but maternal condition is complicated by medical illness, such as hypertension, previous myocardial infarction, or a complication of the surgery has occurred, such as excessive bleeding; (2) the surgery is extensive enough to warrant ICU management; (3) neither the medical condition nor the extent of surgery alone is of major significance, but the disease process may cause major respiratory-hemodynamic alteration (e.g., ruptured tubo-ovarian abscess).

LIMITED GYNECOLOGIC SURGERY

Although life-threatening events are rare after hysterectomies, less serious complications are more common. Vascular injuries are infrequent during a simple abdominal hysterectomy for benign disease. When bleeding does occur, it most commonly comes from the vaginal cuff. Intraoperative bleeding may occasionally be excessive. White reported a series in which 2% of hysterectomies had intra-abdominal hemorrhage of more than 3000 ml. If the vaginal vault is left open, postoperative bleeding may be detected readily from the appearance of vaginal bleeding. Many surgeons, however, advocate closure of the vaginal cuff because of the increase in granulation tissue that occurs if it is left open. Closure, however, may delay detection of active bleeding.

Posthysterectomy hemorrhage may occur quite rapidly. In White's series, 1.3% of the patients developed profound hypovolemic shock. Venous oozing may also be a problem, especially when extensive dissection is done, as in severe endometriosis or chronic pelvic inflammatory disease.

Arterial bleeding usually requires surgical ligation of the bleeding vessels.

Tissue friability, poor exposure, and vessel retraction occasionally make this impossible, and internal iliac artery ligation must be performed to reduce the pulse pressure of the bleeding vessels and allow stable clots to form. Although complications are rare, many types have been reported. These include necrosis of viscera, such as the bladder, as well as of the areas supplied by the posterior branches of the internal iliac artery, including the buttocks and perineum. Other structures such as the external iliac artery and ureter may be incorrectly identified as the internal iliac artery. Injury and thrombosis may occur in the nearby external iliac artery. Selective arterial embolization has also been used in cases of massive pelvic bleeding, with no major complication of the procedure.

Venous oozing may be surgically uncontrollable because of the large areas of generalized bleeding with friable, poorly exposed tissue. Abdominal packs and hemostatic topical agents have been used in these instances. The military antishock trousers (MAST) have been used frequently with success in pelvic hemorrhage. Delayed hemorrhage usually occurs between 7 and 14 days postoperatively as suture and pedicle sloughs. Postoperative hemorrhage after vaginal hysterectomy is usually treated conservatively. Laparatomy is rarely required. Because of the practice of closing the vaginal cuff, early bleeding (within 24 hr) is usually not associated with vaginal bleeding, although usually a pelvic mass can be palpated after significant bleeding.

UROLOGIC INJURIES

Bladder and ureteral injury may occur in patients undergoing nonradical hysterectomy. The reported incidence is approximately 1%. The majority of these are usually unsuspected. Bladder injury unrecognized at the time of surgery may present with unusual abdominal or flank pain or may be associated with distention and ileus. An intravenous pyelogram will show blockage or extravasation.

BOWEL INJURY

Bowel injury is very uncommon during abdominal hysterectomy. When it occurs, it is usually related to lysis of adhesions between the bowel and the pelvic organs, as in the case of endometriosis or chronic pelvic inflammatory disease.

INFECTION

Febrile morbidity is fairly common after vaginal and abdominal hysterectomy. Dicker reported a rate of 15% after vaginal hysterectomy and 32% after abdominal hysterectomy. Pelvic infections accounted for only 1% to 2% of those with febrile morbidity. Bimanual exam may demonstrate tenderness at the surgical site in excess of the expected postsurgical tenderness. Occasionally an abscess will present as a palpable mass.

The pathogens involved are part of the normal microflora of the vagina and cervix. Anaerobes are the most prevalent organisms and include lactobacilli, gram-positive cocci, bacteroides and, rarely, clostridia. The most common facultative bacteria include streptococci, *Staphylococcus epidermidis, Garderella vaginitis* and *Escherichia coli*. Klebsiella, proteus, and enterobacter are less common. The infection is usually polymicrobial.

It is important to recognize that pelvic infection does not occur in the vagina. Therefore, vaginal cultures are not useful. The appropriate specimen is peritoneal fluid obtained by culdocentesis. For a cuff abscess, aspiration of purulent material from the apex of the vagina is acceptable. Specimens should be sent for aerobic and anaerobic cultures. Antimicrobial therapy should include a broad-spectrum cephalosporin for mild to moderate infection and a gentamycin–clindamycin regimen for severe infections. Ampicillin can be added, if response is poor, to cover enterococci. If the patient fails to respond to antimicrobial therapy, drainage of the abscess collection should be done.

Occasional pelvic thrombophlebitis may be a cause of failed therapy. When acute ovarian vein thrombophlebitis is present, a rope-like tender abdominal mass may be palpable in the region of the iliac fossa and extend laterally and cephalad toward the upper abdomen. When other pelvic veins are involved, specific signs are usually absent. There is no definite laboratory test for pelvic vein thrombophlebitis. Laboratory data will be of only ancillary aid. There have been isolated reports using venography, computed tomography scan and ultrasound, but the efficacy of these tests is unknown.

Broad-spectrum antibiotics effective against the common pelvic pathogens should be used together with therapeutic anticoagulation for 7 to 10 days. Surgery should be reserved for patients who remain ill or who have embolization to the lungs. Ovarian and occasionally vena cava ligation is necessary.

RADICAL HYSTERECTOMY

Radical hysterectomy involves removal of the uterus, upper vagina, part of the parametrium, and a pelvic lymphadenectomy. This procedure is used as an alternative to irradiation in the treatment of the early stages (Ib and IIa) of carcinoma of the cervix. Due to extensive dissection of the bladder off the cervix posteriorly, damage to the bladder may occur. Ischemic necrosis of the distal end of the ureters is a problem because of the lymphadenectomy, with a reported incidence of 2% to 3%. Disruption of the lymphatic drainage and extent of surgery often lead to continued loss of intravascular fluid postoperatively. Prophylactic antibiotics have reduced the risk of pelvic cellulitis to approximately 5%. Formation of a pelvic abscess is much less common.

Anticoagulation is advocated by many to reduce the risk of thromboembolic disease, without increasing the risk of bleeding. Packs, hemostatic agents, and the MAST have all been used to control pelvic bleeding.

PELVIC EXENTERATION

Pelvic exenteration is used by the gynecologist to treat radio-resistant or advanced states of cervical carcinoma and, sometimes, for vulval, vaginal, or urethral carcinoma when the disease has extended to the anterior vaginal wall with involvement of the vesicovaginal septum. Frequently these patients have postirradiation changes making surgery very difficult. Complications such as bleeding, infection, fistula formation, and thromboembolism occur more frequently after exenteration than other radical hysterectomy. Postoperative morbidity may be reduced with intensive monitoring and close supervision of these high risk patients.

Respiratory insufficiency frequently occurs and prophylactic ventilatory support, for at least 12 hours, has been advocated by Girtanner. Pulmonary artery catheters are often helpful to facilitate fluid management because extensive dissection results in disruption of lymphatic channels and continued postoperative fluid loss.

POSTABORTAL INFECTION

Severe postabortal infection resulting in maternal death has dramatically decreased with the legalization of therapeutic abortions. Death from abortion, however, still remains a problem, with infection being the leading cause. Risks are increased as gestational age, at the time of termination, increases. Infection is an ascending process, and it usually occurs when there is operative trauma or retained products of conception. Perforation of the uterus and subsequent bowel damage may also occur after termination. Symptoms include signs of sepsis, surgical abdomen, vaginal bleeding, or foul discharge with passage of placental tissue.

Specific questions should be asked about soap douche because this procedure is often accompanied by extensive pelvic tissue necrosis and may be an indication for immediate laparotomy. Endocervical and intrauterine aspirate may aid in identifying the involved or predominant organisms. If gram-positive encapsulated rods are found in Gram stain, an evaluation for intrauterine gas by radiography should be obtained. If free air is seen under the diaphragm, laparotomy should be performed. Gas within the uterus indicates the need for hysterectomy. If no gas is seen, antibiotic therapy (penicillin, gentamycin and clindamycin), should be started on admission and curettage done within 6 to 8 hours. Ultrasound may be used to look for intrauterine tissue to evaluate need for curettage.

Septic shock may sometimes occur. Common organisms are the endotoxin-producing aerobic gram-negative bacilli. *Escherichia coli* is the most common organism involved, with klebsiella, proteus, pseudomonas and enterobacter accounting for the majority of the other cases. As circulatory failure ensues, lactic acidosis develops. Adult respiratory distress syndrome (ARDS) may occur, requiring ventilatory support. Renal failure is another late sequela.

Management involves hemodynamic monitoring and restoration of effective circulating blood volume. Cardiac function is best monitored with a pulmonary artery catheter. Vasoactive drugs may occasionally be necessary after fluid resuscitation. If the patient fails to respond to resuscitation and antibiotic therapy, then hysterectomy should be considered if signs of infection such as foul discharge and tender uterus persist.

RUPTURED TUBO-OVARIAN ABSCESS

Ruptured tubo-ovarian abscess used to be one of the most feared conditions in gynecology. The mortality rate approached 100% 40 years ago. Aggressive surgical therapy with a total abdominal hysterectomy and bilateral salpingo-oophorectomy should be done. Occasionally in young patients, more conservative therapy may be attempted. Antibiotic therapy should be started immediately. As with other pelvic infection, the organ is usually polymicrobial with normal vaginal flora being present. Penicillin, gentamycin, and clindamycin have been a successful combination in these patients. Hemodynamic and respiratory support is often necessary. Fluid requirements, even in the absence of septic shock, may be massive.

For further information, please see Chapter 57 in Civetta JM, Taylor RW, Kirby RR: Critical Care. *Philadelphia: J. B. Lippincott, 1988*

BIBLIOGRAPHY

ACOG: Antimicrobia therapy for gynecologic infection. ACOG *Technical Bulletin No.* 97. Washington, DC, 1986

Creasman WT, Hill BG, Weed JC, et al: A trial of prophylactic Cefamandole in extended gynecologic survey. *Obstet Gynecol* 1982; 59:309

Dicker RC, Greenspan JR, Strauss LT, et al: Complications of abdominal and vaginal hysterectomy among women of reproductive age in the United States. *Am J Obstet Gynecol* 1982; 144:841

Duff P, Cullis RS: Pelvic vein thrombophlebitis: Diagnostic dilemma and therapeutic challenge. *Obstet Gynecol Survey* 1983; 38:365

Girtanner RE, DeCampo T, Alleyn JN, et al: Routine intensive care for pelvic exenterative operations. *Surg Gynecol Obstet* 1981; 159:657

Goldstein HM, Medellin H, Ben–Menachem Y, Wallace S: Transcatheter arterial embolization in the management of bleeding in the cancer patient. *Radiology* 1975; 115:603

Landers DV, Sweet RL: Current trends in the diagnosis and management of tubo-ovarian abscess. *Am J Obstet Gynecol* 1985; 151:1098

Le Cocq F: Internal iliac artery ligation. *Am J Obstet Gynecol* 1966; 95:32

Pearce CS Magrina JF, Finley BE: Use of MAST suit in obstetrics and gynecology. *Obstet Gynecol Survey* 1984; 39:416

Siegel P, Mengert WF: Internal iliac artery ligation in obstetrics and gynecology. *JAMA* 1961; 1978:1059
Sweet RC, Gillis RS (eds): Postabortal infection and septic shock In *Infectious Diseases of the Female Genital Tract.* Baltimore, Williams & Wilkins, 1985
White SC, Wattel LJ, Wade ME: Comparison of abdominal and vaginal hysterectomies: A review of 600 operations. *Obstet Gynecol* 1971; 37:530

21
Bacterial Infectious Disease in the Surgical Patient

Infection following elective or emergency surgical procedures is the leading cause of morbidity and mortality in postoperative patients. Most frequently encountered surgical infections are not particularly difficult to identify and can be found in the operative wound or the urinary and respiratory tracts. Deeper infections in the abdominal and thoracic cavities may present more difficult problems in diagnosis. Many factors, such as the type of surgery, the microflora of the diseased organ, and the choice of antibiotics, contribute to the development of infection.

INCIDENCE OF POSTOPERATIVE INFECTION

The overall incidence of postoperative wound infection following elective surgery was 7.5% in a national study reported two decades ago. The lowest wound infection rates—less than 2%—followed clean, elective operations in which possible sources of wound contamination were solely exogenous and related to the operating team or environment. Clean-contaminated elective operations, that is, those involving potential exposure of operative sites to endogenous bacteria, have infection rates of 10% to 20%. The average hospital stay doubles, and hospitalization costs increase accordingly, when postoperative wound infection develops after commonly performed elective operations in these categories.

Contaminated or grossly dirty surgical procedures, usually performed in emergency or trauma situations, carry the highest infection rates, ranging from 20% to 40%. This fact was demonstrated recently in several studies of penetrating abdominal trauma in which only patients with documented intestinal spillage were included. Gentry and colleagues described 152 such patients: intra-abdominal abscesses were found in 12% of patients receiving cefamandole alone; 6% of those receiving cefoxitin alone; and 6% of those receiving combination ticarcillin and tobramycin. Wound infections occurred in 6%, 0, and 4% of these patients, respectively. Jones and associates studied 257 patients and found major infections (bacteremia and abscesses) in 8%

of those receiving combination clindamycin and tobramycin; 15% of those receiving cefamandole alone; and 7% of those receiving cefoxitin alone. In a study of 145 patients, Nichols and co-workers found overall infection rates of 20% for those receiving cefoxitin alone and 23% for those receiving combination clindamycin and gentamicin; 9% of patients in each group had major infections including abdominal abscesses, septicemia, and peritonitis. Minor infections, almost entirely wound infections, were found in 13% and 15% of the two groups, respectively. In general, patients sustaining blunt or penetrating trauma without contamination by gastrointestinal contents have substantially lower rates of infection.

In addition to spillage from the gastrointestinal tract, factors contributing to the risk of posttraumatic infection include the severity and number of organs injured, degree of bacterial contamination, blood loss, therapeutic delay, and choice of antibiotics. Some authors report a higher incidence of infection following gunshot versus stab wounds, particularly if the colon is involved. Nichols and colleagues found no statistical differences based on mechanism of injury (gunshot versus stabbing), small- versus large-bowel injury, or volume of blood in the peritoneal cavity at exploration. A higher risk of infection was found if a colostomy was performed following left colon injury. Significant individual risk factors included injury to four or more organs, shock upon arrival at the hospital, number of units of blood products transfused, and increasing age.

PRINCIPLES OF SURGICAL ANTIBIOTIC MANAGEMENT

The choice of antibiotic therapy, whether prophylactic or therapeutic, should always be directed empirically to those organisms that usually cause infection unless specific culture and sensitivity results are available. One must be aware of the appropriate route of administration, the dosage necessary to achieve effective tissue and serum levels, and administration timing that offers maximum benefits.

Well-controlled, prospective, blinded studies outline many areas in which antibiotic prophylaxis is of benefit, as well as those clinical settings in which the risks of antibiotic prophylaxis outweigh the expected value. Widespread use of antibiotic prophylaxis in clean surgical procedures, faulty timing of initial antibiotic administration, and continuation of antibiotic therapy beyond the period of maximal benefit (72 hours) are the most common management errors.

In elective surgery, antibiotic prophylaxis refers to empirical preoperative antibiotic administration in the absence of established infection to reduce the risk of postoperative infection. Antibiotic prophylaxis should be limited to patients at high risk for postoperative infection (clean-contaminated cases) and those in whom the development of infection might be catastrophic (clean wounds with insertion of prosthetic material).

CHOICE OF ANTIBIOTICS

No single antibiotic agent or combination provides effective prophylaxis in all surgical situations. Agents should be chosen primarily on the basis of efficacy against bacteria that usually cause infection in each clinical setting. In clean elective operations, the usual causes of postoperative infection are aerobic streptococci or staphylococci. Infections following contaminated and emergency operations are frequently polymicrobial, and the appropriate choice of antibiotics requires knowledge of the endogenous microflora from each site (Table 21-1).

ROUTE OF ADMINISTRATION

Systemic intravenous administration of antibiotics in a relatively small volume of diluent over a short period of time is the preferred route and results in higher serum levels, more rapid tissue entry, and higher early concentrations in wound fluid. Equivalent doses of antibiotics administered by either continuous intravenous infusion or intermittent intramuscular injection produce lower serum levels and retarded entry into wound fluid. Oral administration of relatively poorly absorbed antibiotics plays a major role only in bowel preparation for elective colon surgery.

TABLE 21-1 MICROORGANISMS MOST COMMONLY ISOLATED FROM POSTOPERATIVE INFECTION

	Aerobes	**Anaerobes**
Mouth and esophagus	Streptococci	Bacteroides (other than *B. fragilis*), peptostreptococci, fusobacteria
Stomach	Enteric gram-negative bacilli, streptococci	Bacteroides (other than *B. fragilis* peptostreptococci, fusobacteria)
Biliary tract	Enteric gram-negative bacilli, Group D streptococci	Clostridia
Distal ileum, colon, and female reproductive system*	Enteric gram-negative bacilli	*B. fragilis* peptostreptococci
Bone	Staphylococcci, streptococci	
Chest	Streptococci, pneumococci	Bacteroides (other than *B. fragilis*), peptostreptococci
Cardiovascular system	Enteric gram-negative bacilli	Bacteroides (other than *B. fragilis*)
Urinary tract	Enteric gram-negative bacilli, Group D streptococci	

*Colonic and gynecologic microorganisms are seen in greater numbers.

TIMING OF ADMINISTRATION

In elective surgery, sufficient antibiotic doses should first be administered intravenously 30 minutes before the operative incision is made. This timing is ensured by having the anesthesiologist give antibiotics in the operating room just before the induction of anesthesia. Therapeutic drug levels in the wound and related tissues can be achieved during the operation, without development of bacterial resistance.

Two or three perioperative antibiotic doses are typically used for prophylaxis in elective operations, although a single dose may be sufficient. In general, solely prophylactic antibiotic administration should be continued for no longer than 24 hours after surgery, a period during which the concentration of bacteria may exceed the capacity of unaided tissues to destroy them. Continuation of prophylactic antibiotics beyond this point increases the risk of drug toxicity or bacterial superinfection and does not further reduce the incidence of infection.

Antibiotic prophylaxis administered orally for elective colon resection should be given only during the 24 hours before surgery. Longer periods of oral preoperative bowel preparation are not necessary and have been associated with the isolation of resistant colonic organisms.

CLEAN SURGICAL PROCEDURES

Prophylactic antibiotics in clean elective surgery should be limited to cases in which a prosthetic foreign body will be implanted. The benefit of antibiotic prophylaxis for other clean operations is outweighed by potential harmful effects, including toxic or allergic drug reactions and bacterial or fungal superinfections. Low infection rates in clean cases are best obtained by strict adherence to sound surgical principles. Experimental studies suggest that a single suture in a wound is sufficient to allow suppuration with a bacterial inoculum that would not otherwise result in infection. The presence of a prosthesis or other foreign body disables normal wound defense and healing mechanisms; therefore, fewer bacteria are necessary to cause infection in the presence of a foreign body than in normal tissue.

The risk of patients developing infection in clean surgical procedures requiring prosthetic devices fortunately is low, but such infections can be catastrophic. Prophylactic antistaphylococcal agents may reduce the incidence of postoperative infection in procedures requiring prostheses and are recommended. Penicillinase-resistant penicillins (methicillin, oxacillin, or nafcillin) have traditionally been used for antibiotic prophylaxis in such operations. Increasing numbers of infections by *Staphylococcus epidermidis*, an organism often resistant to semisynthetic penicillins, have been reported recently. For this reason, first-generation cephalosporins that exhibit acceptable activity against all organisms commonly causing postoperative sepsis in these cases are now the drugs of choice.

CLEAN-CONTAMINATED SURGICAL PROCEDURES

GASTRODUODENAL SURGERY

The efficacy of short-term perioperative antibiotic prophylaxis has been confirmed for patients undergoing gastroduodenal surgery for bleeding duodenal or gastric ulcer, obstructing duodenal ulcer, and gastric ulcer or malignancy. Patients undergoing gastric resection for chronic nonobstructing duodenal ulcer rarely experience postoperative infection, an observation leading to the general belief that stomach contents are sterile and antibiotic prophylaxis is not indicated. Postoperative infections are more common today because gastroduodenal operations are performed primarily for complicated duodenal or gastric ulcer and for malignancy. A 10-year review of sepsis after gastroduodenal surgery indicated that patients at high risk for postoperative infection could be identified preoperatively. In a recent clinical trial of 39 high-risk patients undergoing such operations, 7 of 20 patients in the placebo group developed gastric-related infections; in contrast, only 1 of 19 patients receiving a perioperative cephalosporin became infected.

Patients with normal gastric acid output and motility rarely harbor bacteria in the stomach or proximal intestine. A clinical study demonstrated that few, if any, bacteria can be isolated from needle aspirates of stomach contents taken during surgery from patients with normal gastric acid and motility who are not receiving antibiotics; the postoperative infection rate in these patients was correspondingly low. Gastric bacterial colonization occurred almost uniformly in other patients undergoing operation for bleeding or obstructing duodenal ulcer, gastric ulcer, or malignancy. Gastric bacterial overgrowth in these patients is best explained by compromise of the bacterial inhibitory effects of normal gastric acid and motility. Another study found that 22 of 30 patients with infection after gastroduodenal surgery were deficient in one or both gastric inhibitory factors.

When present, gastric bacteria are usually divided equally between oral or proximal intestinal aerobes and oral anaerobes. Patients with gastric colonization at the time of operation have postoperative infection rates greater than 20%. Organisms responsible for postoperative infection are almost always the same as those isolated from the gastric microflora. Cephalosporins are the drugs of choice for antibiotic prophylaxis in this setting.

BILIARY TRACT SURGERY

Antibiotic prophylaxis in chronic calculous cholecystitis is justified for patients with clinical risk factors or a positive intraoperative Gram stain indicating biliary bacteria. Initial antibiotic therapy should be effective against facultative gram-negative coliforms; cephalosporins or aminoglycosides are the drugs of choice. If a gram-positive rod is reported on Gram stain, penicillin should be added. Equal benefit can be expected from antibiotics that produce high serum or bile levels. Routine use of prophylactic antibiotics in patients undergoing cholecystectomy is probably unnecessary.

The healthy human biliary tract rarely harbors significant bacterial concentrations. Bacteria can be isolated, however, in 15% to 30% of cases of chronic calculous cholecystitis. Bacteria isolated from the human biliary tract are primarily gram-negative enteric coliforms. *Escherichia coli,* alone or mixed with another organism, is present in 50% of positive cultures; other coliforms (e.g., *Klebsiella, Enterobacter,* and *Proteus*) are isolated less commonly. *Streptococcus faecalis,* an enterococcus, is also isolated frequently. Anaerobic microorganisms are isolated in fewer than 20% of cases; *Clostridium perfringens* is most common.

Certain patients undergoing elective cholecystectomy without clinical risk factors will, nevertheless, have biliary bacteria. Keighley and colleagues reported on the technique of immediate intraoperative bile Gram staining. The bile sample, usually taken from the gallbladder, should be sent to the microbiology laboratory for Gram staining, culture, and sensitivity testing early in the operation. The overall accuracy of Gram-stained specimens compared to subsequent bile cultures exceeds 75%. This technique allows the surgeon to begin administration of antibiotics during the operation and also allows appropriate alteration of choice of antibiotics when unanticipated organisms are seen.

A 33% postoperative infection rate has been reported in patients undergoing biliary tract surgery in the presence of a positive bile culture. Clinical factors favoring isolation of biliary bacteria and a corresponding increased risk of infection include age greater than 70 years; previous biliary tract operation; jaundice; chills or fever within 1 week of operation; and operation performed within 1 month of an acute cholecystitis attack. Prophylactic antibiotics are indicated when one or more of these clincial risk factors are identified preoperatively.

COLON SURGERY

The human colon contains a greater variety of microorganisms at higher concentrations than any other organ's endogenous microflora. The efficacy of oral neomycin and erythromycin base in preoperative colon preparation has been demonstrated clearly. The importance of anaerobic fecal organisms in the pathogenesis of clinical wound infections is now recognized by most surgeons. Many anaerobes are resistant to antibiotics employed commonly for bowel preparation, so it is unlikely that previously recommended regimens were pharmacologically adequate. Oral antibiotic administration should take place during the 19 hours before surgery. If the operation is planned for later than 8 a.m., the timing of administration should be altered appropriately to produce peak serum and stool levels at the time of surgery.

Effective oral antimicrobial bowel preparation requires knowledge of the normal endogenous colon flora, the capacity of various fecal bacteria to produce infections, and the patterns of antimicrobial sensitivity of these microorganisms. Microflora are sparse in the proximal human gastrointestinal tract but increase significantly in the distal ileum, where concentrations of both aerobes and anaerobes average 10^4/ml and 10^5/ml. *Bacteroides fragilis* and other fecal anaerobes first appear at this level. The most prevalent aerobe in the colon, *E. coli,* is usually isolated in concentrations of 10^6 to 10^8 organisms per gram of stool, *B. fragilis* and other obligate anaerobes are 1,000 to 10,000 times more common than any of the aerobes in all portions of the colon. The normal colonic flora comprise more than 20 species of resident and transient aerobes and over 40 species of anaerobes, most of which are not pathogens. The most common organisms found in septic wounds after colon operations are *E. coli* and *B. fragilis;* other pathogenic organisms are found less frequently. For practical purposes, oral antibiotic therapy directed against *E. coli* (either oral neomycin or kanamycin) and *B. fragilis* (oral erythromycin base, metronidazole, or tetracycline) is effective in the majority of cases.

The first Veterans Administration Cooperative Study demonstrated the effectiveness of preoperative oral neomycin and erythromycin base combined with vigorous purgation in patients undergoing elective colon resection when compared with mechanical preparation and placebo. Septic complications were seen in 43% of the placebo group and 9% of the group given neomycin and erythromycin base. A second study tested the parenteral use of cephalothin, in addition to oral neomycin and erythromycin base for elective preoperative colon preparation. Three groups were compared: intravenous cephalothin alone, oral neomycin and erythromycin base, and a combination of these intravenous and oral antibiotics; all groups received the same mechanical preparation. Addition of patients to the intravenous-cephalothin-only group was stopped after 10 months because sequential data analysis indicated significantly more infections, with an overall incidence of septic complications of 39%. In groups receiving oral neomycin and erythromycin alone or in combination with intravenous cephalothin, the infection rate was less than 9%.

GROSSLY CONTAMINATED AND TRAUMATIC PROCEDURES

Empirical antibiotic therapy following spontaneous gastrointestinal perforation (perforated appendicitis or diverticulitis) or penetrating intestinal trauma is not prophylactic in the same sense as that applied in elective surgery because therapy is initiated after, not before, potential contamination. These patients are similar and have comparable risks of postoperative sepsis. A practical outline of endogenous bacteria that might be expected following contamination from various regions of the gastrointestinal tract is included in Table 21-1.

Rational antimicrobial therapy for emergency abdominal operations should include parenteral antibiotics effective against both aerobic and anaerobic endogenous bacteria (especially *B. fragilis*); cefoxitin alone, or the combination of clindamycin and gentamicin, is used most frequently. Empirical regimens in this setting do not require initial antimicrobial coverage for *Pseudomonas* or enterococci. *Pseudomonas* is rarely isolated as one of the primary organisms, but later may become an opportunistic pathogen in critically ill patients. Enterococcus can be isolated in approximately one third of post-traumatic abdominal infections, but does not require prophylactic therapy because it is rarely the sole pathogen. If isolated in the blood or in pure culture from the infected site, enterococcus should be treated with specific combination therapy.

Until recently, antibiotic protocols in emergency and trauma surgery relied on therapy directed entirely against aerobic bacteria. Early experience with anaerobic isolation techniques in patients with penetrating abdominal trauma demonstrated the advantage of combination therapy with antibiotics effective against both aerobic and anaerobic bacteria. Anaerobes were recovered more frequently from wounds and drain sites in patients receiving cephalothin and kanamycin (aerobic coverage only) than in those receiving clindamycin and kanamycin (anaerobic and aerobic coverage). Major infections in this study occurred in 28% and 11%, of the two groups, respectively, with the difference reflecting fewer mixed aerobic and anaerobic cultures in the latter. Note that major infections today are more frequently reported in studies with cefamandole-treated groups, primarily because of this agent's lack of efficacy against *B. fragilis* isolates.

Effective antibiotic use in emergencies depends on appropriate timing and duration of therapy. Sufficient doses of antibiotics should be given within 1 hour of operation, usually during the intial emergency department evaluation, to yield therapeutic drug levels in the wound and tissues during abdominal exploration. Appropriate tetanus prophylaxis is also given at this time (Table 21-2). After trauma surgery, antibiotic therapy should be continued for 2 to 5 days, depending on the degree of peritoneal contamination and severity of injuries. Antibiotics should be limited to one preoperative dose in the absence of intestinal soilage. The importance of early antibiotic administration is well established, but the ideal duration of therapy after intestinal perforation is still under investigation.

SURGICAL WOUND INFECTION

CLASSIFICATION OF SURGICAL WOUNDS

Surgical wounds are generally classified as clean, clean-contaminated, contaminated, or dirty. Clean wounds are those in which gastrointestinal or respiratory tracts were not entered during the course of operation. The usual cause of postoperative infection in such cases is exogenous aerobic bacteria, such as staphylococci, which enter the wound during surgery. The overall infection rate in clean surgical procedures should be less than 2%.

TABLE 21-2 TETANUS PROPHYLAXIS*

Clean Minor Wound
- Not immunized—Complete immunization per schedule, TT 0.5 ml
- Immunized, 5–10 years—None
- Immunized, > 10 years–TT 0.5 ml

Clean Major Wound
- Not immunized—HTIG 250 units (one arm), TT 0.5 ml (other arm); complete immunization per schedule
- Immunized, 5–10 years—TT 0.5 ml
- Immunized, > 10 years—HTIG 250 units (one arm), TT 0.5 ml (other arm)

Tetanus–prone Wound
- Not immunized—HTIG 250 units (one arm), TT 0.5 ml (other arm); complete immunization per schedule; antibiotics
- Immunized, 5–10 years—TT 0.5 ml; antibiotics
- Immunized, > 10 years—HTIG 250 units (one arm), TT 0.5 ml (other arm); antibiotics

(Adapted from Specific measures for previously immunized patients. In Walt AJ: *Early Care of the Injured Patient,* 3rd ed. Philadelphia, WB Saunders, 1982, p 71)
*TT = Tetanus toxoid; HTIG = human tetanus immune globulin.

Clean-contaminated wounds include elective operations on the gastrointestinal or respiratory tracts. The risk of infection in these cases is higher than in clean surgical procedures, and is generally reported to be between 5% and 10%. Infection in these patients primarily results from the endogenous microflora of the organ that was surgically resected.

Contaminated wounds include those in which acute inflammation (without pus formation) or gross spillage of gastrointestinal contents is encountered at the time of operation. Infections in these cases are also primarily caused by endogenous bacteria, and the infection rate is approximately 20%.

Dirty wounds, in which gross pus following organ perforation is encountered at surgery, have infection rates in excess of 40%, related primarily to the endogenous microflora of the involved organ.

NONANTIBIOTIC FACTORS

A number of factors other than antibiotic use can be shown to influence postoperative infection rates following clean elective operations in which bacterial contamination is absent or minimal. There is no convincing evidence that preoperative scrub technique, surgical glove damage, barrier materials, and "laminar flow" air-blowing systems influence postoperative wound infection; anecdotal experience and commercial interests rather than scientific studies often account for these associations.

For further information, please see Chapter 69 in Civetta JM, Taylor RW, Kirby RR: Critical Care. *Philadelphia: J. B. Lippincott, 1988*

BIBLIOGRAPHY

Barlett JB, Sullivan-Sigler N, Louie TJ, et al: Anaerobes survive in clinical specimens despite delayed processing. *J Clin Microbiol* 1978; 3:133

Bornside GH, Cohn I Jr: The normal microbial flora: Comparative bacterial flora of animals and man. *Am J Digest Dis* 1965; 10:844

Cruse PJE, Foord R: A five-year prospective study of 23,649 surgical wounds. *Arch Surg* 1973; 107:206

Gentry LO, Feliciano DV, Lea AS, et al: Perioperative antibiotic therapy for penetrating injuries of the abdomen. *Ann Surg* 1984; 200:561

Hardin WD, Aran AJ, Smith JW, et al: Aerotolerance of common anaerobic bacteria—Fact or fancy? *South Med J* 1982; 75:1051

Jones RD, Thal ER, Johnson NA, et al: Evaluation of antibiotic therapy following penetrating abdominal trauma. *Ann Surg* 1985; 201:576

Kaiser AB: Antimicrobial prophylaxis in surgery. *N Engl J Med* 1986; 315:1129

Keighley MRB, McLeish AR, Bishop HM: Identification of the presence and type of biliary microflora by immediate gram stains. Surgery 1977; 81:469

Nichols RL: Gas gangrene and similar anaerobic soft tissue infections. In Conn R (ed): *Current Diagnosis,* 7th ed, p 149. Philadelphia, WB Saunders 1984

Nichols RL: Empiric antibiotic therapy for intra-abdominal infections. *Rev Infect Dis* 1983; 5(Suppl):90

Nichols RL, Smith JW: Modern approach to the diagnosis of anaerobic surgical sepsis. *Surg Clin North Am* 1975; 55:21

Nichols RL, Webb WR, Jones JW, et al: Efficacy of antibiotic prophylaxis in high risk gastroduodenal operations. *Am J Surg* 1982; 143:94

Shapiro M, Munoz A, Tager IB, et al: Risk factors for infection at the operative site after abdominal or vaginal hysterectomy. *N Engl J Med* 1982; 307:1661

Tally FP, Stewart PR, Sutter VL, et al: Oxygen tolerance of fresh clinical anaerobic bacteria. *J Clin Microbiol* 1975; 1:61

22 Postoperative Respiratory Considerations

Clinicians use postoperative mechanical ventilation for two primary situations. In many instances, the need for such therapy is anticipated because of underlying abnormal lung function in specific surgical patients. However, patients with normal lung function also are treated with mechanical ventilation or continuous positive airway pressure (CPAP) because of the anesthetic technique and the agents used during the surgical procedure or because the surgical procedure causes ventilatory abnormalities.

Most current literature to guide clinicians in designing the therapeutic approach to the postoperative patient deals with the necessity to ventilate patients with respiratory failure. Although the intraoperative effects of general anesthesia on normal lungs has been well studied, little information is available to guide postoperative therapy.

Postoperative respiratory problems encompass inadequate ventilation and inadequate oxygenation. In either case the underlying disease may necessitate therapy, including mechanical ventilation, or may be aggravated by the anesthetic or surgical procedure.

VENTILATION

Intraoperative barbiturates, narcotics, or inhalational anesthetics can result in respiratory depression at the termination of the operative procedure. These agents must be metabolized or reversed pharmacologically. In the meantime, support of ventilation often is necessary. Ventilatory insufficiency also results from neuromuscular blocking drugs used during the surgical procedure. Their action must also be reversed or mechanical ventilation provided until they are metabolized or excreted.

Operations in and around the brain stem, such as removal of an acoustic neuroma, sometimes require such support. Underlying disease, trauma, neoplasm, or hemorrhage in the medulla often necessitate preoperative mechanical ventilation, and this support must also be provided in the postoperative period. Spinal pathways are interrupted by a high cervical dislocation for which long-term ventilatory support is almost always essential.

Although less common today, anterior horn cell disease, such as occurs with poliomyelitis, may leave the patient in a compromised state. Other neuromuscular diseases such as Guillain–Barré syndrome, myasthenia gravis, or muscular dystrophy may be aggravated by the stress of the surgery and anesthesia. Thoracic cage abnormalities such as flail chest, whether or not underlying pulmonary contusion is present, occasionally are severe enough to require positive-pressure ventilation. Upper airway obstruction associated with neoplasm, trauma, or infection frequently is best handled by intubation of the trachea or a tracheostomy, with subsequent positive airway pressure support.

OXYGENATION

When inadequate oxygenation is anticipated or documented postoperatively, the causes again can be related to specific problems with the anesthetic, the surgical procedure, or the underlying disease. During general anesthesia, for example, inadequate lung volumes, specifically a decrease in functional residual capacity (FRC), occur that are related to the duration of surgery and anesthesia, to maintenance of one position for prolonged periods of time, and to the site of the surgical incision.

During intrathoracic and intra-abdominal surgery and in some trauma cases, large volumes of fluid are administered, and significant translocation of fluid occurs between the intracellular and extracellular compartments. At the conclusion of the surgical procedure, the patient may be unstable hemodynamically with an inadequate cardiac output. Pulmonary edema may result from fluid overload or from the accumulation of extravascular lung water associated with extracorporeal circulation ("pump lung"). Postoperatively on the second or third day, the translocated fluid is mobilized from the areas of sequestration and returned to the circulation, often resulting in volume overload and a need for support of oxygenation.

Acute respiratory insufficiency sometimes follows anesthetic misadventures, including the pulmonary aspiration of gastric or pharyngeal secretions during the induction or maintenance of anesthesia or during emergence following tracheal extubation. Hypothermic patients have reduced metabolism of anesthetic agents or difficulty in maintaining spontaneous ventilation and frequently are ventilated postoperatively until return of their normal body temperature.

Underlying diseases that may influence the decision to provide postoperative respiratory therapy include chronic obstructive lung disease; episodic bronchospasm with acute asthma, which may be induced by the manipulation of the airway during the anesthetic; and respiratory failure not related to the anesthetic or surgical procedure. The last category includes sepsis, posttraumatic pulmonary insufficiency with pulmonary edema, transfusion reactions, and syndromes of aspiration/inspiration such as near-drowning or inhalation of toxic gases. In these situations, tracheal intubation with mechanical ventilation and CPAP is often initiated preoperatively.

VENTILATOR SUPPORT

Overt respiratory failure can be manifested by alveolar hyperventilation or hypoventilation and abnormalities in arterial *p*H and carbon dioxide tension (Pa_{CO_2}). Inadequate lung expansion, whether caused by the length of the procedure, the site of the incision, or the remaining effects of anesthetic agents, decreases FRC and arterial oxygen tension (Pa_{O_2}) and increases physiologic shunting.

These patients breathe with low tidal volumes and have a low inspiratory capacity. The residual effects of inhalational anesthetics, narcotics, and neuromuscular blockers also diminish the peak negative pressure that can be generated against an occluded airway. These simple tests of respiratory mechanics are inexpensive and easy to perform to sort out the abnormalities documented by blood gas analysis. Abnormalities of ventilation and oxygenation may be associated with manifestations of excessive respiratory muscle work. Increased oxygen consumption and carbon dioxide production frequently result from abnormalities of inspired gas distribution and an increase of dead space ventilation. Alterations in ventilatory mechanics also are seen in bronchospastic patients, those with upper airway obstruction, and those with significant alterations in pulmonary compliance or pulmonary edema. Several tests are used to evaluate respiratory muscle strength, abnormalities in ventilatory mechanics, available ventilatory reserve, breathing pattern effectiveness (minute ventilation versus dead space ventilation), and abnormalities in oxygenation (Table 22-1). They are appropriate for many patients in respiratory failure and for postoperative patients for whom a decision on mechanical support of ventilation must be made.

Most ventilators can be used to administer the three currently most popular modes of mechanical ventilation: controlled mechanical ventilation (CMV), assisted (assist-control) mechanical ventilation (AMV), and intermittent or synchronized intermittent mandatory ventilation (IMV/SIMV). Each can be used to provide adequate ventilatory support. The differences that exist include patient comfort and safety, alarm mechanisms, ease of ventilator weaning for individual patients, and cost of the ventilator itself.

Weisman and colleagues and Luce and associates reviewed information with respect to the choice of techniques. In many cases, studies are not comparable owing to differences in the ventilator circuits and the way in which the ventilators were used. Most patients undergoing postoperative mechanical ventilation do not have significant underlying lung disease; hence, equipment requirements are rather simple and do not require a great degree of sophisticated ventilator designs.

TABLE 22-1 "BEDSIDE" PULMONARY FUNCTION SUGGESTING SUCCESSFUL WEANING FROM MECHANICAL VENTILATION

Muscle strength	
PNP	< -20 cm H_2O
Ventilatory mechanics	
FVC	> 15 ml/kg
VT	> 5 ml/kg
C_{lt} (static)	> 30 ml/cm H_2O
Ventilatory reserve (endurance)	
VE	< 10 liters/min
MVV	> 20 liters/min ($> 2 \times \dot{V}E$)
Effectiveness of ventilation	
VD/VT	< 0.60
Pa_{CO2}	< 50 mm Hg
Oxygenation	
Pa_{O2}/FI_{O2}	> 200 mm Hg
$P(A - a)O_2$ ($FI_{O2} = 1.0$)	< 350 mm Hg
Qs/Qt	$< 20\%$

IMV/SIMV

The advantages of IMV/SIMV include the avoidance of asynchoronous breathing and a lower intrathoracic pressure—hence a potentially more stable hemodynamic profile. Reported disadvantages include reliance on spontaneous breathing in patients with fluctuating mental status or altered ventilatory drive, although careful monitoring should detect these abnormalities.

The major issue, debated often in the published literature, centers on the respiratory work that the patient encounters. As Downs suggests, a small endotracheal tube or poorly designed inspiratory circuit can significantly increase the work of breathing. Poor design of the expiratory circuit and the pressurized CPAP exhalation valve compounds the problem. In the face of these circuit defects, IMV/SIMV may actually prolong the weaning process and the cost to the patient. Proponents of IMV/SIMV argue that these considerations do not reflect poorly on the techniques but rather on their application.

AMV

Assisted mechanical ventilation likewise has many proponents. Supporters claim a major advantage is that the entire minute ventilation is provided with minimal work of breathing generated by the patient and suggest that this technique is particularly desirable postoperatively when respiratory muscle function may be a problem. Assisted ventilation is described as patient responsive because minute ventilation can be increased or decreased on demand.

Disadvantages of AMV include significant cardiovascular compromise in some patients, particularly if they are hypovolemic or if PEEP/CPAP is used.

Postoperative patients frequently are agitated with either increased ventilatory drive or a sensation of dyspnea, and often trigger the ventilator excessively, causing mechanical hyperventilation and respiratory alkalemia. Generally, this condition is associated with a leftward shift in the oxyhemoglobin dissociation curve, a decrease in cardiac output, a decrease in cerebral blood flow, and alterations in lung–thorax mechanics. The importance of these dangers postoperatively has not been quantitated.

CMV

Little controversy surrounds CMV, since the clinical indications for its use are apparent. When a patient is heavily narcotized, sedated, or paralyzed, IMV/SIMV and AMV cannot be used appropriately. Most clinicians agree, however, that once the patient regains consciousness and respiratory muscle strength, CMV can be maintained only with additional drug administration to suppress spontaneous breathing. Therefore, AMV or IMV/SIMV during emergence from anesthesia provides a smoother transition to spontaneous ventilation and is more comfortable for the patient.

In summary, the wide array of ventilatory modes is of no great benefit to the postoperative patient. For the most part, these patients have normal lung function, and in most instances ventilatory support involves a period of only a few hours. Of more importance than the ventilatory technique is adequate postoperative monitoring.

For further information, please see Chapter 19 in Civetta JM, Taylor RW, Kirby RR: Critical Care. *Philadelphia: J. B. Lippincott, 1988*

BIBLIOGRAPHY

Anderes C, Anderes V, Gasser D, et al: Postoperative spontaneous breathing with CPAP to normalize late postoperative oxygenation. *Intens Care Med* 1979; 5:15

Aubier M, Trippenbach T, Roussos C: Respiratory muscle fatigue during cardiogenic shock. *J Appl Physiol* 1981; 51:499

Bartlett RH, Gazzaniga AG, Geraghty TR: Respiratory maneuvers to prevent postoperative pulmonary complications. *JAMA* 1973; 224:1017

Bendixen HH, Bullwinkel B, Hedley–Whyte J: Atelectasis and shunting during spontaneous ventilation in anesthetized patients. *Anesthesiology* 1964; 25:297

Bendixen HH, Smith GM, Mead J: Pattern of ventilation in young adults. *J Physiol* 1964; 19:195

Bergman NA: Intrapulmonary gas trapping during mechanical ventilation at rapid frequencies. *Anesthesiology* 1972; 37:626

Bergman NA: Effects of varying respiratory waveforms on gas exchange. *Anesthesiology* 1967; 28:390

Downs JB: Inappropriate applications of IMV. *Chest* 1980; 78:897

Fairley HB, Blenkarn GD: Effect of pulmonary gas exchange of variations in inspiratory flow rate during intermittent positive pressure ventilation. *Br J Anaesth* 1966; 38:320

Ford GT, Guenther CA: Toward prevention of postoperative pulmonary complications. *Am Rev Respir Dis* 1984; 130:4

Fuleihan SF, Wilson RS, Pontoppidan H: Effect of mechanical ventilation with end-inspiratory pause on blood gas exchange. *Anesth Analg* 1976; 55:122

Grimby G, Hedenstierna G, Löfström B: Chest wall mechanics during artificial ventilation. *J Appl Physiol* 1975; 38:576

Guenther CA: Toward prevention of postoperative pulmonary complications. *Am Rev Respir Dis* 1984; 130:4

Jansson L, Janson B: A theoretical study on flow patterns of ventilators. *Scand J Respir Dis* 1972; 53:237

Levine M, Gilbert R, Auchincloss JH: A comparison of the effects of sighs, large tidal volumes, and positive end-expiratory pressure in assisted ventilation. *Scand J Respir Dis* 1972; 53:101

Lichtenthal PR, Wade LD, Niemyski PR, et al: Respiratory management after cardiac surgery with inhalation anesthesia. *Crit Care Med* 1983; 11:603

Luce JM, Pierson DJ, Hudson LD: Intermittent mandatory ventilation. *Chest* 1981; 79:678

Lyager S: Ventilation/perfusion ratio during intermittent positive pressure ventilation—Importance of no-flow interval during the insufflation. *Acta Anaesthesiol Scand* 1970; 14:211

Midell AI, Skinner DB, DeBoer A, et al: A review of pulmonary problems following valve replacement in 100 consecutive patients. *Ann Thorac Surg* 1974; 18:219

Pepe PE, Marini JJ: Occult positive end-expiratory pressure in mechanically ventilated patients with airflow obstruction. *Am Rev Respir Dis* 1982; 126:166

Prakash O, Johnson B, Meij S, et al: Criteria for early extubation after intracardiac surgery in adults. *Anesth Analg* 1977; 56:703

Quasha AL, Loeber N, Feeley TW, et al: Postoperative respiratory care: A controlled trial of early and late extubation following coronary artery bypass grafting. *Anesthesiology* 1980; 52:135

Radford EP: Ventilation standards for use in artificial respiration. *J Appl Physiol* 1955; 7:451

Shackford SR, Virgilio RW, Peters RM: Early extubation vs. prophylactic ventilation for the high risk patient: A comparison of postoperative management in the prevention of respiratory complications. *Anesth Analg* 1981; 29:463

Stock MC, Downs JB, Corkran ML: Pulmonary function before and after prolonged continuous positive airway pressure. *Crit Care Med* 1984; 12:973

Suter PM, Fairley HB, Isenberg MD: Effect of tidal volume and positive end-expiratory pressure on compliance during mechanical ventilation. *Chest* 1978; 73:158

Sykes MK, Young WE, Robinson BE: Oxygenation during anesthesia with controlled ventilation. *Br J Anaesth* 1965; 37:314

Weisman IM, Rinaldo JE, Rogers RM, et al: Intermittent mandatory ventilation. *Am Rev Respir Dis* 1983; 127:641

Young SL, Tierney DF, Clements JA: Mechanism of compliance change in excised rat lungs at low transpulmonary pressure. *J Appl Physiol* 1970; 29:780

23 Postanesthetic Problems

Most problems in the postoperative period are also found in other situations. Acute changes in cardiovascular function (dysrhythmias, hypertension, hypotension, decreased cardiac function), pulmonary function (ARDS, aspiration, barotrauma) and other organ failure occur in critically ill patients and are discussed in other chapters.

The average healthy patient receives eight drugs during hospitalization plus five to ten more drugs during anesthesia. Some drugs used during anesthesia are not commonly used outside the operating room. The side-effects of these drugs and interactions with other drugs can lead to problems peculiar to the postanesthetic period. Important examples of these types of postanesthetic complications are [1] prolonged neuromuscular blockade, [2] malignant hyperthermia, and [3] respiratory depression by epidural and spinal narcotics.

PROLONGED NEUROMUSCULAR BLOCKADE

Patients with prolonged neuromuscular blockade usually present in one of three ways in the immediate postanesthetic period: [1] delayed return to "consciousness," [2] hypoventilation and respiratory distress, or [3] muscle weakness. Oxygenation and ventilation with prevention of aspiration must be maintained while a rapid diagnosis is made. Intubation or constant observation, or both, must occur while the diagnosis is being made.

Most anesthesiologists take precautions to monitor neuromuscular blockade. Despite monitoring and careful use of muscle relaxants, reversal is not always possible, and the diagnosis of residual neuromuscular blockade may not be obvious. Patients initially may appear to have "adequate" neuromuscular reversal and later manifest weakness. Some may present to the recovery room or ICU with apparent delayed return of consciousness as a primary sign of muscle weakness without obvious hypoventilation. Causes of postoperative delayed return to consciousness are diverse (Table 23-1). Testing of neuromuscular function should be part of your diagnostic evaluation.

TABLE 23-1 CAUSES OF POSTOPERATIVE DELAYED RETURN TO CONSCIOUSNESS

Prolonged anesthetic effect
  Premedication
  Benzodiazepines, neuroleptics, barbiturates, natcotics, *etc.*

  Intraoperative anesthetics
    All inhalational anesthetics
    Intravenous drugs (barbiturates, narcotics, *muscle relaxants, prolonged neuromuscular blockade*)
"Other drugs"
  Lidocaine, antihypertensives, MAO inhibitors, "street drugs," cimetidine, drug interactions, etc.
Respiratory insufficiency
Hypothermia
Malignant hyperthermia
Hyperglycemia and hypoglycemia, electrolyte abnormalities
Intraoperative catastrophes
  Cardiovascular
    Hypovolemia, sepsis, anaphylaxis, ischemia

  Intracranial
    Increased intracranial pressure, hypoxia, pneumocephalus, vasospasm, postictal state, hemorrhage

Other patients complain of dyspnea or present with hypoventilation and hypoxia that progresses to agitation, cardiovascular instability, and coma. The causes of postoperative hypoventilation are also numerous (Table 23-2), and the primary diagnosis is easy to miss when you treat the consequences of hypoventilation due to residual neuromuscular blockade. Still others are usually alert and breathing adequately but appear "floppy" and complain

TABLE 23.2 CAUSES OF POSTOPERATIVE HYPOVENTILATION

Central respiratory depression
  Inhalation anesthetic
  IV anesthetics
  Hypothermia
Respiratory muscle dysfunction
  Site of incision (upper abdomen, thorax)
  Prolonged neuromuscular blockade
  Obesity, body casts, tight chest or abdominal dressing
Intraoperative hyperventilation
Increased carbon dioxide production
  Sepsis, shivering, malignant hyperthermia
Acute lung disease
  Aspriation, upper airway obstruction, postintubation croup, secretions, vocal cord paralysis, pneumothorax, ARDS, bilateral carotid artery surgery
Chronic lung disease
  COPD, bronchospasm
Acute cardiovascular disease
  Pulmonary edema

of muscle weakness (difficulty swallowing, opening eyes, lifting head). The diagnosis is usually apparent in this group.

Adequate reversal from neuromuscular blocking drugs usually is present when a patient can maintain adequate ventilation during stresses such as airway obstruction or vomiting. One third of neuromuscular end-plate receptors can be blocked by muscle relaxants without any observable effect. Tests that confirm the reversal of neuromuscular blockade include those which require patient cooperation and others that directly assess neuromuscular function. The ability to open one's eyes, cough effectively, and sustain head lift for 5 seconds is associated with a vital capacity of at least 15 to 20 ml/kg and a peak negative pressure of at least −20 to −25 cm H_2O. These values generally are thought to demonstrate adequate reversal.

The adequacy of reversal in anesthetized, sedated patients or in those unable to respond to commands is assessed by normal tidal volume, by peak negative pressure of at least −25 cm H_2O, and by use of a neuromuscular stimulator. The last mentioned delivers an electrical stimulus to a peripheral nerve (ulnar, facial, or peroneal). The force of contraction of the appropriate muscle group is observed. Sustained tetanic contraction for 5 seconds after a stimulus of 50 Hz and equal twitch response to four stimuli of 0.2 msec duration at 0.5-second intervals ("train of four") correlate with adequate neuromuscular reversal. A decline in the force of contraction to a 5-sec tetanus ("fade") or a decrease in the force of the fourth twitch compared to the first in the train-of-four stimulus is evidence for neuromuscular blockade.

If full reversal cannot be acomplished quickly, the patient should be reintubated. Once the airway has been protected, the cause can be ascertained and specific management of the problem can proceed in an orderly manner. Causes of prolonged neuromuscular blockade are listed in Table 23-3.

Most cases of prolonged neuromuscular blockade involve the nondepo-

TABLE 23.3 CAUSES OF PROLONGED NEUROMUSCULAR BLOCKADE

Depolarizing muscle relaxants (succinylcholine)
- Failure to metabolize succinylcholine
  - (1) ↓ effective pseudocholinesterase (genetic deficiencies, pregnancy, liver disease)
  - (2) Antagonism of pseudocholinesterase (ecothiophate, insecticides, neostigmine, pyridostigmine, edrophonium)
- Phase II block

Nondepolarizing muscle relaxants
- Intensity of block
- Inadequate dose of reversal agents
- Failure to excrete (renal, liver diseases)
- Acid–base status
- ↓ K^+, ↑ Mg^{2+}, ↓ Ca^{2+}
- Hypothermia
- Drug interactions (see Table 17–4)
- Diseases that may alter muscle relaxant interaction

larizing muscle relaxants (curare, pancuronium, metubine, vecuronium, atracurium). Some other drugs also affect the duration of blockade (Table 23-4). Residual blockade can be demonstrated (tetanic fade to 5-sec stimulus, fourth/first twitch height of less than 70% using train-of-four stimulation). An attempt should be made to reverse the blockade with neostigmine (0.035 to 0.07 mg/kg); pyridostigmine (0.175 to 0.35 mg/kg); or edrophonium (0.5 to 1.0 mg/kg), along with an anticholinergic agent (atropine 0.02 mg/kg or glycopyrrolate 0.01 mg/kg). Profound neuromuscular blockade before reversal (90–100% twitch height suppression) requires as much as 30 minutes or more before full recovery. Neostigmine is a better reversal agent for profound block. One hour should elapse before more anticholinesterase is given because excessive anticholinesterase paradoxically can lead to increased blockade.

MALIGNANT HYPERTHERMIA

Malignant hyperthermia (MH) is a rare pharmacogenetic disease in which skeletal muscles develop a fulminant hypermetabolic response to certain anesthetic agents, other drugs, or stress. The fulminant episode (Table 23-5) is associated with a 10% mortality. Temperature may increase up to 44°C in 20 minutes. Because the shortest reported time-interval from induction to death is 20 minutes, immediate diagnosis and therapy are mandatory. Malignant hyperthermia can occur preoperatively, intraoperatively, and postoperatively and constitutes an acute, potentially lethal, crisis with unusual presentations in the intensive care unit.

MH should be distinguished from other causes of fever and hypermetabolism (Table 23-6). Once the diagnosis is made or other etiologies ruled out, rapid treatment is imperative (Table 23-7). Dantrolene should be administered because it directly decreases intramyoplasmic stores of calcium and is responsible for the recently decreased mortality from 80% to 10%. Most experts recommend 2.5 mg/kg as an intravenous bolus because there is no acute toxicity and the mean effective dose is 2.4 mg/kg. All signs of MH should be resolved within 45 minutes after appropriate therapy. However, if the patient fails to respond, the dose can then be increased to a maximum

TABLE 23-4 DRUG INTERACTIONS AFFECTING DURATION OF NEUROMUSCULAR BLOCKADE

Antibiotics
  Aminoglycosides, polymyxins, clindamycin, tetracycline, erythromycin
Local anesthetics
Cardiovascular drugs
  Propranolol, quinidine, bretylium, trimethaphan, nitroglycerin
Furosemide
Dantrolene

TABLE 23-5 PRESENTING SIGNS OF MALIGNANT HYPERTHERMIA

Tachycardia
Tachypnea
Respiratory acidosis
Metabolic acidosis
Fever
Rigidity
Electrolyte derangement
Cyanosis
Unstable blood pressure

of 10 mg/kg. Because dantrolene is an antipyretic, other causes of increased temperature and hypermetabolism will be slightly improved by its use.

Recrudescence occurs in 10% of fulminant cases and presents with increased signs of MH after initial therapy. It is more common if MH symptoms and signs have not been completely eradicated and have occurred as long as 36 hours after the initial episode. Intensive observation and dantrolene therapy, therefore, is recommended for at least 48 hours.

Late complications of MH are cardiac failure, pulmonary edema, cerebral edema, renal failure, disseminated intravascular coagulopathy, muscle edema, and muscle necrosis. These complications are mostly secondary to

TABLE 23-6 DIFFERENTIAL DIAGNOSIS OF HYPERMETABOLIC STATE AND FEVER DURING ANESTHESIA

Increased ↑ heat production
Excessive shivering
Thyrotoxicosis
Pheochromocytoma
Osteogenesis imperfecta
Infection
Endotoxin
Transfusion reaction
Increased ↑ external heating
Heat lamps
Warming blankets
Room temperature
Decreased ↓ heat loss
Excessive drapes
Decreased ↓ central regulation
Intracranial hypothalamic lesion
Serotonin
Drug reaction
Glutethimide, MAO inhibitors, amphetamine, neuroleptics (neurolept malignant syndrome), tricyclic antidepressants, atropine, ketamine
Monitoring-machine malfunction
Heating blanket
Temperature probe

TABLE 23-7 TREATMENT OF MALIGNANT HYPERTHERMIA

1. Stop anesthesia and surgery immediately
2. Hyperventilate patient with 100% oxygen
3. Dantrolene, 2.5 mg/kg bolus
4. Change anesthesia machine to "clean machine"
5. Correct acidosis and electrolyte abnormalities (↑ K^+, ↑ Ca^{2+})
6. Cooling (surface, intravenous, body cavities)
7. Monitor (arterial lines, CVP, Foley, two temperature probes, capnograph)
8. Maintain urine output
9. Intensively monitor 48 to 72 hours, observe for recrudescence
10. Continue dantrolene 48 to 72 hours
11. Observe for late complications

the derangement in skeletal muscle metabolism but may be partly due to a generalized membrane defect in MH-susceptible patients. The severe demands of increased cardiac output, acidosis, hypoxia, and fever, as well as the effects of the increased fluids administered, can lead to cardiac or pulmonary failure and cerebral edema. Renal failure is attributable to myoglobinuria. The coagulopathy in part is related to an intrinsic platelet defect, although this relationship is by no means clear.

EPIDURAL AND SPINAL NARCOTICS

The use of epidural and spinal narcotics to relieve the pain associated with major trauma; abdominal, thoracic, orthopedic, and obstetric surgery; and chronic cancer pain is well documented. Rare respiratory depression compared to intravenous narcotics, and profound and prolonged analgesia makes this technique particularly advantageous in patients who are obese, have respiratory compromise, or who are undergoing thoracic or upper abdominal procedures. These postoperative surgical patients may develop respiratory complications because of splinting (inadequate analgesia) but often hypoventilate if enough intravenous narcotics are given. They are excellent candidates for epidural or spinal narcotics.

TABLE 23-8 SPINAL AND EPIDURAL NARCOTICS

Technique	Drug	Dose (mg)	Onset (min)	Duration (h)
Spinal	Morphine (preservative-free)	0.5–1.0	15–45	12–24
Epidural	Morphine (preservative-free)	5–10	15–60	5–36
	Meperidine	30–100	5–15	4–18
	Fentanyl	0.1	5–10	2.6–4
	Methadone	5	10–20	6–8

The advantages of narcotics placed close to opiate receptors located in the substantia gelatinosa of the dorsal horns of the spinal cord, thus effectively blocking pain perception, must be balanced against narcotic spread to other areas of the spinal cord (urinary retention) and brain stem (respiratory depression, pruritis, and nausea). Respiratory depression, when it occurs, is biphasic and can be seen within the first hour after administration or up to 24 hours later. Treatment includes assisted ventilation or intravenous naloxone (5 μg/kg/h).

The onset and the duration of action of spinal and epidural narcotics (Table 23-8) correlate with their pKa and lipid solubility. A polar hydrophilic drug like morphine, when given intraspinally, passes slowly into the spinal cord, and its onset of action is delayed. However, because most of the narcotic remains in the CSF and is slowly absorbed by the arachnoid granulations, its duration of action is long. Morphine is also transported in the CSF to brain-stem respiratory centers, where it causes delayed respiratory depression. Fentanyl is less ionized, hence much more lipid-soluble than morphine. Subarachnoid fentanyl quickly leaves the CSF and penetrates the spinal cord. Onset of action is rapid, and transport from the CSF to the respiratory centers is less likely. It also leaves the CNS quickly and thus has a short duration of action. Epidural narcotics must penetrate the dura in order to gain access to the CSF and spinal cord. Larger doses can produce significant blood levels in the epidural veins, and systemic effects may contribute to the initial analgesia. They reach the CSF quickly through direct dural penetration and by uptake into spinal segmental artery branches, thus accounting for the similar onset times of spinal and epidural narcotics.

Spinal and epidural narcotics can induce profound respiratory depression, nausea and vomiting, urinary retention, pruritis, and dysphoria, most of which can be reversed by intravenous naloxone.

For further information, please see Chapter 17 in Civetta JM, Taylor RW, Kirby RR: Critical Care. *Philadelphia: J. B. Lippincott, 1988*

BIBLIOGRAPHY

Amaranath L, Lavin TJ, Trusso RA, et al: Evaluation of creatinine phosphokinase screening as a predictor of malignant hyperthermia. *Br J Anaesth* 1983; 55:531

Britt BA: Malignant hyperthermia. *Can Anaesth Soc J* 1985; 32:666

Britt BA: Dantrolene—A review. *Can Anaesth Soc J* 1984; 31:61

Cousins MJ, Mather LE: Intrathecal and epidural administration of opioids. *Anesthesiology* 1984; 61:276

Giger U, Kaplan RF: Halothane-induced ATP depletion in platelets from patients susceptible to maligant hyperthermia and from controls. *Anesthesiology* 1983; 58:347

Grinberg R, Edelist G, Gordon A: Postoperative malignant hyperthermia episodes in patients who received "safe" anaesthetics. *Can Anaesth Soc J* 1983; 30:273

Gronert GA: Malignant hyperthermia. *Anesthesiology* 1980; 53:395

Kaplan RF, Feinglass N, Webster W, et al: Phenelzine overdose treated with dantrolene sodium. *JAMA* 1986; 255:642

May DC, Morris SW, Stewart RM, et al: Neuroleptic malignant syndrome: Response to dantrolene sodium. *Ann Intern Med* 1983; 98:183

Miller RD (ed): *Anesthesia,* 2nd ed, p 871. New York, Churchill Livingstone, 1986

Miller RD, Savarese JJ: Pharmacology of muscle relaxants and their antagonists. In Miller RD (ed): *Anesthesia,* 2nd ed, p 889. New York, Churchill Livingstone, 1986

Rawal N, Scott V, Bengt D, et al: Influence of naloxone infusion on analgesia and respiratory depression following epidural morphine. *Anesthesiology* 1986; 64:194

Rawal N, Sjostrand UH, Bengt D, et al: Epidural morphine for postoperative pain relief: A comparative study with intramuscular narcotic and intercostal nerve block. *Anesth Analg* 1983; 61:93

Shnider SM: Extradural and intrathecal narcotics. *Atlanta, American Society of Anesthesiologists Annual Meeting,* 1985, lecture 503, p 1

III. The Obstetrical Patient

24
Systemic Disease

Pregnancy, labor, delivery, and the immediate postpartum period cause profound physiologic changes that may result in exacerbations of chronic illnesses or death from an acute obstetric pathologic process. Major obstetric conditions include hypertensive disorders, amniotic fluid embolism, peripartum cardiomyopathy, and hemorrhagic and septic shock from placenta previa, abruptio placentae, uterine atony, inversion or rupture, and chorioamnionitis. The major nonobstetric conditions during pregnancy include respiratory disorders, mainly asthma, and cardiac disease, including rheumatic and congenital abnormalities.

PHYSIOLOGIC CONSIDERATIONS

RESPIRATORY SYSTEM

The upper respiratory tract (nares, nasopharynx, oropharynx, larynx, and trachea) are congested from capillary engorgement of the mucosa.

Minute ventilation is increased by 50% during pregnancy, with a greater rise during labor and delivery. Tidal volume increases to a greater extent than respiratory rate. Functional residual capacity (FRC) is decreased by about 20% with a fall in both expiratory reserve volume and residual volume. However, total lung capacity is unchanged. Oxygen consumption in pregnancy is increased about 20% with a further 60% increase during active labor.

Orotracheal intubation should be considered prior to nasotracheal intubation for general anesthesia or any other emergent conditions to prevent epistaxis. Small endotracheal tubes (6.0–7.0 mm) should be used.

Arterial blood gas partial pressures reveal a mild alkalemia with a decreased Pa_{CO2} (average 32 mm Hg) and a compensatory decrease in serum bicarbonate (average 20 meq/liter). Arterial P_{O_2} is increased approximately 10 mm Hg during pregnancy. However, during late pregnancy, especially with the patient supine, mild hypoxemia may occur because of the decrease in FRC and increase in oxygen consumption. The importance of adequate preoxygenation prior to rapid sequence induction of anesthesia cannot be overemphasized. Induction of anesthesia with the potent inhalation agents is rapid because of the decrease in FRC and increase in minute ventilation, rendering the patient more susceptible to deep levels of anesthesia.

CARDIOVASCULAR SYSTEM

Maternal blood volume increases throughout pregnancy and peaks to about 40% above nonpregnant levels at term. The increase in plasma volume (45–55%) is greater than the increase in red blood cell (RBC) volume (20–30%), resulting in a relative anemia of pregnancy. This increase in blood volume is associated with an increase in cardiac output, which begins early in gestation and peaks at levels 30% to 40% over nonpregnant values between 20 and 30 weeks. It then plateaus until term. The increase in cardiac output results from an increase in heart rate and stroke volume. During labor, cardiac output rises another 15% to 45% above prelabor values with an additional increase of 10% to 25% during uterine contractions. In the immediate postpartum period, cardiac output increases 30% to 40% over the labor period.

As a consequence of some of these cardiovascular changes, normal symptoms during pregnancy include fatigue, dyspnea, decreased exercise capacity, and light-headedness. Cardiac signs include distended neck veins, peripheral edema, widely split first heart sound, loud third heart sound, systolic ejection murmurs, and continuous murmurs (cervical venous hums and mammary souffle). Normal chest radiographs demonstrate increased lung markings and a horizontal position of the heart caused by diaphragmatic elevation. Electrocardiographic (EKG) changes may include a left QRS axis deviation and nonspecific ST segment and T-wave changes.

Despite an average 200- to 500-ml blood loss for routine, uncomplicated vaginal deliveries and 800- to 1000-ml blood loss for cesarean section deliveries, blood transfusions are seldom necessary because of the increased blood volume and the autotransfusion of approximately 500 ml of blood from the contracted uterus in the postpartum period. Although this increase in blood volume protects against blood loss at delivery, pulmonary congestion and cardiac failure can result in patients with underlying cardiac dysfunction. Patients with minimal cardiac reserve may tolerate early pregnancy and subsequently decompensate from increasing blood volume and cardiac output in the late second trimester and early third trimester. Patients with moderate cardiac reserve may tolerate pregnancy well until labor and delivery or the puerperium.

Uterine displacement by maternal position (lateral decubitus), bed position (left lateral tilt), or uterine displacement devices is imperative, especially in the last trimester, to avoid aortocaval compression. Moreover, maternal hypotension and placental hypoperfusion from aortocaval compression can be compounded by regional anesthesia that interferes with compensatory sympathetic nervous system mechanisms.

ASTHMA

The most common respiratory disease during pregnancy is asthma. Other respiratory ailments such as cystic fibrosis, tuberculosis, and sarcoidosis are rare and will not be discussed. Approximately 1% of pregnant women have asthma, and 10% to 15% of these women require hospitalization for acute, severe attacks. The overall effects of pregnancy on asthma are mixed (9 studies involving 1059 pregnancies). Forty-nine percent of patients remained unchanged, 29% of patients improved, and 22% worsened. Hormonal changes that may ameliorate the disease during pregnancy include increased elaboration of progesterone and cortisol. However, exacerbation of the disease may be promoted by the increase in prostaglandin $F_{2\alpha}$. Moreover, the increase in upper airway congestion, oxygen consumption, and decreased pulmonary reserve may further complicate any acute exacerbations. Asthma may increase the incidence of prematurity and increases perinatal and maternal mortality.

Management includes optimization of nondrug treatment before starting medication, which should be withheld during the first trimester if possible. Patients with chronic symptoms should continue taking medications that are considered safe during pregnancy (theophylline, beta-adrenergic agonists, anticholinergic agents, cromolyn, and corticosteroids). Treatment of an acute asthmatic episode includes oxygen, inhaled bronchodilators, or subcutaneous epinephrine. If no improvement is seen, intravenous aminophylline should be added, followed, if necessary, by intravenous corticosteroids. Arterial blood gas measurements and spirometry should be used to assess the effects of therapy.

Preventive measures and aggressive management of acute asthma symptoms during pregnancy are imperative to avoid perinatal and maternal mortality. Moreover, patients with benign courses during gestation may still have exacerbations of their disease during labor and delivery owing to increased stress, anxiety, ventilatory pattern, and hormonal changes.

NONCARDIAC PULMONARY EDEMA

Noncardiac pulmonary edema can have multiple etiologies in pregnancy, including amniotic fluid, thrombotic or air emboli, abruptio placentae, aspiration of gastric contents, beta-adrenergic agonist therapy, with or without corticosteroids for premature labor, blood transfusion reactions, dead fetus syndrome, septicemia, and shock (Table 24-1). Unfortunately, in the absence of known cardiac lesions, clincial differentiation between cardiac and noncardiac pulmonary edema may be quite difficult, often necessitating the use of a PA catheter. The hemodynamic changes of pregnancy can easily mimic a cardiogenic etiology, rendering a clinical diagnosis without invasive monitoring very difficult. Treatment of cardiac and noncardiac pulmonary edema differs. Cardiogenic edema requires inotropic, vasodilatory, or diuretic therapy, whereas respiratory failure necessitates aggressive ventilatory support.

Although amniotic fluid embolism is an uncommon event, the maternal mortality rate is reported as high as 86%. Following membrane rupture, amniotic fluid enters the maternal circulation through uteroplacental sinusoids or endocervical veins. This entity most commonly occurs during labor and vaginal or cesarean delivery and has been reported in early pregnancy during abortive procedures. Ensuing events include pulmonary embolism, uterine atony, and DIC. The clinical picture includes a sudden onset of respiratory distress, cyanosis, cardiovascular collapse, or coma. Other early signs include chills, sweating, hemorrhage, hyperreflexia, and seizures.

The diagnosis is made by the presence of fetal elements in the maternal circulation, which can be obtained from the right side of the heart through a central venous or PA catheter. The differential diagnosis includes other types of pulmonary emboli (thrombotic or air), eclampsia, intracranial hemorrhage, aspiration pneumonia, hemorrhagic or anaphylactic shock, and acute heart failure. Invasive monitoring should include an intra-arterial catheter for blood pressure and serial blood gas determinations and a PA catheter for diagnosis and treatment.

Treatment includes cardiopulmonary resuscitation with tracheal intubation to provide 100% oxygen, expeditious surgical evacuation of the uterus, vasopressor agents, digitalization and diuresis if ventricular failure is present, and, possibly, hydrocortisone (1–2 g bolus) to decrease endothelial edema and chemical irritation. Packed RBCs and other blood products should be used to treat the bleeding diathesis.

If cardiopulmonary resuscitation is indicated, be sure to displace the uterus by placing the patient in a left tilt position or using a uterine displacement device to prevent aortocaval compression. Evacuation of the uterus should be expedited because delivery of the fetus may relieve inferior vena cava compression and increase venous return.

CARDIAC DISEASE

MITRAL STENOSIS

Mitral stenosis accounts for approximately 90% of the rheumatic valvular lesions in pregnancy. Clinical symptoms are nonspecific and include fatigue and dyspnea. Physical examination of the heart includes a mid diastolic–presystolic murmur, heard best in the left lateral decubitus position. Chest radiographs and the EKG may be normal early in the course of the disease; however, signs of chamber enlargement and pulmonary congestion are present with progression. Mitral stenosis is characterized by left ventricular filling impairment. Avoidance of tachycardia, increased PA pressure, decreased systemic vascular resistance, and increased central blood volume are therefore essential in patient management. Pregnancy aggravates mitral stenosis because of the increased blood volume and heart rate, leading to a high incidence of pulmonary edema and atrial fibrillation.

TABLE 24-1 RESPIRATORY DISEASE IN PREGNANCY

Nonobstetric causes
Asthma
Obstetric causes (Noncardiac pulmonary edema)
Abruptio placentae
Amniotic fluid–air–thrombotic embolism
Beta-adrenoreceptor agonists for premature labor
Blood transfusions
Dead fetus syndrome
Preeclampsia/eclampsia
Pulmonary aspiration of gastric contents
Septic or hemorrhagic shock

AORTIC STENOSIS

Aortic stenosis is a rare valvular lesion during pregnancy. Clinical manifestations include congestive failure, syncope, angina, and a systolic ejection murmur, heard best at the second right intercostal space and radiating to the neck. The pathophysiology of aortic stenosis includes left ventricular systolic pressure overload. As in mitral stenosis, a decrease in systemic vascular resistance is poorly tolerated. Moreover, because of the fixed stroke volume, decreases in heart rate and venous return are also detrimental.

MITRAL INSUFFICIENCY

Mitral insufficiency is the second most common valvular lesion in pregnancy and is manifested by left ventricular volume overload. Severe mitral insufficiency is associated with left ventricular failure and a pansystolic murmur at the apex of the heart which radiates to the axilla. Increases in systemic vascular resistance, decreased heart rate, atrial dysrhythmias, and myocardial depressants are poorly tolerated. Mitral insufficiency is better tolerated during pregnancy than are stenotic lesions.

AORTIC INSUFFICIENCY

Aortic insufficiency also is relatively rare in pregnancy and is manifested by left ventricular volume overload. Symptoms are related to left ventricular failure. Clinical signs include an early diastolic murmur along the left sternal border. As in mitral regurgitation, increases in systemic vascular resistance, decreased heart rate, and myocardial depressants are undesirable. Aortic insufficiency also is reasonably well tolerated during pregnancy.

CONGENITAL HEART DISEASE

Approximately 25% of heart disease in pregnancy is congenital. It can be categorized as left-to-right shunt, right-to-left shunt, and valvular lesions.

Left-to-Right Shunt

The most common congenital heart lesions are atrial and ventricular septal defects, which are usually well tolerated in pregnancy. Nevertheless, the risk of left ventricular failure in pregnancy is increased. Major considerations include avoidance of increases in systemic vascular resistance, increases in heart rate, and supraventricular dysrhythmias.

Right-to-Left Shunt

The high-risk congenital disorders in pregnancy include right-to-left shunts, as seen in tetralogy of Fallot and the Eisenmenger's syndrome (any congenital heart lesion with a bidirectional or right-to-left shunt at the atrial, ventricular, or aortic level). In these disorders, termination of pregnancy should be considered. Decreases in systemic vascular resistance, blood volume, and venous return should be avoided. Increases in pulmonary vascular resistance promote right-to-left shunting; therefore, hypercapnia and hypoxia also are to be avoided.

Aortic Disease

Coarctation of the aorta and aortic manifestations of Marfan's syndrome pose significant problems in pregnancy. Aortic dissection is associated with pregnancy. Although histologic changes involving the aortic intima and media are controversial, physiologic changes during pregnancy, including increased blood volume and increased blood pressure during labor and delivery, may promote aortic dissection.

Mitral Valve Prolapse

Mitral valve prolapse is a common valvular lesion occurring in 5% of the general population and up to 17% of young, childbearing-age women. A wide range of clinical and echocardiographic manifestations are possible. It is characterized by floppy mitral valve leaflets and may result from mucinous changes in the connective tissues of the valve leaflets. It also may involve regional dysfunction of the mitral annulus fibrosus. Auscultatory findings include a mid-to-late systolic click, which is often accompanied by a mid-to-late systolic murmur.

The majority of patients with mitral valve prolapse are asymptomatic, and such patients tolerate pregnancy well, with no evidence of cardiac complications. Moreover, the incidence of antepartum and intrapartum complications or signs of fetal distress are no different when compared with pregnant patients with no known cardiac disorders. These patients should be treated in a routine fashion, except for the possibility of bacterial endocarditis prophylaxis during labor and delivery if an accompanying systolic murmur of mitral regurgitation is present.

A very small subset of patients, especially with severe redundant mitral valve leaflets, may develop the known complications of mitral valve prolapse, which include dysrhythmias, mitral insufficiency, infective endocarditis, and sudden death. As in mitral regurgitation, increases in systemic vascular resistance, and decreases in preload are not well tolerated in patients with associated mitral valvular incompetence.

For further information, please see Chapter 118 in Civetta JM, Taylor RW, Kirby RR: Critical Care. *Philadelphia: J. B. Lippincott, 1988*

BIBLIOGRAPHY

Bonica JJ: *Principles and Practice of Obstetric Analgesia and Anesthesia,* vol 1, p 17. Philadelphia, Davis, 1969

Hernandez E, Angell CS, Johnson JWC: Asthma in pregnancy: Current concepts. *Obstet Gynecol* 1980; 55:739

Hutchins GM, Moore GW, Skoog DK: The association of floppy mitral valve with disjunction of the mitral annulus fibrosus. *N Engl J Med* 1986; 314:535

James CF, Banner T, Levelle JP, et al: Noninvasive determination of cardiac output throughout pregnancy. *Anesthesiology* 1985; 63(3A):A434

Keefer JR, Strauss RG, Civetta JM, et al: Noncardiogenic pulmonary edema and invasive cardiovascular monitoring. *Obstet Gynecol* 1981; 58:46

Marx GF: Cardiopulmonary resuscitation of late-pregnant women (Letter). *Anesthesiology* 1982; 56:156

Morgan M: Amniotic fluid embolism. *Anaesthesia* 1979; 34:20

Nishimura RA, McGoon MD, Shub C, et al: Echocardiographically documented mitral-valve prolapse: Long-term followup of 237 patients. *N Engl J Med* 1985; 313:1305

Pernoll ML, Metcalf J, Kovach PA, et al: Ventilation during rest and exercise in pregnancy and postpartum. *Respir Physiol* 1975; 25:295

Rayburn WF, Fontana ME: Mitral valve prolapse and pregnancy. *Am J Obstet Gynecol* 1981; 141:9

Sangoul F, Fox GS, Houle GL: Effect of regional analgesia on maternal oxygen consumption during the first stage of labor. *Am J Obstet Gynecol* 1975; 121:1080

Schaerf RHM, de Campo T, Civetta JM: Hemodynamic alterations and rapid diagnosis in a case of amniotic-fluid embolus. *Anesthesiology* 1977; 46:155

Szekely P, Snaith L: *Heart Disease and Pregnancy.* Edinburgh, Churchill Livingstone, 1974

Turner ES, Greenberger PA, Patterson R: Management of the pregnant asthmatic patient. *Ann Intern Med* 1980; 93:905

Ueland K: Maternal cardiovascular dynamics. VII. Intrapartum blood volume changes. *Am J Obstet Gynecol* 1976; 126:671

Ueland K, Hansen JM: Maternal cardiovascular dynamics. II. Posture and uterine contractions. *Am J Obstet Gynecol* 1969; 103:1

25 Hemorrhagic Disorders

Hemorrhage is a leading cause of maternal mortality and morbidity. Although abortion and ectopic pregnancy are hemorrhagic disorders, this chapter focuses primarily on abruptio placentae, placenta previa, and postpartum bleeding disorders. It is in these third trimester events that special concerns for the pregnant patient are most relevant. Hence, a review of changes pertinent to the cardiovascular and hematologic system is important.

PHYSIOLOGIC CHANGES OF PREGNANCY

CARDIOVASCULAR SYSTEM

Blood volume increases 30% to 50% during pregnancy, resulting in an additional 1000 to 2000 ml. Because red blood cell volume increases somewhat less than does plasma volume, a dilutional anemia may result. Cardiac output increases by 30% to 50%, predominantly as a result of increased stroke volume, although the heart rate also increases 10 to 12 beats per minute (bpm). During labor, cardiac output increases even further, both progressively and with each contraction, and may be as much as 80% to 90% above normal during the immediate 10 to 15 minutes following birth. Total peripheral resistance is decreased approximately 15%, as is mean arterial blood pressure (MAP). Although central venous pressure (CVP) is unchanged, venous pressure in the lower extremities is elevated because of vena caval compression by the gravid uterus.

Aortocaval compression by the uterus when the patient is supine reduces venous return and cardiac output significantly. Thus, the optimal position for the hemorrhaging obstetric patient is one in which the uterus has little or no possibility of impeding venous return. Resuscitative efforts in pregnant women may be seriously hampered by the supine position.

Blood loss at the time of delivery is another important "physiologic" phenomenon. Accurately measured loss at vaginal delivery averages 500 ml and is normal for most patients. At cesarean section, a 1000-ml loss is normal.

Since blood volume increases by 1000 to 2000 ml during pregnancy, these physiologic alterations complement one another appropriately. In fact, if blood loss is not severe, little decrease in hematocrit is seen even after cesarean delivery.

HEMATOLOGIC AND COAGULATION CHANGES

Because blood volume increases during pregnancy, predominantly in the plasma component, a hemoglobin decrease of about 1 g/dl is common. Therefore, if 12 to 12.5 g/dl is normal, a level less than 11 g/dl cannot be attributed to the dilutional effects of the expanded blood volume. Furthermore, if the patient has received appropriate prenatal care and that care has included iron supplementation, the hemoglobin level may not drop at all.

Coagulation is enhanced during pregnancy, presumably to inhibit blood loss at the time of delivery. Fibrinogen of 400 to 650 mg/dl is normal in late pregnancy, whereas levels of 200 to 450 mg/dl are normal in the nonpregnant state. Factors IV, VII, VIII, and X are also increased; prothrombin is elevated slightly. Factors XI and XIII decrease minimally. The prothrombin time and partial thromboplastin time are shortened minimally. Plasminogen also increases.

Most recent studies indicate a progressive decline in platelet count. However, the value usually remains within the normal range. This decline is often accompanied by a rise in platelet size, indicating the platelets are younger, and increased destruction may be present. Finally, the average life span of platelets during pregnancy is shortened slightly.

The most important difference between the pregnant and nonpregnant patient is the fetus. Because significant increases in perinatal morbidity and mortality occur in patients with antepartum bleeding, an important aspect of therapy is directed toward fetal preservation. The status of the fetus, including gestational age and the presence or absence of fetal distress, signficantly influences the management at any given time.

DISORDERS

PLACENTA PREVIA

Diagnosis

Four categories of placenta previa exist (Table 25-1). The condition occurs in approximately 1 of 150 to 200 pregnancies. Bleeding classically is painless as opposed to that in abruptio placentae, which usually is accompanied by painful uterine contractions. However, approximately 20% of patients with placenta previa will also have pain. Usually, the first bleeding episode is not severe and is rarely fatal. However, repeat episodes are common, often more severe, and necessitate hospitalization.

Bleeding in placenta previa is thought to result from gradual disruption of

TABLE 25-1 CATEGORIES FOR PLACENTA PREVIA

Low lying placenta (type I)—The placenta is implanted in the lower uterine segment, but placental tissue does not encroach upon or cover the internal os of the cervix.
Marginal placenta previa (type II)—The placenta lies very low in the lower uterine segment and actually impinges upon the internal os.
Partial placenta previa (type III)—The internal os is partially but not completely covered by placental tissue.
Total placental previa (type IV)—Placental tissue covers the entire cervical os.

the placenta from the lower uterine segment as it thins and stretches in preparation for labor. The normal hemostatic mechanism, uterine contraction, does not occur, and bleeding ensues from maternal vessels at the placental site.

Treatment

Severity of bleeding and stage of gestation are the principal determinants of management. Usually, the patient enters the hospital and remains at bed rest. Evaluation continues as blood is sent for typing and cross-matching. If bleeding is moderately severe, large-bore intravenous cannulas are placed, and volume replacement is begun with Ringer's lactate or normal saline. A central venous catheter may be indicated as well as a Foley catheter to monitor urine output accurately. Fetal assessment should be performed immediately. An estimation of gestational age also is indicated.

In most instances, time permits ultrasound evaluation to determine placental location. In those rare cases where hemorrhage is so severe that maternal or fetal life is in jeopardy, cesarean section may be indicated immediately. If so, critical care management is the same as for any other hemorrhaging patient, always keeping in mind the normal physiologic changes of pregnancy.

Once the diagnosis is confirmed, if the fetus is at or beyond 35 weeks' gestation, and if bleeding persists, termination of pregnancy is appropriate. Prior to cesarean section, some obstetricians perform a double setup examination. The patient is taken to the operating room, prepared, and draped. An anesthesiologist is in attendance. The obstetrician performs a speculum examination to rule out other causes of vaginal bleeding and a digital examination to estimate dilation of the cervix and to confirm the presence or absence of the placenta previa. If a significant hemorrhage occurs, rapid induction of general anesthesia is followed by cesarean section.

ABRUPTIO PLACENTAE

Diagnosis

In this condition, the placenta separates prematurely from its attachment to the uterine wall. It occurs in 1 in 90 to 1 in 250 births. Maternal mortality is approximately 2% if grade 0 patients are excluded. The perinatal mortality rate is as high as 36.5% for all infants and 25% for those weighing 1000 g or more. Anatomically, there are three types of abruptio placentae, and these are illustrated in Figure 25-1. Clinically, four grades of placental abruption exist and are listed in Table 25-2.

Because a significant portion of bleeding may occur within the uterus and not be manifested externally, hypovolemia and shock may be grossly out of proportion to the observed blood loss. Maternal hypertension is the most consistently identified factor predisposing to placental abruption. It is particularly common in grade 3 abruption and may occur in 40% to 50% of cases.

External maternal trauma, although uncommon as an etiology, does contribute a small percentage of the total; therefore, the potential for abruptio placentae following abdominal trauma should always be considered.

Treatment

Management of hemorrhage is similar to that for any other bleeding patient. Immediate typing and cross-matching of blood are necessary. Large-bore intravenous cannulas and perhaps central venous catheters are indicated. Clotting studies should be performed. Before blood is available, replacement therapy should be initiated with Ringer's lactate.

Gestational age is important in determining management. For the patient with a term fetus in whom the bleeding can be controlled and no significant fetal distress is present, labor is allowed and may even be initiated or augmented with the expectation that vaginal delivery will occur. If blood replacement cannot keep pace with blood loss or if fetal distress becomes apparent, cesarean section is indicated. In the patient with a preterm fetus, termination of pregnancy is delayed unless conditions force the obstetrician's hand. If the fetus is dead, vaginal delivery is always preferred and usually can be accomplished.

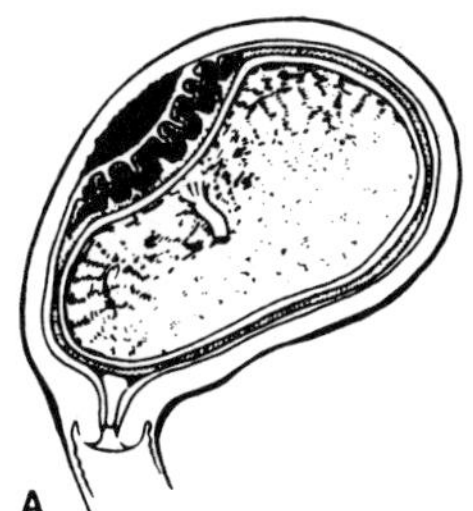

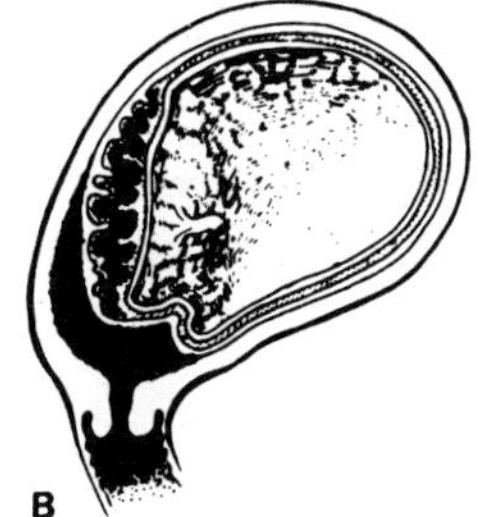

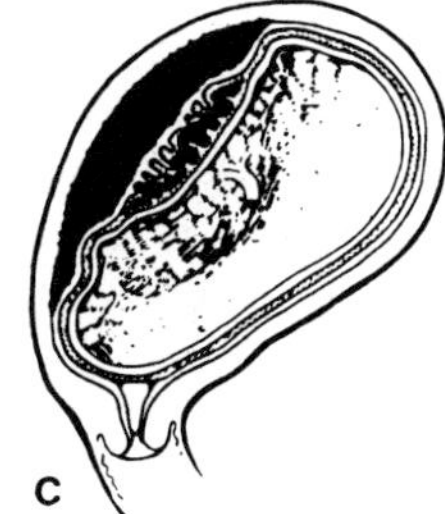

Figure 25-1 Anatomic classification of abruptio placenta: mild abruption with some concealed hemorrhage (*A*), severe abruption with external hemorrhage (*B*), severe abruption with concealed abruption (*C*). (Hayashi RH, et al: Bleeding in pregnancy. In Knuppel RA, Drukker J (eds): *High-Risk Pregnancy: A Team Approach*, p 419. Philadelphia, WB Saunders, 1986)

TABLE 25-2 GRADING SYSTEM FOR ABRUPTIO PLACENTAE

Grade 0	The patient is asymptomatic, and there is no evidence of hemorrhage. However, at delivery, the abruption is obvious when the placenta is examined, and an adherent clot is found on its surface.
Grade 1	Vaginal bleeding is present but not excessive. Uterine tetany and tenderness may be present. The fetus is not affected.
Grade 2	Vaginal bleeding is present and may or may not be external. Uterine tenderness and tetany are usually evident, as are signs of fetal distress. Maternal cardiovascular symptoms are minimal.
Grade 3	Vaginal bleeding may or may not occur, and there is obvious uterine tetany with marked tenderness of the uterus. Maternal hypotension is frequent, and fetal death may have occurred. Clotting abnormalities are also frequent.

At the time of cesarean section or after vaginal delivery, patients may continue to hemorrhage as a result of uterine atony. In some instances, blood from the retroplacental clot extravasates into and between the muscle fibers of the myometrium, preventing effective uterine contractions (Couvelair uterus). Bleeding may be severe enough to necessitate hysterectomy. This procedure frequently is associated with major blood loss.

DISSEMINATED INTRAVASCULAR COAGULATION

Diagnosis

In the obstetric population, disseminated intravascular coagulation (DIC) is seen in several different disease states, including placental abruption, the dead fetus syndrome, amniotic fluid embolism, gram-negative sepsis, saline abortions, and severe preeclampsia/eclampsia. In abruptio placentae release of thromboplastin in the damaged placental tissue triggers the extrinsic clotting pathway. Also contributing is consumption of coagulation factors by the retroplacental clot. Finally, placental abruption causes activation of circulating plasminogen, which destroys circulating fibrinogen and promotes fibrinolysis.

The diagnosis depends on the manifestations of widespread bleeding, hypofibrinogenemia, platelet deficiency, and decreased factors V and VIII as well as increased fibrin degradation products. As the clotting test results are evaluated, keep in mind that normal values in pregnancy are not those of the nonpregnant state. A normal fibrinogen concentration in the third trimester is 450 mg/dl; thus a value of 300 mg/dl may be associated with coagulation abnormalities. If it is less than 150 mg/dl, a significant deficit exists.

Treatment

As is true of any patient who has received considerable amounts of bank blood, the most likely clotting abnormality is thrombocytopenia resulting from the dilutional effect of platelet-poor blood. Thus, fresh whole blood or platelet concentrates should be administered once patients receive more than 5 to 7 units of bank blood.

Definitive treatment of DIC in the obstetric patient with abruption is delivery of the fetus and removal of the placenta. Neither heparin nor fibrinogen, both of which were in vogue in the past, is indicated in these patients. The problem almost always resolves once the pregnancy has been terminated and the placenta removed.

POSTPARTUM HEMORRHAGE

The mechanism primarily responsible for hemostasis in the immediate postpartum period is uterine contractility. When the placenta separates, many vessels in the decidua are sheared off. These maternal vessels, which meander through the uterine musculature, are enlarged during pregnancy. However, because they course through the uterine musculature, contraction of the intertwining muscle fibers compresses them and prevents continued hemorrhage.

Postpartum hemorrhage results from uterine atony, retained placental fragments, injury to pelvic soft tissues, incomplete episiotomy repair, and uterine inversion. It occurs in 3% to 5% of all pregnancies; approximately 20% of patients with antepartum hemorrhage also have postpartum hemorrhage.

The greatly enlarged veins and arteries that course in and between uterine muscle fibers bleed freely until squeezed shut by the contracting musculature. Treatment of postpartum hemorrhage is aimed at improving the efficiency of this mechanism. Manual massage usually causes a relaxed and boggy uterus to contract and "firm up" into a tight ball. If bleeding continues despite a firmly contracted uterus, inspection of the birth canal for other causes is indicated. Vaginal and cervical lacerations and bleeding episiotomies can be diagnosed only by visual inspection. They are not controlled by uterine contractions; treatment is surgical repair. Retention of placental fragments is best diagnosed by exclusion or by examination of the placenta, which reveals large portions missing. Treatment is curettage.

Although all drugs that contract the uterus are oxytocic, the term is usually reserved for agents that possess characteristics of oxytocin secreted by the posterior pituitary gland. Clinically useful synthetic agents are not tainted by the actions of pitressin, a potent vasoconstrictor particularly of the coronary arteries. They do have other cardiovascular effects, however, and when given by intravenous "push" can induce significant hypotension. Thus, they should always be administered as a dilute solution, 20 to 40 U/liter of Ringer's lactate or normal saline.

These agents also have some antidiuretic hormone effect. Even in dilute concentrations, they should not be administered for long periods of time in electrolyte-free solutions. Hyponatremia, with all its attendant complications, can result when oxytocin is administered in such a manner.

The ergot alkaloids ergonovine (ergotrate and methylergonovine) and methergine are also potent uterine stimulants. Because they are direct vasoconstrictors and can produce marked and sustained elevations in blood pressure, they should not be used in patients with known chronic or pregnancy-related hypertension. They potentiate the actions of other vasoconstrictors and have been associated with cerebral hemorrhage.

Prostaglandins also are useful in the treatment of postpartum hemorrhage and act as oxytocic agents. Usually, they are a third choice behind oxytocin and the ergot drugs. Prostaglandin $F_{2\alpha}$ is helpful when injected intramyometrially. The recommended dose is 1 mg. Following vaginal delivery, this route is accessible transabdominally or paracervically. Recently, 15-methyl prostaglandin F_2 administered intramuscularly has been shown to be effective in a dose of 0.25 mg repeated every 1 to 2 hours. These agents can produce nausea and vomiting and are capable of producing hypertension, although to a lesser extent than that produced by the ergot alkaloids. Hence, caution and appropriate monitoring should always be used, particularly in the hypertensive patient.

When pharmacologic methods fail, surgical intervention is necessary. As described previously, inspection of the birth canal is essential when uterine massage and oxytoxic drugs fail. If no local causes are found, retained placental fragments should be suspected. If they are present, curettage is indicated. Should bleeding continue, some obstetricians recommend packing the uterus; this procedure is controversial at best. Others would proceed with uterine artery or hypogastric artery ligation and even hysterectomy. Anesthesiologists should avoid the use of anything except analgesic concentrations of the inhalation agents halothane, enflurane, and isoflurane, which in higher doses relax the uterus.

For further information, please see Chapter 117 in Civetta JM, Taylor RW, Kirby RR: Critical Care. *Philadelphia: J. B. Lippincott, 1988*

BIBLIOGRAPHY

Anderson TW, Padua CB, Stenger V, et al: Cardiovascular effects of rapid intravenous injection of synthetic oxytocin during elective cesarean section. *Clin Pharmacol Ther* 1965; 6:345

Benedetti TJ: Obstetric hemorrhage. In Gabbe SG, Niebyl JR, Simpson JL (eds): *Obstetrics: Normal and Problem Pregnancies,* p 485. New York, Churchill Livingstone, 1986

Biehl DR: Antepartum and postpartum hemorrhage. In Shnider SM, Levinson G (eds): *Anesthesia for Obstetrics,* p 281. Baltimore, Williams & Wilkins, 1987

Brenner WE, Edelman DA, Hendricks CH: Characteristics of patients with placenta previa and results of "expectant management." *Ann J Obstet Gynecol* 1978; 132:180

Casady GN, Moore DC, Bridenbaugh LD: Postpartum hypertension after use of vasoconstrictor and oxytocic drugs: Etiology, incidence, complications and treatment. *JAMA* 1960; 172:101

Hayashi RH, Castillo MS: Bleeding in pregnancy. In Knuppel RA, Drukker JE (eds): *High-Risk Pregnancy: A Team Approach,* p 419. Philadelphia, WB Saunders, 1986

Hayashi RH, Castillo MS, Noah ML: Management of severe postpartum hemorrhage due to uterine atony using an analogue of prostaglandin $F_{2\alpha}$. *Obstet Gynecol* 1981; 58:426

Hurd WW, Miodovnik M, Hertzberg V, et al: Selective management of abruptio placentae: A prospective study. *Obstet Gynecol* 1983; 61:467

Kanb DR: Abruptio placentae: An assessment of the time and method of delivery. *Obstet Gynecol* 1978; 52:625

Marx GF: Cardiopulmonary resuscitation in late-pregnant women. *Anesthesiology* 1982; 56:156

Naeye RL, Harkness WL, Utts J: Abruptio placentae and perinatal death: A prospective study. *Am J Obstet Gynecol* 1977; 128:740

Pritchard JA: Genesis of severe placental abruption. *Am J Obstet Gynecol* 1970; 108:22

Pritchard JA, Baldwin RM, Dickey JC: Blood volume changes in pregnancy and the puerperium. *Am J Obstet Gynecol* 1962; 84:1271

Pritchard JA, Hunt CF: A comparison of the hematologic responses following the routine prenatal administration of intramuscular and oral iron. *Surg Gynecol Obstet* 1958; 106:516

Pritchard JA, MacDonald PC, Gant Norman F: Obstetric hemorrhage. In Pritchard JA, MacDonald PC, Gant NF (eds): Williams Obstetrics, 17th ed, p 389. East Norwalk, CT, Appleton-Century-Crofts, 1985

Rizos N, Doran TA, Miskin M, et al: Natural history of placenta previa ascertained by diagnostic ultrasound. *Am J Obstet Gynecol* 1979; 133:287

Sagi A, Creter D, Goldman J, et al: Platelet functions before, during and after labor. *Acta Haematol* (Basel) 1981; 65:67

Stirling Y, Woolf L, North WRS, et al: Haemostasis in normal pregnancy. *Thromb Haemost* 1984; 52:176

Tomkinson J, Turnbull A, Robson G, et al: *Report on Confidential Enquiries into Maternal Deaths in England and Wales 1979–81. London, Her Majesty's Stationery Office*

Vroys N, Ullery JC, Hanusek GE: The cardiac output changes in various positions in pregnancy. *Am J Obstet Gynecol* 1961; 83:1312

26
Hypertensive Disorders: Preeclampsia and Eclampsia

Approximately 250,000 American women become hypertensive during their pregnancies each year. A large proportion of these women will have preeclampsia, the complications of which contribute significantly to maternal and neonatal morbidity and mortality. The pathophysiology and therapy of the complications of severe preeclampsia are challenging and controversial. The primary focus of this chapter will be the intensive care of the severely preeclamptic patient.

DEFINITIONS

Hypertensive disorders of pregnancy are classified into three categories (Table 26-1), and the degree of hypertension and proteinuria during pregnancy is categorized (Table 26-2). Severe preeclampsia is defined as severe hypertension and proteinuria greater than 5 g/24 hr (3–4 +), and one or more of the following : oliguria less than 400 ml/24 hr, cerebral or visual symptoms, epigastric pain, pulmonary edema, or cyanosis. By definition, preeclampsia is not manifested before the 20th week of gestation. Eclampsia is preeclampsia with convulsions.

INCIDENCE

Preeclampsia occurs in approximately 5% to 7% of all pregnancies and is more frequently a disease of primigravidas. Severe preeclampsia occurs in only 10% of all preeclamptic patients. The incidence of eclampsia is approximately 0.2%, but wide regional variations occur.

MATERNAL MORTALITY

Causes of maternal death associated with preeclampsia or eclampsia are variable (Table 26-3). Cerebral hemorrhage consistently is reported as the

TABLE 26-1 CLASSIFICATION OF HYPERTENSIVE DISORDERS DURING PREGNANCY

- Pregnancy-induced hypertension
  - Without proteinuria or generalized edema (gestational hypertension)
  - With proteinuria or generalized edema (preeclampsia)
    - Mild
    - Severe
  - Eclampsia (preeclampsia with convulsions)
- Chronic hypertension
- Pregnancy-aggravated hypertension
  - Chronic hypertension with superimposed preeclampsia or eclampsia

most common cause of death, although renal failure and pulmonary edema are also frequent. A delay in diagnosis and treatment was documented in over 50% of fatal cases. Inadequate treatment of hypertension is critical in many fatal cases. Porapakkham reported a 22% maternal fatality rate when systolic blood pressure was higher than 200 mm Hg compared with an overall maternal death rate of 4.7%. Although most eclamptic patients are primiparas, fatal eclampsia is more often a problem of multiparas.

DIAGNOSIS

The diagnosis of severe preeclampsia is relatively straightforward. Pregnancy must be past the 20th week of gestation, but the disease rarely is seen before the 24th week of gestation unless a hydatidiform mole is present. Patients usually have a history of rapid weight gain in the preceding month and have significant peripheral edema, especially around the hands and face. Proteinuria is inevitably present. Without it, the diagnosis probably is gestational

TABLE 26-2 DEFINITION OF HYPERTENSION AND PROTEINURIA DURING PREGNANCY

- Hypertension
  - Two blood pressures (BP) taken at least 6 hr apart
  - Mild
    - Systolic BP $\geq$ 140 mm Hg or a rise of 30 mm Hg over baseline
    - Diastolic BP $\geq$ 90 mm Hg or a rise of 15 mm Hg over baseline
  - Severe
    - Systolic BP $>$ 150 mm Hg (or)
    - Diastolic BP $>$ 110 mm Hg
- Proteinuria
  - 300 mg or more per 24-hr collection (or)
  - 1 g/liter in two random urine specimens (1–2+)
  - Severe preeclampsia ($>$ 5 g every 24 hr, 3–4+)

TABLE 26-3 CAUSES OF DEATH ASSOCIATED WITH PREECLAMPSIA OR ECLAMPSIA*

Cause of Death	Donnelly et al* (1946–1953)	Hibbard* (1957–1979)	Lopez-Llera* (1963–1979)	Massachusetts Committee on Maternal Welfare (Evans et al)* (1954–1982)
Cerebral				
Hemorrhage	180(34%)	21 (31%)	62 (72%)	14 (29%)
Edema	—	13 (19%)	—	6 (12%)
Pulmonary				
Edema	133 (25%)	3 (5%)	—	3 (6%)
Insufficiency	29 (5%)	4 (6%)	10 (12%)	—
Hepatic				
Rupture	—	—	1 (1%)	3 (6%)
Necrosis	—	10 (6%)	—	2 (4%)
Renal				
Uremia	30 (6%)	2 (3%)	—	7 (14%)
Necrosis	—	5 (8%)	1 (1%)	—
Coagulopathy	39 (7%)	6 (9%)	7 (8%)	6 (12%)
Anesthesia	12 (2%)	—	—	—
Sepsis	18 (3%)	—	2 (2%)	—
Drug overdose	—	2 (3%)	—	—
Not determined	92 (17%)	1 (2%)	3 (4%)	8 (16%)
Total	533	67	86	49

(Modified from Evans S, Frigoletto FD, Jr Jewett JF: *N Engl J Med* 1983; 309:1644.)
*See bibliography.

hypertension or chronic hypertension. Severe preeclampsia is characterized by hypertension and one or more of the other signs and symptoms listed in Table 26-4. Patients occasionally present with pulmonary edema, cyanosis, or a history of seizures.

TREATMENT

The *only* definitive treatment of severe preeclampsia or eclampsia is delivery of the fetus and placenta. Symptoms almost always resolve within 48 to 72 hours of delivery. Exceptions include the catastrophic complications of cerebral hemorrhage, renal cortical necrosis, and cardiac failure.

Symptoms should be treated until expeditious delivery is accomplished. Successful induction of labor is often possible despite a clinically unfavorable cervix. Supplemental maternal oxygen is recommended for parturients in labor since fetal distress is common. Unsuccessful induction, a remote term date, and fetal distress are frequent indications for cesarean section. Primary treatment principles include control of and prophylaxis against seizures, control of severe hypertension, and expeditous delivery. Primary treatment of severe preeclampsia usually is successful. However, exacerbations may necessitate admission to the intensive care unit.

TABLE 26-4 SIGNS AND SYMPTOMS OF PREECLAMPSIA

Abnormality	Mild	Severe
Diastolic blood pressure	< 100 mm Hg	≥ 110 mm Hg
Proteinuria	Trace to 1+	2+ −4+
Headache	Absent	Present
Visual disturbances	Absent	Present
Upper abdominal pain	Absent	Present
Oliguria	Absent	Present
Convulsions	Absent	Present
Serum creatinine	Normal	Elevated
Thrombocytopenia	Absent	Present
Elevated liver enzymes	Absent-minimal	Present
Pulmonary edema	Absent	Present
Fetal growth retardation	Absent	Present

(Modified from Cunningham FC, Pritchard JA: *Med Clin North Am* 1984; 68:505.)

Seizures

Eclamptic seizures usually are preventable or at least controllable. Magnesium sulfate is the most common drug used for prophylaxis and control in the United States. It probably exerts its anticonvulsant action on the cerebral cortex and has minimal sedative and no analgesic properties in therapeutic doses. Diazepam is used in much of the rest of the world, and chlormethiazole (a sedative/hypnotic drug) is used in the United Kingdom. These agents cause generalized central nervous system (CNS) depression in the mother and fetus. Other undesirable neonatal effects of diazepam are hypotonia, depression of thermal regulation, and possible respiratory depression.

The diagnosis of severe preeclampsia mandates immediate seizure prophylaxis with magnesium sulfate (Table 26-5). Therapeutic plasma magnesium levels range from 4 to 8 meq/liter (Table 26-6). Overdosage can result in significant maternal and fetal respiratory or cardiac embarrassment. When

TABLE 26-5 MAGNESIUM SULFATE DOSAGE

1. Give 4 g magnesium sulfate as a 20% solution intravenously at a rate of 1 g/min during eclamptic seizures or over 10–15 min for seizure prophylaxis.
2. Start a continuous intravenous infusion of magnesium sulfate at the rate of 1–3 g/hr and continue the infusion for at least 24 hr after delivery.
3. If convulsions persist after 15 min give 2–4 g Mg intravenously at a rate no faster than 1 g/min.
4. Monitor the patient's Mg level
   a. The patellar reflex is present (as long as this reflex is present, the patient does not have an overdose of magnesium sulfate).
   b. Respirations are not depressed.
   c. Urine output is at least 30 ml/hr the previous 3 hr.
   d. Measurement of serum Mg level
      —if seizures occur despite normal administration rates.
      —after prolonged infusions (> 8 hr).

TABLE 26-6 EFFECTS OF PLASMA MAGNESIUM LEVELS

Plasma Mg (meq/liter)	Effects
1.5–2.0	Normal plasma level
4.0–8.0	Therapeutic range for seizure prophylaxis
5.0–10.0	EKG changes: widened PR interval and QRS complex
10.0	Loss of deep tendon reflexes
12.0	Skeletal muscle relaxation
15.0	SA and AV block
15–20	Respiratory paralysis (patient conscious)
25	Cardiac arrest

severe respiratory impairment occurs, it is treated with calcium chloride or calcium gluconate, 1 g intravenously, and by prompt tracheal intubation and positive-pressure ventilation if necessary. Magnesium primarily is cleared by renal excretion; thus urine output must be followed closely. Deep tendon reflexes should be monitored hourly. If they disappear, the infusion rate should be markedly reduced. Therapy must be continued at least 24 hours after delivery until all symptoms have abated. Pritchard reported that only 5 of 245 eclamptic women needed supplemental medication to control seizures. In these cases, slow intravenous administration of sodium amobarbital (up to 250 mg) was effective.

Hypertension

Severe acute hypertension is the most dangerous symptom of preeclampsia and is implicated in a large number of fatal complications. Diastolic blood pressures above 110 mm Hg require immediate treatment. Hydralazine, 5 to 10 mg intravenously, should be administered every 15 to 20 minutes until the diastolic blood pressure is below 110 mm Hg. If hydralazine does not reduce maternal mean arterial pressure (MAP) more than 20% to 30%, placental blood flow is preserved or increased. Reduction of the parturient's blood pressure to normal levels is not desirable because placental perfusion may be compromised and result in fetal distress.

Intravenous hydralazine therapy is almost always successful. However, if 40 to 60 mg has been given over 2 hours and the diastolic blood pressure is still above 110 mm Hg, more potent drugs are needed. Small doses of intravenous propranolol, 0.5 to 2 mg, may be efficacious in the parturient who has increased her heart rate significantly in compensation for the vasodilatory effects of hydralazine. Intravenous labetalol is a possible second-line drug. However, despite a history of safety when given orally to hypertensive pregnant patients, intravenous therapy has not been studied in preeclamptic patients. Severely hypertensive preeclamptic patients who are refractory to hydralazine should be admitted to the ICU.

Intravenous diazoxide is accompanied by adverse effects in the pregnant patient. It inhibits uterine contractions, may cause hyperglycemia in the mother and infant, causes sodium, water, and uric acid retention, and is associated with severe hypotension when it is administered after other antihypertensive agents.

Long-term use of potent vasodilators during labor has not been studied, so delivery should be expedited after the hypertension has been controlled. Their safe use requires intra-arterial pressure monitoring and sometimes pulmonary artery (PA) catheterization. The most useful intravenous drugs in these circumstances include nitroglycerin (NTG), sodium nitroprusside (SNP), and trimethaphan.

Nitroglycerin has a rapid onset and short duration of action. No toxic maternal or fetal effects are known, and uterine blood flow may improve with NTG administration. In higher doses (greater than 1 μg/kg/min), NTG has both venous and arteriolar dilating properties. In severe preeclamptic patients, the antihypertensive effects primarily result from a reduction of right ventricular preload and consequent lowering of cardiac output and blood pressure. Resistance to the antihypertensive effects of NTG is more common in patients receiving fluid therapy (improved venous return).

Sodium nitroprusside is a potent vasodilator. Fetal cyanide toxicity has been reported in sheep with large doses or when significant prolonged maternal hypotension is induced. Hence, use of SNP in pregnant women is limited. However, studies of SNP in pregnant ewes, where less than a 30% reduction in MAP was induced, failed to document fetal cyanide toxicity. Short-term use may be life-saving when other vasodilators fail and significant maternal hypertension persists. Nitroprusside also improves uterine blood flow in sheep.

Trimethaphan is a ganglionic blocker and is used to control severe acute hypertension in preeclampsia. It has a relatively high failure rate and tachyphylaxis can occur. The combination of increased arterial blood pressure, cerebral edema, and possible intracerebral hemorrhage is associated with increased intracranial pressure (ICP) in the severely preeclamptic patient. If increased ICP is suspected, trimethaphan is the drug of choice when potent vasodilation is needed. It does not increase ICP as much as does NTG or SNP. Whether the increase in ICP from acute hypertension is worse than the increase that results from NTG or SNP is unknown. However, intracerebral hemorrhage is still the most likely cause of death. Hence, control of severe hypertension takes precedence, even though the risk of ICP exacerbation is present.

For further information, please see Chapter 116 in Civetta JM, Taylor RW, Kirby RR: Critical Care. *Philadelphia: J. B. Lippincott, 1988*

BIBLIOGRAPHY

Borges LF, Gucer G: Effect of magnesium on epileptic foci. *Epilepsia* 1978; 19:81

Cotton DB, Longmire S, Jones MM, et al: Cardiovascular alterations in severe pregnancy-induced hypertension: Effects of intravenous nitroglycerin coupled with blood expansion. *Am J Obstet Gynecol* 1986; 154:1053

Cunningham FG, Pritchard JA: How should hypertension during pregnancy be managed? *Med Clin North Am* 1984; 68:505

Donnelly JF, Lock FR: Causes of death in five hundred thirty-three fatal cases of toxemia of pregnancy. *Am J Obstet Gynecol* 1954; 68:184

Ellis SC, Wheeler AS, James FM III, et al: Fetal and maternal effects of sodium nitroprusside used to counteract hypertension in gravid ewes. *Am J Obstet Gynecol* 1982; 143:766

Evans S, Frigoletto FD Jr, Jewett JF: Mortality of eclampsia: A case report and the experience of the Massachusetts maternal mortality study, 1954–1982. *N Engl J Med* 1983; 309:1644

Hibbard LT: Maternal mortality due to acute toxemia. *Obstet Gynecol* 1973; 42:263

Hood DD, Dewan DM, James FM III, et al: The use of nitroglycerin in preventing the hypertensive response to tracheal intubation in severe preeclampsia. *Anesthesiology* 1985; 63:329

Hood DD, Dewan DM, Rose JC, et al: Control of norepinephrine induced hypertension in gravid ewes with propranolol and sodium nitroprusside. Abstract of a paper presented at the Annual Meeting of the Society for Obstetric Anesthesia and Perinatology (SOAP), May 10, 1985

Hypertensive disorders of pregnancy. In Pritchard JA, MacDonald PC, Gant NF (eds): *Williams Obstetrics,* 17th ed, p 525. East Norwalk, CT, Appleton-Century-Crofts, 1985

Lopez-Llera M: Complicated eclampsia: Fifteen years' experience in a referral medical center. *Am J Obstet Gynecol* 1982; 142:28

Naulty J, Cefalo RC, Lewis PE: Fetal toxicity of nitroprusside in the pregnant ewe. *Am J Obstet Gynecol* 1981; 139:708

Porapakkham S: An epidemiologic study of eclampsia. *Obstet Gynecol* 1979; 54:26

Pritchard JA, Cunningham FG, Mason RA: The Parkland Memorial Hospital protocol for treatment of eclampsia: Evaluation of 245 cases. *Am J Obstet Gynecol* 1984; 148:951

Stempel JE, O'Grady JP, Morton MJ, et al: Use of sodium nitroprusside in complications of gestational hypertension. *Obstet Gynecol* 1982; 60:533

Wheeler AS, James FM III, Meis PJ, et al: Effect of nitroglycerin and nitroprusside on the uterine vasculature of gravid ewes. *Anesthesiology* 1980; 52:390

27

Pregnancy: Trauma and the Acute Abdomen

The pregnant patient will arrive in the intensive care unit (ICU) when an acute severe condition is due to the pregnancy (*e.g.*, preeclampsia, amniotic fluid embolus) or to an illness in which the pregnancy is coincidental (*e.g.*, trauma, acute abdomen, postoperative). This chapter will deal with the latter conditions.

The pregnant patient presents a unique clinical situation because the physician is responsible for two patients simultaneously. Often diagnostic and therapeutic modalities do not mutually benefit both patients and therefore risk–benefit considerations are of paramount importance.

ASSESSMENT AND DIAGNOSIS

Initial assessment of the patient should be similar in the pregnant and non-pregnant patient. Immediate attention should focus on respiratory and cardiovascular functions. A decrease in the functional residual capacity (FRC) secondary to the diaphragmatic elevation which occurs in pregnancy makes the pregnant patient more susceptible to the anoxic effects of apnea.

Hemodynamic management must take into account that normal blood pressure falls in pregnancy by approximately 10 mm in the midtrimester and is accompanied by a fall in hemoglobin because of hemodilution. Care must therefore be taken that blood loss is not overestimated and the patient overtransfused.

If cardiopulmonary arrest occurs, resuscitation should be started immediately, with the uterus displaced by an assistant tilting the abdomen. If a strong pulse cannot be obtained after several thoracic compressions with this maneuver, a cesarean section should be carried out within 4 minutes. Emptying the uterus relieves the aortocaval compression and may lead to dramatic improvements in the stroke volume. The time factor is important for maternal as well as fetal reasons. Most fetal survivors of maternal cardiopulmonary arrest are delivered within 5 minutes, and there are only rare cases of surviving healthy infants delivered more than 10 minutes after cardiopulmonary arrest.

Cardiopulmonary resuscitation should be continued during and after the procedure. Precious minutes should not be wasted with attempts to prepare a sterile field or in moving the patient to an operating room. This procedure should be considered only in the third trimester of pregnancy because significant vena cava compression and fetal survival are both unlikely earlier in pregnancy. From the maternal standpoint, this time interval is extremely important because brain damage and death may occur if reperfusion is not attained within 5 minutes.

After rapid maternal assessment and resuscitation, attention can then be focused on other diagnostic procedures on the mother and fetus. Fetal studies include establishing and dating the pregnancy and assessing fetal well being. Measuring a subunit of beta human chorionic gonadotropin (HCG) produced by the placenta is specific for pregnancy and is positive in the blood as early as 1 to 2 weeks and in the urine 2 to 4 weeks after conception. Fetal heart activity can easily establish the diagnosis of pregnancy and can be detected by real-time ultra-sound as early as 6 to 8 weeks after the last menstrual period. Other instruments use the doppler principle to detect fetal heart action at approximately 12 to 14 weeks. Auscultation with a stethoscope is positive by 17 to 20 weeks, although obesity may make this difficult and detectable only later. Normally the fetal heart rate is between 120 and 160 beats/min (bpm), distinctly different from the maternal pulse and easily distinguished by auscultation. Maternal tachycardia or fetal bradycardia may lead to diagnostic error. Visualization of the fetus can be done radiologically or by real-time ultrasound. Ultrasound offers the added advantage of visualizing fetal heart activity. The fetal skeleton can be distinguished radiologically between 16 and 24 weeks.

Dating the pregnancy is best done by ultrasound. Various parameters have been measured to assess gestational age by diagnostic ultrasound. Gestational sac size, crown–rump length, biparietal diameter, head circumference, femur length, and abdominal circumference are among the methods most commonly used today. Compiled charts from normal pregnancies are then used to date the pregnancy.

Special monitors using doppler technology can detect fetal heart activity and record fetal heart rate patterns to confirm not only signs of life but also fetal well being. Signs of fetal well being include a normal baseline heart rate (120–160 bpm), good variability (5–25 bpm), and acceleration without deceleration (Fig. 27-1).

Absence of fetal heart sounds should not be interpreted as fetal death when using doppler technology because the detection of heart movement is dependent on proper placement. Transmission of sound may also be affected by obesity, and errors may be made in interpreting fetal heart rate as being maternal if the rates are similar. Diagnosis of fetal death should be confirmed by real-time ultrasound to observe the absence of fetal heart motion. Ultrasound can also be used to assess signs of fetal well being such as fetal breathing, active fetal movement with flexion and extension of the limbs, and normal amniotic fluid volume. In addition, ultrasound may detect fetal pa-

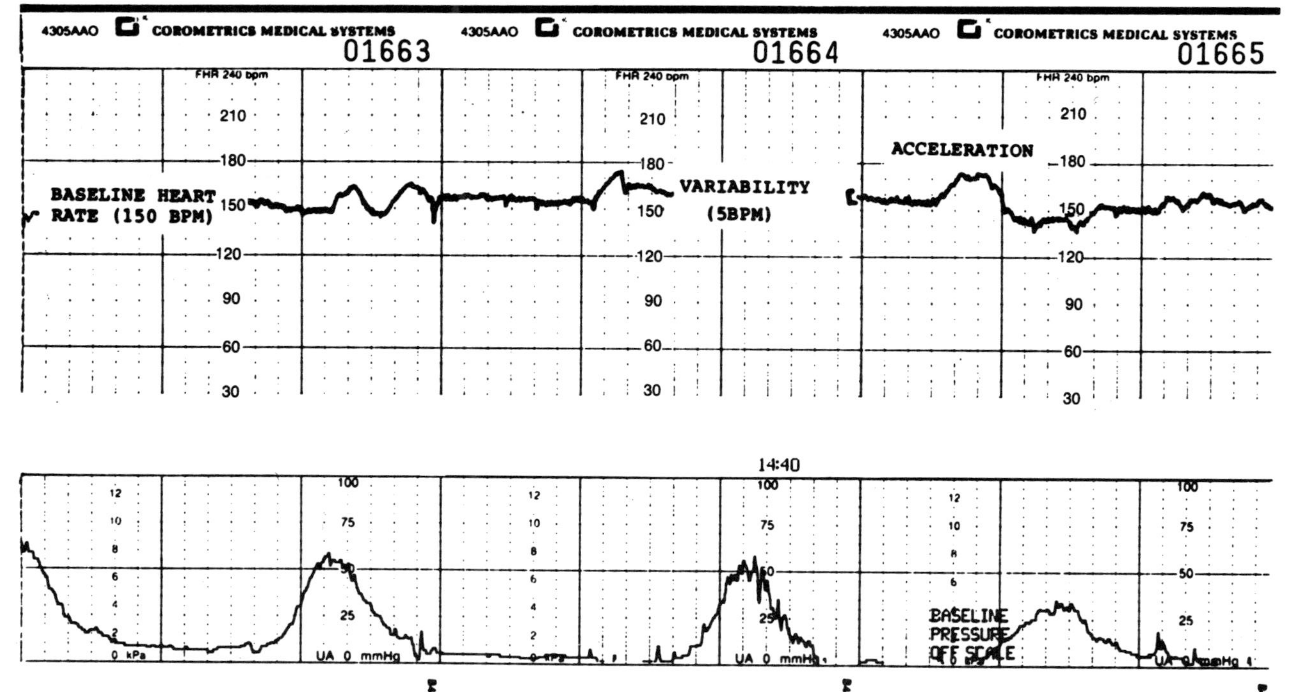

Figure 27-1 Fetal heart tracing showing normal baseline (120–160), normal variability (5–25), and acceleration without deceleration.

thology. Intracranial hemorrhage, which may occur after severe trauma such as pelvic fracture, may be detected *in utero* by ultrasound.

If fetal distress is diagnosed, then efforts should be made to improve uterine perfusion by correcting hypotension and by positioning the patient in a lateral position to decrease vena caval compression. Hypoxemia should also be corrected as maternal hypoxia leads to progressive fall in fetal umbilical arterial and venous P_{O_2} (Fig. 27-2). If evidence of fetal distress persists despite these measures, then a cesarean section should be done if the fetus is potentially viable. At tertiary care centers, fetal survival is approximately 50% at 26 weeks with the majority of these survivors being free of major morbidity. Below 23 weeks, survival approaches zero and therefore cesarean section before this gestational age should almost never be done. Cesarean section should be considered between 23 and 28 weeks, and beyond 28 weeks, should almost always be done for fetal indications. The maternal mortality associated with cesarean section is less than 1:1000, although it remains more hazardous than vaginal delivery by a factor of 2 to

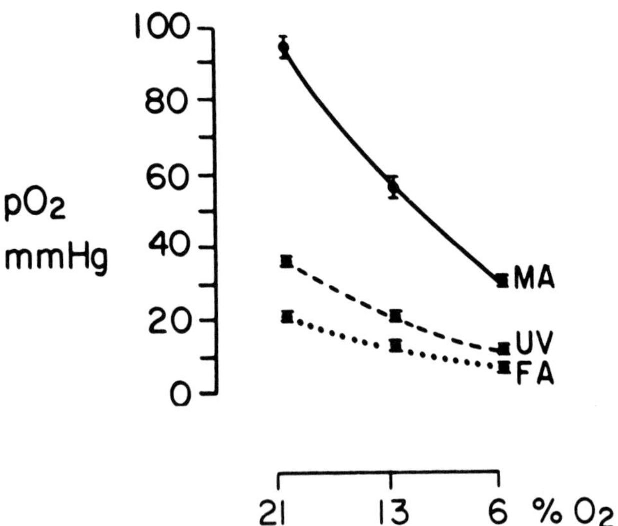

Figure 27-2 Mean values, ± standard error of the mean (SE), for blood oxygen (P_{O_2}) during 21% O_2 (room air), 13% O_2 (mild hypoxia), and 6% O_2 (severe hypoxia) respiration for a series of near-term pregnant ewes, and the effects on their fetuses. *MA*, maternal arterial blood; *UV*, fetal umbilical venous blood; *FA*, fetal arterial blood. (Modified from Brinkman CR III, et al: *Gynecol Invest* 1970; 1:115. Used with permission.)

11 times. Maternal mortality rates of zero in large series of cesarean sections have been achieved in some settings. Infection is the most common cause of morbidity after cesarean section, although this is usually less than 10%.

If fetal death is confirmed, attempts at delivery may be delayed for up to 4 weeks. The majority of women will deliver within 2 weeks of fetal death. Serial weekly coagulation studies should be monitored to detect coagulopathy which may develop. If spontaneous delivery does not occur, the pregnancy may be terminated by oxytocin infusion or prostaglandin suppositories. If the pregnancy is beyond 28 weeks, only oxytocin should be used because of the danger of uterine rupture with prostaglandin.

OTHER DIAGNOSTIC MEASURES

PERITONEAL LAVAGE

The indications for a lavage or laparotomy are similar to those in the nonpregnant patient. The indications should not be restricted but rather expanded because of the additional risk of uterine damage. The semi-open technique may be used in the first half of pregnancy although the "mini-laparotomy" is preferable later in pregnancy.

RADIOGRAPHY

Radiography should be avoided whenever possible. Other diagnostic modalities such as ultrasound and magnetic resonance imaging (MRI) should be considered first. Whenever the examination is felt to be necessary and no satisfactory alternative is available, the radiologist should complete these without hesitation. Discussion should include the patient's family whenever possible to consider the risks of radiation to the fetus as well as the potential dangers of misdiagnosis or delay of diagnosis to the mother without the benefit of using radiographs. The patient should be positioned and shielded in such a manner that the fetus is exposed to a minimum of radiation. The two most important factors determining the fetal effects are the dose of radiation absorbed by the fetus (Tables 27-1 and 27-2) and the gestational age.

In pregnancies less than 2 weeks, radiation death may occur with doses as low as 10 rad while other risks appear small or nonexistent. Between 2 and 15 weeks, the fetus appears most vulnerable to the nonlethal effects of radiation, although the risk of fetal abnormality when the dose is less than 5 rad is felt to be negligible. At higher levels the risk of malformations is increased, especially when it exceeds 15 rad. Other risks include childhood cancer, the relative increase per rad being 2.5 times. These risks placed in proper perspective, however, mean that the risk of developing childhood cancer after *in utero* exposure of 5 rad is less than 1%. Beyond 15 weeks, the risk of radiation-induced abnormality, mental retardation, or childhood cancer is low at levels below 50 rad.

TABLE 27-1 EXAMPLES OF UPPER LIMIT DOSE FROM X-RAY EXAMINATIONS

Examination	Dose
Routine head	50 mrad
Routine thoracic and neck	
Chest	50 mrad
Cervical spine	50 mrad
Thoracic spine	50 mrad

ULTRASOUND

Ultrasound has been used with increasing frequency in pregnancy. The American Institute of Ultrasound in Medicine concluded that no confirmed biologic effects on patients or instrument operators caused by exposure at intensities typical of present diagnostic ultrasound instruments have ever been reported. Although the possibility exists that such biologic effects may be identified in the future, current data indicate that the benefits of the prudent use of diagnostic ultrasound outweigh the risks, if any, to the patients.

MAGNETIC RESONANCE IMAGING

Only limited information is available on the use of MRI on pregnant patients. The MRI techniques have been used in pregnancy without any identifiable risks to the fetus.

MANAGEMENT

PREGNANCY RELATED CONDITIONS

When assessing the acute abdomen in pregnancy, it is important to recognize pregnancy-related conditions which may occur. These include abruptio placenta, ruptured uterus, and red degeneration of a uterine fibroid. Abruptio placenta is the partial or total separation from the uterine wall of the normally implanted placenta. These patients may have acute abdominal pain and a contracted tender uterus. Vaginal bleeding may be absent if the blood remains completely retroplacental. Rebound is usually absent.

Treatment includes fluid or blood resuscitation, correction of coagulopathy, and delivery of the fetus and placenta. If the fetus is dead, this may be accomplished vaginally. If the fetus is alive, cesarean section should be done in cases of fetal distress and should be considered if there are no facilities for immediate delivery because additional placental separation is a constant threat.

TABLE 27-2 ESTIMATED DOSE TO UTERUS FROM ABDOMINAL EXAMINATION

Examination	Range (mrad)
Upper GI	5–1230
IVP	70–5480
Barium enema	28–12600
Abdomen	25–1920
Pelvis	55–2190

Uterine rupture is much less common and is usually seen after severe trauma. Occasionally rupture occurs in patients with previous cesarean section with or without labor. The patient may complain of a sensation of "tearing" and severe pain, although this may subside somewhat after the rupture. The patient may show signs of shock, and the fetus is often expelled from the uterus into the peritoneal cavity. Management includes immediate laparotomy and hysterectomy. Rarely can repair be done.

Fibroids occasionally undergo red degeneration when hemorrhagic infarction occurs within the fibroid. The symptoms and signs are localized pain and tenderness sometimes accompanied by fever and leukocytosis. The treatment is conservative with rest, hydration, and analgesia.

Nausea and vomiting are the most common symptoms of pregnancy, but in the second or third trimester, they should arouse suspicion. Chronic constipation is also common, but absolute constipation is not normal. Distention is often difficult to assess, especially in late pregnancy.

When considering the diagnosis of appendicitis, the upward and lateral displacement of the appendix caused by the enlarging uterus must be considered. Surgical management is similar to that in the nonpregnant patient.

Adler's sign may be used to differentiate uterine from extrauterine complications of pregnancy. The pain is first localized with the patient in the supine position. The patient then turns to the left lateral position, and the pain is reassessed. With uterine lesions, the positioning usually shifts the uterus and the associated point of pain.

TRAUMA

Trauma remains the most common cause of death in pregnant women, when the cause of death is not directly related to pregnancy. Motor vehicle accidents caused death more frequently than other accidents in women of childbearing age. Death is most often caused by head injury. Internal injuries are usually multiple, and death often results from hemorrhagic shock.

Two potentially serious complications of trauma must be considered. With severe collisions, placental separation resulting in fetal death was found in 3% of patients who survived. The majority of patients with pelvic fracture will have placental separation. All pregnant patients with viable fetuses should have fetal monitoring after trauma. Rothenberger and coworkers categorized injuries as major, minor and insignificant, which may guide the physician on the need for fetal monitoring (Table 27-3). Higgins and Garite suggested continuous monitoring of women with major injuries for at least 48 hours. After minor or insignificant injury, they recommended continuous monitoring for a few hours only.

Uterine rupture is another complication of severe trauma.

Postoperative Period

The postoperative period presents similar problems for the pregnant and the nonpregnant patient. The major difference is the need to assess the pregnancy-related problems.

Up to 13% of patients operated on in the second and third trimester go into premature labor within a week of operation. Risks are increased if sepsis is present.

Premature labor is detectable by the alert patient, but may go unnoticed by the intubated, narcotized patient or by those whose mental status is depressed for other reasons, (*e.g.*, traumatic, metabolic). Uterine contractions are palpable abdominally, although this may not be possible with large abdominal dressings. Repeated pelvic examination to detect a dilating cervix may be necessary in the immediate postoperative period to detect premature labor.

Monitors, referred to as external tocotransducers, allow uterine activity to be monitored. These are placed on the patient's abdomen and held in place by an elastic belt. When the uterus contracts, the change in shape and hardness of the uterus depresses a plunger which moves a slight distance and causes a change in the voltage of a small electric current passing through, and this change is displayed by a recorder as a waveform. Today, monitors for this purpose are small and mobile and can be placed by the

TABLE 27-3 DIVISION OF TRAUMA INTO THREE CATEGORIES

Major injuries	Documentation of shock at the time of admission, skull fracture, cerebral contusion or intracerebral hemorrhage, spinal column fracture, or a spinal cord injury, chest injury necessitating thoracotomy or tube thoracostomy, injury of the abdominal viscera or genitourinary tract treated operatively, or a pelvic fracture
Minor injuries	All other injuries of the head, chest, abdominal and genitourinary injuries plus deep lacerations, long bone fractures, and facial fractures
Insignificant injuries	Soft-tissue injuries, superficial lacerations, and fractures of the bones of the hands and feet

bedside. They are not obstructive to the care of the critically ill patient. If large abdominal dressings are used, there may be problems of placement. Movement of the plunger may also be dampened by obesity or by the loosening of the elastic belt.

No trials to date have defined the role of prophylactic therapy to prevent uterine contractions. Treatment of premature labor is more established in the medical literature. Drugs in common usage include beta-sympathomimetics and magnesium sulphate. Beta-mimetics are not specific for the uterine musculature, so other beta-effects occur. Tachycardia and hypotension are common side-effects. Pulmonary edema is a serious complication of its use although the mechanism is unclear. Magnesium sulphate is excreted in the urine so it should be used cautiously in oliguric patients. Toxic effects include respiratory and cardiac depression. Calcium glucconate IV will usually reverse respiratory depression.

NUTRITIONAL NEEDS

Specific indications for total parenteral nutrition are unclear although it has been used in many instances. Theoretical risks from total parenteral nutrition include effects of maternal hyperglycemia which may lead to congenital anomalies and macrosomia. During pregnancy, plasma glucose levels should be kept below 120 mg/dl. High phenylalanine levels that occur with amino acid administration may also possibly cause fetal damage.

Analgesics

Morphine use is not associated with major or minor malformations. Like all narcotics, placental transfer is rapid. Prolonged use may lead to neonatal withdrawal, but this is usually seen only in addicts. Other narcotics, such as Demerol, have also been used in pregnancy. They have been reported to cause less respiratory depression in newborns, although others have found no difference when equianalgesic doses were used.

Antibiotics

Penicillin and its derivatives have been widely used in pregnancy without apparent sequelae. Erythromycin can also be used safely. Cephalosporin use during pregnancy has been infrequent, but no major effects on the fetus have been reported. Kanamycin and streptomycin use during pregnancy have been associated with eighth nerve damage in the fetus, so aminoglycosides should be used cautiously. Antibiotics such as clindamycin, useful in anaerobic infection, have not been associated with fetal problems. Antifungal agents have not been linked with adverse fetal effects.

For further information, please see Chapter 57 of Civetta JM, Taylor RW, Kirby RR: Critical Care. *Philadelphia: J. B. Lippincott, 1988*

BIBLIOGRAPHY

AIUM (American Institute of Ultrasound in Medicine): AIUM statement on clinical safety. *J Ultrasound Med* 1984; 3:R10

Alders N: A sing for differentiating uterine from extrauterine complications of pregnancy. *Br Med J* 1951; 2:1194

American College of Obstetricians and Gynecologists: Diagnosis and management of fetal death, ACOG, Technical Bulletin 98, Washington, DC, ACOG, 1986

BEIR (Committee on the Biologic Effects of Ionizing Radiations): The effects on populations to exposure to low levels of ionizing radiations: 1980, Washington, DC, National Academy Press, 1980

Bondurant S, Boehm FH, Fleischer AC, Machin JE: Antepartum diagnosis of fetal intracranial hemorrhage by ultrasound. *Obstet Gynecol* 1984; 63:255

Brent RL, Corson RO: Radiation exposure in pregnancy. *Curr Problem Radiol,* 1972a; 2:1

Brinkman CR III, Kirschbaum TH, Assali NS: The role of the umbilical sinus in the regulation of placental vascular resistance. *Gynecol Invest* 1970; 1:115

Buchsbaum HJ, Cruikshank DP: Postmortem Cesarean section. In Buchsbaum HJ (ed): *Trauma in Pregnancy,* Philadelphia, WB Saunders, 1979

Crosby WM: Traumatic injuries during pregnancy. *Clin Obstet Gynecol* 1983; 26:902

Crosby WM, Costiloe JP: Safety of lap belt restraint for pregnant victims of automobile collisions. *N Engl J Med* 1977; 284:632

Goldenberg RL, Nelson KG, Davis RO, Kaski J: Delay in delivery: Influence of gestational age and the duration of delay on perinatal outcome. *Obstet Gynecol* 1984; 64:480

Graham D, Saunders RC: Assessment of gestational age in the second and third trimesters. In Saunders RC, James AE (eds): *Ultrasonography in Obstetrics and Gynecology,* 3rd ed, Norwalk, Appleton-Century-Crofts, 1985

Hage ML: Interpretation of nonstress tests: Clinical section. *Am J Obstet Gynecol* 1985; 153:490

Higgins SD, Garite TJ: Late abruptio placenta in trauma patients: Implications for monitoring. *Obstet Gynecol* 1984; 63:105

Johnson IR, Symonds EM, Kean OM, et al: Imaging of the pregnant human uterus with nuclear magnetic resonance. *AJOG* 1984; 148:1136

Katz FL, Dotters DJ, Droegemueller W: Perimortem Cesarean delivery. *Obstet Gynecol* 1986; 68:571

Manning FA, Morrison I, Lange IR, et al: Fetal assessment based on fetal biophysical profile scoring: Experience in 12,620 referred high risk pregnancies. *Am J Obstet Gynecol* 1985; 151:343

National Council on Radiation Protection and Measurements (NCRP): Medical radiation exposure on pregnant or potentially pregnant women. NCRP Report No. 54, Washington, DC, 1977

O'Brien GD, Queenan JT: Dating gestation in the first 20 weeks. In Saunders RC, James AE (eds): *Ultrasonography in Obstetrics and Gynecology,* 3rd ed, Norwalk, Appleton-Century-Crofts, 1985

Petitti DB: Maternal mortality and morbidity in Cesarean section. *Clin Obstet Gynecol* 1985; 28:763

Rothenberger D, Quattlebaum FW, Peiry JF, et al: Blunt maternal trauma: A review of 103 cases. *J Trauma* 1978; 18:173

Spernoff L, Glass RH, Kase NG: Clinical Assays. In Glass RH (ed): *Clinical Gynecologic Endocrinology and Infertility,* Baltimore, Williams & Wilkins, 1983

The amount of radiation absorbed by the conceptus. In Wagner LK, Lester RG, Saldana LR (eds): *Exposure of the Pregnant Patient to Diagnostic Radiation,* Philadelphia, JB Lippincott, 1985

Weingold AB: Appendicitis in pregnancy. *Clin Obstet Gynecol* 1983; 26:801

28 Fetal Monitoring

Although physicians know a great deal about fetal life, we use only a part of the information available for clinical management. Problems stem from the persistence of an old and pervasive idea that the placenta has only a limited capacity to transfer nutrients. This concept, in its most extreme form, implies that the fetus exhausts the capacity of the placenta by term, exposing it to the fearsome option of death *in utero* or birth. According to this view, the metabolite in shortest supply is oxygen, a conviction that continues to have tremendous impact on patient management today. This chapter critically reviews the basis for these views and discusses their implications for today's clinician.

BASIC CONSIDERATIONS

Based in part on outdated information, tradition demands that every term infant be considered in a precarious position and that maternal management should proceed accordingly. In today's litigious society, this viewpoint constitutes a heavy burden and also goes against recent information that suggests the fetus has reserves enabling it to cope with all but the most serious conditions.

Obviously the difficulty lies in our inability to evaluate fetal status precisely. At present we deal fairly well with the normal fetus and the one already severely stressed. Problems come with infants between these extremes, those who may be stressed to the point that they have evoked but not yet exhausted their adaptive mechanisms. Current methods lack the sensitivity and specificity to detect these circumstances. As a result, we deal with our uncertainty by treating all infants as if they are on the edge of disaster. If this approach poses no problems for mother and infant, it can be justified. In many circumstances, however, it does. Accordingly, we must ask if we can do better. How can we avoid being rushed into an unwise course of action?

Part of the clinical dilemma stems from our rigid adherence to oxygen deprivation as an explanation for intrauterine stress. Virtually all methods for evaluating and treating the unborn child assume that this molecule is the metabolic substrate in shortest supply. Given the multitude of factors that affect fetal condition and viability, no justification exists for such a myopic approach. Unless fetal physiology differs greatly from that of adults, we must assume that severe hypoglycemia wreaks no less havoc on the brain than does acute hypoxia. Do observations of fetal heart rate or measurements of scalp *p*H detect acute hypoglycemia? Unlikely! Yet we continue to rely on these measurements to evaluate fetal condition and, in so doing, fail to develop a substitute technology that takes into account all that we already know about fetal glucose metabolism. Throughout adult and pediatric medicine, batteries of tests are used to evaluate each organ system; clinical skills include the selection of appropriate measurements. In no other specialty do physicians assume that one or two tests, in this case electrocardiography (EKG) and scalp *p*H, are sufficient to identify the various clinical problems threatening their patients.

At the same time, we do not use fetal EKG monitoring to its full extent. The possibility exists that acute fetal electrolyte abnormalities cause problems, perhaps even death. We have considerable insight concerning the effects of high and low concentrations of potassium and ionized calcium on various components of the EKG. Yet we have not used this information in the management of obstetric patients. These circumstances would simply be curiosities if the clinician were not forced to act. Unfortunately, many common problems require him or her to weigh the risks to the mother against those to the fetus when deciding on a course of action or therapy.

Any physician dealing with pregnant women has experienced a situation in which he or she has had to modify care of the mother out of concern for the presumed effect on the child. For example, vasopressors with pure alpha-adrenergic action may be the therapy of choice when treating hypotension. Nevertheless, the clinician hesitates for fear that vasoconstriction of the uterine vasculature may place the infant at some unreasonable, yet undefined, risk. Or, because of a diagnosis of "acute fetal bradycardia," an anesthesiologist may feel pressured to induce anesthesia by a rapid sequence technique in a woman for whom prudence dictates a slower, but safer, awake intubation because of some anatomic peculiarities of the upper airway.

Both examples illustrate situations in which the preferred mode of management of the mother may be modified out of concern for its effect on the infant. Usually such decisions are strongly influenced by the assumption that the term fetus is at risk, even in the best of circumstances, or that the fetal EKG or scalp *p*H is sensitive and specific enough to detect problems. Laboratory data and clinical experience suggest that both assumptions are open to question. The time is ripe to develop a new perspective on the management of the pregnant patient and her passenger.

CHRONIC ADAPTATIONS

With better methods of study, investigators have learned that the environment of the unstressed fetus is remarkably stable with respect to oxygen, glucose, and every metabolite tested during the last part of gestation (Table 28-1). Oxygen does not decrease nor does hematocrit rise as was previously thought. The stability even exists at high altitude, where the mother is chronically hypoxic, an observation that prompted more detailed studies of placental function. Subsequently, the functional capacity of the placenta was found to be increased throughout pregnancy, even though its weight remains constant. Structural and functional changes within the placenta cause a systematic increase in its *diffusion capacity* for oxygen, urea, and other compounds that keep pace with the fetal weight and, *pari passu,* metabolic activity.

Individual factors governing placental diffusion capacity are the same as those affecting this measurement in the lung and include surface area, diffusion distance, the physiochemical characteristics of intervening tissue, and the transplacental concentration gradient of the substance in question (Table 28-2). *Surface area,* normally measured in square meters, refers to the total area of all microscopic villi, similar to the alveolar surface area of the lung. *Diffusion distance* refers to the mean distance that substances must traverse when they move between maternal and fetal blood. Factors governing the *concentration gradient* include the mean concentration of substances on either side of the placenta (or partial pressure in the case of gases) and the rate of delivery of the substance to or from either side of the placenta. *Rate of delivery* is determined by the rates of flow of uterine and umbilical blood and by the carrying capacity of blood, which in the case of oxygen is related directly to hemoglobin concentration. The close relationship between fetal weight (and metabolic activity) and diffusion capacity throughout pregnancy reflects adjustments in each of these components. For example, as pregnancy advances, fetal capillaries in placental villi move toward the surface, decreasing the diffusion distance; microvilli become convoluted, increasing the surface area; and uterine blood flow increases, maintaining the concentration gradients. Of course, these placental characteristics also affect the movement of drugs.

The delivery system for essential substrates also shows remarkable flexibility. In the event of any inadequacy, compensatory changes occur elsewhere. An experimentally induced fall in maternal hemoglobin stimulates increased rates of uterine blood flow so that oxygen delivery, the product of

TABLE 28-1 EVIDENCE FOR STABILITY OF THE INTRAUTERINE ENVIRONMENT UNTIL ONSET OF LABOR

Stable concentration of blood constituents (e.g., hematocrit, P_{O_2}, glucose concentrations)
A consistent relationship between weight of the fetus and various structural and functional characteristics of the placenta (e.g., surface area, diffusion capacity)
A consistent relationship between weight of the fetus and flow/kg tissue of umbilical and uterine circulations
Appropriate adaptive changes in the event of maternal or fetal stress, which may involve either structural or functional change

TABLE 28-2 DIFFUSION CAPACITY

Defining the amount of material transferred per unit time per unit difference of concentration gradient (DC):

$$DC = \frac{k\,(SA)\,(\Delta C_1 - C_2)}{d}$$

k	=	constant that varies with the physiochemical properties of the intervening tissue
SA	=	surface area of the membrane
d	=	mean diffusion distance
$\Delta C_1 - C_2$	=	mean concentration gradient between maternal and fetal blood

flow and oxygen concentration, remains stable. Limitation of placental growth induces higher rates of uterine blood flow and overdevelopment of the remaining placental tissue. Similar adaptions occur clinically in women with anemia and heart disease and in infants afflicted with anemia from a hemolytic disorder.

It is clear, then, that far from representing the inflexible system originally conceived by clinicians, the placenta shows a considerable ability to adapt to special circumstances. Perhaps the most remarkable examples of this adaptability are cases in which the placenta implants on the omentum, or the liver or other abdominal organs, rather than the uterine mucosa. Despite the unfavorable site, the fetus often achieves normal weight, apparently because it has the capacity to extract the necessary nutrients from whatever maternal tissues are available.

Clinical observations suggest that factors limiting the delivery of oxygen to the fetus stimulate, by mechanisms not yet identified, compensatory change in placental morphology or physiology. Placental size, relative to the fetus, tends to be greater when some maternal factor, hypoxemia, or anemia limits availability of oxygen to the fetus. Placental surface area also is greater than normal in proportion to the severity of anemia in cases of erythroblastosis fetalis. In other instances higher than normal rates of uterine blood flow compensate for disruptions of placental development or decreased maternal oxygen-carrying capacity, maintaining fetal homeostasis in the face of disruption from within or without.

It is difficult to appreciate the extent to which the aforementioned observations contradict prevailing thought or the extent to which they have been ignored in clinical practice. Present-day clinical literature is rife with allusions to the developmental incompetence of the placenta. For example, we ascribe morphologic changes in the placenta during pregnancy to "aging" or "senescence" and not to "maturation." We assume, *de rigueur,* that placental infarcts compromise function even though we lack the evidence necessary to prove this thesis. We interchange words such as "neonatal depression" and "hypoxia" even though we know the former may be caused by many factors completely unrelated to the availability of oxygen.

ACUTE ADAPTATIONS

The foregoing examples illustrate adaptations to chronic stress. Clinicians may rejoin saying that they must also consider the capacity of the fetus to deal with acute stress, as encountered in pregnant women who are trauma victims, acutely ill with a medical disease, or in labor. But even here clinical concepts contradict current information. The normal fetus has several mechanisms that enable it to survive acute stress (Table 28-3).

Fluctuation of metabolic rate constitutes an important acute adaptive response. Whereas the normal rate of oxygen consumption of the unstressed fetus varies from 10 to 15 ml/kg/min, it may decrease to 4 ml/kg/min or less during acute stress. In fact, the very low rate that early investigators mistook for normal metabolic activity probably exemplifies this response. Presumably this change occurs when the fetus stops growing (growth being a process that requires high rates of energy consumption) and uses only the energy necessary to sustain body homeostasis. Rates of 4 ml/kg/min are typical for a nongrowing adult. Viewed in this light, infants who fail to grow *in utero* evince an effective adaptive response. They keep their metabolic requirements low by two mechanisms: first by virtue of their total size, and second by the cessation of growth. Acute stress may evoke this response quite rapidly.

The placenta metabolizes lactate as another response to stress. During periods of hypoxia the fetus may revert to anaerobic metabolism. Should lactate be produced, it is metabolized by the placenta, traverses the placenta to be metabolized by the mother, or remains in the fetal circulation. The route taken appears to depend on the severity of hypoxia. Two of the three pathways are protective; only in the latter circumstance is there a tendency for development of a metabolic acidosis.

Fetal bradycardia also may be a manifestation of an adaptive response and not hypoxic myocardial depression. A *diving reflex* in human neonates and in adult aquatic birds and mammals consists of bradycardia and peripheral vasoconstriction. This reflex preserves circulation to the heart and brain at the expense of peripheral tissue perfusion during water immersion and prolongs the time that these two essential organs can survive without damage. The reflex is especially prominent in premature infants; in term infants

TABLE 28-3 ADAPTATIONS TO HYPOXIA

Structural changes within the placenta (e.g., increased surface area, decreased diffusion distance)
Increased flow/kg of uterine or umbilical blood flow
Increased fetal hematocrit
Decreased growth rate decreasing fetal requirements
Decreased fetal movement
Placental metabolism of lactate
Redistribution of fetal cardiac output to the brain and heart
Premature labor

it tends to disappear during the first few days of life. It may be elicited by vagal stimulation as well as by hypoxia. Presumably it is no less protective for human infants *in utero* than for free-living diving animals, but it does create a diagnostic problem. The clinican reading fetal heart rate tracings cannot distinguish with certainty the bradycardia of severe myocardial depression from reflex bradycardia. The one may warrant immediate cesarean section; the other may simply be a sign of a healthy response to stress.

The tendency to decrease spontaneous movements during hypoxia is related to the diving reflex and is seen in fetuses and some newborns. This response is exactly opposite to that which occurs in hypoxic adults who respond by struggling and attempting to escape. The flaccid response diminishes fetal oxygen requirements during periods of deprivation, thus prolonging the time of survival without damage to the brain and heart. Some evidence suggests that the fetal central nervous system of many species appears to have greater capacity than the adult central nervous system to withstand periods of oxygen deprivation.

For further information, please see Chapter 119 in Civetta JM, Taylor JW, Kirby RR: Critical Care. *Philadelphia: J. B. Lippincott, 1988*

BIBLIOGRAPHY

Barron DH, Metcalfe J, Meschia G, et al: Adaptations of Pregnant Ewes and Their Fetuses to High Altitude p 115. Oxford, Pergamon Press, 1963

Beischer NA, Sivasamboo R, Vohra S, et al: Placental hypertrophy in severe pregnancy anaemia. *Am J Obstet Gynecol* 1970; 77:398

Caton D, Crenshaw C, Wilcox CJ, et al: O_2 delivery to the pregnant uterus: Its relationship to O_2 consumption. *Am J Physiol* 1979; 237:R52

Caton D, Henderson J, Wilcox J, et al: Oxygen consumption of the uterus and its contents and weight at birth of lambs. In Longo LD, Reneau (eds): Fetal and Newborn Cardiovascular Physiology, p 123. New York–London, Garland STPM Press, 1976

Clavero JA, Botilla Llusia J: Measurement of the villous surface in normal and pathologic placentas. *J Obstet Gynaecol Br Commonw* 1963; 86:234

Comline RS, Silver M: Daily changes in foetal and maternal blood of conscious unbilical and uterine vessels. *J Physiol* 1970; 209:567

Himwich HE, Bernstein AO, Herrlich H, et al: Mechanisms for the maintenance of life in the newborn during anoxia. *Am J Physiol* 1942; 135:387

Huckabee WE, Metcalfe J, Prystowsky H, et al: Movements of lactate and pyruvate in pregnant uterus. *Am J Physiol* 1962; 202:193

Huckabee WE, Metcalfe J, Prystowsky H, et al: Insufficiency of O_2 supply to pregnant uterus. *Am J Physiol* 1962; 202:198

Irving L: Respiratory reflexes in diving mammals. *Physiol Rev* 1939; 19:112

Makowski EL, Battaglia FC, Meschia G, et al: Effect of maternal exposure to high altitude upon fetal oxygenation. *Am J Obstet Gynecol* 1968; 100:852

Meschia G, Cotter JR, Brethmach CS, et al: The diffusibility of oxygen across the sheep placenta. *Q J Exp Physiol* 1965; 50:466

IV. Cardiovascular Disorders

29
Shock

Shock and respiratory failure are the most important problems encountered by intensive care physicians. Unfortunately, despite decades of research, the mortality for each remains excessively high. Our incomplete understanding of the underlying pathophysiology is undoubtedly a major reason for the poor clinical outcome associated with shock. Because of this lack of knowledge, virtually every aspect of shock, from definition to treatment, is controversial. Such uncertainty is understandably frustrating, and this frustration is compounded by the knowledge that untreated shock inevitably leads to death. As a result, the ICU physician must often initiate management immediately, before an adequate database has been collected or an etiology has been determined.

Nevertheless, well-founded principles of therapy should improve the outcome of shock. Ultimately, however, success depends on treatment of the underlying cause; the general management of shock outlined here must be accompanied by a rapid and determined attempt to diagnose and treat a specific etiology. The detailed approach to such specific causes is discussed elsewhere in the book; Table 29-1 provides an outline of shock classification.

DEFINITION

Although some authors define shock as a metabolic defect, a more traditional definition incorporates a perfusion abnormality as central to the pathophysiology. Therefore, shock is an acute clinical syndrome initiated by hypoperfusion and severe dysfunction of organs vital to survival. It is important to note the emphasis on shock as a syndrome, that is, a relatively constant set of signs and symptoms that predictably result from well-described pathophysiologic events of diverse etiology. Because shock always involves multiple vital organ systems, it is a systemic disorder. The clinical picture, therefore, reflects the sum of the effects on each system and will vary because each organ system is affected differently, depending on the severity of the perfusion defect, the underlying etiology, and the presence or absence of prior organ

TABLE 29-1 CLASSIFICATION OF SHOCK

- I. Hypovolemic
  - A. Hemorrhagic
    - 1. Gastrointestinal causes
    - 2. Trauma
    - 3. Internal bleeding
      - a. Blunt trauma
      - b. Long bone or pelvic fractures
      - c. Ruptured aortic aneurysm
      - d. Retroperitoneal bleeding (any cause)
  - B. Nonhemorrhagic
    - 1. Gastrointestinal losses
      - a. Vomiting
      - b. Diarrhea
    - 2. Renal losses
      - a. Excessive diuretic effect
      - b. Osmotic diuresis
      - c. Diabetes insipidus
    - 3. Other
      - a. Burns
      - b. Pancreatitis
      - c. Peritonitis
- II. Cardiogenic
  - A. Failure of contractile mechanism
    - 1. Myocardial infarction
    - 2. Cardiomyopathy
  - B. Impedance to ventricular outflow
    - 1. Intrinsic
      - a. Aortic stenosis
      - b. Idiopathic hypertrophic subaortic stenosis
    - 2. Extrinsic
      - a. Massive pulmonary embolism
      - b. Pulmonary hypertension with cor pulmonale
      - c. Aortic dissection
  - C. Impedance to ventricular outflow
    - 1. Intrinsic
      - a. Mitral stenosis
      - b. Atrial myxoma
      - c. Atrial thrombus
    - 2. Extrinsic
      - a. Pericardial tamponade
      - b. Restrictive pericarditis
  - D. Valve failure
    - 1. Acute mitral regurgitation
    - 2. Acute aortic regurgitation
  - E. Dysrhythmia
    - 1. Tachydysrythmias
    - 2. Bradydysrhythmias
  - F. Myocardial rupture
    - 1. Myocardial infarction
    - 2. Trauma

TABLE 29-1 *(continued)*

III. Mixed*
  A. Sepsis
  B. Toxic shock
  C. Neurogenic
  D. Anaphylaxis
  E. Drug overdose
  F. Trauma without hypovolemia

*Usually involves a combination of mechanisms, including hypovolemia, myocardial depression, or an abnormal distribution of the circulation.

dysfunction. Because shock is a "final common pathway" for pathophysiologic events common to various causes, management must be directed toward interrupting the downward spiral of events that serve to continue and to amplify shock, and toward treating the specific initiating cause.

Hypoperfusion is a key concept for both understanding and recognizing the shock state. Organ dysfunction initiated by other causes is not shock. Organ perfusion can be compromised by an overall decrease in cardiac output or by a maldistribution of cardiac output. A maldistribution of blood flow within the organ can further aggravate organ dysfunction. Finally, tissues may be incapable of utilizing what substrate is supplied, mimicking the effects of hypoperfusion.

The mechanisms controlling regional organ blood flow are of central importance to the pathophysiology of shock. Blood flow to an organ is a function of both the perfusion pressure and the vascular resistance of the vessels supplying the organ. Hypoperfusion and dysfunction will occur if vascular resistance cannot compensate for low systemic perfusion pressure, or if systemic pressures cannot overcome high levels of resistance within the vessels supplying an organ. The former cause of organ hypoperfusion occurs in the brain and heart with severe systemic hypotension; the latter cause is often important in the kidneys. With marked changes in interregional blood flow distribution, as may occur in sepsis, multiple organ dysfunction can occur despite "normal" levels of systemic pressure. Factors affecting the microcirculation (*i.e.*, perfusion at a cellular level) may also contribute to organ dysfunction. Such factors might include microvascular compression due to cellular edema or abnormal vasoregulation due to the release of various vasoactive substances. The common denominator, however, at least initially, is inadequate perfusion (*i.e.*, perfusion that is not adequate to meet tissue metabolic needs).

CLINICAL RECOGNITION

Shock may be difficult to define, but translating any definition into measurable parameters that can aid clinical recognition is more difficult still. For instance, how severe is "severe"? What actually constitutes "organ dysfunction"? These are questions that plague both the shock literature and the clinician faced with a patient exhibiting less than the full shock syndrome (Table 29-2).

The vital organs most often affected by shock are the brain, heart, and kidneys. The brain is able to autoregulate its perfusion despite moderate changes in perfusion pressure (in this case, systemic arterial pressure minus the intracerebral pressure). Eventually, however, cerebral perfusion decreases if mean arterial pressure falls below 60 to 70 mm Hg. Cerebral perfusion falls at even higher levels of arterial pressure in previously hypertensive patients. Although this fall in cerebral perfusion can affect all levels of brain function, the most common clinical manifestation is an acute change in mental state, varying from mild changes in mental acuity to frank coma.

The heart is particularly important because cardiac dysfunction due to shock can perpetuate shock, leading to further coronary hypoperfusion and a cycle of ever-worsening cardiac dysfunction. This type of adverse feedback loop or "vicious cycle" is common in the pathophysiology of shock; interrupting it is often a key aspect of management.

TABLE 29-2 THE CLINICAL RECOGNITION OF SHOCK*

Organ System	Symptom or Sign	Causes
CNS	Mental status changes	↓ Cerebral perfusion
	Pinpoint pupils	Narcotic overdose
Circulatory		
Heart	Tachycardia	Adrenergic stimulation, depressed contractility
	Other dysrhythmias	Coronary ischemia
	Hypotension	Depressed contractility secondary to ischemia or MDFs, right ventricular failure
	New murmurs	Valvular dysfunction, VSD
Systemic	Hypotension	↓ SVR, ↓ venous return
	↓ JVP	Hypovolemia, ↓ venous return
	↑ JVP	Right heart failure
	Disparate peripheral pulses	Aortic dissection
Respiratory	Tachypnea	Pulmonary edema, respiratory muscle fatigue, sepsis, acidosis
	Cyanosis	Hypoxemia
Renal	Oliguria	↓ Perfusion, afferent arteriolar vasoconstriction
Skin	Cool, clammy	Vasoconstriction, sympathetic stimulation
Other	Lactic acidosis	Anaerobic metabolism, hepatic dysfunction
	Fever	Infection

*MDF = myocardial depressant factors; VSD = ventricular septal defect; SVR = systemic vascular resistance; JVP = jugular venous pulsations.

Cardiac dysfunction manifests itself in several ways. The most common presentation, tachycardia, is primarily due to a reflex neurohumoral response to decreased myocardial performance. The pulse is frequently "thready," indicating a low cardiac stroke volume. With coronary ischemia, more complex rhythm disturbances may occur, and these can also impair cardiac function. Systemic arterial hypotension increases coronary ischemia and worsens cardiac dysfunction. As the heart fails, left ventricular end-diastolic pressure rises, ultimately causing pulmonary edema and respiratory failure. The impairment in gas exchange causes hypoxemia, exaggerating tissue hypoxia. The most common clinical symptoms of coronary hypoperfusion are chest pain and dyspnea; physical signs include the appearance of a dyskinetic apical cardiac impulse, a new third or fourth heart sound, a new murmur of mitral regurgitation (representing papillary muscle dysfunction), and pulmonary crackles. Electrocardiographic signs (ST-T wave changes) of myocardial ischemia can also be expected.

Renal function is also critically dependent on perfusion. The kidney, like the brain and heart, autoregulates its perfusion over a moderate range of arterial pressure. When hypoperfusion does occur, the glomerular filtration rate (GFR) falls. Oliguria is, therefore, a common manifestation of shock. As with other organs, the perfusion deficit may be absolute or relative; that is, it may reflect either an overall decrease of blood flow or an unfavorable redistribution of flow. In the kidney, redistribution of blood flow from the renal cortex toward the renal medulla occurs as perfusion decreases.

These three organs—brain, heart, and kidneys—are virtually always affected by shock. The severity of organ dysfunction and clinical presentation, however, varies with previous levels of organ function, compensatory mechanisms, and the etiology of the shock syndrome. Although other organ systems are affected, they are less important for clinical recognition or outcome.

When the skin is poorly perfused, its temperature falls and its color changes, so that it is often pale and dusky, representing both oligemia and venous pooling of blood desaturated of oxygen. With concomitant hypoxemia, frank cyanosis can be present. Sympathetic nervous system stimulation, a compensation for hypotension, causes sweat gland hypersecretion. The result is the frequently observed cool, clammy skin of shock. However, shock can occur in the absence of such features. Activation of the coagulation system is common, although disseminated intravascular coagulation (DIC) is not often clinically evident at initial presentation. Liver failure is occasionally prominent. When shock is due to an infectious cause, hyperglycemia and fever are usually present; paradoxically, hypothermia can also occur.

SYSTEMIC MANIFESTATIONS

Two common systemic manifestations of shock are metabolic acidosis and arterial hypotension. Metabolic (lactic) acidosis is due to tissue hypoxia and anaerobic metabolism, often complicated by hepatic function inadequate to metabolize the increased lactate. The severity of acidosis varies greatly and is poorly correlated with outcome when all forms of shock are considered. Systemic arterial hypotension is also common during shock. Marked decreases in systemic blood pressure inevitably lead to hypoperfusion and vital organ system dysfunction. However, changes in regional vascular resistance can compensate for modest decreases in perfusion pressure thereby maintaining perfusion to vital organs. Thus, a fall in arterial pressure can be a harbinger of potential shock, as well as a common manifestation of shock itself. Indeed, arterial hypotension can often be treated before vital organ dysfunction is clinically obvious—presumably preventing irreversibility of organ dysfunction, or at least ameliorating its severity. Common hemodynamic patterns in shock are summarized in Table 29-3.

An accurate blood pressure measurement is necessary when treatment is initiated, especially to avoid falsely low readings. Normally, blood pressure can be measured by cuff and stethoscope because Korotkoff sounds arise from turbulent blood flow distal to the point of vessel occlusion by the blood pressure cuff. Conditions that decrease such turbulence, however, may cause the pressure to be underestimated. These include peripheral vascular disease, tachycardia with a small pulse pressure, and irregular rhythms such as atrial fibrillation. Doppler devices improve detection of pressure but do not always reliably resolve the problem. In many, if not most, instances, direct arterial pressure measurement by an indwelling catheter is preferable, especially when hypotension on auscultation is not accompanied by evidence of organ dysfunction (e.g., if mental status is normal).

TABLE 29-3 SOME COMMON HEMODYNAMIC PATTERNS IN SHOCK*

Cause	CO	SVR	PAOP	CVP	$S\bar{v}_{O_2}$
Hypovolemic shock	↓	↑	↓	↓	↓
Left ventricular MI	↓	↑	↑	nl–↑	↓
Right ventricular MI	↓	↑	nl–↓†	↑†	↓
Pericardial tamponade	↓	↑	↑‡	↑‡	↓
Massive pulmonary embolism	↓	↑	nl–§	↑	↓
Septic shock					
Early	↓,nl,↑	↑,nl,↓	nl	nl–↑	↓
Early, after fluid administration	↑	↓	nl–↑	nl–↑	↓,nl,↑
Late	↓	↑	nl	nl	↓ (rarely ↑)

* CO = cardiac output; CVP = central venous pressure; $S\bar{v}_{O_2}$ = mixed venous oxygen saturation; MI = myocardial infarction; nl = normal.
† Occasionally, equalization of pressures suggestive of pericardial tamponade may be present.
‡ Equalization (± 3 mm Hg) of pressures, including pulmonary artery diastolic and right ventricular end-diastolic pressures, is characteristic.
§ May be clinically unobtainable or uninterpretable.

SUMMARY

Shock is present when an acute generalized disturbance in the normal circulatory pattern results in hypoperfusion and severe dysfunction of critical organs. Confusion, tachycardia, arterial hypotension, and oliguria are the most common early manifestations of brain, cardiac, and kidney dysfunction, respectively. More severe degrees of shock result in coma, myocardial ischemia, and pulmonary edema. Metabolic acidosis and arterial hypotension are frequent, especially when shock is severe, but are not prerequisites for recognition of the syndrome. Other physical signs depend on the underlying etiology, the level of organ function before the onset of shock, and the presence of compensatory mechanisms (see Table 29-2).

For further information, please see Chapter 74 in Civetta JM, Taylor RW, Kirby RR: Critical Care. *Philadelphia: J. B. Lippincott, 1988*

BIBLIOGRAPHY

Aubier MT, Trippenbach T, Roussos C: Respiratory muscle fatigue during cardiogenic shock. *J Appl Physiol* 1981; 51:499

Bone RC, Fisher CJ, Clemmer TP, et al: A controlled clinical trial of high-dose methylprednisolone in the treatment of severe sepsis and septic shock. *N Engl J Med* 1987; 317:653-658

Eisenberg PR, Jaffe AS, Schuster DP: Clinical evaluation compared to pulmonary artery catheterization in the hemodynamic assessment of critically ill patients. *Crit Care Med* 1984; 12:349

Hess ML, Hastillo MA, Greenfield LJ: Spectrum of cardiovascular function during gram negative sepsis. *Prog Cardiovasc Dis* 1981; 23:279

Monafo WW: Volume replacement in hemorrhage, shock and burns. *Adv Shock Res* 1980; 3:47

Moss GS, Saletta JD: Traumatic shock in man. *N Engl J Med* 1974; 290:724

Parillo JE, Burch C, Shelhammer J, et al: A circulating myocardial depressant substance in humans with septic shock: Septic shock patients with a reduced ejection fraction have a circulating factor that depresses myocardial cell performance. *J Clin Invest* 1985; 76:1539

Parker MM, Shelhammer JH, Bacharach SL, et al: Profound but reversible myocardial depression in patients with septic shock. *Ann Intern Med* 1984; 100:483

Rackley CE, Russell JO Jr, Mantle KA, et al: Cardiogenic shock: Recognition and management. *Cardiovasc Clin* 1975; 7:251

Veteran's Administration Systemic Sepsis Cooperative Study Group: Effect of high-dose glucocorticoid therapy on mortality in patients with clinical signs of systemic sepsis. *N Engl J Med* 1987; 317:659-665

30
Acute Myocardial Infarction

No area of contemporary cardiology is changing as dramatically as the approach to acute myocardial infarction. Understanding therapeutic options in this clinical setting is important because acute myocardial infarction and its sequelae result in more than 400,000 deaths in the United States annually. Progressive heart failure and sudden cardiac death are the two major categories of mortality. Both problems are more likely to be seen when large amounts of myocardium have been destroyed during the infarction. Necrotic myocardial cells are incapable of regeneration, so that prevention of cell death seems the logical key to reducing mortality from acute myocardial infarction. In the 1970s, emphasis was placed on therapies designed to decrease myocardial oxygen demand. The 1980s heralded a new era in which the therapeutic emphasis is on increasing myocardial oxygen supply. This chapter addresses this change in emphasis and summarizes current knowledge regarding the appropriate approach to acute myocardial infarction.

INTERVENTION STRATEGIES

THROMBOLYSIS

The last decade has seen a tremendous change in the management of acute myocardial infarction. The safety of cardiac catheterization in the first hours of acute myocardial infarction has been established, the pathophysiology has been defined, and the benefits of thrombolytic therapy have been documented.

A landmark study in this evolution was that of DeWood and colleagues. Patients underwent cardiac catheterization during acute myocardial infarction, less than 4 hours after the onset of chest pain. Total occlusion of the infarct-related artery was found in 87% of those cases. Further, the vast majority of patients had high-grade atherosclerotic coronary stenosis in the infarct-related artery, upon which thrombus was superimposed. These observations were made primarily in patients with ST segment elevation who went on to develop Q waves; that is, patients with transmural infarction. The documentation of coronary thrombosis during the early hours of acute myocardial infarction led to an expanded investigation of thrombolytic therapy to effect early reperfusion of the infarct-related artery, potentially saving jeopardized myocardium. The thrombolytic agents used in these trials was streptokinase, given either intravenously or by the intracoronary route.

Studies of acute myocardial infarction in animal models indicate that myocardial necrosis is nearly complete 6 hours after ligature of a coronary artery. Therefore, strategies of acute thrombolytic intervention that prolong the time to delivery of effective therapy decrease the likelihood of preserving myocardium, thereby reducing the chances of lessening mortality. In studies performed by leading medical centers and universities, the choice of the intracoronary route of administration resulted in an additional 2-hour delay before the initiation of thrombolytic therapy. A second observation from these data is the need for adequate public education urging people with chest pain to seek early medical attention for definitive diagnosis and therapy, because hours are usually wasted before arrival at emergency rooms.

The practical emphasis in thrombolytic therapy has shifted from intracoronary to intravenous administration because of the clear advantages of the latter. Intravenous thrombolytic therapy can be given rapidly and, because of its simplicity of administration, is available to the majority of patients with acute myocardial infarction who present to emergency rooms within 4 hours of the onset of chest pain. Of primary importance is the fact that intravenous therapy can be delivered earlier than intracoronary treatment. It is estimated that intravenous therapy saves 2 hours of ischemic time, which is the minimal time it takes to mobilize a cardiac catheterization laboratory team, perform the catheterization, and deliver therapy to the infarct-related artery. The intravenous route is therefore preferred, provided an agent is available that, when given by this route, achieves adequate reperfusion in the majority of patients.

The large body of literature regarding both intravenous and intracoronary streptokinase can be summarized with a few important observations: First, the earlier the administration, whether intravenous or intracoronary, the more likely that reperfusion will be achieved. Second, studies claiming that thrombolysis led to an improvement in regional or global left ventricular function were usually limited to patients in whom thrombolytic therapy was successfully delivered within 4 hours. Finally, clinical reinfarction occurs frequently (20%–40%) in the early months following successful thrombolysis, an observation indicating that additional therapy is necessary.

The importance of early diagnosis followed by treatment with an effective thrombolytic agent emphasizes the potential to save lives and identifies a major challenge to health professionals to establish an effective public awareness program emphasizing the prompt recognition and evaluation of chest pain syndromes. It is also clear that a delay of thrombolytic therapy exceeding 6 hours probably results in a situation with little potential therapeutic benefit but all the potential risks of thrombolytic therapy. These risks are related to the systemic fibrinolytic effects that result in bleeding (gastrointestinal, intravenous puncture site, and, rarely, intracerebral bleeding). Therefore, thrombolytic therapy is contraindicated in patients with a history of bleeding disorders, gastrointestinal bleeding, or stroke.

Coronary Angioplasty After Thrombolytic Therapy

The potential value of percutaneous transluminal coronary angioplasty (PTCA) following successful thrombolysis is based primarily on two observations. First, the majority of patients with total thrombolytic coronary occlusion still have tight residual coronary stenosis, despite successful thrombolysis. Second, routine cardiac catheterization before hospital discharge in patients with initially successful thrombolysis shows a high reocclusion rate. The clinical consequence associated with these observations is that a substantial portion of patients who receive successful thrombolytic therapy have recurrence of myocardial infarction within a few months.

It seems logical that coronary angioplasty might result in a more widely patent coronary artery than the use of either intravenous or intracoronary thrombolytic agents, since angioplasty also treats the underlying atherosclerotic lesion. However, it shares with intracoronary administration of thrombolytic agents the disadvantage of requiring cardiac catheterization before achieving reperfusion, with the inherent delays mentioned previously. The clinical importance of achieving the earliest possible reperfusion cannot be overemphasized.

LIDOCAINE PREVENTION OF PRIMARY VENTRICULAR FIBRILLATION

Although this is a controversial area, there is an important target population in whom lidocaine prophylaxis should be considered. The following recommendations are designed to achieve maximal benefit with the least toxicity, providing no contraindications to lidocaine exist.

1. Lidocaine prophylaxis should be considered only in patients who present with less than 6 hours of chest pain.
2. The initial bolus of lidocaine should be 50 mg, followed by two subsequent 50-mg boluses 5 minutes apart, for a total intravenous bolus of 150 mg over 15 minutes. (This dose must be adjusted downward in the elderly, patients weighing less than 60 kg, and those with severe liver function impairment or congestive heart failure.)
3. The intravenous infusion of lidocaine should be limited to 2 mg/min.
4. Lidocaine prophylactic infusions should be limited between 12 and 24 hours.
5. Lidocaine prophylaxis should be especially considered in small community hospitals without coronary care units or 24-hour in-house staff physician coverage.

MECHANICAL COMPLICATIONS

It is not surprising that myocardial ischemia severe enough to cause muscle necrosis can create hemodynamic alterations that precipitate heart failure and cardiogenic shock, with subsequent high mortality. Clinical heart failure in this setting can be caused by a variety of events, and it is important to understand the pathophysiologic processes associated with left ventricular dysfunction in patients with acute myocardial infarction. Table 30-1 lists the common etiologies of congestive heart failure associated with acute myocardial infarction.

In addition to extensive muscle necrosis, lack of structural integrity may also cause failure. Papillary muscle dysfunction or rupture can cause mitral regurgitation and heart failure of varying severity. If significant necrosis occurs in the region of the posteromedial papillary muscle, rupture of this support structure is possible. This development can produce massive mitral regurgitation, resulting in sudden pulmonary edema, subsequent shock, and death. The murmur accompanying papillary muscle rupture or dysfunction is variable in relation to duration in systole, and its radiation is dependent on the leaflet involved and the extent of regurgitation. If the patient is in pulmonary edema and cardiogenic shock, a new systolic murmur may not even be appreciated. If this complication is suspected, right heart catheterization and echocardiography are required to establish the correct diagnosis. The pulmonary artery occlusion tracing may show regurgitant waves or an increased V wave—a nonspecific finding seen in all conditions leading to a noncompliant, infarcted ventricle. Still, an elevated occlusion pressure with pulmonary hypertension and a large V or regurgitant wave in the face of a new systolic murmur and low forward output state strongly suggest papillary muscle dysfunction or an acute ventricular septal defect. Echocardiography can be helpful by demonstrating flailing motion of the mitral leaflet during systole, and doppler echocardiographic techniques can diagnose and quantify regurgitation into the left atrium.

TABLE 30-1 CAUSES OF HEART FAILURE DURING ACUTE MYOCARDIAL INFARCTION

Causes
Massive muscle necrosis
Severe muscle ischemia with dysfunction ("stunning")
Ventricular free wall rupture
Acute mitral regurgitation
Papillary muscle dysfunction from ischemia
Papillary muscle rupture from necrosis
Formation of ventricular septal defect
Pericardial effusion with cardiac tamponade
Right ventricular involvement in infarction
Unstable rhythms (e.g., sustained ventricular tachycardia, rapid atrial fibrillation)

Rupture of the ventricular septum also may cause severe heart failure and shock. As opposed to congenital ventricular septal defects, which are in the membranous septum, interventricular rupture most frequently occur at the junction of the septum and the anterior or posterior left ventricular free wall, where collateral blood flow is sometimes attenuated. This fact also explains why septal rupture occurs most often in patients experiencing their first transmural myocardial infarction. These patients generally have less collateral blood flow than those who have had prior infarcts. Like papillary muscle rupture or severe papillary muscle dysfunction, rupture of the intraventricular septum produces dramatic clinical deterioration, characterized by new systolic murmurs, heart failure, and cardiogenic shock. Right heart failure becomes apparent early, with subsequent pulmonary edema. The murmur is variable in quality, with or without a systolic thrill, and is clinically indistinguishable from acute papillary muscle rupture or dysfunction. This condition must be differentiated from acute mitral regurgitation by right heart catheterization; an inappropriate increase in oxygen saturation is observed when passing the catheter from the right atrium through the right ventricle to the pulmonary artery.

Ventricular free wall rupture during myocardial infarction generally occurs several days after the acute event, is more common in women, and is seen in patients with extensive anterior or inferior-posterior wall infarcts. Sudden catastrophic hemodynamic deterioration occurs. Blood may leak vigorously into the pericardial space, and cardiac tamponade can rapidly occur. Occasionally, a fibrinous exudate will form over the defect and blood will clot (pseudoaneurysm formation) without subsequent tamponade. Two-dimensional echocardiography is again helpful in making a correct diagnosis.

Pericardial effusion and cardiac tamponade can be seen independently of cardiac rupture in patients with acute myocardial infarction. When an infarct extends to the pericardial surface, it may produce pericarditis. Significant effusions sometimes occur several days after infarction, with the peak incidence at 1 week. If a large effusion develops, hemodynamic compromise may ensue. Most often, however, effusions are small and the pericarditis is associated with transient, but at times severe, chest pain, atelectasis, and electrocardiographic (EKG) changes. Therapy with aspirin, indomethacin, or oral corticosteroids is generally used. Anticoagulants are contraindicated because of the risk of bleeding into the pericardial space, enlarging the effusion, and producing further hemodynamic compromise.

RIGHT VENTRICULAR INFARCTION

The diagnosis of significant right ventricular involvement carries important implications. The presence of an acute inferior or inferior-posterior wall myocardial infarction, distended neck veins with systemic hypotension, and clear lung fields should suggest this diagnosis. Although the incidence of right ventricular infarction assessed by noninvasive methods is high (30%–60%), full clinical expression of the syndrome as described is less frequent.

The classical hemodynamic findings of right ventricular infarct include a normal pulmonary artery pressure with low left ventricular filling pressure, low cardiac output, and elevated right ventricular end-diastolic and right atrial pressures. Although acute and chronic cor pulmonale or pericardial disease can produce a similar clinical picture, the hemodynamic abnormalities of right ventricular infarction are improved with rapid volume expansion. Inotropic agents may be required when hypoperfusion due to hypotension persists despite adequate restoration of left ventricular filling pressure; this suggests concomitant left ventricular dysfunction. Echocardiography and radionuclide blood pool scans are helpful in these patients, revealing not only right ventricular dilation and wall motion abnormalities but also left ventricular dysfunction. If hypotension can be corrected, the prognosis in right ventricular infarction is good because the left ventricle often has adequately preserved function. The prognosis worsens with increasing concomitant left ventricular dysfunction.

Digitalis preparations have minimal inotropic effect in the setting of acute myocardial infarction and may increase systemic vascular resistance. Patients with acute infarcts, therefore, do not benefit from these agents unless they are used to control the ventricular response in atrial fibrillation or actually convert atrial dysrhythmias to more stable rhythms.

MEDICAL THERAPY DURING AND AFTER MYOCARDIAL INFARCTION

β-BLOCKER THERAPY

Several important questions may be asked regarding β-blocker therapy following myocardial infarction. First, who will benefit? A positive effect is most likely in those patients with a recurrent or complicated myocardial infarction, provided they do not have congestive heart failure. Benefits are less clear in the patient with a small, uncomplicated Q-wave infarction or in patients with relatively normal myocardial function after a non-Q wave infarction.

Second, how soon after myocardial infarction should β-blockers be administered? Review of acute trials shows that there is a small initial incremental benefit in the acute administration of intravenous β-blockers. If the clinician chooses to initiate therapy during the first hours of acute myocardial infarction, he is doing so with the idea of potentially salvaging ischemic myocardium. Thus, treatment should begin as soon as possible. Whether acute intravenous therapy with β-blockers has an additional incremental benefit to the initiation of chronic oral β-blocker therapy late in hospitalization is controversial. However, it is clear that initiation of oral nonselective β-blockers after myocardial infarction is effective before hospital discharge.

Third, what dose of β-blockers should be used? Full β-blocking doses of a non-selective β-blocker are necessary to achieve the beneficial reduction in mortality seen in the clinical trials.

Finally, should β-blockers be given to all risk groups after acute myocardial infarction? This is a more complicated question, in that there has never been a clinical trial large enough to assess whether β-blockers have a specific therapeutic benefit in the low-risk population. This would require a very large clinical trial selecting only low-risk patients. The results of both the Norwegian timolol trial and the BHAT suggest that the primary benefit will be in patients with a previous myocardial infarction or a complicated myocardial infarction. A reasonable approach to the patient with an initial small, uncomplicated, myocardial infarction is to perform noninvasive testing, assessing residual ischemia and ventricular dysrhythmia and then individualizing therapy based on these results.

CALCIUM CHANNEL BLOCKERS

Although clinical trials have been performed with nifedipine, verapamil, and diltiazem, only the diltiazem reinfarction study showed benefit of calcium channel blockade during evolving infarction. Heart rate is probably the most important determinant of myocardial oxygen consumption after myocardial infarction.

The diltiazem reinfarction study focused on patients with non-Q-wave myocardial infarctions. These patients were given either placebo or oral diltiazem (up to 90 mg every 6 hours) in the period between 24 and 72 hours after the onset of myocardial infarction. Therapy was continued throughout the hospitalization. The primary end-point was reinfarction, as defined by an abnormal recurrent evaluation of MB-CK in the plasma within the 14 days. The results showed that reinfarction was reduced by 51.2% in the diltiazem group compared to placebo ($p = 0.0297$). In addition, diltiazem reduced the frequency of refractory post-infarction angina and was well tolerated despite the concurrent treatment with β-blockers in over 60% of the patients.

This study is the first to demonstrate a specific benefit of calcium channel blockade after myocardial infarction and is important in that it focused on patients in whom other therapies have been shown (*i.e.*, those with non-Q-wave infarction). It should be emphasized, however, that this study dealt with end-points at 14 days, and one cannot speculate regarding long-term effects on morbidity and mortality.

NITRATES

Nitrates are effective antianginal agents and are frequently used in the post-infarction setting. Intravenous nitroglycerin is useful for the control of recurrent angina after myocardial infarction or unstable angina syndromes. Intravenous nitroglycerin infusions are usually begun at a dose of 10 μg/min followed by 10 μg increments every 5 to 10 minutes while blood pressure and clinical response are observed. The average infusion of intravenous nitroglycerin to control rest angina in patients unresponsive to standard nitrate therapy is approximately 140 μg/min. In unstable angina syndromes, the intravenous technique appears to offer advantages over oral therapy in that there is a more consistent control of ischemic episodes. Thus, although oral and intravenous nitroglycerin therapy have not been shown to reduce mortality after myocardial infarction, they are extremely useful, especially in the setting of recurrent and unstable angina pectoris.

For further information, please see Chapter 75 in Civetta JM, Taylor RW, Kirby RR: Critical Care. *Philadelphia: J. B. Lippincott, 1988*

BIBLIOGRAPHY

Beta-Blocker Heart Attack Trial Research Group: Randomized trial of propranolol in patients with acute myocardial infarction. *JAMA* 1982; 247:1707

Chesebro JH, Knatterud G, Roberts R, et al: Thrombolysis in myocardial infarction (TIMI) trial, phase I: A comparison of intravenous tissue plasminogin activator and intravenous streptokinase. *Circulation* 1987; 76:142

Curfman GD, Heinsimer JA, Lozner EC, et al: Intravenous nitroglycerin in the treatment of spontaneous angina pectoris: A prospective randomized trial. *Circulation* 1983; 67:276

DeWood MA, Spores J, Notske R, et al: Prevalence of total coronary occlusion during the early hours of transmural myocardial infarction. *N Engl J Med* 1980; 303:897

Dioguardi N, Mannucci PM, Lotto A, et al: Controlled trial of streptokinase and heparin in acute myocardial infarction. *Lancet* 1971; 2:891

Gibson RS, Boden WE, Theroux P, et al: Diltiazem and reinfarction in patients with non-Q-wave myocardial infarction. *N Engl J Med* 1986; 315:423

Gruppo Italiano Per Lo Studio Della Streptochinasi Nell'infarto Miocardico (GISSI): Effectiveness of intravenous thrombolytic treatment in acute myocardial infarction. *Lancet* 1986; 1:397

Kaplan K, Davison R, Parker M, et al: Intravenous nitroglycerin for the treatment of angina at rest unresponsive to standard nitrate therapy. *Am J Cardiol* 1983; 51:694

Multicenter International Study Group: Reduction in mortality after myocardial infarction with long-term beta-adrenoceptor blockade. *Br Heart J* 1977; 2:419

Raizner AE, Tortoledo FA, Verani MS, et al: Intracoronary thrombolytic therapy in acute myocardial infarction: A prospective, randomized, controlled trial. *Am J Cardiol* 1985; 55:301

Sharpe DM, Botvinick EH, Shames DM: Noninvasive diagnosis of right ventricular infarction. *Circulation* 1978; 57:483

The Norwegian Multicenter Study Group: Timolol-induced reduction in mortality and reinfarction in patients surviving acute myocardial infarction. *N Engl J Med* 1981; 304:801

The Thrombolysis in Myocardial Infarction (TIMI) Study Group: Special report: The thrombolysis in myocardial infarction (TIMI) trial, Phase I findings. *N Engl J Med* 1985; 312:932

31 Cardiogenic Shock

As discussed in Chapter 30, one of the potential complications of an acute myocardial infarction is the development of cardiogenic shock. This clinical syndrome is manifested by hypotension in the presence of a low cardiac output and an elevated left ventricular filling pressure. The causes of cardiogenic shock are many, involving both primary myocardial and secondary mechanical factors, but the syndrome is most commonly encountered following a myocardial infarction. This chapter focuses on cardiogenic shock in the setting of acute myocardial infarction. Cardiogenic shock occurring in other clinical situations is discussed briefly.

Approximately 15% of patients with an acute myocardial infarction develop cardiogenic shock. There is no way to predict which patients will develop this complication, because it is not definitively related to the patient's age, location of the infarction, or duration of symptoms before presentation. Despite great strides in pharmacologic and mechanical therapy, mortality has remained unacceptably high. Effective therapy necessitates an understanding of the basic pathophysiologic process. Only by early and aggressive intervention is survival improved.

ETIOLOGY

Many classification schemes have been proposed for this syndrome, each having a particular advantage. The system used here separates cardiogenic shock into nonmechanical and mechanical causes (Table 31-1). This system has proved beneficial because therapy and prognosis are directly related to the presence or absence of a mechanical defect. Types of shock other than cardiogenic are important in the differential diagnosis, and are discussed more fully in Chapter 29.

PATHOPHYSIOLOGY

The total amount of muscle infarcted appears to be the most important determinant in the evolution of the shock state. In the setting of an acute

TABLE 31-1 CAUSES OF CARDIOGENIC SHOCK

Nonmechanical causes
- Acute myocardial infarction
- Low cardiac output syndrome
- Right ventricular infarction
- End-stage cardiomyopathy

Mechanical causes
- Acute mechanical disorders (rupture of septum or free wall, mitral or aortic insufficiency)
- Papillary muscle rupture or dysfunction
- Critical aortic stenosis
- Pericardial tamponade

myocardial infarction, the severity of left ventricular dysfunction is related to the amount of myocardium that is damaged. A critical mass of contractile heart muscle is necessary to maintain adequate pump function, and the clinical syndrome of cardiogenic shock usually develops when necrosis to the left ventricle exceeds 45% of the muscle mass. This may be the result of one massive myocardial infarction or the cumulative effect of several smaller events. In the absence of a right ventricular infarct, most patients who develop cardiogenic shock have three-vessel coronary artery disease, with particularly severe disease of the left anterior descending coronary artery.

CLINICAL MANIFESTATIONS

Cardiogenic shock is present when there is decreased blood flow to vital organs, as evidenced by decreased urine output, impaired mental function, extremities that are cool, clammy, and cyanotic, and pulmonary vascular congestion. These features usually correspond with hypotension (systolic blood pressure < 90 mm Hg), a cardiac index less than 1.84 liter/min/m^2, and a pulmonary artery occlusion pressure (PAOP) greater than 20 mm Hg.

Although a thorough initial clinical exam and chest radiograph are the cornerstones of primary assessment, these findings may manifest a temporal lag. A more accurate assessment of systolic function and volume status can be made with the use of a flow-directed pulmonary artery catheter or by radionuclide ventriculography. Hemodynamic monitoring is usually indicated when hypotension does not respond to an adequate fluid challenge or pulmonary congestion is resistant to diuretic therapy.

THERAPY

IN THE SETTING OF ACUTE MYOCARDIAL INFARCTION

In benign or slowly progressive diseases, therapy can often be postponed until a full diagnostic evaluation is completed. Cardiogenic shock, however, is life-threatening and evolves rapidly, so that diagnostic and therapeutic interventions should proceed virtually simultaneously. Once this clinical entity is recognized, the physician must act intelligently and swiftly to maximize the patient's chances for survival.

Therapy is determined by the underlying pathophysiology. Inotropic agents, diuretics, and vasodilators are the main drugs used in managing these patients. However, these agents all have potentially deleterious as well as beneficial effects on the heart and blood supply to target organs. Intra-aortic balloon counterpulsation may also be used in selected patients. Practical indications for this modality are listed in Table 31-2. In severe coronary artery disease, any attempt to improve pump function must balance oxygen supply and demand. Some agents may increase myocardial contractility at the expense of increasing myocardial oxygen requirements, with a net detrimental effect on pump function.

Efforts To Limit Infarct Size

The immediate and long-term prognosis following acute myocardial infarction is largely determined by the extent of muscle damage. Limitation of the absolute loss of myocardium following an infarction to less than 40% would theoretically prevent cardiogenic shock. Infarct extension occurs when an imbalance between oxygen supply and demand exists in a jeopardized area in the periinfarction zone. Oxygen consumption ($M\dot{V}_{O_2}$) of the myocardium is determined primarily by three factors: heart rate, left ventricular contractility, and left ventricular wall tension, which, in turn, is related to the ventricular radius, the systemic blood pressure (afterload), and the filling pressure (preload). The neurohumoral response to an acute myocardial infarction is mediated by the sympathoadrenal axis, and includes increases in heart rate, blood pressure, and contractility. Each of these may unfavorably alter the delicate balance between oxygen supply and demand in the jeopardized area at the periphery of an infarct. This cycle can then be perpetuated, leading to a further decline in left ventricular function and culminating with the hypotension, low cardiac output, and pulmonary edema that characterize cardiogenic shock.

The concept that early intervention may limit infarct size was introduced in 1970. If therapy is begun within 3 hours (after an acute myocardial infarction), the incidence of subsequent cardiogenic shock is 4%; if therapy is delayed longer than 3 hours, the incidence of acute pump failure may increase to

TABLE 31-2 PRACTICAL INDICATIONS FOR THE INTRA-AORTIC BALLOON PUMP

Failure of conventional therapy after all contributing factors have been corrected (e.g., hypovolemia, hypoxemia, acidosis, dysarrhythmias)
Short-term inotropic support with reassessment at 12–24 hours
Search for surgically correctable lesions
Possible prophylactic use

13%. Studies with β-blockers and calcium antagonists show that these agents may reduce cardiac work and thus limit infarct size. However, because of their negative inotropic effects, routine use of these drugs in cardiogenic shock is not warranted.

Initial Management

Once cardiogenic shock is suspected, appropriate therapy should be instituted immediately. If the patient is profoundly hypotensive, attempts to raise the blood pressure should be simultaneous with the insertion of a pulmonary artery catheter. Pain should be relieved with intravenous morphine sulfate (2–4 mg), with doses based on the patient's blood pressure. Mechanical ventilation should be considered early, as the work of breathing is markedly increased in a patient with cardiogenic shock. If the PAOP is less than 15 mm Hg, it should be raised to 15 to 18 mm Hg with rapid volume infusion. The goal of pharmacologic support is to maximize coronary blood flow and reduce myocardial work, while improving systemic perfusion. Despite aggressive and appropriate medical care, patients in cardiogenic shock treated with drugs alone have a mortality rate approaching 90%.

OTHER TYPES OF CARDIOGENIC SHOCK

LOW OUTPUT SYNDROME

One of the most serious complications resulting from cardiac surgery is postoperative pump failure. The decreased cardiac output may result from a disruption of the normal interplay among the energy source (the heart), the responsiveness of the arterial system (systemic vascular resistance), the capacitance of the venous system (venous tone), the volume of flowing blood (preload), and the effectiveness of respiration (oxygenation). The clinical state resulting from derangements in these five factors may help to categorize the pathologic process. In the presence of adequate ventilation and a normal blood volume, severe myocardial failure produces the syndrome referred to as "low cardiac output syndrome." This myocardial failure may be the result of acute infarction (perioperative), persistent myocardial ischemia during the immediate postoperative period, or a preoperative diffuse myocardial disease.

Many inotropic drugs have been advocated for the treatment of low cardiac output after open-heart surgery including isoproterenol, dopamine, dobutamine, amrinone, glucagon, and others. Therapy of this syndrome must be individualized, and strict guidelines as to indications for invasive measures (e.g., the IABP) versus pharmacologic support are difficult to establish. Measurement of filling pressures and other hemodynamic variables by a flow-directed pulmonary artery catheter is essential. The next step is to ensure an adequate preload, and if blood pressure, urine output, and cardiac output fail to respond to blood volume replacement, inotropic support is indicated.

RIGHT VENTRICULAR INFARCTION

The entity of right ventricular infarction has only recently been appreciated. The clinical presentation of a right ventricular infarct may simulate cardiogenic shock secondary to a left ventricular infarction or cardiac tamponade. Correct diagnosis is imperative because treatment of this problem is quite different. These patients almost invariably have a concomitant infarction of the interventricular septum and a portion of the posterior wall of the left ventricle. Clincially, they can present with jugular venous distention, hypotension, and bradydysrhythmias. The electrocardiogram reveals evidence of an inferior or inferoposterior infarction. A pulmonary artery catheter demonstrates elevations in the right atrial and right ventricular pressures, and the PAOP is normal or slightly increased. The hemodynamic and clinical diagnosis can be confirmed with two-dimensional echocardiography, which shows dilation and hypokinesis of the right ventricle.

Once the diagnosis of a right ventricular infarction is established, intravascular volume expansion is usually indicated. If the blood pressure does not respond to a fluid challenge (PAOP = 12–15 mm Hg), a dopamine or dobutamine infusion should be started in the hope of improving left and right ventricular contractility. Should the patient fail to respond to fluids and inotropic agents, the combination of the IABP and dobutamine therapy has been successful in reversing the shock state.

MECHANICAL DEFECTS

The mechanical defect category includes a group of conditions that often complicate an acute myocardial infarction and result in cardiogenic shock. However, the defect is local and secondary to a mechanical problem rather than a diffuse lack of pump function. With early diagnosis and a definitive surgical procedure, survival rates approach 40%.

Ventricular Septal Defect (VSD). Acute VSDs following myocardial infarction are most commonly seen 3–5 days after the event, and are equally divided between anterior and inferior infarcts. Cardiogenic shock develops in over 50% of patients with an acute VSD and is probably due to impairment of the right ventricle. The clinical examination reveals a pansystolic murmur, often accompanied by a thrill, at the left lower sternal border, and clinical signs of biventricular failure. A step-up in the oxygen saturation of more than 10% between the right atrium and right ventricle is diagnostic, and therapy involves stabilization and early surgical repair.

Acute Mitral Regurgitation. Acute mitral regurgitation may occur with severe papillary muscle dysfunction, papillary head or tip rupture, or complete rupture of a papillary muscle. Hemodynamically signficant acute mitral insuficiency is rare, occurring in less than 0.1% of all myocardial infarctions. It usually occurs 2 to 4 days after a myocardial infarction that has destroyed an average of 20% of the left ventricular wall. The posteromedial muscle is most often involved. This clinical syndrome results in regurgitation of blood into a relatively normal sized, noncompliant left atrium, producing giant V waves (70–100 mm Hg) and acute pulmonary edema. The overall mortality from acute papillary muscle rupture approaches 90%.

Clinically, these patients often present with an episode of chest pain, followed by the rapid onset of hypotension and pulmonary congestion. Physical examination reveals a loud systolic murmur at the apex, and invasive monitoring confirms the elevated PAOP with a large V wave. Initial management involves the usual measures for the treatment of congestive heart failure, including sodium restriction and diuretics. For patients with a mean aortic pressure greater than 70 mm Hg, the next line of therapy includes the use of afterload-reducing agents. The physiological basis for this is a reduction of impedance, defined as the load resisting left ventricular ejection. Some additional improvement may be obtained with the use of the IABP, but this beneficial effect is often short-lived. Although many patients with acute mitral insufficiency and secondary left ventricular decompensation can be medically stabilized, most require surgery within 1 year.

Tepe and Edmunds described 11 patients who required emergency valve replacement for severe mitral insufficiency and cardiogenic shock in the early postinfarction period. They suggested that the circulatory insufficiency represented the addition of two lesions (valvular and myocardial) that may impair the circulation independently. The overall survival rate was 45% (5 of 11). The prognosis was more favorable in patients operated on sooner after the infarction (a mean of 3 days versus 15 days). Preoperative estimates of left ventricular function or the need for concomitant CABG were not predictive of outcome. In conclusion, acute mitral insufficiency can be a highly lethal condition, with the outcome dependent on early diagnosis, medical stabilization, and, often, early valve replacement.

Acute Aortic Insufficiency. Severe acute aortic insufficiency is seen most frequently as a complication of infective endocarditis. The physical examination is notable in that many of the signs of chronic aortic insufficiency are absent. Since this condition is one of acute volume overload, the chest radiograph may not show evidence of ventricular enlargement. M-mode echocardiography is quite valuable in showing the premature closure of the mitral valve before the onset of the QRS complex. This occurs because of the massive diastolic regurgitation into a normally compliant left ventricle, raising the left ventricular end-diastolic pressure above the left atrial pressure prior to systole. Therapy for acute aortic valvular insufficiency is quite similar to that for acute mitral regurgitation. Hemodynamic stability can occasionally be achieved, at least briefly, with inotropic agents or vasodilators to increase forward flow. If this proves unsuccessful, the patient should be placed on the IABP before aortic valve is surgically replaced.

Left Ventricular Free Wall Rupture and Pericardial Tamponade. Rupture of the left ventricle following an acute myocardial infarction is a catastrophic and usually fatal event. Risk factors for this infrequent complication include female sex, age above 60 years, hypertension, anterior infarction, and a first-time infarction. Clinically, these patients present with the jugular venous distention, hypotension, and distant heart sounds that characterize pericardial tamponade. The presence of a pulsus paradoxus (defined as a drop in systolic blood pressure greater than the normal 10 mm Hg during inspiration) should be sought. The physiological basis for tamponade is elevation of intrapericardial pressure, which limits diastolic filling of the ventricles and venous return. This results in a reduction in cardiac output. The definitive therapy for tamponade is pericardial drainage, although the use of intravenous fluids, catecholamines, and vasodilators may provide temporary support. In the setting of a left ventricular free wall rupture, death is the usual outcome; a few patients may develop an adherent clot over the rupture site, allowing time for diagnosis and definitive surgical procedures.

Left Ventricular Aneurysm/Wall Dyskinesia. A left ventricular aneurysm complicates myocardial infarction in approximately 10% to 15% of cases. The true incidence is probably directly related to how carefully it is looked for. In about 80% of cases, the aneurysm is located on the anterior or apical wall; it is usually associated with an anterior myocardial infarction. The aneurysm may develop early in the postinfarction period and can be asymptomatic or present with cardiogenic shock, congestive heart failure, recurrent ventricular dysrhythmias, or thromboembolic events.

The natural history of a left ventricular aneurysm or regions of akinesis is often the development of progressive pump failure. Schlichter and colleagues evaluated this problem in a retrospective analysis and found that 73% of patients were dead by 3 years, and only 12% were alive by 5 years. The usual causes of death included refractory heart failure, myocardial infarction, and peripheral embolic events.

The surgical approach to this problem was first accomplished in 1958 by Cooley, who used cardiopulmonary bypass to excise a left ventricular aneurysm. Since that time, this procedure has found wide clinical application, with an acceptably low operative mortality rate. If possible, the surgery should be delayed for at least 3 months after an infarction to allow the scar tissue to mature and demarcate from the adjacent myocardium. The clinical results have been quite encouraging. Favaloro and colleagues reported a series of 130 patients who underwent ventricular aneurysm resection between 1959 and 1967. Detailed follow-up, extending up to 7 years, was available for 68 of these patients. Of these, 49 were alive and 41 were symptom-free. As is true for all types of surgery related to coronary artery disease, the resection of a left ventricular aneurysm is only a palliative procedure. The ultimate effect on mortality is directly related to the underlying disease.

For further information, please see Chapter 76 in Civetta JM, Taylor RW, Kirby RR: Critical Care. *Philadelphia: J. B. Lippincott, 1988*

BIBLIOGRAPHY

Chatterjee K, Parmler WW: Vasodilator therapy for acute and chronic heart failure. *Br Heart J* 1977; 39

Cooley DA, Collins HA, Morris GC, et al: Ventricular aneurysm after myocardial infarction: Surgical excision with the use of temporary cardiopulmonary bypass. *JAMA* 1958: 167:557

Favaloro RG, Effler DB, Groves LK, et al: Ventricular aneurysm—clinical experience. *Ann Thorac Surg* 1968; 6:227

Gafford FH, Ayers SM: Shock associated with myocardial infarction: Pathophysiology, diagnosis, treatment and prevention. *Baylor College of Medicine Cardiology Series* 1985; 8:6

Keung EC, Siskind SJ, Sonnenblick EH, et al: Dobutamine therapy in acute myocardial infarction. *JAMA* 1981; 245:144

LeJemtel TH, Davis R, Schwartz W, et al: Amrinone: A new non-glycosidic, non-adrenergic agent effective in the treatment of intractable myocardial failure in man. *Circulation* 1979; 59:1098

Lvoff R, Wilcken DEL: Glucagon in heart failure and in cardiogenic shock. Experience in 50 patients. *Circulation* 1972; 45:534

Mueller HS, Ayres SM, Giannelli S, et al: Effect of isoproterenol, l-norepinephrine, and intra-aortic counterpulsation on hemodynamics and myocardial metabolism in shock following acute myocardial infarction. *Circulation* 1972; 45:335

Resenkov L: Cardiogenic shock. *Chest* 1983; 83:893

Richard C, Ricone JL, Rimailho A, et al: Combined hemodynamic effects of dopamine and dobutamine in cardiogenic shock. *Circulation* 1983; 67:620

Schlichter J, Hellerstein HK, Katz LN: Aneurysm of the heart: A correlative study of one hundred and two proved cases. *Medicine* 1954; 33:43.

Tepe NA, Edmunds LH: Operation for acute post infarction mitral insufficiency and cardiogenic shock. *J Thorac Cardiovas Surg* 1985; 89:525

32
Heart Failure

Impaired ventricular performance caused by a variety of cardiac disorders manifests clinically in a common syndrome of congestive heart failure. It is estimated that 2.4 million Americans suffer from heart failure, and approximately 400,000 new cases are added each year. Diagnosis of heart failure carries a grim prognosis—almost half of the patients die within the first 2 years.

WHAT IS HEART FAILURE?

To the physiologist, heart failure means inability of the heart to pump blood at a rate commensurate with the requirements of the metabolizing tissues, irrespective of whether the cardiac output is high, normal, or low. Clinicians recognize the syndrome from symptoms and signs of pulmonary or systemic venous congestion, with or without the effects of depressed cardiac output at rest.

Clinical manifestations of heart failure depend on the rapidity with which the decompensation occurs and whether enough time has elapsed for compensatory mechanisms to partially alleviate the consequences of reduced cardiac output. Thus, heart failure may be acute or chronic. Patients with chronic failure may develop acute exacerbations with the advent of precipitating events such as infections or dysrhythmias. Refractory heart failure indicates the persistence of significant failure despite intensive medical therapy. Intractable heart failure is resistant to all known therapeutic measures.

Evaluation of a patient presenting with symptoms of heart failure includes (1) a correct diagnosis, (2) an attempt at identifying the underlying structural cause, (3) an understanding of the pathophysiologic basis for the develoment of decompensation in order to organize a rational therapeutic approach, (4) detection of any acute precipitating events, and, finally (5) a subjective and objective assessment of cardiac performance at the time of presentation.

DIAGNOSIS

A careful history and physical examination is mandatory. The clinical diagnosis of heart failure is based on a combination of symptoms and signs (Table 32-1). Each of the clinical manifestations, taken singly, may be due to causes other than heart failure. Clinical diagnosis can be substantially aided by a good chest radiograph film taken in posteroanterior and lateral views. Common causes of heart failure are listed in Table 32-2.

PRECIPITANTS OF ACUTE HEART FAILURE

About half of all acute episodes of heart failure are caused by acute precipitating events (Table 32-3). Recognition of those events is as important as diagnosis of the underlying cause in planning appropriate therapy.

Dietary indiscretions are extremely common, and every effort should be made to obtain a detailed dietary history. Patients frequently fail to appreciate that a favorite food or beverage may contain excessive salt. Similarly, reduction, discontinuation, or intermittent intake of medicines frequently leads to trouble.

Factors that tend to increase the work of the heart, such as physical activity

TABLE 32-1 CLINICAL AND RADIOGRAPHIC MANIFESTATIONS

	Symptoms	Signs
Reduced cardiac output	Fatigue Tiredness Dizziness Syncope	Cold, blue extremities Malar flush Muscular wasting Cachexia
Pulmonary venous congestion	Dyspnea Orthopnea Paroxysmal nocturnal dyspnea	Tachypnea Shallow breathing Pulsus alternans Gallop sounds 3 and 4 Pulmonary basal crackles Bronchospasm (rare)
Systemic venous congestion	Right hypochrondrial pain and tenderness (hepatic congestion) Ankle swelling Abdominal swelling	Hepatojugular reflux Jugular venous distension Right-sided gallop sounds Hepatomegaly Ankle/sacral edema
	Chest radiograph: Reversal of vascular distribution, dilated upper lobe veins (in acute left ventricular failure, mitral stenosis and occasionally COPD*), interstitial pulmonary edema (perihilar haze, perivascular and peribronchial cuffing, septal lines, Kerley A-hilum B-basal [common]); alveolar pulmonary edema (bilateral hilar clouding, butterfly pattern); pleural effusions (right > left), hydrothorax; cardiomegaly, enlargement of individual heart chambers.	

*COPD = chronic obstructive pulmonary disease.

TABLE 32-2 CAUSES OF HEART FAILURE

Coronary artery disease
Cardiomyopathy
Hypertensive heart disease
Valvular heart disease (rheumatic)
Congenital heart disease

in excess of the ventricular reserve, emotional stress, or extremes of heat or cold, can provoke acute heart failure. The sympathetic nervous system is activated in congestive heart failure and, as expected, peripheral vascular beds containing a rich population of α-adrenergic receptors (kidneys, viscera, and skin) suffer the greatest reduction in flow. Patients are susceptible to heart failure in hot and humid climates because they cannot dilate their skin vessels in response to heat stress.

Dysrhythmias can often worsen heart failure and in certain situations may even precipitate severe heart failure. The onset of atrial fibrillation in patients with severe left ventricular hypertrophy and significant diastolic dysfunction (as in hypertrophic cardiomyopathy) can have dire consequences and may be solely responsible for the onset of pulmonary edema. Ventricular dysrhythmias are frequent in patients with dilated cardiomyopathy and cause significant impairment of ventricular function. Since stroke volume is relatively fixed in most patients with heart failure, adequacy of heart rate is important to maintaining cardiac output. Onset of bradydysrhythmias can have adverse effects by further reducing cardiac output.

A number of drugs with negative inotropic properties or an ability to cause retention of salt and water may be responsible for a significant depression of ventricular function.

Systemic infection, bacterial endocarditis, and pulmonary embolism are complications that may be more frequent in patients with heart disease. A careful search for these complications can be rewarding in the effort to control symptoms of failure. Acute ischemic events, including myocardial infarction, can precipitate heart failure in patients with valvular heart disease. Unrelated illness can put demands on the heart. Renal failure, prostatic obstruction in males, excessive volume overload in postoperative patients, and liver disease can all contribute to development of heart failure in patients with myocardial dysfunction.

ASSESSMENT OF SEVERITY

The initial evaluation of patients with heart disease must include subjective and objective assessment of functional capacity so that appropriate treatment and follow-up can be planned. Conventional subjective assessment uses the functional classification adopted by the New York Heart Association:

Class I. Normal cardiac output without systemic or pulmonary congestion: patients are asymptomatic at rest and on heavy exertion.

TABLE 32-3 ACUTE PRECIPITATING EVENTS IN HEART FAILURE

- Patient induced
  - Noncompliance with therapy
  - Dietary indiscretions
  - High alcohol intake
  - Physical activity in excess of cardiac reserve
  - Emotional stress
- Environmental stress
  - Excessive heat or cold
- Conditions common in patients with heart failure
  - Respiratory and systemic infections
  - Bacterial endocarditis
  - Pulmonary embolism
- Unrelated illnesses
  - Acute myocardial infarction in valvular heart disease
  - Renal failure
  - Liver disease
  - Postoperative intravenous volume loading
- Conditions increasing demand on limited cardiac reserve
  - High-output states
- Drugs
  - Negative inotropic agents
    - β-Adrenergic receptor antagonists
    - Calcium channel blockers
    - Antidysrhythmic agents—disopyramide
  - Drugs producing salt and water retention
    - Corticosteroids
    - Nonsteroidal antiinflammatory agents
      - Indomethacin
      - Ibuprofen
      - Phenylbutazone
      - Others
  - Direct myotoxic effects
    - Adriamycin
    - Daunorubicin
  - Hormones
    - Estrogens and androgens
  - Tricyclic compounds
  - Chlorpropamide (may increase antidiuretic hormone)
  - Digitialis intoxication
- Acute ischemic events in patients with chronic coronary artery disease

Class II. Normal cardiac output maintained with moderate increase in pulmonary/systemic congestion: symptomatic on heavy exertion.

Class III. Normal cardiac output maintained with marked increase in pulmonary/systemic congestion: symptomatic on mild exercise.

Class IV. Cardiac output reduced at rest with marked increase in pulmonary/systemic congestion: symptomatic at rest.

Despite numerous theoretical limitations, the most convenient approach to the objective assessment of cardiac function continues to be based on measurement of intravascular and intracardiac pressure, cardiac output and, perhaps, ventricular volume or dimensions. In evaluating principal determinants of cardiac performance, it has been possible to precisely measure the following:

1 Ventricular preload (end-diastolic pressure or volume).
2 Heart rate.
3 Afterload (the product of left ventricular radius and pressure divided by wall thickness). For practical purposes, calculated systemic vascular resistance (mean aortic pressure minus mean right atrial pressure, divided by cardiac output) may be substituted for left ventricular calculations.
4 Left ventricular wall motion.

Noninvasive methods can also make a significant contribution to the assessment of cardiac function. Such methods are particularly suited for serial evaluation of cardiac performance, such as assessment of the acute and chronic effects of drug therapy. Indices that previously could be derived only by cardiac catherization can now be obtained from echocardiographic and radionuclide angiographic examinations. Ejection fraction and wall motion abnormalities can be ascertained from echocardiographic studies. Ejection fraction, ventricular volumes and wall motion abnormalities also can be obtained from radionuclide studies, which have the added advantages of including an exercise protocol and examining abnormalities of diastolic filling. Heart failure due to systolic dysfunction is usually clinically evident when the ejection fraction is reduced to less than 40%.

TREATMENT

Other than removing an underlying cause or treating a precipitating event, therapeutic approaches to heart failure are based on improving the four determinants of cardiac performance (preload, afterload, contractility, and heart rate) so as to allow the failing heart to deliver a normal or near-normal cardiac output. Treatment strategies include use of inotropic agents, diuretics, and vasodilators. Principles in the treatment of heart failure are outlined in Table 32-4. Commonly used pharmacologic agents are detailed in Tables 32-5 and 32-6.

HIGH-OUTPUT HEART FAILURE

Conditions that impose heavy demands on cardiovascular system (Table 32-7) can cause or contribute to heart failure. The ability of the normal heart to vary its output in response to external demands allows it to accept with impunity the additional hemodynamic burden imposed by hypermetabolic states, provided that the onset of hemodynamic load is gradual and the

TABLE 32-4 PRINCIPLES OF TREATMENT OF HEART FAILURE

Clinical Finding	Treatment Approach
Decreased contractility	Digitalis glycosides and other positive inotropic agents
Increased preload	Salt restriction Diuretics Venodilators Mechanical removal of fluid Phlebotomy Thoracentesis Paracentesis
Low cardiac output and high vascular resistance	Arteriolar vasodilators
Rapid heart rate (atrial fibrillation or sinus tachycardia)	Improve left ventricular performance Increase atrioventricular block with digitalis

compensatory mechanisms (dilatation and hypertrophy) have had time to come into play. If the onset is sudden or if there is preexisting myocardial disease, the heart is unable to adapt to the new hemodynamic situation and fails. In most instances, the high-output states are precipitating factors rather than causes in producing heart failure.

Patients with high-output heart failure present with typical clinical manifestations. They differ hemodynamically in having a normal or high cardiac output with normal or low arteriovenous oxygen content difference. In addition to conventional treatment for heart failure, these patients require management of the specific underlying disease state.

CARDIAC TRANSPLANTATION

In just under two decades, cardiac transplantation has progressed from an experimental procedure to an accepted and effective therapy for patients with end-stage heart disease. Through refinement of surgical techniques, effective immunosuppressive therapy—particularly the availability of Cyclosporin A—and improved postoperative care, survival rates exceed 70% for the first year and a significant number of patients are alive at 5 years. All patients with intractable heart failure should be assessed for cardiac transplantation if they fulfill the following criteria: (1) end-stage cardiac disease, with estimated life expectancy of less than 12 months; (2) age under 55 years in most cases; (3) normal or reversible renal and hepatic function; and (4) compliance with medical regimens, psychosocial stability, and the presence of a supportive social environment.

TABLE 32-5 PHARMACOLOGIC AGENTS USED TO TREAT HEART FAILURE*

	Route of Adminis-tration	Hemodynamic Effects			Dose	Onset of Action	Duration of Action	Indications	Adverse Effects and Remarks
		CI	PAOP	SVR					
Direct Smooth Muscle ***Relaxants***									
Nitrates	Sublingual	↓—	↓	↓	0.4–0.8 mg	2–5 min	10–30 min	To reduce preload: Acute myocardial infarction: Nitrates may be preferable to diuretics	Headaches (sometimes debilitating), dizziness, nausea, syncope, occasionally paradoxical bradycardia and hypotension in acute myocardial infarction (empty-heart syndrome)
	Buccal	↓—	↓	↓	3–5 mg	1–5 min	4–6 hr		
	Topical 2%	↓—	↓	—	0.5″–2″	35–60 min	4–8 hr		
	Inhalation	↓—	↓	↓	0.4 mg/puff	1–5 min	10–30 min		
	Oral (isosorbide dinitrate)	↑↓	↓	↓	10–40 mg qid	15–30 min	120–180 min	Chronic heart failure with pulmonary congestion: Use nitrates in combination with hydralazine	Skin irritation with topical preparations Methemoglobinemia Tolerance can develop Avoid in right ventricular infarction, significant diastolic dysfunction, hypertrophic cardiomyopathy, hypovolemia, pericardial effusion or constriction, glaucoma, increased intracranial pressure. IV: Given by infusion pump using polyethylene tubing. Polyvinyl chloride
	Intravenous	↓↑	↓	↓↓	3–10 mg/hr by infusion	1 min	Continuous titration		
	Nitro discs	↓	↓	↓	10–20 mg	30–60 min	Up to 24 hr		

									tubing adsorbs up to 80T of nitroglycerin.
Nitroprusside	Intravenous	↑↑	↓	↓↓	50 mg in 500 ml 5% dextrose = 100 μg/ml 0.5-5 μg/kg/min 0.005-0.05 ml/kg/min Protect from light; avoid extravasation.	1–2 min	Continuous titration	Acute myocardial infarction with pulmonary edema and normal blood pressure Chronic heart failure (acute exacerbation)	Accumultion of thiosulphates, increase in renal insufficiency. Blood thiosulphate level should not exceed 6 mg/100 ml. Thiosulphate toxicity: Psychosis, convulsions, hypothyroidism, muscle twitching, abdominal pain dizziness Methemoglobinemia, vitamin B 12 deficiency
Hydralazine	Oral Intravenous	↑↑	↓↑	↓↓↓	100–300 mg 10–20 mg	15–30 min 10–20 min	4–6 hr 3–4 hr	Afterload reducing agent In low cardiac output states with normal blood pressure, may combine with nitrates	Vascular headache, flushing, nausea, vomiting, drug fever, skin rash, positive ANF Drug-induced systemic lupus erythematosus (usually over 400 mg/day, slow acetylators) Pyridoxine deficiency
Adrenergic Blocking Agents									
Phentolamine	Intravenous	↑↑	↓↓	↓↓	0.3–2 mg/min by IV infusion	1 min	Titrated	Refractory congestive heart failure Pulmonary edema	Hypotension, tachycardia, nausea, vomiting, abdominal pain

(continued on page 256)

TABLE 32-5 *(continued)*

	Route of Adminis-tration	Hemodynamic Effects			Dose	Onset of Action	Duration of Action	Indications	Adverse Effects and Remarks
		CI	PAOP	SVR					
Prazosin	Oral	↑↑	↓↓	↓↓	1–10 mg bid	30 min	6 hr	Chronic congestive heart failure requiring balanced dilatation May have acute dysrhythmic effect	"First dose" phenomenon: faintness, dizziness, palpitation and (rarely) syncope after first dose Transient rashes, dry mouth, mental depression, polyarthralgia Salt and water retention on chronic use due to activation of reninangiotensin axis; increase diuretic dose
β-Adrenergic Receptor Agonists									
Dopamine	Intravenous infusion								
	Low dose	↑↑	–	↓ –	2.5–5 μg/kg/min	1 min	Titrated	Normotensive cardiac failure (combined with dobutamine)	Cardiac dysrhythmias, gangrene of digits in patients with peripheral vascular disease (seen on high-dose dopamine)
	High dose	↑↓	↓	↓ –	5–15 μg/kg/min	1 min	Titrated	Hypotension (combined with nitroprusside)	
Dobutamine	Intravenous	↑↑	↓	↓ –	5–15 μg/kg/min	Immediate	Titrated		
Salbutamol	Oral	↑↑	↓	↓↓	2–4 mg tid	30–45 min	6 hr	Dilated cardiomyopathy associated with COPD	Cardiac dysrhythmias, hypokalemia (from β_2 stimulation), tachycardia, tremor, and (rarely) diabetic ketoacidosis
Pirbuterol	Oral	↑↑	↓	↓↓	20 mg tid				

Drug	Route	CI	PWP	SVR	Dose	Onset	Duration	Indication	Side effects/Comments
Converting Enzyme Inhibitors									
Captopril	Oral	↑↑	↓↓	↓↓	12.5–50 mg tid	30–45 min	4–6 hr	Low-ouput chronic failure	Hypotension, proteinuria, skin rashes, loss of taste, worsening of renal function in preexisting renal disease (rare), pancytopenia (in patients with collagen vascular disease)
Enalapril	Oral	↑↑	↓↓	↓↓	2.5–20 mg/day	60 min	24 hr	Low-output chronic failure	Hypotension, hyperkalemia, angioedema, syncope, palpitations, insomnia, nervousness, abdominal pain, dyspepsia
Phosphodiesterase III Inhibitors									
Amrinone	Intravenous	↑↑	↓↓	↓	0.75–1.5 mg/kg bolus in 3–5 min; 0.75 mg/kg 2nd bolus in 15–30 min; maintenance infusion 5–10 μg/kg/min	5–10 min	Continuous titration	Low-output chronic failure	Nausea, vomitting, diarrhea, anorexia (0.5%–2%), thrombocytopenia (2.4%), hypotension, liver function abnormalities, increase in ventricular ectopic activity Can be used in combination with dobutamine, nitrates, and nitroprusside

* CI = Cardiac index; PWP = pulmonary wedge pressure; SVR = systemic vascular resistance; ↓ = reduced; ↓↓ = markedly reduced; ↑ = increased; ↑↑ = markedly increased; – = no effect.

TABLE 32-6 DIURETICS IN HEART FAILURE

	Dose					
	Oral (mg)	**IV (mg)**	**Onset of Action**	**Peak Effect Duration**	**Site of Action**	**Adverse Effects and Remarks**
Thiazides						
Chlorothiazide	50–1000		1 hr	4 hr (6–12)	Distal convoluted tubule (DCT)	Hypokalemia, metabolic acidosis, hyperuricemia, hyponatremia, carbohydrate intolerance, hypercalcemia, agranulocytosis, thrombocytopenia, pancreatitis, hepatic coma in liver insufficiency
Hydrochlorothiazide	50–100		2 hr	4 hr (> 12)	DCT	
Chlorthalidone	50		2 hr	6 hr (> 24)	DCT	
Metolazone	2.5–5		1 hr	2–4 hr (24–48)	DCT	
Cyclopenthiazide	0.5–1		1 hr	2–4 hr (> 12)	DCT	Thiazides may have synergistic effects with loop diuretics. Metolazone does not reduce renal blood flow and glomerular filtration rate so may be particularly suitable.
Loop						
Furosemide	40–80	20–80	Oral—1 hr IV—5 min	Oral—1–2 hr (6) IV—30 min (1–2 hr)	Loop and ascending limb of Henle	Glucose intolerance, deafness, thrombocytopenia

Ethacrynic acid	50–100	50 in 50 ml 5% dextrose or saline	Oral—30 min IV—15 min	Oral—2 hr (6–8) IV—45 min (3 hr)		Synergistic effects with thiazide or potassium-sparing diuretics
Potassium-sparing						
Spironolactone	50–100		2 hr	1–2 days (2–3)	DCT, collecting duct system	Hyperkalemia, gynecomastia, impotence, diminished libido: do not use in acute or chronic renal failure.
Triamterene	50–100		2 hr	6–8 hr (12–16)	DCT, collecting duct system	Azotemia, muscle cramps, renal calculi; do not combine with indomethacin. Potassium-sparing diuretics should always be combined with loop duretics.
Amiloride	5–10		2 hr	6–8 hr (12–16)	DCT, collecting duct system	
Carbonic Anhydrase Inhibitor						
Acetazolamide	250 tid for 2–4 days		1 hr	2–4 hr (8)	Proximal tubule	Metabolic acidosis, hyperchloremia, renal calculi. Weak diuretic action lasts for 3–4 days. Useful in patients with heart failure who have developed hypochloremic metabolic alkalosis in presence of normal serum potassium.

TABLE 32-7 HIGH-OUTPUT STATES

Anemia
Pregnancy
Arteriovenous fistulae
Thyrotoxicosis
Paget's disease
Beriberi heart disease
Fibrous dysplasia (Albright's syndrome)
Pulmonary disease
Polycythemia vera
Carcinoid syndrome
Exfoliative dermatitis
Psoriasis
Hypernephroma with bone metastasis

For further information, please see Chapter 77 in Civetta JM, Taylor RW, Kirby RR: Critical Care. *Philadelphia: J. B. Lippincott, 1988*

BIBLIOGRAPHY

Davis R, Ribner HS, Keung E, et al: Treatment of chronic congestive heart failure with captopril; an oral inhibitor of angiotensin converting enzyme. *N Engl J Med* 1979; 301:117

Fowler MB, Schroeder JS: Current status of cardiac transplantation. *Mod Conc Cardiovasc Dis* 1986; 55:37

Furburg CD, Yusuf S, Thom TJ: Potential for altering natural history of congestive heart failure: Need for large clinical trials. *Am J Cardiol* 1985; 55:45A

Goldberg LI, Hsieh YY, Resenkov L: New catecholamines for treatment of heart failure and shock: An update on dopamine and a first look at dobutamine. *Prog Cardiovasc Dis* 1977; 19:327

Killip T: Epidemiology of congestive heart failure. *Am J Cardiol* 1985; 56:2A

Koch-Wesser J: Hydralazine. *N Engl J Med* 1976; 295:320

Lowenstein J, Steele J Jr: Prazosin. *Am Heart J* 1978; 95:262

Mancini D, Lejemtel T, Sonnenblick E: Intravenous use of amrinone for the treatment of the failing heart. *Am J Cardiol* 1984; 56:8B

Miller RR, Awan NA, Mason DT: Pharmacologic mechanisms for left ventricular unloading in clinical congestive heart failure. *Circ Res* 1976; 39:127

Ross J Jr: Left ventricular function and the timing of surgical treatment in valvular heart disease. *Ann Intern Med* 1981; 94:498

Smith WM: Epidemiology of congestive heart failure. *Am J Cardiol* 1985; 55:3A

Sonnenblick EH, Frishman WH, Lejemtel TH: Dobutamine: A new synthetic cardioactive sympathetic amine. *N Engl J Med* 1979; 300:17

33
Cardiac Dysrhythmias

Cardiac dysrhythmias are conveniently grouped as supra-ventricular or ventricular, and as bradycardic or tachycardic. Dysrhythmias may be due to a number of causes, including enhanced automaticity, reentry, triggered automaticity, and abnormal conduction.

GENERAL DIAGNOSTIC CONSIDERATIONS

The ability to diagnose a dysrhythmia is based on determination of the basic rhythmic pattern; each pattern has a specific differential diagnosis. The eight basic patterns are listed in Table 33-1; Table 33-2 presents a partial differential diagnosis list for each pattern.

Once the rhythm pattern is determined one should proceed to evaluate the QRS complex in an attempt to determine whether it is initiated by a supraventricular impulse or is ectopic. In general, this reduces to an analysis of the QRS duration because ventricular complexes $\leq$ 120 msec are virtually always caused by supraventricular mechanisms. Wider ventricular complexes may be ectopic or due to a supraventricular beat with aberrant ventricular conduction. There are several criteria one may use to decide whether wide ventricular complexes are more likely to be aberrantly conducted or ectopic (Table 33-3). Occasionally, however, invasive monitoring techniques may be required for definitive diagnosis.

Once the origin of the QRS is determined, the P waves should be identified and their site(s) of origin established if possible. Next, the relationship between the P wave and QRS should be examined to determine which site is controlling cardiac activity. Finally, one should identify the *primary* underlying dysrhythmia since several may be present—for example, atrial flutter with complete heart block or atrial fibrillation with ventricular tachycardia. Failure to determine the primary problem could lead to difficulties in treatment.

TABLE 33-1 EIGHT BASIC RHYTHM PATTERNS

Regular rhythm at normal rates	Early beats
Unexpected pauses	Regular bradycardia
Regular tachycardia	Bigeminal rhythms
Group beating	Chaotic irregularity

(Adapted from Marriott HJL: *Practical Eletrocardiography,* 7th ed. Baltimore, Williams & Wilkins, 1983)

TABLE 33-2 Causes of the Eight Basic Rhythm Patterns

Regular rhythm at normal rates
- Normal sinus rhythm
- Accelerated junctional rhythm
- Accelerated idioventricular rhythm
- Atrial flutter with 4:1 conduction
- Atrial tachycardia with block

Early beats
- Extrasystole
- Parasystole
- Capture beats
- Intermittent improved conduction during heart block
- Rhythm resumption after inapparent bigeminy

Pauses
- Nonconducted PACs (most common)
- Second-degree AV block (types I and II)
- Second-degree SA exit block
- Concealed conduction
- Concealed junctional extrasystoles

Bradycardia
- Sinus bradycardia
- Nonconducted atrial bigeminy
- Second- and third-degree AV block
- Second- and third-degree SA block

Bigeminy
- PACs and PVCs
- 3:2 SA and AV block
- Atrial tachycardia or fluttér with alternate 4:1 and 2:1 conduction
- Nonconducted atrial trigeminy
- Reciprocal beating
- Concealed junctional extrasystoles

Chaos
- Artial fibrillation
- Atrial flutter with variable conduction
- Multifocal atrial tachycardia
- Wandering pacemaker
- Multifocal PVCs
- Parasystoles
- Combinations of the above

TABLE 33-2 *(continued)*

Regular tachycardia
Sinus tachycardia
Paroxysmal atrial tachycardia
Atrial flutter
Ectopic atrial tachycardia
Junctional tachycardia
Ventricular tachycardia
Group beating
Nonconducted extrasystoles
SA nodal Wenckebach exit block
AV nodal Wenckebach block

(Adapted from Marriott JHL: *Practical Electrocardiography,* 7th ed. Baltimore, Williams & Wilkins, 1983)

DIAGNOSTIC MANEUVERS

In addition to the electrocardiogram (EKG), there are several diagnostic techniques that are quite helpful in defining dysrhythmias. Most can be rapidly performed at the bedside, and they often allow rapid diagnosis when EKG analysis has been inconclusive.

Physical examination can be helpful but is often not considered in the diagnosis of dysrhythmias. Attention to the jugular venous wave may demonstrate flutter waves in atrial flutter or fibrillation waves in atrial fibrillation.

TABLE 33-3 DIFFERENTIATION OF ABERRANT VENTRICULAR CONDITION FROM VENTRICULAR ECTOPY

Characteristics favoring aberrant ventricular conduction
Right bundle-branch block with R′>R
Rate > 170
Initial QRS vector same as conducted QRS
QRS duration < 140 msec
Normal axis
Preceding P′
Ashman's phenomenon
Characteristics favoring ventricular ectopy
Left axis deviation
QRS > 140 msec
Monophasic or diphasic in V_1
Fusion or capture beats
Rate <170
AV dissociation
R>R′ in V_1
Concordant precordial pattern
! NOTHING IS ABSOLUTE !

Intermittent cannon A waves may be seen with PVCs or with complete heart block or AV dissociation. Auscultation may reveal a variable first heart sound in AV dissociation, complete heart block, or atrial fibrillation.

Vagal maneuvers, such as the Valsalva maneuver or carotid sinus massage, may be diagnostic in patients with difficult tachycardias. Table 33-4 lists common responses of several dysrhythmias to vagal maneuvers.

Special surface leads, such as the Lewis lead, may be useful in delineating atrial activity in selected patients but rarely yield more information than might be obtained by standard leads 2 and V_1. Recording of simultaneous atrial electrograms and EKG can be quite useful in demonstrating atrial and ventricular rhythms and their relationships. Atrial electrograms can be recorded from epicardial leads after cardiovascular surgery, from esophageal electtrodes, or from transvenous intra-atrial electrodes.

Occasionally, even though adequate tracings can be obtained, a dysrhythmia remains undiagnosed. Atrial electrograms may demonstrate a 1:1 atrial-ventricular relationship, but the exact physiology remains unclear. For example, if a patient has a narrow-complex SVT at 150/min, EKG and atrial recording may show simultaneous activation of the atrium and ventricle without revealing whether the dysrhythmia is sinus tachycardia, PAT, ectopic atrial tachycardia (EAT), or nonparoxysmal junctional tachycardia. By pacing the atrium at a rate faster than the dysrhythmia, information can be gained that may make the diagnosis. If the dysrhythmia is sinus tachycardia, the sinus node will likely return at an initially slower rate (overdrive suppression), and the first spontaneous activity after cessation of pacing will be atrial. If the dysrhythmia is PAT, it will either be terminated by pacing or be unchanged following the cessation of pacing. Ectopic atrial tachycardias may still be difficult to delineate from sinus tachycardia but may be successfully interrupted. With nonparoxysmal junctional tachycardia, the junctional pacemaker will also display overdrive suppression, but the first spontaneous beat after cessation of pacing will be a QRS complex.

TABLE 33-4 RESPONSE OF DYSRHYTHMIAS TO VAGAL MANEUVERS

Sinus tachycardia	Slows gradually, returns to intrinsic rate when maneuver is ended
Ectopic atrial tachycardia	Stepwise decrease in AV conduction, may develop 2:1 or 3:1 conduction
PAT	No response or breaks suddenly to sinus rhythm
Atrial flutter	Decrease in AV conduction, may go from 2:1 to 3:1 or 4:1 conduction
Atrial fibrillation	Gradual decrease in ventricular rate, returns to original rate after termination of maneuver
MAT	No response or may cause some P waves to be nonconducted
Ventricular tachycardia	No response

MANAGEMENT

GENERAL PRINCIPLES

The initial step in determining appropriate management after a dysrhythmia is recognized is to determine the hemodynamic consequences and the patient's tolerance of the dysrhythmia. In addition, a careful search for reversible causes of dysrhythmias (*e.g.*, hypoxemia, hypokalemia, digitalis toxicity, myocardial infarction) must be made. Too often, dysrhythmias in the critically ill patient are treated with antidysrhythmic drugs when the patient is not at any particular risk from the dysrhythmia or when correction of a related threatening problem would be preferable. Given that the incidence of serious adverse reactions, including life-threatening prodysrhythmic effects, with antidysrhythmic drugs is 8% to 20%, and that patients can and do die from unrecognized causes of dysrhythmias, the need to search thoroughly for such abnormalities is apparent.

SPECIFIC DYSRHYTHMIAS

Atrial

Sinus tachycardia is almost always an indicator of an underlying problem and rarely requires specific treatment. Occasionally, hyperadrenergic patients with accelerated hypertension, myocardial infarction, or thyrotoxicosis may benefit from specific therapy. The drugs of choice in these cases are β-blockers, which may be given intravenously (propranolol 1–3 mg every 5 min to a total of 0.1 mg/kg) or orally. Care must be taken not to treat patients with poor left ventricular function with β-blockers. Pulmonary disorders with airflow obstruction are strong relative contraindications to β-blockers.

Sinus bradycardia, first-degree AV block and type I second-degree AV block require treatment only when hemodynamically significant. Type II second-degree AV block and third-degree AV block should always be treated. Pharmacologic treatment, when appropriate, can include atropine, 0.5 to 1.0 mg IV, which can be repeated as needed to a maximum of 2 mg. When pharmacologic therapy is ineffective for sinus or junctional bradycardias or for type I second-degree AV block, external or transvenous pacing may be instituted. Even if pharmacologic interventions result in improvement, patients with type II second-degree AV block or complete heart block should have transvenous pacing established. It is worth noting that the currently available external pacemakers are quite effective and are well tolerated. They can frequently be very helpful in stabilizing a patient so that placement of a transvenous pacemaker can be done under controlled circumstances.

Premature atrial beats and premature junctional beats are almost never an independent indication for drug therapy but frequently mark the emergence of an underlying problem. Paroxysmal atrial tachycardia, paroxysmal junctional tachycardia, and reciprocating tachycardias utilizing an accessory pathway can be considered under the general heading of *supraventricular tachycardia* (SVT). In the critical care setting, these should virtually always be treated. Unstable SVT (*e.g.*, with hypotension, angina, or congestive heart failure) requires emergency cardioversion. The drug of choice for stable SVT is verapamil, 5 mg IV, followed in 15 to 20 minutes by 10 mg IV if needed. One should remember that verapamil can shorten the refractory period of accessory pathways, leading to increases in ventricular rates and possible ventricular fibrillation if the patient should develop atrial fibrillation. Therefore, immediate availability of a defibrillator is imperative. If therapy with verapamil is unsuccessful, elective cardioversion, digoxin, β-blockers, and therapeutic pacing can be considered.

Fortunately, EAT is relatively rare—it can be particularly difficult to treat and often responds very poorly to therapy. If EAT is due to digoxin toxicity and the patient is stable, one can discontinue the digitalis preparation and give support. Unstable patients with digitalis toxicity may respond to treatment with Fab fragments of digoxin-specific antibody. When the dysrhythmia is due to heart failure, it may respond to treatment of the failure. In idiopathic EAT, very little seems to work well, although there are some reports that flecainide is useful. Atrial overdrive pacing at a rate higher than the intrinsic rate is sometimes successful. This generally produces 2:1 or 3:1 AV conduction at pacing rates of 200/min to 250/min, effectively slowing the ventricular rate from 150–200/min to 75–100/min. This is, of course, only a short-term treatment. Some patients with EAT have been paced into atrial fibrillation, with better control of ventricular rates. Occasional patients respond only to surgical therapy with excision of the atrial focus or ablation of the AV node and placement of a VVI pacemaker.

Multifocal atrial tachycardia is more common than EAT, but treatment can also be quite difficult. The mainstay of treatment is aggressive therapy of the underlying, usually pulmonary, disease. Verapamil works well in many patients, not only controlling the ventricular response but occasionally reducing the frequency of the atrial activity. One should, of course, avoid verapamil in patients who have significant left ventricular dysfunction.

Atrial flutter should be treated by cardioversion if the patient is unstable. When the patient is stable, the treatment proceeds in two stages. First, control of the ventricular response is obtained with verapamil, digoxin, or β-blockers. Once this is accomplished, treatment with a type 1a antidysrhythmic (quinidine or procainamide) can be started to effect conversion to sinus rhythm. Alternatively, elective cardioversion can be performed. Another option that can be used at any time is atrial overdrive pacing.

Atrial fibrillation should be treated with cardioversion when the patient is unstable. Patients with a rapid (>200/min) wide-complex ventricular response to atrial fibrillation should be assumed to have a participating accessory pathway. Drug therapy can be two-staged, identical to that used with atrial flutter, or can be directed only toward control of the ventricular rate if conversion to sinus rhythm is not desired. In addition to intermittent therapy with verapamil, β-blockers, or digoxin, recent investigations have demonstrated the efficacy of continuous infusion of verapamil for rate control.

Nonparoxysmal junctional tachycardia is most commonly seen in the critically ill as a manifestation of digitalis toxicity and should be treated as such. Attempts at cardioversion should be avoided since patients with digitalis toxicity who are cardioverted have a tendency to develop unresponsive ventricular fibrillation.

Ventricular

Isolated *PVCs* require treatment only if they are frequent enough to cause a significant effective bradycardia. For example, if the sinus rate is 80 and the patient develops ventricular bigeminy, the effective rate may be 40. Evidence that increasing numbers of PVCs are an independent cause of more complex ventricular dysrhythmias is unconvincing. Rather, the patient with increasing PVC frequency should be considered to have an underlying unstable condition that is likely to cause more complex dysrhythmias. Therapy, therefore, should ideally be directed toward the underlying cause. Specific treatment for PVCs, when appropriate, could include lidocaine or procainamide.

Ventricular couplets may be considered as a more pressing example of ventricular ectopy. A search for the precipitating cause is still imperative, but most authorities recommend that suppressive therapy with lidocaine or procainamide be started.

Sustained and nonsustained ventricular tachycardia should always be treated by lidocaine, procainamide, or cardioversion as indicated. Ventricular fibrillation and ventricular flutter should be treated with emergency defibrillation. Asystole is particularly difficult to treat. Success is often predicated not on specific cardiac therapy but on the discovery and correction of a severe underlying physiological abnormality, such as profound acidosis or hypoxemia. Epinephrine in 0.5–1.0 mg boluses is the drug of choice.

For further information, please see Chapter 79 in Civetta JM, Taylor RW, Kirby RR: Critical Care. *Philadelphia: J. B. Lippincott, 1988*

BIBLIOGRAPHY

Baker JT: Recognition and management of arrhythmias. In Bone RC (ed): *Critical Care: A Comprehensive Approach,* p 304. Park Ridge, IL, ACCP, 1984

Chou TC: Part II: The cardiac arrhythmias. In Chou TC (ed): *Electrocardiography in Clinical Practice.* New York, Grune & Stratton, 1979

Del Negro AA, Fletcher RD: Supraventricular tachycardia emergencies: Diagnosis and management. In Rackley CE (ed): *Advances in Critical Care Cardiology,* p 101. Philadelphia, FA Davis Co, 1986

Jackson LK: Sustained and nonsustained ventricular tachycardia: Genesis, significance and management, In Rackley CE (ed): *Advances in Critical Care Cardiology,* p 83. Philadelphia, FA Davis Co, 1986

Lundberg GD: Standards and guidelines for cardiopulmonary resuscitation (CPR) and emergency cardiac care (ECC). JAMA 1986; 255:2843

Marriott, HJL: *Practical Electrocardiography,* 8th ed. Baltimore, Williams & Wilkins, 1981

34
Infective Endocarditis

Infective endocarditis is defined as an infection of the endothelial surface of the heart with microorganisms present in the lesion. The usual sites of infection are the heart valves, although vegetations can be found with mural thrombi or around septal defects in rare cases. The term "infective endocarditis" has replaced the previous designation of "bacterial endocarditis" because fungi, chlamydiae, and rickettsiae are known to be causative organisms in addition to bacteria.

Two forms of infective endocarditis were described in the earlier literature. The term "subacute" denoted a more insidious onset, less toxicity, and a longer clinical course; previous heart damage was present in a high percentage of patients. The acute form was associated with a more rapid onset, increased toxicity, and shorter duration of clinical findings and was seen in patients who often lacked a history of heart disease. In addition, the microbiology differed between the two forms. Organisms of low virulence (*i.e., Streptococcus viridans)* were most frequently cultured from cases of subacute endocarditis. In acute forms, more pathogenic organisms (*i.e., Staphylococcus aureus*) were commonly isolated. Although the bacteriologic distinctions remain helpful, there is sufficient overlap of the syndromes to make the clinical separation less important.

With the introduction of penicillin therapy, the mortality rate from infective endocarditis decreased from almost 100% to 30% to 40%. However, since that time, there has been no further significant decrease in the mortality rate. The frequency of occurrence of this relatively uncommon infection has not changed appreciably since before the antibiotic era. Nevertheless, the morbidity in those who survive and the impact on health costs remain sufficient to warrant continued studies of improved prophylaxis and therapy.

In the past decades, there have been changes in the target populations, the clinical presentation, the microbiology, and therapeutic interventions associated with infective endocarditis. An increased frequency of endocarditis has been noted in intravenous drug abusers, after procedures performed in the hospital, after prosthetic valve placement, and in the elderly. The decrease in rheumatic heart disease underlying infective endocarditis has been documented. An increase in more virulent organisms, especially among intravenous drug abusers, has become important over the past 15 to 20 years. Combination therapies, shortened total course of antibiotics, and increasing surgical intervention are now recognized as necessary in the management of these patients. These changes are discussed in some detail in the following sections.

CLINICAL MANIFESTATIONS

The signs and symptoms of infective endocarditis can involve any organ system and are often confused with other medical conditions. Fever and heart murmur are the most frequently detected symptom and sign, respectively. With renal failure, congestive heart failure or advanced age, fever may be absent. No specific pattern of fever is pathognomonic, but temperatures rarely exceed 103°F. With right-sided endocarditis, a heart murmur may not be heard. It is only in the minority of cases that a changing murmur or onset of a new murmur is described.

Peripheral manifestations are present in approximately 50% of cases. Splinter hemorrhages are uncommon and may be secondary to trauma. If the disease is of long duration, clubbing may be found. Petechiae are common if looked for and occur secondary to local vasculitis or emboli. Detailed examination of the conjunctivae, extremities, and mucous membranes of the mouth will usually reveal these petechiae. In addition, a close examination may disclose the less common Osler's nodes and Janeway lesions. Osler's nodes may be found in patients with nonbacterial thrombotic endocarditis, gonococcal infections, and hemolytic anemia. Unlike the painless macular Janeway lesions of embolic origin, Osler's nodes are usually painful and nodular. Roth's spots are hemorrhagic retinal lesions that occur in a small percentage of endocarditis patients and have also been described with severe anemia, leukemias, and systemic lupus erythematosus.

The frequency of nonspecific symptoms such as chills, weakness, weight loss, and fatigue may cause the physician to consider other systemic problems or chronic diseases. Symptoms and signs referable to the musculoskeletal system are common as an initial or concomitant complaint. Arthralgias, arthritis, low back pain, and diffuse myalgias are reported to be common.

A wide variety of neurologic conditions are associated with infective endocarditis. These neurologic manifestations may be the initial presentation or may occur among the complications seen in these infections. Cerebral emboli may lead to hemiplegia, ataxia, aphasia, or change in mental status. A young person with an acute stroke should be evaluated for possible endocarditis. Subarachnoid hemorrhage secondary to mycotic aneursyms is unusual and is correlated with a high mortality rate.

Patients with right-sided endocarditis usually have signs and symptoms referable to the pulmonary system. Intravenous drug addicts have an increased incidence of tricuspid valve endocarditis. Pleuritic chest pain and dyspnea are common complaints. Chest radiographs may reveal infiltrates compatible with septic pulmonary emboli.

LABORATORY TESTS

Although laboratory test abnormalities are commonly found in cases of endocarditis, most are not diagnostic. Anemia and elevated erythrocyte sedimentation rates are found in $> 75\%$ of cases. Other hematologic abnormalities, such as thrombocytopenia and leukocytosis, are detected less often. Monocytosis has been reported in cases of endocarditis but is also found in other infectious diseases, such as tuberculosis and typhoid fever. Less frequent abnormalities include microscopic hematuria, proteinuria, hypergammaglobulinemia, hypocomplementemia, and positive rheumatoid factor.

The detection of circulating immune complexes may be helpful in diagnosis and management. Although a third of patients with septicemia and 10% of normal controls have circulating immune complexes, these are present in high titer in most patients with definite infective endocarditis. With appropriate treatment, the levels decrease. Blood cultures are usually positive in patients with bacterial endocarditis. However, under certain circumstances (Table 34-1), blood cultures may be negative.

MICROBIOLOGY

The etiology of infective endocarditis is still predominantly bacterial. Over the past 40 years, the relative frequencies of bacterial isolates in endocarditis cases have changed. Approximately a third of cases today are still due to the ungroupable streptococci, *Streptococcus viridans*. The incidence of endocarditis caused by streptococci has not changed over this span of time. However, there have been increases in the percentage of cases caused by staphylococci, gram-negative bacilli, and fungi. The distribution of organisms varies considerably depending on specific host factors, such as age, history of intravenous drug abuse, or prosthetic valve placement.

TABLE 34-1 DIFFERENTIAL DIAGNOSIS OF CULTURE-NEGATIVE ENDOCARDITIS

Recent antibiotic treatment prior to blood cultures
"Fastidious" bacteria with special growth requirements
Fungi that grow poorly in blood cultures
Nonbacterial causes:
Q fever
Chlamydia
Viruses

TABLE 34-2 TREATMENT OF INFECTIVE ENDOCARDITIS

Clinical Situation	Antibiotic Regimen	Duration
Empirical Situation		
Acute	Nafcillin (6–12 g/day) + ampicillin (6–12 g/day) + gentamicin (3–5 mg/kg/day)	Based on microbiologic results
Subacute	Ampicillin (6–12 g/day) + gentamicin (3–5 mg/kg/day)	Based on microbiologic results
Specific Pathogens		
Viridans streptococci and nonenterococcal group D steptococci	Penicillin G alone (12–20 million units/day), or procaine penicillin (4.8 million units/day) + streptomycin (1 g/day), or penicillin G (12–20 million units/day) + streptomycin (1 g/day)*	4 weeks 2 weeks 2 weeks 4 weeks 2 weeks
Groups D streptococci (enterococcus)	Penicillin G (20 million units/day) Gentamicin (3–5 mg/kg/day)	6 weeks 4 weeks
Staphylococcus aureus†	Nafcillin‡ (6–12 g/day) ± gentamicin (3–5 mg/kg/day)	4–6 weeks 1 week
Staphylococcus epidermidis	Nafcillin *(6–12 g/day) or vancomycin (2g/day)*	*4–6 weeks*
Streptococcus pneumoniae	Penicillin G (12–20 million units/day)	4 weeks
Gram-negative bacilli	Antipseudomonal penicillin + aminoglycoside	Based on microbiologic results
Fungi§	Amphotercin B (0.5–1.0 mg/kg/day)	10 weeks
Penicillin-allergic patient	Vancomycin (2 g/day)	4–6 weeks, depending on pathogen

* Gentamicin can be subtituted for streptomycin in combinations listed.
† Methicillin-sensitive *S. aureus*. Patients with methicillin-resistant *S. Aureus* should receive vancomycin.
‡ Oxacillin or methicillin could be substituted for nafcillin.
§ Surgery is needed with amphotericin B.

THERAPY

Treatment of infective endocarditis requires bactericidal antibiotics given parenterally for several weeks. Because of the location of the infection in an area of impaired host resistance and the large number of bacteria present in the vegetation, eradication takes weeks of therapy, and relapse is not uncommon. Combinations of antibiotics that rapidly kill the bacteria have been shown to increase recovery. The choice of antibiotics is based on antimicrobial susceptibility tests. Whether monitoring of serum bactericidal concentrations and antimicrobial blood levels alters the outcome of treated infective endocarditis remains controversial. Antibiotic treatment of infective endocarditis is shown in Table 34-2, and indications for surgical intervention in Table 34-3. Recommendations for antibiotic prophylaxis of endocarditis are given in Table 34-4.

TABLE 34-3 SURGICAL INTERVENTION IN ACTIVE ENDOCARDITIS: CRITERIA AND INDICATIONS

Major criteria: Any single criterion necessitates early operation
- Progressive heart failure
- Significant heart failure*
- Multiple embolic episodes
- Persistent bacteremia despite appropriate antibiotics
- Fungal endocarditis
- Extravalvular foreign body
- Development of heart block, bundle-branch block, or purulent pericarditis†
- Prosthetic valve dehiscence or obstruction
- Relapse following "adequate" trial‡

Minor criteria: Any three criteria predict a high rate of antibiotic failure with resultant (often sudden and major) complications; surgery should be considered in certain patients if only two criteria are met.
- Congestive heart failure resolved with medical therapy
- Single embolus
- Definite left-sided vegetations seen on M-mode echocardiography
- Early mitral valve closure or flail valve leaflets
- Early prosthetic endocarditis caused by other than highly penicillin-sensitive streptococci
- Gram-negative rod tricuspid endocarditis
- Persistent fever without other identifiable cause
- New regurgitant murmur in aortic prosthetic endocarditis
- Lack of appropriate cell wall antibiotic

(Adapted from Dinubile MJ: Surgery in active endocarditis. *Ann Intern Med* 1982; 96:656)

* Symptoms and signs of heart failure fail to resolve after "simple" medical therapy. If heart failure predated endocarditis, "resolution" would imply a return to baseline.

† Conduction defects should be persistent and unrelated to drug therapy or ischemic cardiac disease; these should occur in the setting of aortic valve involvement

‡ "Adequate" here implies the use of the best available antibiotics in the maximum tolerated dosage for a minimum of 6 to 8 weeks.

TABLE 34-4 SUMMARY OF RECOMMENDED ANTIBIOTIC REGIMENS FOR ENDOCARDITIS PROPHYLAXIS

Dental/Respiratory Procedures*	
Standard Regimen	
For dental procedures that cause gingival bleeding, and oral/respiratory tract surgery	Penicillin V 2.0 g PO 1 hour before procedure, then 1.0 g 6 hours later. For patients unable to take oral medications, 2 million units of aqueous penicillin G IV or IM 30–60 minutes before procedure and 1 million units 6 hours later may be substituted.
Special Regimens	
For use when maximal protection desired, e.g., for patients with prosthetic valves	Ampicillin 1.0–2.0 g IM or IV plus gentamicin 1.5 mg/kg IM or IV, one half hour before procedure, followed by 1.0 oral penicillin V 6 hours later. Alternatively, the parenteral regimen may be repeated once 8 hours later.
For penicillin-allergic patients	
Oral regimen	Erythromycin 1.0 g PO 1 hour before procedure, then 500 mg 6 hours later.
Parenteral regimen	Vancomycin 1.0 g IV *slowly* over 1 hour, starting 1 hour before. No repeat dose is necessary.
Gastrointestinal/Genitourinary Procedures†	
Standard Regimen	
For genitourinary/gastrointestinal tract procedures listed in the text	Ampicillin 2.0 g IM or IV plus gentamicin 1.5 mg/kg IM or IV, given one half to 1 hour before procedure. One follow-up dose may be given 8 hours later.
Special Regimen	
For minor or repetitive procedures in low-risk patients	Amoxicillin 3.0 g PO 1 hour before procedure and 1.5 g 6 hours later.
For penicillin-allergic patients	Vancomycin 1.0 g IV *slowly* over 1 hour, plus gentamicin 1.5 mg/kg IM or IV given 1 hour before procedure. May be repeated once 8–12 hours later.

(Adopted from Shulman ST, Amren DP, Bisno AL, et al: Prevention of bacterial endocarditis. *Circulation* 1984; 70:1123A)

* Pediatric doses: ampicillin, 50 mg/kg per dose; erythromycin, 20 mg/kg for first dose then 10 mg/kg; gentamicin, 2.0 mg/kg per dose; penicillin V, full adult dose if weight is greater than 60 pounds (27 kg), one half adult dose if less than 60 pounds; aqueous penicillin G, 50,000 units/kg (25,000 units/kg for follow-up); vancomycin, 20 mg/kg per dose. The intervals between doses are the same as for adults. Total doses should not exceed adult doses.

† Pediatric doses: ampicillin, 50 mg/kg per dose; gentamicin, 2.0 mg/kg per dose; amoxicillin, 50 mg/kg per dose; vancomycin, 20 mg/kg per dose. The intervals between doses are the same as for adults. Total doses should not exceed adult doses.

For further information, please see Chapter 80 in Civetti JM, Taylor RW, Kirby RR: Critical Care. *Philadelphia: J. B. Lippincott, 1988*

BIBLIOGRAPHY

Bayer AS: Staphylococcal bacteremia and endocarditis. State of the art. *Arch Intern Med* 1982; 142:1169

Come PC: Infective endocarditis: Current perspectives. *Compr Ther* 1982; 8:57

Pelletier LL, Petersdorf RG: Infective endocarditis: A review of 125 cases from the University of Washington Hospitals, 1963-1972. *Medicine* 1977; 56:287

Reyes MP, Lerner AM: Current problems in the treatment of infective endocarditis due to *Pseudomonas aeruginosa*. *Rev Infect Dis* 1983; 5:314

Rubenstein E, Noreiga ER, Simberkoff MS, et al: Fungal endocarditis: Analysis of 24 cases and review of the literature. *Medicine* 1975; 54:331

Sande MA, Scheld WM: Combination antibiotic therapy of bacterial endocarditis. *Ann Intern Med* 1980; 92:390

Serra P, Brandimarte C, Martino P, et al: Synergistic treatment of enterococcal endocarditis. *Arch Intern Med* 1977; 137:1562

Shulman ST, Amren DP, Bisno AL, et al: Prevention of bacterial endocarditis. *Circulation* 1984; 70:1123A

Tsao MMP, Katz D: Central venous catheter-induced endocarditis: Human correlate of the animal experimental model of endocarditis. *Rev Infect Dis* 1984; 6:783

Venezio FR, Westenfelder GO, Cook FV, et al: Infective endocarditis in a community hospital. *Arch Intern Med* 1982; 142:789

Weinstein L, Schlesinger JJ: Pathoanatomic, pathophysiologic, and clinical correlations in endocarditis: Part I. *N Engl J Med* 1974; 291:832

35
Acute Pericarditis and Cardiac Tamponade

ACUTE PERICARDITIS

Inflammation of the pericardial sac results in acute pericarditis. Exudation of inflammatory fluid into the pericardium can increase the fluid content to a greater than normal level and results in pericardial effusion. This effusion is caused by an inflammatory exudation and occlusion of the normal drainage of epicardial venous and lymphatic systems by the inflammatory process. Pericardial effusion can also occur in the absence of pericardial inflammation, for example, in a hemorrhagic effusion. Common causes of acute pericarditis are shown in Table 35-1. Most often, clinically recognizable pericarditis in the adult is idiopathic. In these cases, a variety of viruses are often suspected causes; an etiologic agent is rarely demonstrated. The most commonly demonstrated virus is the Coxsackie B group which tends to elicit myopericarditis in children and pleuropericarditis in adults (also called Bornholm disease).

Pericarditis caused by infectious organisms other than viruses is less frequent now than it was in the preantibiotic era. Bacterial and tuberculous pericarditis are now more frequent, especially in children or in immunocompromised patients. In adults, *Staphylococcus aureus* is still the most common organism, and there is an apparent decline in streptococcal and pneumococcal infections. Pus should be evacuated promptly from the pericardium, usually by operative intervention, because of the need to establish a definitive diagnosis, eradicate the infection, and prevent constrictive pericarditis. Tuberculous pericarditis was once a common cause of acute and constrictive pericarditis but is now rare, although mycobacterial infection must be ruled out in any case of suspected purulent pericarditis. A constellation of high fever, pericardial effusion, and pericardial rub should suggest infection with gram-negative organisms in the immunocompromised host and *Haemophilus influenzae* in children. Antibiotics have influenced purulent pericarditis in the following ways: the incidence has decreased; survivial has increased; drainage is still necessary; resistant organisms have appeared; some cases are masked; there are more hospital-acquired cases; and there is a greater incidence after cardiac surgery.

TABLE 35-1 COMMON CAUSES OF PERICARDITIS

Idiopathic
Viral
Tuberculous
Bacterial
Mycotic
Parasitic
Neoplastic
Primary
Metastatic
Contiguous spread
Myxedema
Uremia
Rheumatologic diseases
Rheumatoid arthritis
Systemic lupus erythematosus
Scleroderma
Postmyocardial infarction
Postpericardiotomy
Trauma
Radiation
Drug-Induced
Procainamide
Hydralazine
Quinidine
Isoniazid
Methysergide
Daunorubicin
Penicillin
Streptomycin
Phenylbutazone

Pericarditis can also be caused by lymphoma, leukemia, melanoma, and other malignancies when there is direct invasion of the pericardium by the offending neoplasm. Pericarditis is also seen in systemic lupus erythematosus, rheumatoid arthritis, and scleroderma. Hemodialysis and renal failure can induce acute pericarditis that can be very refractory. Renal-failure-induced pericarditis usually appears shortly before or after beginning dialysis and probably is not related to the serum blood urea nitrogen level. Associated constrictive pericarditis is now a real problem because of the prolonged survival of patients receiving dialysis. Radiation pericarditis often follows a mediastinal dose of 4000 rads or more and can also lead to acute cardiac tamponade. The long-term effects of radiation can also lead to constrictive pericarditis.

Iatrogenic pericarditis is primarily drug-related. Procainamide, either directly or by the drug-induced "lupus syndrome," can produce acute pericarditis. Hydralazine and other therapeutic agents can also cause acute pericarditis.

Acute pericarditis following transmural myocardial infarction can mimic recurrent angina pectoris and, if the patient is receiving anticoagulants, can lead to cardiac tamponade. This condition is directly associated with myocardial infarction and is currently thought to be caused by visceral epicardial irritation.

CLINICAL FINDINGS

Symptoms of acute pericarditis are characteristic and include sharp and usually persistent chest pain that is generally pleuritic. The pain is typically so severe that only the most shallow breathing is tolerated. It is somewhat improved, but not relieved, by sitting upright and can radiate to the trapezius ridges. Signs of acute pericarditis include a three-component friction rub that is evanescent. This usually occurs in early diastole, presystole, and systole. A pleuropericardial rub may also be heard. The laboratory may report positive acute phase reactants (especially the erythrocyte sedimentation rate) and an elevated white blood cell count. The chest radiograph shows an enlarged cardiac silhouette when over 200 ml of fluid has accumulated in the pericardial sac. Acute pericarditis can also present silently or with any combination of the signs and symptoms mentioned above. Thus, a high index of suspicion is needed to avoid missing the diagnosis.

The electrocardiogram (EKG) has been characterized as having four different stages in acute pericarditis; these can evolve over hours to days and weeks. Stage I includes classic diffuse ST elevations with a concave ST segment and significant PR segment depression. Stage II includes normalization of the EKG. Stage III is the development of diffuse T-wave inversion that may persist or normalize; the latter defines Stage IV. The EKG may include all stages or none in the evolution of acute pericarditis. Electrocardiographic differential diagnosis includes acute myocardial infarction, variant angina, hypertrophic cardiomyopathy, and pulmonary embolism—all of which can mimic the EKG changes described above. The key to diagnosis is the diffuse nature of these changes, the absence of localization to a particular EKG area, PR segment depression, and the absence of ST depression except in lead aVR.

The triad of typical chest pain, pericardial friction rub, and the aforementioned EKG changes confirms the diagnosis of acute pericarditis. This diagnosis must be differentiated from acute myocardial infarction and pulmonary embolism because treatments for these problems vary considerably, as do prognoses. The use of creatinine kinase isoenzymes (CK-MB), lactate dehydrogenase isoenzyme, and nuclear scanning can help rule out myocardial infarction. However, CK-MB isoenzymes can be positive in acute myopericarditis and may confuse the diagnosis. The EKG and other confirmatory tests should support myocardial infarction before this diagnosis is made. Pulmonary embolism can be ruled out with arterial blood gases, ventilation-perfusion lung scan, and, if indicated, pulmonary angiography.

Several studies demonstrate that dysrhythmias are rare but do occur in acute pericarditis. Atrial dysrhythmia in particular can occur as a first manifestation of acute pericarditis. Frequent and signifcant dysrhythmias should suggest myocardial or valvular involvement in addition to the pericardial disease process.

TREATMENT

Acute pericarditis is usually treated with antiinflammatory drugs. These include high-dose salicylates (300–900 mg acetylsalicylates *q.i.d.*) and all the nonsteroidal antiinflammatory agents, especially indomethacin (25–50 mg *q.i.d*). These drugs should be given on a full stomach to prevent adverse gastrointestinal effects. Some patients may be refractory to these agents and may require a course of corticosteroids. Corticosteroid therapy should be reserved for nonsteroidal drug nonresponders. The side-effects of corticosteroid treatment include peptic ulcer disease, sodium retention, hypokalemia, hyperglycemia, Cushing's syndrome, suppression of the adrenal axis, and reactivation of infection. When an acute bacterial infection has been excluded and the patient's gastrointestinal status and cardiovascular status have been properly assessed, corticosteroids can be given. Prednisone is usually given in a dose of 60 mg/day for 5 days, then 40 mg/day for 5 days, then 20 mg/day for 5 days with a continued tapering of the dose by 5 mg/week until the drug has been withdrawn.

The presence of acute pericarditis in acute myocardial infarction necessitates caution with the use of intravenous heparin. This drug is not, however, absolutely contraindicated, as suggested by some authors. Intravenous streptokinase has been reported to cause cardiac tamponade and should not be used in the patient with acute myocardial infarction and acute pericarditis.

Recurrence of acute pericarditis is also common and often requires long-term corticosteroid therapy along with other antiinflammatory drugs. This aggressive therapy often relieves symptoms and prevents chronic scarring and constriction of the pericardium.

CARDIAC TAMPONADE

Cardiac tamponade is a serious ICU problem that can be rapidly fatal. If the correct diagnosis is made in a timely fashion, treatment may be lifesaving.

The pericardium resists sudden stretching but gradually expands in response to a chronic distending force. This allows the separation of cardiac tamponade into acute and chronic syndromes. Fowler describes tamponade as the accumulation of pericardial contents to the extent that hemodynamically significant cardiac chamber compression occurs. Shabetai defines it as the equalization of the intrapericardial pressure and the right ventricular diastolic pressure. Acutely, this occurs with rapid fluid entrance into the pericardium, causing a marked and rapid elevation of intrapericardial pressure. The causes of such an event are diverse. Intrapericardial hemorrhage may occur from trauma, ischemic myocardial rupture, or aortic dissection and rupture. This may happen in the postoperative patient, especially when anticoagulants are used. In this acute syndrome, the triad of increased central and pulmonary venous pressure, systemic hypotension, and a normal heart contour is present. Pulsus paradoxus and a large pericardial effusion can also be seen.

CLINICAL FINDINGS

The patient with pericardial tamponade is often confused, agitated, and restless. Tachycardia and tachypnea are present. Breathing may become labored as accessory muscles are activated for respiration. This condition may on occasion be more occult; the patient presents with a low-output state, right upper quadrant pain due to swelling of the hepatic capsule, or even ascites and edema. Other symptoms may relate to the underlying etiology of the acute tamponade. In this setting, it usually takes less than 200 ml of fluid to compromise the heart, and the intrapericardial pressure rises from a normal of −3 mm Hg to 20 to 30 mm Hg.

Classic clinical signs include an increased jugular venous pulse demonstrating a rapid X descent but no Y descent because of the inability of the heart to fill in early diastole. Compression of the heart throughtout the entire cardiac cycle causes this sign and distinguishes acute tamponade. An accentuated pulsus paradoxus is also present and can be ascertained by inspection of the arterial pressure tracing, by palpation of an artery, or with a sphygmomanometer. This finding represents an accentuation of the normal fluctuation of the arterial pressure caused by changes in intrathoracic pressure. Normally, arterial pressure falls with inspiration and rises with expiration. The amount of paradox is gauged by measuring the systolic blood pressure and observing the difference in the level at which the Korotkoff sounds are heard only during expiration and the level at which they are heard throughout the respiratory cycle. A paradoxical pulse greater than 10 mm Hg is abnormal but may not be seen in tamponade when severe aortic insufficiency or atrial septal defect is also present. Pulsus paradoxus can be seen with severe chronic obstructive pulmonary disease and asthma, however, and is rarely present with constrictive pericarditis. In acute cardiac tamponade, hypotension is often present and the pulse may be unobtainable or may disappear completely with inspiration.

Other clinical signs of acute cardiac tamponade are distant and muffled heart sounds and an often quiet precordium. Compensatory cathecholamine release, caused by a decreased cardiac output, leads to sinus tachycardia and often to peripheral vasoconstriction. The EKG usually shows signs of acute pericarditis, sinus tachycardia, including PR depression, and abnormal T-wave changes. Electrical alternans involving the P, QRS, and T vectors of the EKG is almost pathognomonic of pericardial effusion. However, QRS alternans alone is the most common finding, and is probably due to the movement of the heart in a large volume of fluid. It is not always present in cardiac tamponade.

The hemodynamic profile of acute cardiac tamponade is characteristic and can be assessed by placement of a pulmonary artery catheter. The right-sided cardiac pressures are elevated and the diastolic pressures equilibrate. The right atrial mean pressure, right ventricular diastolic pressure, pulmonary artery diastolic pressure, pulmonary artery occlusion pressure, and the left ventricular diastolic pressure are elevated and are within 2 to 3 mm Hg of each other. This pressure contour does not show a "dip plateau" sign, and pulsus paradoxus can be seen on an arterial pressure tracing. This finding must be differentiated from congestive heart failure. The pressures in chronic congestive heart failure are elevated but do not equilibrate in diastole. These measurements can often be made rapidly in the ICU setting to confirm the diagnosis of cardiac tamponade. Chronic tamponade develops more slowly and, therefore, passively stretches the pericardium to large volumes before significant compression of the heart chamber occurs. The patient's underlying illness may be symptomatically manifest. The most common causes of chronic tamponade include bronchogenic carcinoma, carcinoma of the breast, lymphoma, renal failure during dialysis, tuberculosis, and idiopathic pericarditis.

The physical findings in chronic tamponade include an accentuated pulsus parodoxus, an absent Y descent, and decreased heart sounds; the systemic blood pressure is usually maintained, and the cardiac silhouette is enlarged on chest radiograph.

TREATMENT

Pericardiocentesis should be performed in any patient with acute tamponade and a reduction in systolic pressure of more than 30 mm Hg from the baseline level. The patient should be positioned supine at a 45° angle, and the area between the processus xiphoideus and the left costal arch should be sterilized. A 3-inch aspiratory needle (16–18 gauge) with a short bevel should be directly attached to a three-way stopcock and a 50-ml syringe and the needle advanced at an angle of 45° to the abdominal wall and oriented in a posterocephalad direction. Once the needle enters the subcutaneous tissue, it should be connected to the V lead of the electrocardiogram. As the needle punctures the pericardium, gentle suction usually yields freely flowing fluid.

If the tip of the needle contacts the epicardium, the EKG suddenly demonstrates ST segment elevation. The needle should then be withdrawn until the changes disappear. Complications of this procedure include pneumothorax and myocardial laceration, as well as coronary artery laceration. Many authors have pointed out the high risk of this lifesaving procedure, which should be approached with experience and caution.

If the patient in acute cardiac tamponade can be stabilized by volume expansion and by inotropic therapy, then a safer and equally effective drainage of pericardial fluid can be accomplished by surgical subxiphoid or open pericardial resection and drainage. Subxiphoid resection can be performed in a sterile environment under local anesthesia; pericardial fluid can be removed and pericardial tissue obtained for biopsy and culture. Subxiphoid or open surgical resection of the pericardium is the recommended treatment of pericardial tamponade unless the situation is life-threatening and immediate action is essential to save the patient's life.

For further information, please see Chapter 81 in Civetta JM, Taylor RW, Kirby RR: Critical Care. *Philadelphia: J. B. Lippincott, 1988*

BIBLIOGRAPHY

Fowler NO: Physiology of cardiac tamponade and pulsus paradoxus. *Mod Concept Cardiovasc Dis* 1978; 48:115

Guberman BA, Fowler NO, Engel PJ, et al: Cardiac tamponade in medical patients. *Circulation* 1981; 64:633

Santos GH, Frater RW: The subxiphoid approach in the treatment of pericardial effusion. *Ann Thorac Surg* 1977:23:468

Shabetai R: The Pericardium, p 224. New York, Grune and Stratton, 1981

Spodick DH: The normal and diseased pericardium: Current concepts of pericardial physiology, diagnosis, and treatment. *J Am Coll Cardiol* 1983; 1:240

Spodick DH: Diagnostic electrocardiographic sequences in acute pericarditis. *Circulation* 1973; 48:575

Spodick DH: Electric alternation of the heart. *Am J Cardiol* 1962; 10:155

36 Hypertensive Emergencies

Situations requiring rapid reduction of blood pressure may be divided into emergencies, those situations requiring reduction of blood pressure within 1 hour, and urgencies, those situations requiring reduction of blood pressure within 24 hours (Table 36-1). It is best to think of a hypertensive emergency as severe hypertension producing acute damage to the central nervous system (CNS), the cardiovascular system, or the kidneys. Traditional terms such as malignant hypertension (severe hypertension associated with grade IV retinopathy) and hypertensive encephalopathy (severe hypertension associated with altered mental status, transient neurologic signs, and headache) are narrow and will be discarded.

CLINICAL ASSESSMENT

Most patients with a hypertensive emergency have a previous history of hypertension. Blacks, men, and patients with chronic renal disease appear to be at higher risk than others. Central nervous system damage is suggested by symptoms of headache, weakness, visual disturbances, and confusion. Headaches are steady, anterior, and most severe in the morning. Substernal chest pain suggests hypertension-induced myocardial ischemia or infarction. It may be difficult at times to differentiate between myocardial ischemic-induced hypertension and hypertension-induced myocardial ischemia. However, in reality, the treatments are similar and differentiation is not absolutely necessary. The sudden onset of severe tearing chest pain is reported by more than 90% of patients with acute dissection of the thoracic aorta.

The blood pressure must be interpreted in context. Although a diastolic blood pressure greater than 140 mm Hg is seen in most patients requiring acute reduction, children or patients who were previously normotensive may have CNS damage at diastolic blood pressures as low as 110 mm Hg. Any diastolic blood pressure greater than 90 mm Hg is of concern in a patient with aortic dissection or intracranial hemorrhage. Some patients with chronic hypertension may have diastolic blood pressures greater than 120 mm Hg

TABLE 36-1 SITUATIONS REQUIRING BLOOD PRESSURE REDUCTION

Hypertensive emergencies
- Severe hypertension* with acute end-organ damage
  - Central nervous system
  - Myocardial ischemia
  - Left ventricular failure
  - Renal insufficiency
- Severe hypertension with:
  - Eclampsia
  - Head trauma
  - Extensive burns
  - Postoperative bleeding
  - Pheochromocytoma
- Any degree of hypertension† with:
  - Intracranial hemmorhage
  - Dissecting aortic aneurysm

Hypertensive urgencies
- Accelerated hypertension
- Perioperative hypertension

* Diastolic blood pressure > 120 mm Hg
† Diastolic blood pressure > 90 mm Hg

without evidence of acute end-organ damage or symptoms. Grade IV (papilledema) retinal changes, if present, are diagnostic of increased intracranial pressure in patients with severe hypertension and a hypertensive emergency. Grade III retinal changes (cotton-wool exudates and flame-shaped hemorrhages) represent ischemic injury to retinal nerve fibers and rupture of retinal blood vessels and a diagnosis of hypertensive urgency. Grade III changes may also be associated with other CNS or cardiac findings, rendering a diagnosis of hypertensive emergency. Other fundus changes such as arteriolar narrowing and arteriovenous (AV) nicking are not specific for acute CNS damage. Mental status changes and a myriad of neurologic findings (often transient) may be present with hypertension-induced CNS injury, including nystagmus, weakness, Babinski's sign, and lateralizing defects.

Rales, a third heart sound, and tachycardia suggest acute left ventricular failure, whereas pulse deficits, paraplegia, aortic insufficiency, and pericardial friction rub suggest acute aortic dissection.

Acute renal dysfunction may be associated with minimal physical examination abnormalities. The cardinal sign of acute hypertensive nephropathy is a previously unrecognized elevation of serum creatinine in the presence of severe hypertension. The urinalysis may show an active sediment with microscopic or gross hematuria. Anemia suggests preexisting renal disease. Microangiopathic hemolysis is common. Mild hypokalemia is frequently seen and is usually secondary to high renin levels. Red cell casts suggest acute glomerulonephritis and renal-induced hypertension.

Many chronically hypertensive patients have evidence of left ventricular hypertrophy on the electrocardiogram (EKG). The EKG is most useful in ruling out acute myocardial ischemia or infarction.

The chest radiograph is best compared to previous films. Acute pulmonary edema (perihilar acinar filling pattern) in association with a severely elevated diastolic pressure is the hallmark of acute cardiac end-organ damage. A widened mediastinum is suggestive of aortic dissection, but contrast angiography or computed tomography (CT) scanning is required to confirm this diagnosis.

MANAGEMENT OF HYPERTENSIVE EMERGENCY

The ideal management of a hypertensive emergency includes admission to an intensive care unit (ICU) and continuous arterial pressure monitoring. This allows titration of medication and close observation of the patient for development of new symptoms and medication side-effects. If ICU admission must be delayed, it is acceptable to monitor patients with frequent cuff pressures, but certain drugs with rapid onset of action (sodium nitroprusside and trimethaphan camsylate) should probably be avoided. The goal of therapy is to arrest and hopefully reverse the progression of end-organ damage. Agents used must quickly lower blood pressure to acceptable levels yet have few deleterious effects. Rapid reduction of blood pressure is not without risk. In normotensive patients autoregulation prevents cerebral blood flow (CBF) from falling until the mean arterial blood pressure drops below 60 mg Hg. In chronically hypertensive patients autoregulation is altered. Cerebral blood flow may fall at mean blood pressures as high as 120 mm Hg with resultant cerebral ischemia. Indeed, many cases of cerebral and cardiac damage due to excessive blood pressure lowering have been documented. Although renal function may transiently deteriorate during treatment, this should not deter the clinician. Long-term renal function is better maintained with aggressive antihypertensive treatment.

Parenteral therapy is preferred for hypertensive emergencies (Table 36-2). Reducing blood pressure over 1 to 2 hours to a mean blood pressure of 120 mm Hg is a reasonable goal. Oral medications are begun after 12 to 24 hours, and the blood pressure is reduced to the normal range over the next several days.

HYPERTENSIVE URGENCY

Accelerated hypertension, traditionally defined as severe hypertension and grade III retinopathy (flame-shaped hemorrhages but no papilledema), may progress to hypertensive emergency if untreated but does not require immediate lowering or parenteral therapy. Hypertension in the preoperative patient should also be lowered gradually with oral agents if the diastolic

TABLE 36-2 PARENTERAL ANTIHYPERTENSIVE AGENTS

Drug	Dose and Route of Administration	Mechanism	Onset of Effect	Duration of Effect	Comments
Sodium nitroprusside (Nipride)	Continuous IV infusion Initial rate: 0.5–1.0 μg/kg/min Titrate to desired blood pressure	Direct vasodilation	Immediate	Minutes	Requires ICU and arterial pressure monitoring Side-effects: hypotension, cyanide and thiocyanate toxocity, nausea Concentration of continuous infusion: 0.2 mg/ml
Trimethaphan camsylate	Continuous IV infusion 1–5 mg/min	Ganglionic blockade	Immediate	Minutes	Requires ICU and arterial pressure monitoring Side effects: urinary retention, ileus, orthostatic hypotension, cycloplegia Concentration of continuous infusion 1 mg/ml

Diazoxide (Hyperstat)	Minibolus 100 mg every 5 min Continuous IV infusion 30 mg/min	Direct arteriolar dilation	2–5 min	4–12 hr	ICU, arterial line optional Variable duration of action Side-effects: tachycardia, angina, vomiting, hypotension, hyperglycemia
Labetalol	20 mg test dose then 40–80 mg every 10 min Maximum 300 mg Continuous IV infusion 0.5–2.0 mg/min	Combined alpha- and beta-blockade	5–15 min	2–12 hr	ICU, arterial line optional Avoid in uncompensated heart failure and hypertension secondary to a low output state Contraindicated in heart block, severe sinus bradycardia, and asthma Concentration of continuous infusion: 1 mg/ml
Phentolamine mesylate	IV bolus 5–20 mg IM injection 10–20 mg	Alpha-blockade	Immediate	2–10 min	ICU, arterial line optional Side-effects: hypotension, tachycardia, vomiting, angina, nausea
Hydralazine	IM or IV injection 5–10 mg	Direct arteriolar dilation	15–30 min	2–4 hr	ICU, arterial line optional Side-effects: tachycardia, flushing, angina

TABLE 36-3 ORAL ANTIHYPERTENSIVE AGENTS

Drug	Dose and Route of Administration	Mechanism	Onset of Action	Duration of Effect	Comments
Clonidine	Initial dose 0.2 mg then 0.1 mg every hour as needed Maximum dose 0.7 mg	Central alpha-agonist	30–60 min	12–20 hr	Side-effects: hypotension, sedation, dry mouth Monitor BP for 4 hrs after last dose
Nifedipine	10 mg po or sublingual May repeat every 10 min as needed	Calcium antagonist	10 min	3–8 hr	Side effects: tachycardia, fluid retention, dizziness, angina (rare)
Minoxidil	Initial dose: 20 mg then 10–20 mg every 4 hrs as needed	Direct arteriolar dilation	30–120 min	12–24 hr	Side-effect: tachycardia, fluid retention Diuretics and beta-blockers used to counter fluid retention and reflex tachycardia, respectively
Captropril	10–50 mg po	Angiotensin-converting enzyme inhibitor	15 min	2–8 hr	Side-effects: Rash, proteinuria, acute renal failure

blood pressure exceeds 110 mm Hg. There is no evidence that severe hypertension in the asymptomatic patient who has no end-organ damage need be treated urgently. These patients are best treated with conventional antihypertensive regimens with close follow-up (Table 36-3).

For further information, please see Chapter 82 in Civetta JM, Taylor RW, Kirby RR: Critical Care. *Philadelphia: J. B. Lippincott, 1988*

BIBLIOGRAPHY

Alpert MA, Bauer JH: Hypertensive emergencies: Management. *Cardiovasc Rev Rep* 1985; 6:602

Case DB, Atlas SA, Sullivan PA, et al: Acute and chronic treatment of severe and malignant hypertension with the oral angiotensin converting enzyme inhibitor captopril. *Circulation* 1981; 64:765

Cohen IM, Katz MA: Oral clonidine loading for rapid control of hypertension. *Clin Pharmacol Ther* 1978; 24:11

Cohn JN, Burke LP: Nitroprusside. *Ann Intern Med* 1979; 91:752-757

Cressman MD, Vidt DO, Gifford RW, et al: Intravenous labetalol in the management of severe hypertension and hypertensive emergenices. *Am Heart J* 1984; 107:980

Hricik DE, Browning PJ, Kopelman R, et al: Captopril-induced functional renal insufficiency in patients with bilateral renal artery stenoses or renal-artery stenosis in a solitary kidney. *Engl J Med* 1983; 308:373

Joint National Committee on Detection, Evaluation and Treatment of High Blood Pressure: The 1984 report of the Joint National Committee. *Arch Intern Med* 1984; 144:1045

Ram CV: Calcium antagonists in the treatment of hypertension. *Am J Med Sci* 1985; 290:118

Wheat MW: Current status of medical therapy of acute dissecting aneurysms of the aorta. *World J Surg* 1980; 4:563

V. Respiratory Disorders

37
Pulmonary Edema

Pulmonary edema results from the accumulation of excess water in the lungs. It is not an independent disease entity but rather a result of a variety of disease processes. The mechanisms usually responsible for its appearance are increased hydrostatic pressure (*i.e.*, congestive heart failure [CHF]) and increased permeability (*i.e.*, the adult respiratory distress syndrome [ARDS]).

Pulmonary edema is potentially life-threatening because it impairs lung function to the point that gas exchange fails. The associated high mortality, nevertheless, is due more to the underlying disease than to the actual gas exchange abnormalities. Despite multiple etiologies, the clinical presentation is rather uniform. Recognition of risk factors for its development as well as its early diagnosis are imperative, since current therapeutic modes, achieved by better supportive therapy, may be very effective.

DIAGNOSIS

The diagnosis of pulmonary edema and its differentiation into hydrostatic or permeability categories combines the history, physical examination, chest radiograph, and arterial blood gas analysis. The problem often is underdiagnosed because, in most cases, fluid is confined to the interstitial space and may have few associated early clinical signs.

MEDICAL HISTORY

Pulmonary edema is nearly always associated with some preexisting disease or insult. Congestive heart failure and ischemic or hypertensive heart disease point to a cardiac (hydrostatic pressure) origin. Permeability pulmonary edema is precipitated by many factors (Table 37-1).

PHYSICAL EXAMINATION

As water accumulates, the lungs become heavy and noncompliant, resulting in an increase in the work of breathing. Lung volume at the end of normal

TABLE 37-1 DISORDERS ASSOCIATED WITH PERMEABILITY PULMONARY EDEMA

Direct lung injury	Blood-borne
Pulmonary contusion	Sepsis
Blast injury	Multiple trauma
Lung infection	Multiple tranfusions
Through the airway	Air embolism
Inhalation	Fat embolism syndrome
Toxic fumes	Surface burn
Heat	Amniotic fluid embolism
Aspiration	Cardiopulmonary bypass
Acid	DIC
Blood	Uremia
Near drowning	Pancreatitis
Drugs	Anaphylaxis
Heroin	Reperfusion
Tricyclic antidepressants	Abnormal pressures(?)
Naloxone	Neurogenic
Salicylates	High altitude
	Reexpansion of pneumothorax
	Upper airway obstruction

expiration (functional residual capacity [FRC]) is greatly decreased. The loss of volume and increase in extravascular lung water (EVLW) provide potent stimuli to interstitial stretch receptors; a marked rise in respiratory rate follows. The tachypnea of pulmonary edema is not relieved when the partial pressure of arterial blood oxygen (Pa_{O_2}) is restored to normal by the administration of oxygen.

Discoordinate thoracoabdominal movement, intercostal retractions, and the use of accessory respiratory muscles are evident. Pulmonary edema is often accompanied by signs of stress such as hypertension, tachycardia, and sweating. When edema is excessive and the alveoli are flooded, frothy sputum is expectorated. Hypoxemia is manifested by cyanosis in extreme cases.

Auscultatory findings may include coarse crackles (alveolar edema), fine moist crepitations, or normal breath sounds (early ARDS). Heart size often is increased in hydrostatic pulmonary edema, and an S_3 or S_4 gallop, high central venous pressure (CVP), and jugular venous distension are frequently observed.

CHEST RADIOGRAPH

A careful analysis of the chest radiograph can be important (Figs. 37-1 and 37-2). "Cephalization" of the pulmonary vasculature and hilar opacification and enlargement are characteristic of CHF. Other signs of fluid accumulation include septal lines, peribronchial and perivascular cuffs, accentuation of the interlobar fissure, and diffuse infiltrates that eventually acquire a homogenous appearance.

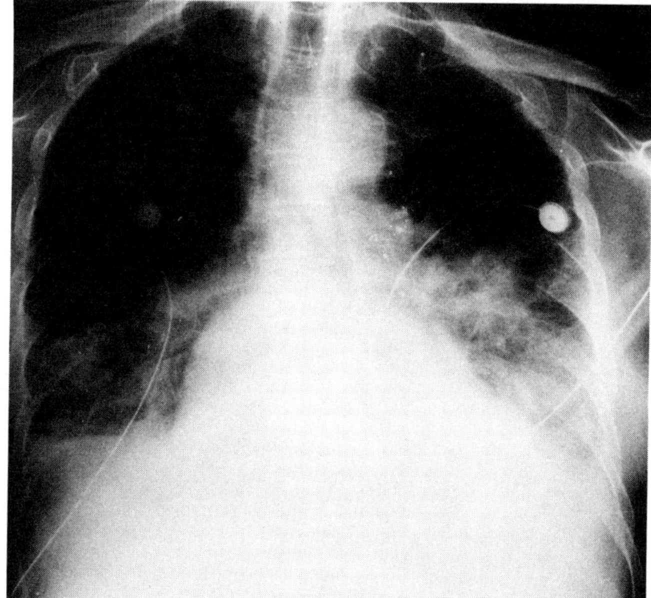

Figure 37-1 Hydrostatic (cardiogenic) pulmonary edema. Note large heart and basilar distribution of edema.

Radiographic assessment may detect early interstitial pulmonary edema before the onset of clinical signs. Quite often, however, the radiographic picture is "slow" to appear, and its correlation with the physiologic derangement is poor.

ARTERIAL BLOOD GASES

The analysis of arterial blood gas partial pressures is vital to both the initial diagnosis and the management of pulmonary edema. Hypoxemia results mainly from ventilation/perfusion ($\dot{V}/\dot{Q}$) abnormalities and right-to-left intrapulmonary shunting, although signficant pulmonary edema may be present before any change in oxygenation occurs.

The normal Pa_{O_2}/FI_{O_2} value is roughly 500 mm Hg over the FI_{O_2} range of 0.21 to 1.0. A Pa_{O_2} of 75 mm Hg when a patient breathes a FI_{O_2} of 1.0 may be "adequate," (*i.e.*, prevent cellular hypoxia) but signifies severe pulmonary dysfunction since the Pa_{O_2}/FI_{O_2} is only 75 mm Hg. When a large right-to-left shunt is present, the Pa_{O_2} is affected by any changes in the central venous oxygen content. Any decrease in cardiac output or increase in oxygen consumption lowers the Pa_{O_2} further.

The arterial P_{CO_2} (Pa_{CO_2}) can be initially low because of tachypnea and

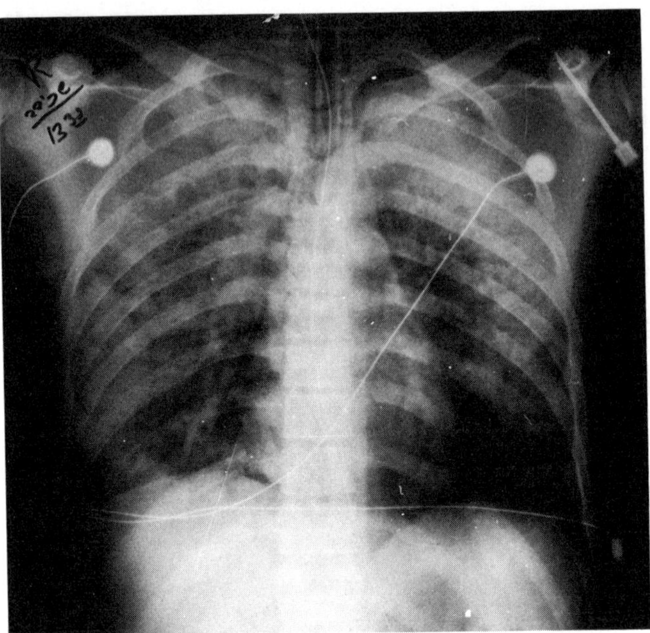

Figure 37-2 Permeability pulmonary edema following head injury. Note normal heart size and diffuse infiltrates. (Courtesy of M. Horev, M.D., Department of Radiology, Hadassah Hospital, Jerusalem)

the high associated minute ventilation ($\dot{V}$). It may be normal, signifying an elevated dead space to tidal volume ratio (V_D/V_T) in the presence of a high minute ventilation. Finally, as a result of muscle fatigue, advanced stages of ARDS, or chronic obstructive pulmonary disease (COPD), Pa_{CO_2} may also be high. Metabolic acidosis due to hypoxemia is unusual, and the *p*H usually reflects the change in Pa_{CO_2}. However, pulmonary edema also can be accompanied by lactic acidosis due to low cardiac output, poor perfusion, or sepsis.

HEMODYNAMIC ASSESSMENT

Congestive heart failure usually is characterized by high CVP and pulmonary artery occlusion pressure (PAOP) and a low cardiac output. Systemic vascular resistance often is high. In contrast, permeability pulmonary edema frequently is associated with a high cardiac output. The PAOP usually is normal or low, but may be elevated due to fluid overload or underlying heart disease. Central venous pressure can be elevated because of fluid overload or selective right heart failure associated with increased pulmonary vascular resistance. Significant pulmonary hypertension frequently is present in severe ARDS.

INITIAL MANAGEMENT

Pulmonary edema is a medical emergency. Management must include treatment of the underlying disease and support of other failing organ systems. The immediate therapeutic goal is to optimize oxygen delivery rather than oxygenation *per se*.

POSITIONING

The low FRC characteristic of pulmonary edema is a major factor in the deranged lung mechanics and right-to-left shunt. The first measure to be taken, when possible, is to place the patient in a sitting position. The resulting increase in FRC improves compliance and reduces the work of breathing. Preload of the heart is reduced as more blood is pooled in the dependent portions of the body. Pulmonary microvascular hydrostatic pressure, one of the main driving forces in the production of pulmonary edema, is thereby decreased. When procedures such as the insertion of a central venous catheter are performed, preparation with the patient sitting is advisable. A supine configuration should be used only for the actual insertion, followed immediately by return to the upright position.

OXYGEN

A high flow of 100% oxygen administered by mask should be instituted in every case of pulmonary edema not associated with chronic carbon dioxide retention. Possible deleterious effects of oxygen appear only after prolonged exposure. If relief of hypoxemia is not achieved, and if a high FI_{O_2} must be used for longer periods of time, more aggressive respiratory support is indicated.

FLUID BALANCE

Fluid administration should be kept to a minimum unless the patient is hypovolemic. In the presence of high cardiac filling pressures, or normal filling pressures and cardiac output, diuretics are indicated to minimize pulmonary microvascular hydrostatic pressure. Increase in the volume of capacitance vessels and decrease in left atrial pressure precede the diuresis. A preliminary 10-mg dose of furosemide, may induce considerable diuresis in patients with an elevated hydrostatic pressure.

POSITIVE END-EXPIRATORY PRESSURE

Positive end-expiratory pressure (PEEP) increases the effectiveness of ventilatory assistance in the treatment of pulmonary edema and ARDS. Such therapy can be applied in conjunction with any mechanical ventilatory mode.

TABLE 37-2 EFFECTS OF CPAP MASK IN FOUR PATIENTS WITH ACUTE PULMONARY EDEMA AND CARBON DIOXIDE RETENTION

	Before CPAP Mask	**After CPAP Mask***
Systolic BP (mm Hg)	191 ± 40	140 ± 28
Diastolic BP (mm Hg)	107 ± 23	81 ± 10
Heart rate (beats/min)	134 ± 13	96 ± 11
Respiratory rate (breaths/min)	35 ± 5	24.5 ± 2.5
Pa_{O_2}/FI_{O_2} (mm Hg)	121 ± 12	175 ± 9
Pa_{CO_2}	59.8 ± 17.9	43.0 ± 4.7
pH	7.26 ± 0.10	7.36 ± 0.05

* Data recorded within 30 min of CPAP mask institution. All differences are statistically significant ($p < 0.05$).

Since many patients with pulmonary edema have adequate minute ventilation, it also can be used for spontaneously breathing patients.

CONTINUOUS POSITIVE AIRWAY PRESSURE

Positive airway pressure is easily applied to a conscious, spontaneously breathing patient with a continuous positive airway pressure (CPAP) mask. Such therapy increases FRC, relieves hypoxemia, and reduces the work of breathing without tracheal intubation. It significantly improves the clinical picture of permeability and hydrostatic pulmonary edema. The best sign of CPAP mask effectiveness is patient acceptance and reduced dyspnea. More objective signs include decreased heart rate, blood pressure, and respiratory rate which may precede the improvement in oxygenation (Table 37-2).

Candidates for a CPAP mask trial should be chosen carefully. Altered consciousness, severe cardiovascular instability, or clear signs of respiratory fatigue with carbon dioxide retention are absolute contraindications to such therapy. However, in patients with preexisting COPD and superimposed pulmonary edema, hypercapnia may result from decreased compliance of the edematous lungs and lead to low tidal volume and high V_D/V_T ratios. Through improvement in lung mechanics, a CPAP mask may decrease the Pa_{CO_2} in selected patients (see Table 37-2).

For further information, please see Chapter 85 in Civetta JM, Taylor RW, Kirby RR: Critical Care. *Philadelphia: J. B. Lippincott, 1988*

BIBLIOGRAPHY

Bourland WA, Day DK, Williamson HE: The role of the kidney in the early nondiuretic action of furosemide to reduce elevated left atrial pressure in the hypervolemic dog. *J Pharmacol Exp Ther* 1977; 202:221

Cheney FW, Colley PS: The effect of cardiac output on arterial blood oxygenation. *Anesthesiology* 1980; 52:496
Kudoh I, Segawa Y, Numata K, et al: Pa_{O_2} change during progressive pulmonary edema in dogs. *Crit Care Med* 1985; 13:1020
Perel A, Williamson DC, Modell JH: Effectiveness of CPAP by mask for pulmonary edema associated with hypercarbia. *Intensive Care Med* 1983; 9:17
Pistolesi M, Miniati M, Milne ENC, et al: The chest roentgenogram in pulmonary edema. *Clin Chest Med* 1985; 6:315
Sibbald WJ, Cunningham DR, Chin DN: Non-cardiac or cardiac pulmonary edema? A practical approach to clinical differentiation in critically ill patients. *Chest* 1983; 83:452
Suter PM: Assessment of respiratory mechanics in ARDS. In Zapol WM, Falke KI (eds): *Acute Respiratory Failure, Lung Biology in Health and Disease,* vol 24, p 507. New York, Marcel Dekker, Basel, 1985
Zapol WM, Snider MT: Pulmonary hypertension in severe acute respiratory failure. *N Engl J Med* 1977; 296:476

38 The Adult Respiratory Distress Syndrome

The patient with dyspnea, hypoxemia, diffuse bilateral pulmonary infiltrates, and stiff lungs has the adult respiratory distress syndrome (ARDS). This condition demands rapid recognition and skillful intervention to minimize mortality that is still estimated at a 50% rate. The syndrome is caused by diffuse lung injury that leads to an increase in extravascular lung water (EVLW), and it usually occurs after a catastrophic event in individuals with no previous lung disease (Table 38-1).

Although ARDS may be caused by or associated with a large list of conditions or diseases (Table 38-2), most patients demonstrate similar clinical and pathologic features irrespective of the cause of the acute lung injury. Most of our therapy for ARDS is supportive; however, in some cases, specific treatment for the inciting cause is necessary. Why one individual with an acute illness develops ARDS, and another with the same apparent illness does not, remains unexplained. Risk factors for development of ARDS have been identified (Table 38-3). Age does not appear to be an important risk factor. Aspiration of gastric contents and sepsis are highly associated with ARDS. Risk factors appear to be additive. Pepe reported the incidence of ARDS with one risk factor was 25%, two risk factors was 42%, and three risk factors was 85%.

DIAGNOSIS

After the inciting event, several hours to a day may pass before clinically apparent respiratory failure ensues. Based on work by Gomez, the clinical findings in ARDS may be roughly grouped into four phases (Table 38-4). Tachypnea and tachycardia usually develop during the first 12 to 24 hours. The skin may appear moist and cyanotic. Intercostal and accessory respiratory muscles become actively involved in supporting ventilation. A dramatic increase in work of breathing can be appreciated at a glance from the bedside. High-pitched end-expiratory crackles are heard throughout all lung

TABLE 38-1 CRITERIA FOR DIAGNOSING ARDS

Clinical setting
- Catastrophic event
  - Pulmonary
  - Nonpulmonary (e.g., shock)
- Exclusions
  - Chronic pulmonary disease
  - Left heart abnormalities
- Respiratory distress (judged clinically)
  - Tachypnea > 20, usually greater
  - Labored breathing

Chest radiograph: diffuse pulmonary infiltrates
- Interstitial (initially)
- Alveolar (later)

Physiologic
- $Pa_{O_2} < 50$ mm Hg with $FI_{O_2} > 0.6$
- Overall compliance < 50 ml/cm H_2O (usually 20–30 ml/cm H_2O)
- Increased shunt fraction ($\dot{Q}s/\dot{Q}t$) and dead space ventilation V_D/V_T

Pathologic
- Heavy lungs, usually > 1,000 g
- Congestive atelectasis
- Hyaline membranes
- Fibrosis

(Petty TL: Adult respiratory distress syndrome: Definition and historical perspective. *Clin Chest Med* 1982; 3:3. Used with permission of WB Saunders Company.)

fields. Increasing agitation, lethargy, then obtundation may occur as the syndrome progresses. Because these clinical findings may become apparent long after hypoxemia develops, careful attention to blood gas analysis is warranted in patients at risk for ARDS.

The radiographic changes in ARDS are characteristic but nonspecific and rarely reveal the etiology of the syndrome. Acutely, pulmonary edema is seen. Interstitial infiltrates progress to a diffuse, fluffy, panacinar pattern (Fig. 38-1). Although it may be difficult to differentiate from cardiogenic pulmonary edema, there is generally an absence of pulmonary vascular redistribution, pleural effusion, or cardiomegaly. The panacinar infiltrates may consolidate and with time take on a patchy or nodular pattern. If the patient improves, the radiograph may revert to normal. If the disorder progresses, a pattern of diffuse interstitial fibrosis may ensue (Fig. 38-2).

Therapeutic interventions may alter the radiographic findings. Pulmonary infiltrates may increase with injudicious fluid administration. Positive-pressure ventilation and positive end-expiratory pressure may lead to hyperinflation, subcutaneous, mediastinal, retroperitoneal, and intraperitoneal emphysema, or pneumothorax. Main stem bronchus intubation may lead to ipsilateral pneumothorax or contralateral lung collapse (Fig 38-3).

TABLE 38-2 CONDITIONS ASSOCIATED WITH ARDS

Shock
- Hemorrhagic
- Septic
- Cardiogenic
- Anaphylactic

Trauma
- Burns
- Fat emboli
- Lung contusion
- Nonthoracic trauma (especially head trauma)
- Near-drowning

Infection
- Viral pneumonia
- Bacterial pneumonia
- Fungal pneumonia
- Gram-negative sepsis
- Tuberculosis

Inhalation of toxic gases
- Oxygen
- Smoke
- NO_2, NH_3, Cl_2
- Cadmium
- Phosgene

Aspiration of gastric contents (especially with a pH < 2.5)

Drug ingestion
- Heroin
- Methadone
- Barbiturates
- Ethchlorvynol
- Thiazides
- Fluorescein
- Propoxyphene
- Salicylates
- Chlorodiazepoxide
- Colchicine
- Dextran 40

Metabolic
- Uremia
- Diabetic ketoacidosis

Miscellaneous
- Pancreatitis
- Postcardiopulmonary bypass
- Postcardioversion
- Multiple transfusions
- DIC
- Leukoagglutinin reaction
- Eclampsia
- Air or amniotic fluid emboli
- Bowel infarction
- Carcinomatosis

(Taylor RW, Duncan CA: The adult respiratory distress syndrome. *Res Medica* 1983; 1:17)

TABLE 38-3 RISK FACTORS ASSOCIATED WITH DEVELOPMENT OF ARDS

Definite Risk Factors	Probable Risk Factors
Systemic sepsis	Severe pancreatitis
Pulmonary contusion	Diffuse pneumonia
Aspiration	Multiple emergency blood transfusions
Inhalation of toxic substances	
Near drowning	
Fractures of long bones	

(Norwood SH, Civetta JM: Ventilatory support in patients with ARDS. *Surg Clin North Am* 1985; 65:895. Used with permission of WB Saunders Company.)

TABLE 38-4 PROGRESSION OF CLINICAL FINDINGS IN ARDS

Phase 1: Acute Injury
Normal physical examination and chest radiograph
Tachycardia, tachypnea, and respiratory alkalosis develop
Phase 2: Latent Period
Lasts approximately 6–48 hr following injury
Patient appears clinically stable
Hyperventilation and hypocapnia persist
Mild increase in work of breathing
Widening of the alveolar-arterial oxygen gradient
Minor abnormalities on physical examination and chest radiograph
Phase 3: Acute Respiratory Failure
Marked tachypnea and dyspnea
Decreased lung compliance
Diffuse infiltrates on chest radiograph
High-pitched crackles heard throughout all lung fields
Phase 4: Severe Abnormalities
Severe hypoxemia unresponsive to therapy
Increased intrapulmonary shunting
Metabolic and respiratory acidosis

(Taylor RW: The adult respiratory distress syndrome. In Kirby RR, Taylor RW [eds]: *Respiratory Failure* pp 208–244. Chicago, Year Book Medical Publishers, 1986. Adapted from Gomez.)

TREATMENT

Treatment of the underlying etiology (if possible) is essential in the management of ARDS. Unfortunately no therapeutic modality exists at this time that will halt or reverse either the capillary leak or the pulmonary fibrosis. Although corticosteroids have theoretical benefit they have not proven efficacious in this setting.

Classic criteria for the initiation of ventilatory support include a respiratory rate greater than 40 breaths per minute, a dead space/tidal volume ratio (V_D/V_T) greater than 0.6:1, hypercapnia, cyanosis, and infiltrative changes on the chest radiograph. These findings are consistent with late respiratory failure and that support should be strongly considered if the respiratory rate is greater than 30 breaths per minute or the Pa_{O_2} is less than 55 mm Hg (FI_{O_2} = 0.21). The most sensitive and important indicator is progressive diminution of arterial oxygen tension. In the early stages the Pa_{CO_2} is usually low so that even a normal level raises concern about impending ventilatory failure and lends support to intervention.

The first priority must always be reversal of life-threatening hypoxemia. If the disease process is not discovered until late in its course, high inspired oxygen concentrations (> 0.5) may be necessary as a temporary measure to maintain an acceptable Pa_{O_2}. As soon as possible, however, this level

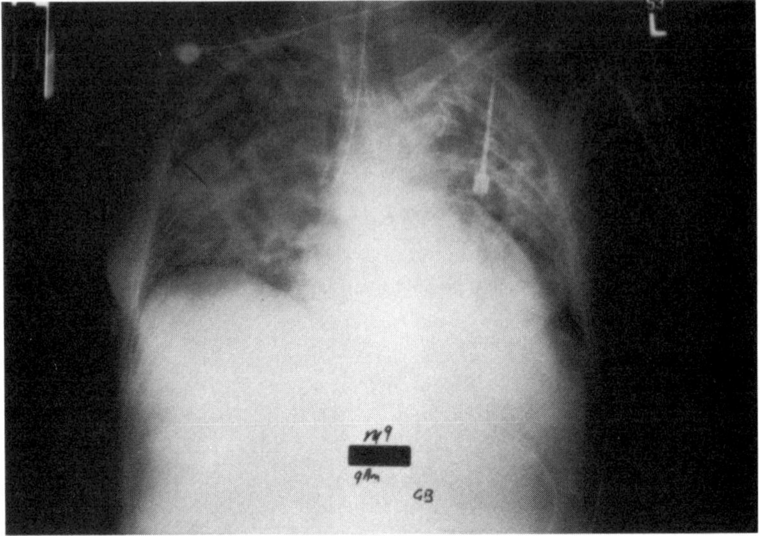

Figure 38-1 Diffuse interstitial and panacinar infiltrates are seen in a 36-year-old patient with ARDS. Note also one of the complications of our respiratory support—a right mainstem intubation.

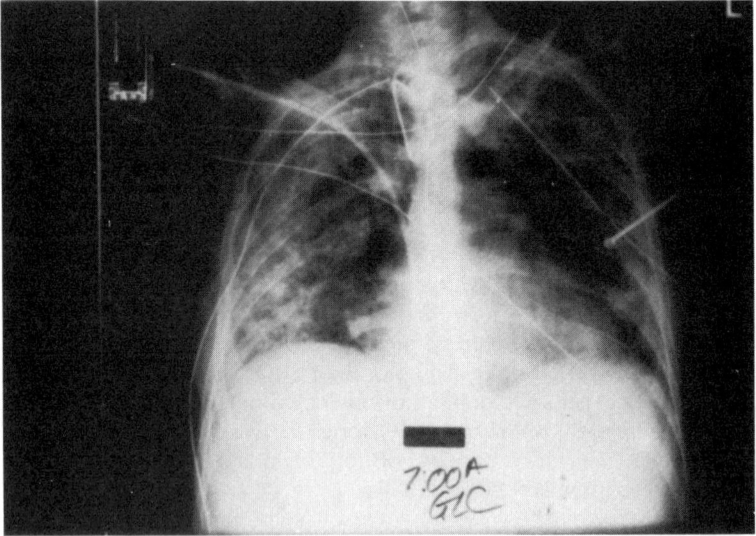

Figure 38-2 A pattern of diffuse interstitial fibrosis has developed in this 52-year-old patient with ARDS.

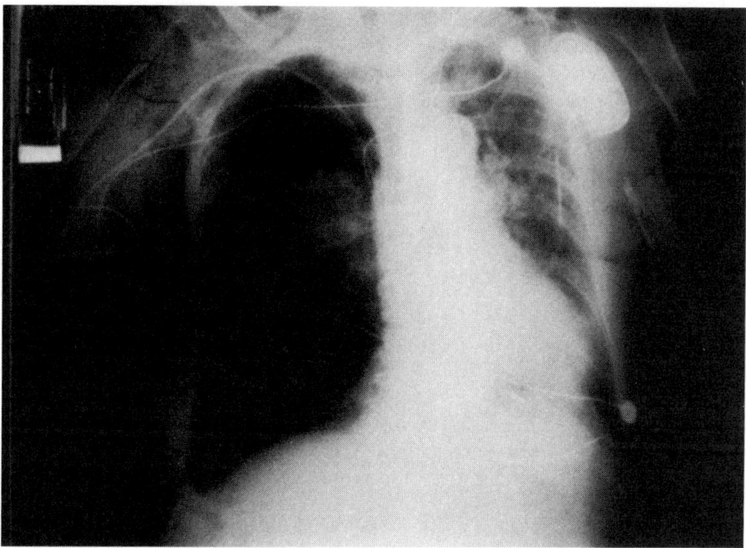

Figure 38-3 This 70-year-old patient with ARDS has a right tension pneumothorax and right mainstem intubation.

should be reduced to less than 0.5 (perhaps < 0.4) to prevent oxygen toxicity and absorption atelectasis.

Positive end-expiratory pressure (PEEP) is the most effective supportive therapy for ARDS. It improves the reduced FRC, usually reverses the hypoxemia associated with ARDS, and often allows downward titration of inspired oxygen concentration to nontoxic levels. The "modern" application of PEEP is 20 years old, yet the "optimal" level of PEEP is still controversial. In general, PEEP should be increased gradually with measurements made to prevent deleterious effects on cardiac output or oxygen transport. Hemodynamic monitoring and augmentation of cardiac output by increasing preload or adding inotropic agents has been advocated. The fact remains, the optimal level of PEEP in terms of the patient's overall physiologic state and outcome is not known.

A reasonable approach to therapy with PEEP is best understood in light of total patient management. Adequate vital organ perfusion with oxygenated blood is a primary goal in treating patients with ARDS. PEEP should be titrated in increments of 2 to 3 cm H_2O approximately every 15 minutes, with frequent reassessment of arterial oxygen tension, intrapulmonary shunt fraction, and oxygen transport. The therapeutic end-point is a level of PEEP that allows reduction of F_{IO_2} to a nontoxic level (< 0.5) while an adequate arterial oxygen tension and oxygen transport are maintained. Although the lung should be kept as "dry" as possible, a reduction in cardiac output by positive pressure ventilation (PPV) or PEEP may be effectively reversed by volume expansion. Fluid is titrated in quantities just sufficient to ensure adequate cardiac output and tissue perfusion. If hemodynamic performance is acceptable, judicious diuresis may help to decrease lung water and improve oxygenation. Excessive diuresis, however, especially when coupled with PPV and PEEP, may markedly reduce preload, cardiac performance and worsen oxygen transport.

For further information, please see Chapter 86 of Civetta JM, Taylor RW, Kirby RR: Critical Care. *Philadelphia, J. B. Lippincott, 1988*

BIBLIOGRAPHY

Fowler AA, Hamman RF, Good JT, et al: Adult respiratory distress syndrome: Risk with common predispositions. *Ann Intern Med* 1983; 98:593

Gomez AC: Pulmonary insufficiency in non-thoracic trauma (discussion, Moore F). *J Trauma* 1968; 8:666

Gong H: Positive pressure ventilation in the adult respiratory distress syndrome. *Clin Chest Med* 1982; 3:69

Pepe PE, Potkin RT, Reus DH, et al: Clinical predictors of the adult respiratory distress syndrome. *Am J Surg* 1982; 144:124

Pontoppidan H, Laver MB, Geffin B: Acute respiratory failure in the surgical patient. *Adv Surg* 1970; 4:163

Skillman JJ, Malhotra IV, Pallot JA, et al: Determinants of weaning from controlled ventilation. *Surg Forum* 1971; 22:198

Weisman IM, Rinaldo JE, Rogers RM: Positive end-expiratory pressure in adult respiratory failure. *N Engl J Med* 1982; 307:1381

39 Aspiration Syndromes

Aspiration pneumonia was a clinical problem as early as 400 BC when Hippocrates recognized "Dangers of Aspiration." In 1946, Mendelson presented a series of parturients suspected of having aspirated stomach contents during labor or anesthesia induction. Subsequently, his laboratory investigations led him to the conclusion that two entirely separate clinical entities existed. One followed the aspiration of solid food and produced the picture of laryngeal or bronchial obstruction, whereas the other resulted from direct acid injury to the lung and produced the "asthmalike" syndrome which now carries his name.

CLINICAL PRESENTATION

Signs and symptoms depend on the quality and quantity of the aspirate. Since most aspirations involve gastric contents, be aware of those situations in which patients are at higher risk for this problem (Table 39-1).

PARTICULATE OBSTRUCTIVE

Food particles large enough to cause complete obstruction usually have not yet passed into the stomach. The "cafe coronary" is caused by an obstructed airway from partially masticated food that is aspirated during swallowing. Patients are unable to breathe or speak and rapidly become cyanotic; if the obstruction continues, they become comatose and die of hypoxemia. Five of Mendelson's 66 patients suffered this type of aspiration, and 2 died. Partial tracheal or bronchial obstruction may result from gastric aspiration of intermediate-sized particles and lead to the symptoms common to any foreign body aspiration. Stridor, tachypnea, coughing, and wheezing frequently are present, with radiographic findings of atelectasis, expiratory emphysema, and pneumonia. Occasionally, a history of recurrent pneumonia is elicited with an associated choking spell preceding the symptoms. Foreign bodies such as food, bones, or coins also can lodge in the trachea, resulting in respiratory distress with stridor, wheezing, and tachypnea and can be fatal.

TABLE 39-1 RISK FACTORS IN GASTRIC ASPIRATION

Perioperative
Parturition
Emergencies
Obesity
Outpatients
Gastrointestinal dysfunction
Hiatal hernia
Scleroderma
Intestinal obstruction
Esophageal diverticulae
Gastroesophageal reflux
Depressed level of consciousness
Head injury
Drug overdose
Metabolic coma
CNS infections
Seizures
Hypothermia
Sepsis
Laryngeal incompetence
CNS disease causing bulbar dysfunction
Guillain–Barré syndrome
Multiple sclerosis
Brain stem cerebrovascular accidents
Posterior fossa tumors
Muscular dystrophy
Myasthenia gravis
Amyotrophic lateral sclerosis
Traumatic vocal cord paralysis
Extensive surgery of the pharynx and hypopharynx
Nasogastric feeding
Artificial airways
Tracheostomy tube
Endotracheal tube
Gastrointestinal hemorrhage

PARTICULATE NONOBSTRUCTIVE

Particulate gastric aspiration of neutral materials not sufficiently large to cause airway obstruction often causes a prolonged inflammatory process similar in many respects to acid aspiration. Patients manifest tachypnea, cyanosis, wheezing, cough, sputum production, and occasionally shock. Although 96% of the patients become symptomatic within the first hour after aspiration, 4% have a delayed onset of up to 2 hours. The intitial presentation may be mild with gradual worsening as the inflammatory response develops.

ACIDIC LIQUID (*p*H LESS THAN 2.5)

Inhalation of any amount of fluid with a *p*H less than 2.5 is likely to damage lung tissue extensively. Larger quantities result in more severe sequelae, sometimes causing pulmonary edema within minutes. Tachypnea, dyspnea, cyanosis, wheezing, and hypotension may be the presenting signs. Smaller volumes cause more subtle changes initially but ultimately produce a similar picture. Arterial blood gas analysis reveals hypoxemia and increasing alveolar-to-arterial oxygen gradient. Hypoxemia occurs within seconds of acid aspiration, and decreasing pulmonary compliance follows shortly thereafter. Patients may hyperventilate initially until the work of breathing increases enough to result in hypoventilation.

WATER ASPIRATION—NEAR DROWNING

The pulmonary lesion in near drowning depends on the amount of water aspirated. Because of laryngospasm and breath-holding, 12% of patients do not aspirate. For those who do, tachypnea, wheezing, cyanosis, and pulmonary edema depend on the amount aspirated. Pulmonary compliance is decreased. These changes are seen with either fresh or salt water. However, the pulmonary findings usually are short-lived, and those who survive the initial insult generally have no long-term alteration in pulmonary function. Gastric dilatation often leads to vomiting and aspiration of gastric contents during resuscitation.

BLOOD

Inhalation of blood may occur as a consequence of hematemesis, intrapulmonary hemorrhage, and surgical procedures involving the upper airway, pharynx, or maxillofacial areas. Immediately following blood aspiration, patients have an increased pulse and respiratory rate and may become cyanotic if the amount inhaled is sufficient to cause intrapulmonary shunting. The acute phase often mimics acid aspiration, but the symptoms usually disappear rapidly, and patients suffer sequelae only if large quantities are aspirated. Animal experiments document the benign lesion produced by blood aspiration.

HYDROCARBON

Ingestion of hydrocarbons such as kerosene, furniture polish, lighter fluid, gasoline, and other petroleum solvents accounts for 18% of accidental poisoning in children. Pulmonary toxicity occurs only if the hydrocarbon is aspirated either during ingestion or after it is regurgitated. The clinical presentation appears to be independent of the type of hydrocarbon ingested. An initial burning sensation of the mouth and oropharynx is accompanied by choking, coughing, and gagging. The characteristic hydrocarbon odor is usually detected on the patient's breath. Respirations become rapid and labored, and cyanosis follows. Central nervous system (CNS) irritability is manifested by dizziness, weakness, lethargy, twitching, and rarely, convulsions. This last problem may be due to or enhanced by hypoxemia. When present, respiratory symptoms usually worsen over the first 24 hours. Those patients who aspirate substantial quantities may develop pulmonary edema, hemoptysis, and respiratory failure. Those who aspirate small to moderate amounts usually improve over the next 2 to 5 days. In the first 24 to 48 hours most patients have fever, which is not infectious in origin.

INITIAL DIAGNOSIS

Success in diagnosing pulmonary aspiration depends on maintaining a high index of suspicion for its occurrrence in at-risk patients. In 63% of cases, regurgitation is witnessed. Frequently the diagnosis is confirmed by the visualization of gastric contents in the airway or hypopharynx during tracheal intubation or by tracheal suction retrieval of gastric contents. However, 37% of patients have either silent or unwitnessed aspirations.

When clinical findings suggest pulmonary aspiration, further evaluation is essential. Arterial blood gas and *p*H analysis affords the most useful initial laboratory test. Oxygen tensions ranging from 30 to 70 mm Hg when the patient breathes room air are a ubiquitous finding with significant aspiration. Since the initial physical findings and blood gas values may be identical in acid and nonacid aspiration, determination of the *p*H of any remaining gastric or pharyngeal fluid can be helpful. If the fluid is highly acidic, anticipate a worsening course. However, a finding of nonacidic fluid may be factitious because of dilution with secretions and is not of much help. The clinical course and response to therapy provide important information regarding the extent and type of aspiration.

Approximately 88% to 94% of individuals who aspirate gastric contents eventually demonstrate pulmonary infiltrates on chest radiographs. Thus a normal chest film does not exclude the possibility of aspiration. The radiographic findings often lag behind the clinical symptoms for 12 to 24 hours. In severe aspiration, diffuse bilateral infiltrates and pulmonary edema may be present (Fig. 39-1). Lack of cardiac enlargement and congested pulmonary veins distinguish this condition from heart failure. Less severe lesions initially cause atelectasis followed by alveolar infiltrates. Since the right main stem bronchus offers the most direct accessible path for aspirated material, the right lower lobe is the most frequently and severely afffected when only one lobe is involved (60%); the left lower lobe is next (42%), followed by the right middle lobe (32%).

Aspiration of particulate material may cause bronchial obstruction. Initially the chest radiograph sometimes appears normal, but expiratory emphysema may be present. Subsequently, the blocked segment loses volume. Aspiration

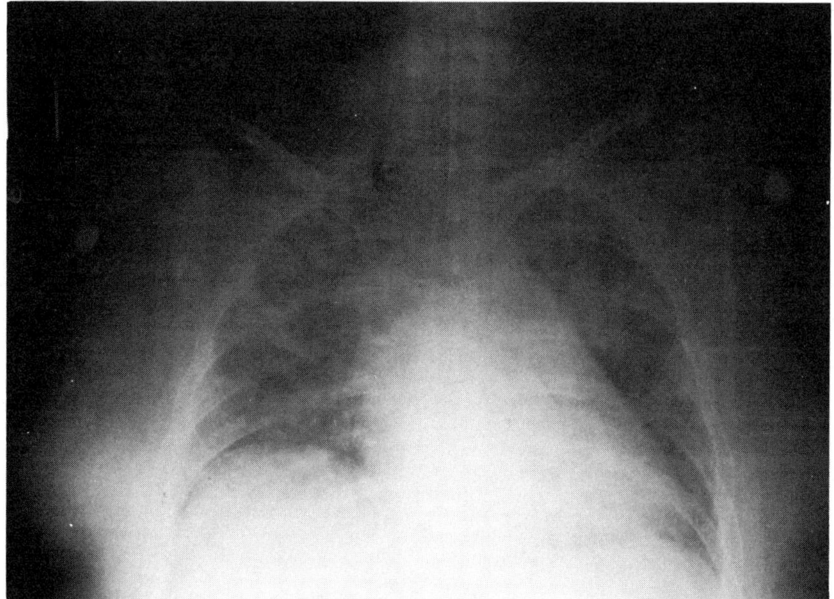

Figure 39-1 Diffuse, bilateral pulmonary infiltrates in a pediatric patient with pulmonary aspiration of gastric contents.

of water occurs in 88% of near-drowning patients. In one series, 20 of 90 near-drowning victims (22%) had normal chest radiographs at hospital admission. The other 70 had lesions ranging from lobar infiltrates to extensive bilateral pulmonary edema.

Chest radiographic abnormalities may be seen within 30 minutes of direct hydrocarbon aspiration. If aspiration occurs following ingestion, patients develop infiltrates within 12 hours (Fig. 39-2). Hypoxemia and respiratory acidosis occur rapidly.

INITIAL THERAPY

AIRWAY PROTECTION

Initial management depends on whether aspiration is imminent, occurring, or completed. When regurgitation occurs in an obtunded patient, clear the airway and tilt the patient's head down and to the side. Be sure to have suction equipment available and ready to use in areas where this problem is likely to occur (operating, delivery, emergency, and recovery rooms as well as the intensive care unit. Oxygen should be administered immediately to all patients suspected of pulmonary aspiration. Next, secure the airway by in-

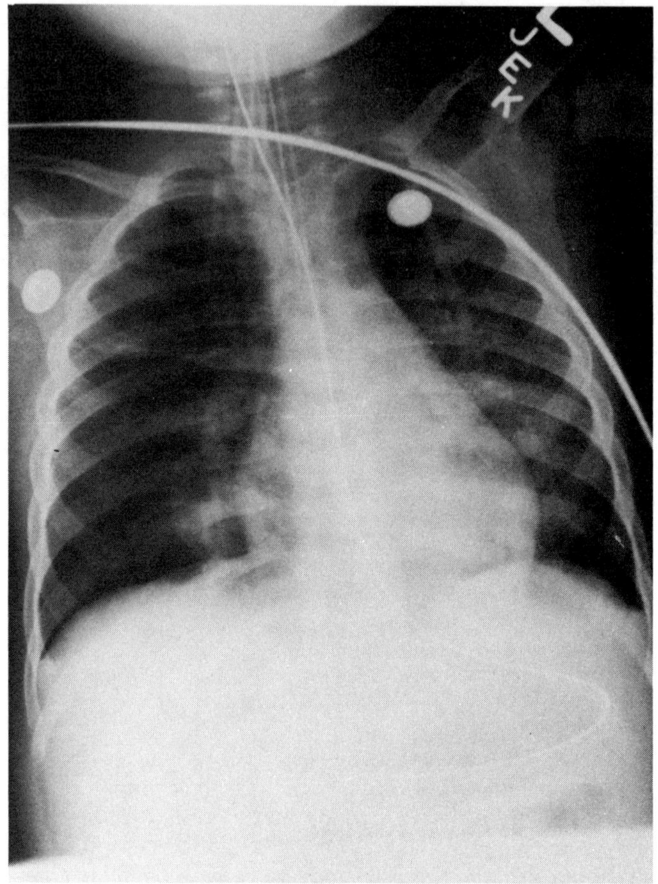

Figure 39-2 Delayed radiographic manifestations of hydrocarbon ingestion.

tubating the trachea, then suction any particulate aspirate. This action will have no beneficial effect with acid aspiration since the injury is immediate. No benefit is derived from alkaline tracheal lavage; the practice actually is detrimental. Removal of large particulate matter necessitates rigid bronchoscopy. Fiberoptic techniques permit the removal of only very small particles.

RESPIRATORY SUPPORT

Further therapy is designed to support the patient during the injury and healing phases and to prevent further damage. Face mask oxygen increases oxygen tension and may be all that is necessary in very mild cases. However, if symptoms worsen, the patient becomes obtunded, or hypoxemia persists despite supplemental oxygen, tracheal intubation and mechanical support of ventilation are often indicated.

The value of early intervention is debated. Some experts feel that as long as the patient is not hypoxemic ($Pa_{O_2} \geq 60$ mm Hg when the FI_{O_2} is ≤ 0.50) and is alert, tracheal intubation is unnecessary. Others feel that intubation and continuous positive airway pressure (CPAP) shorten the course of the disease. Aspiration causing severe intrapulmonary shunting and hypoxemia must be treated aggressively. Positive-pressure ventilation with and without CPAP improves arterial blood gas values and may improve survival. If the patient is alert, cooperative, and not at risk for further aspiration, face mask CPAP to a maximum of 14 mm Hg is sometimes useful. Higher levels exceed the lower esophageal sphincter tone and can promote gastric distention and further emesis.

CORTICOSTEROIDS

Corticosteroids are of no benefit in any of the aspiration syndromes and may interfere with healing.

ANTIBIOTICS

Clinical and laboratory studies show no benefit of antibiotic therapy early in the course of aspiration of noncontaminated fluid. Leukocytosis and fever are frequent findings, often within 30 minutes of hydrocarbon aspiration, but prophylactic antibiotics are not beneficial. Prophylaxis may be useful when the aspirate is feculent or otherwise infected.

BRONCHODILATORS

Wheezing and air trapping are common findings in the various aspiration syndromes. Aerosolized bronchodilators may be beneficial, followed by intravenous bronchodilators if a therapeutic response is observed.

FLUIDS

Fluid management is difficult in severe aspiration. Intravascular volume is depleted because of diffusely increased pulmonary capillary permeability (except possibly early in fresh water aspiration). Therapy may be further complicated by high levels of CPAP with the attendant compromise in cardiac filling. Careful monitoring of urinary output and vital signs is adequate in guiding therapy in mild to moderate cases; invasive hemodynamic monitoring with central venous or pulmonary artery catheters is sometimes indicated for more severe lesions. The controversy over which type of fluid is best for volume repletion exists with this condition as in many others. Some authors feel colloid administration is beneficial; others show a detrimental effect of such therapy. No convincing evidence supports the use of colloids or indicates improvement in outcome when they are used.

EMESIS/LAVAGE

Gastric lavage or induced emesis following ingestion of large amounts of hydrocarbon may well lead to subsequent aspiration. The major life-threatening lesion is caused by pulmonary aspiration, not gastrointestinal absorption. Such therapy should be used only if a cuffed endotracheal tube is in place.

For further information, please see Chapter 38 in Civetta JM, Taylor RW, Kirby RR: Critical Care. *Philadelphia: J. B. Lippincott, 1988*

BIBLIOGRAPHY

Bynum K, Pierce AK: Pulmonary aspiration of gastric contents. *Am Rev Respir Dis* 1976; 114:1129

Chadwick J, Mann WN: *Medical Works of Hippocrates.* Oxford, England, C & J Adlard, 1950

Dice WH, Ward B, Kelly J, et al: Pulmonary toxicity following gastrointestinal absorption of kerosene. *Ann Emerg Med* 1982; 11:138

Downs JB, Chapman RL, Modell JH, et al: An evaluation of steroid therapy in aspiration pneumonitis. *Anesthesiology* 1974; 40:129

Mendelson CL: The aspiration of stomach contents into the lungs during obstetric anesthesia. *Am J Obstet Gynecol* 1946; 52:191

Mittleman M, Perik J, Kolkov Z, et al: Fatal aspiration pneumonia caused by an esophageal foreign body. *Ann Emerg Med* 1985; 14:365

Modell JH, Graves SA, Ketover A: Clinical course of 91 consecutive near-drowning victims. *Chest* 1976; 70:231

Modell JH, Moya F: Effects of volume of aspirated fluid during chlorinated fresh water drowning. *Anesthesiology* 1966; 27:662

Wynne JW, Modell JH: Respiratory aspiration of stomach contents. *Ann Intern Med* 1977; 87:466

Wynne JW, Reynolds JC, Hood CI, et al: Steroid therapy for pneumonitis induced in rabbits by aspiration of foodstuff. *Anesthesiology* 1979; 51:11

40 Pulmonary Embolization Syndrome

Acute pulmonary embolism (PE) is a common complication in patients hospitalized for other medical or surgical problems. Although reported to be the third most common cause of death in the United States, the true incidence of clinically signficant and fatal PE is not accurately known. There are several reasons for this paradox. The diagnosis of PE is often difficult to make on clinical grounds alone; there are no specific laboratory tests diagnostic for PE; and clinically silent PE may occur in patients with asymptomatic venous thromboembolic disease.

Despite its protean nature, the incidence of PE is approximately 600,000 cases per year in the United States. The annual mortality from PE is estimated to exceed 200,000; in half the cases, PE is the primary cause of death, and in the others, it is a major contributory factor. Ten percent of victims die within 1 hour; in this group of patients, time is insufficient for definitive diagnosis and therapy. Ninety percent of patients with PE will survive more than 1 hour, but the diagnosis is not made in two thirds of these. In those patients in whom the diagnosis is made and therapy instituted, 8% die, but in the larger group with unrecognized PE, the mortality rate approaches 30%.

Pulmonary embolism is a respiratory complication of venous thrombosis that originates in the deep veins of the legs in over 90% or more of cases. Since many patients die before a diagnosis can be made or treatment started, reduction in mortality from PE requires the identification and prophylactic treatment of patients at risk for developing venous thromboembolic disease.

DIAGNOSIS

CLINICAL MANIFESTATIONS

The signs and symptoms of PE are nonspecific, particularly in the presence of underlying cardiopulmonary disease. Frequently the disease is clinically silent. The manifestations and prognosis of PE are dependent on the size and number of emboli, the patient's cardiopulmonary status, the rates at which clot fragmentation and lysis occur, and on whether there is a source from which further embolism may occur. The presentation can be abrupt and catastrophic, suggestive of pneumonia or pleurisy, or may be subtle. Acute massive PE in a previously healthy patient can result in right heart failure with only mild pulmonary hypertension, because the normal thin-walled right ventricle is incapable of generating high pressures when acutely overloaded. The degree of pulmonary hypertension in this situation correlates significantly with the extent of vascular occlusion on angiography. On the other hand, a small embolus may be associated with signs of moderately severe pulmonary hypertension, if there is underlying chronic cardiac or pulmonary disease, or recurrent PE causing chronic right ventricular overload.

The classical triad of dyspnea, pleuritic pain, and hemoptysis is present in only 20% of patients with major PE. In general, PE presents as one of three syndromes: unexplained dyspnea, acute right ventricular failure and shock, and the pulmonary infarction syndrome. Patients with PE may complain only of sudden dyspnea. Tachycardia, tachypnea, and low-grade fever may be evident. In acute cor pulmonale, there is usually a sudden onset of dyspnea, cyanosis, right ventricular failure, and systemic hypotension. Patients with pulmonary infarction usually complain of dyspnea, pleuritic pain, and hemoptysis. A pleural friction rub may be present. These conditions are determined by the extent of the embolic process and the presence or absence of underlying cardiopulmonary disease. Acute cor pulmonale is caused by massive embolization; acute PE presenting as infarction or dyspnea usually indicates a lesser degree of embolization. Pulmonary infarction tends to occur in patients with underlying heart disease as a result of hemorrhage secondary to obstruction of the distal pulmonary arteries.

In the intensive care unit (ICU), PE should be included in the differential diagnosis of shock. Benotti and Dalen describe subtle manifestations of PE that may occur in ICU patients:

1 Worsening arterial hypoxemia and respiratory alkalosis in the spontaneously ventilating patient;

2 Persistent dyspnea and hypoxemia unresponsive to bronchodilators despite a reduction of arterial PCO_2 in the patient with chronic lung disease and known CO_2 retention;

3 Unexplained fever, atelectasis, or pleural-based pulmonary infiltrate;

4 Sudden development of pulmonary hypertension in hemodynamically monitored patient;

5 Sudden elevation of central venous pressure (CVP) in conjunction with evidence of impaired organ perfusion;

6 Unexplained tachycardia or tachypnea; and

7 Worsening hypoxemia, hypercapnia, and respiratory acidosis in the sedated patient on controlled mechanical ventilation.

The physical examination in acute PE also tends to be nonspecific (Table 40-1). Sinus tachycardia is common, and if unexplained, should lead one to

TABLE 40-1 PHYSICAL FINDINGS IN PE*

Tachypnea	85%
Tachycardia	40%
Fever	45%
Increased second heart sound	50%
Rales (localized)	60%
Thrombophlebitis	40%
Supraventricular dysrhythmias	15%

* Based on a summary of data compiled from the medical literature.

suspect PE. Tachypnea (respirations > 20/min) occurs in about 75% to 85% of patients. Fever may be found in 40% to 50% of patients and lacks the spiking nature of systemic infection. Blood pressure and peripheral perfusion are usually well maintained except in cases of massive embolization. Signs of a pleural effusion or a pleural friction rub may be found. When pleuritic pain is present, splinting of the chest wall, with reduced ventilation of the affected side, is characteristic. A pulmonary infarction syndrome has been described, consisting of fever, pleural effusion, and pericarditis. Breath sounds are usually normal, although rhonchi are occasionally heard. The presence of rales signifies CHF and occurs almost exclusively in patients with a history of cardiopulmonary disease. Accentuation of the second heart sound (pulmonary valve closure) occurs in about 50% of patients and may indicate the presence of massive embolic obstruction. The presence of S_3 and S_4 gallop heart sounds is a reflection of abnormal right ventricular hemodynamics which result from the sudden elevation of pulmonary arterial pressure. Their right ventricular origin can be confirmed at the bedside by their variation with phasic respiration. In patients with recurrent PE, signs of pulmonary hypertension may be more prominent.

Symptomatic thrombophlebitis is an uncommon finding, occurring in only 35% to 50% of patients. However, asymptomatic deep venous thrombosis (DVT) is not, and is of clinical importance since most pulmonary emboli arise from thrombi in the deep veins of the legs.

In massive PE, the patient may present in shock. Since many patients with PE have underlying cardiopulmonary disease, shock resulting from massive PE must be differentiated from that due to acute myocardial infarction (AMI) or cardiac tamponade. In each circumstance, signs of peripheral hypoperfusion may be present and occur in conjunction with common symptoms such as dyspnea and chest pain.

When shock is due to AMI, electrocardiographic (EKG) evidence of infarction (transmural or subendocardial) is usually seen. In PE, the EKG is frequently nonspecific unless right ventricular strain is evident, which in the presence of shock is virtually diagnostic of PE. The EKG shows low-voltage or electrical alternans in patients with tamponade.

The pulmonary artery (PA) catheter may help identify PE, tamponade, or AMI as the cause of shock. In massive PE, the right atrial and right ventricular diastolic pressures are elevated (> 10 mm Hg). There is moderate pulmonary hypertension (mean pressure 35–45 mm Hg), and a normal or low pulmonary artery occlusion pressure (PAOP). In patients with shock due to AMI and left ventricular failure, the right atrial pressure is normal and only modest elevations in PA and right ventricular pressures may be evident. However, the PAOP is markedly elevated.

The chest radiograph (Fig. 40-1) is an important part of the pulmonary evaluation, but it is neither sensitive nor specific for the diagnosis of PE. Many of the radiographic changes thought characteristic of PE, such as elevated hemidiaphragm, atelectasis, infiltrates, hyperlucency, pleural effusion, pleural-based opacity, acute dilatation of pulmonary arteries, and relative hypovolemia, are frequently seen in patients with other diseases.

Electrocardiographic abnormalities in PE are generally nonspecific. These include various dysrhythmias, QRS abnormalities, and ST–T wave changes. The most frequently encountered dysrhythmias are ventricular and atrial ectopic activities, and the most common sustained dysrhythmia is paroxysmal

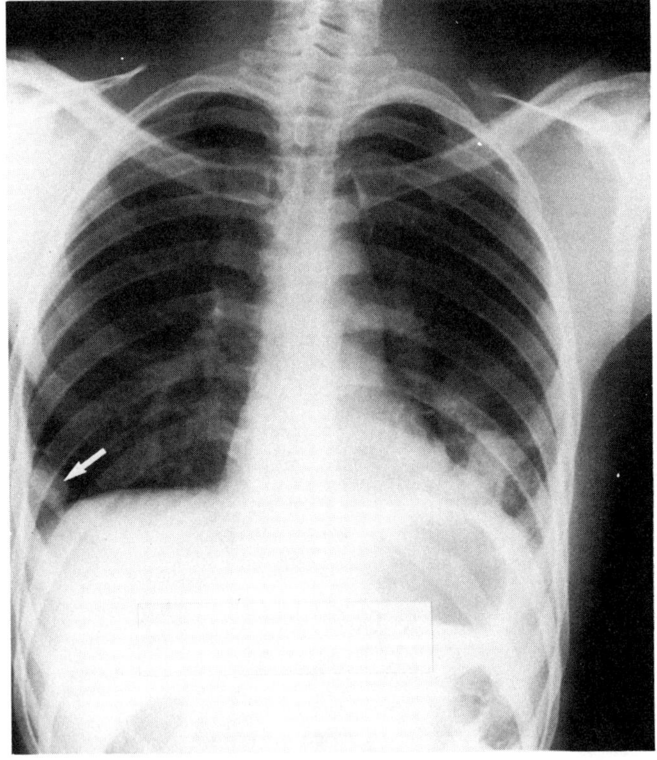

Figure 40-1 A pleural-based infiltrate secondary to pulmonary infarction is seen at the arrow (Hamptom's hump).

atrial fibrillation. Acute right heart strain as manifested by right axis deviation, incomplete right bundle branch block, or the triad of deep S wave in lead I, Q wave in lead I, and an inverted T wave in lead III is seen only in patients with massive PE. These findings indicate acute right ventricular dilation and failure as a result of pulmonary hypertension from pulmonary vascular embolic obstruction.

PULMONARY ANGIOGRAPHY

Pulmonary angiography (Fig. 40-2) continues to be the gold standard for the diagnosis of PE. The two findings considered diagnostic are the presence of an intraluminal filling defect and an arterial vessel cutoff. The procedure is associated with low morbidity and mortality, but it is invasive and requires considerable expertise in performance and interpretation.

LUNG SCANNING

The perfusion lung scan is an integral part of the evaluation of suspected PE. A normal multiple-view perfusion lung scan performed within a few days of the clinical event reliably rules out PE with a nearly 100% certainty. Abnormalities on the perfusion lung scan can result from mechanisms other than intraluminal vascular obstruction. Thus, the perfusion lung scan has a low diagnostic specificity for intravascular thromboemboli; detected abnormalities may require further evaluation to assess the probability of PE.

Ventilation lung scanning was introduced in an effort to increase the diagnostic specificity of perfusion lung scanning. Usually performed with ^{133}Xe, the test is based on the assumption that vascular obstruction due to an embolus will cause a perfusion defect without interrupting ventilation ($\dot{V}/\dot{Q}$ mismatch), wheras most other processes causing perfusion abnormalities will produce ventilation defects in the same area ($\dot{V}/\dot{Q}$ match). This is seen in Figures 40-3 and 40-4.

TREATMENT

Heparin has proven effective in treating PE. It alters the conformation of AT III, allowing this inhibitor to combine with and inactivate thrombin (factor II) and factor X. Its effect on platelet function is less striking, and thus it is only maximally active in the presence of AT III. Intravenous injection produces immediate anticoagulation and a half-life of about 90 minutes. The inhibition of thrombin also interferes with thrombin-induced platelet aggregation and release of platelet factors including serotonin, an effect thought to be important in modifying the bronchoconstrictor and vasomotor consequences of PE. The presence of extensive clot in the circulation accelerates heparin clearance; larger doses may be required early in the course of therapy. Since the

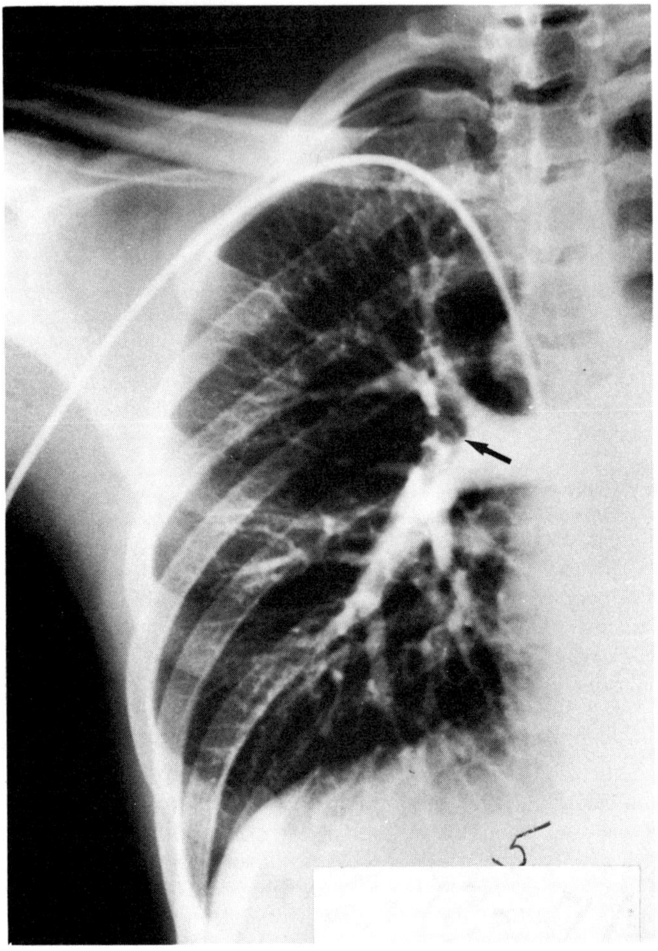

Figure 40-2 Pulmonary arteriogram demonstrating an intraluminal filling defect *(arrow)* secondary to pulmonary embolism.

anticoagulant effect of heparin varies between individuals, laboratory monitoring, usually with the partial thromboplastin time (PTT), is advisable.

Heparin therapy may be started with a loading dose of 5,000 to 10,000 U followed by a dose of 500 to 1500 U/hr by continuous infusion. The maintenance dose is titrated to maintain the PTT at least 1.5 to 2 times control values; a few hours should elapse before checking the PTT following an adjustment in dose to allow sufficient time for stabilization. Administered in this fashion, Salzman observed only a 1% incidence of major bleeding.

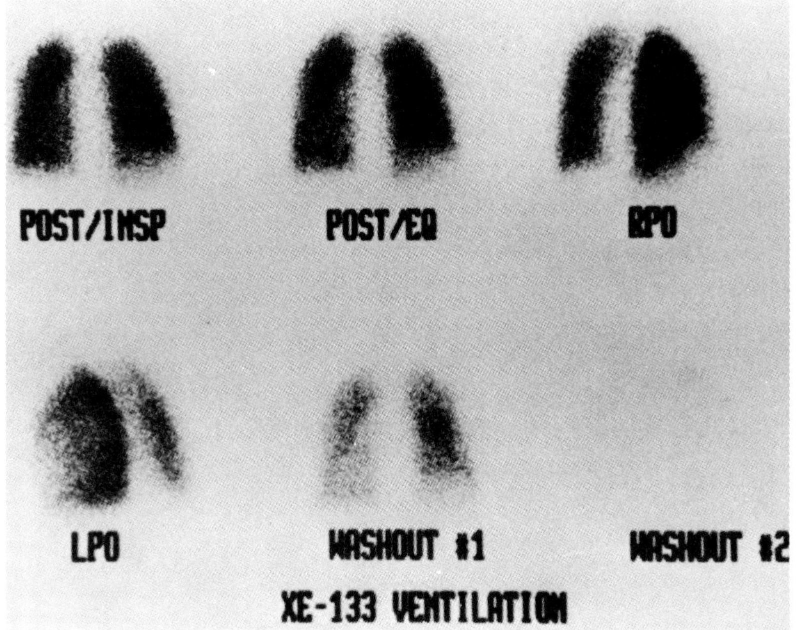

Figure 40-3 Xenon-133 lung demonstrating normal ventilation.

Thrombolytic therapy with streptokinase or urokinase is designed to promote more rapid resolution of PE, thereby increasing pulmonary perfusion and gas exhange and alleviating pulmonary hypertension (Table 40-2). Benefits of thrombolytic therapy compared to anticoagulation with heparin include a marked increase in the rate at which thrombi are lysed and more rapid resolution of abnormal pulmonary hemodynamics. In another study, restoration of the pulmonary microcirculation as measured by the diffusion capacity was greater in long-term survivors of PE treated with thrombolytic agents compared to heparin. It is important to emphasize that though thrombolytic therapy improved the resolution rate of PE, this has not been associated with improved survivial or a reduction in morbidity (*i.e.*, postphlebitic syndrome or chronic pulmonary hypertension).

The standard treatment regimen for streptokinase includes a loading dose of 250,000 U administered intravenously over 30 minutes followed by a constant infusion of 100,000 U/hr. Therapy usually is maintained from 12 to 72 hours, but the optimal duration of therapy has yet to be established. When therapy is discontinued, maintenance heparin is resumed after an hour's delay or when the PTT has returned to two times the control or less. Standard

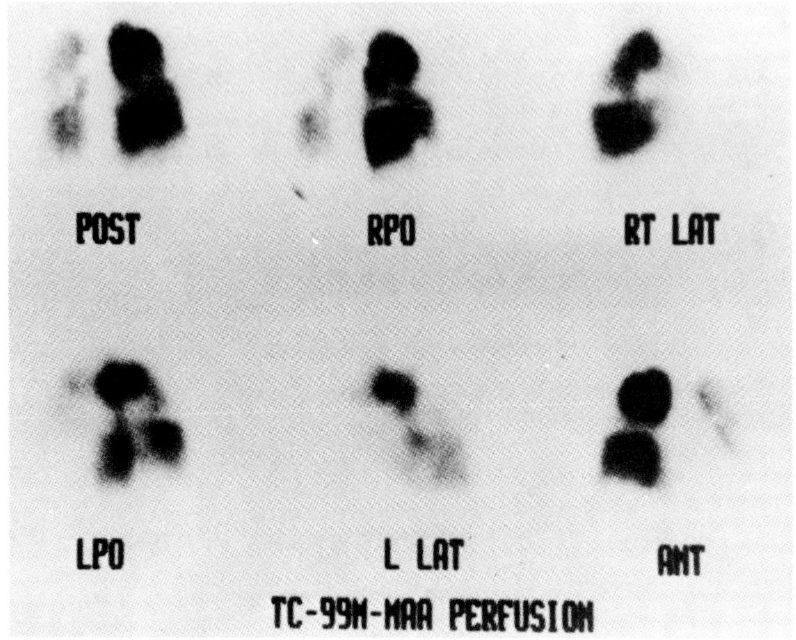

Figure 40-4 Technetium-99m macroaggregated albumin lung scintigram demonstrating segmental and subsegmental defects due to multiple pulmonary emboli.

therapy with urokinase includes a loading dose of 2,000 U/lb administered over 10 minutes, followed by a constant infusion of 2,000 U/lb/hr.

MASSIVE EMBOLISM

The evaluation and treatment of PE manifesting itself as collapse, syncope, acute right ventricular failure, and cardiogenic shock are more complicated. Full anticoagulation should be started as soon as diagnosis of massive PE is suspected.

Management of vascular collapse as a result of PE should include the rapid administration of crystalloid or synthetic colloid solution to elevate right ventricular preload. This permits more effective right ventricular emptying against the acute increase in afterload that occurs following PE. Persistent hypotension and organ hypoperfusion are indications for sympathetic agents. Isoproterenol, norepinephrine, and dopamine are the preferred agents. If hypotension persists after right atrial pressure has been elevated to at least 15 mm Hg by fluid administration, norepinephrine or dopamine in high dose is indicated. Isoproterenol may be used if blood pressure is adequate yet

TABLE 40-2 THROMBOLYTIC THERAPY FOR THROMBOEMBOLIC DISEASE

Disease suspected
- Heparin bolus 5,000–10,000 U
- Check thrombin time, PT, PTT
- Order diagnostic tests—venogram, pulmonary angiogram

Disease confirmed
- Stop heparin and show dissipation of anticoagulant effect; PT or thrombin time within 10 sec of baseline or control valve
- Thrombolytic infusion (12–72 hrs); make sure no contraindications to thrombolytic therapy are present

DVT	*PE*
Streptokinase (24–72 hr)	Streptokinase (24 hr)
250,000 U load; 100,000 U/hr	250,000 U load; 100,000 U/hr

After 4 hr of therapy, check thrombin time or PTT for evidence of lytic state

Restarting anticoagulant
- Stop thrombolytic agent and restart heparin (no loading dose), when thrombin time is less than twice baseline

cardiac output remains low, and tissue perfusion remains insufficient. Heparin (10,000 U) should be given as soon as diagnosis of massive PE is suspected. A flow-directed PA catheter should be placed to substantiate the diagnosis of low cardiac output and right ventricular failure consequent to pulmonary vascular obstruction and precapillary pulmonary hypertension. Hemodynamic findings in patients with massive PE will often demonstrate a normal or low PAOP with moderate elevation of mean PA (> 25 mmHg) and right atrial (> 8 mmHg) pressures. Hemodynamic monitoring is imperative as a guide to vasopressor therapy. The results of arterial blood gas measurements determine the need for supplemental oxygen, intubation, and mechanical ventilation.

Pulmonary angiography rather than perfusion lung scanning is the immediate diagnostic procedure of choice in this clinical setting. Performed early in the course, it rapidly provides information regarding the extent of embolic obstruction and its hemodynamic impact. This eliminates delay in proceeding to potentially life-saving therapeutic options such as pulmonary embolectomy or thrombolytic therapy should the shock syndrome fail to respond to fluids and pressors. Right heart catheterization in conjunction with pulmonary angiography provides the information required to confirm the diagnosis and direct therapy. The identification of massive PE suggests the need for definitive prophylaxis against recurrent embolism and may be an indication for placement of a mechanical filtering device in the inferior vena cava. After a caval filter is placed, anticoagulant therapy with heparin followed by warfarin may be continued until local evidence of DVT resolves.

As discussed previously, thrombolytic therapy has been recommended for patients with hemodynamically significant PE who have not responded to medical management with fluids and pressors. The invasive methods required to diagnose and manage massive PE may subject patients to an increased risk of bleeding from sites of vascular access during the lytic state induced by thrombolytic therapy. Patients should be monitored closely and invasive measures kept to a minimum if this form of treatment is used.

For further information, please see Chapter 89 in Civetta JM, Taylor JW, Kirby RR: Critical Care. *Philadelphia: J. B. Lippincott, 1988*

BIBLIOGRAPHY

Barritt DW, Jordan SC: Anticoagulant drugs in the treatment of pulmonary embolism. *Lancet* 1960; 1:1309
Bell WR, Meek AG: Guidelines for the use of thrombolytic agents. *N Engl J Med* 1979; 301:1266
Benotti JR, Dalen JE: Pulmonary Embolism. In Rippe JM, Irwin RS, Alpert JS, Dalen JE (eds): *Intensive Care Medicine,* p 129. Boston, Little, Brown & Co, 1985
Cook WW, Coller FA. Some epidemiologic considerations of thromboembolism. *Surg Gynecol Obstet* 1959; 109:487
Dalen JE, Haffajee CI, Alpert JS, et al: Pulmonary embolism, pulmonary hemorrhage and pulmonary infarction. *N Engl J Med* 1977; 296:1431
Genton E: Thrombolytic therapy of pulmonary thromboembolism. *Prog Cardiovasc Dis* 1979; 21:333
Genton E, Wolf PS: Urokinase therapy in pulmonary thromboembolism. *Am Heart J* 1968; 76:628
Greenspan RH, Raven CE, Polansky SM, et al: Accuracy of the chest radiograph—Diagnosis of pulmonary embolism. *Invest Radiol* 1982; 17:535
Hirsch J, McDonald IG, Hale GA, et al: Comparison of the effects of streptokinase and heparin on the early rate of resolution of major pulmonary embolism. *Can Med Assoc* 1971; 104:488
Moser K. Pulmonary embolism. State of the art. *Am Rev Respir Dis* 1977; 115:829
Salzman EW, Teykin T, Shaprio RM, et al: Management of heparin therapy: Controlled, prospective trial. *N Engl J Med* 1975; 292:1046
Sharma GVRK, Burleson VA, Sashara AA: Effect of thrombolytic therapy on pulmonary–capillary blood volume in patients with pulmonary embolism. *N Engl J Med* 1980; 303:842
Stein PD, Dalen JE, McIntyre KM, et al: The electrocardiogram in acute pulmonary embolism. *Prog Cardiovasc Dis* 1975; 17:247
Tibutt DA, Davies JA, Miller GAH, et al: Comparison between streptokinase and heparin in life-threatening pulmonary embolism. *Br J Haematol* 1973; 25:275
Wenger NK, Stein PD, Willis PW: Massive acute pulmonary embolism. The deceivingly nonspecific manifestations. *JAMA* 1972; 220:843
Williams JR, Wilcox WC: Pulmonary embolism: Roentgenography and angiographic considerations. *Am J Radiol* 1963; 89:333

41 Pneumonia

Pneumonia remains a major clinical problem. More than 1.2 million cases are estimated to occur annually in the United States. In persons over age 65, pneumonia and influenza together constitute the leading infectious causes of death. The frequency and mortality rates associated with pneumonia remain alarmingly high despite significant advances in the epidemiology, control, and treatment of serious pulmonary infections. In addition, during the past decade, patients, pathogens, and the environment in which infectious diseases occur have changed dramatically. Most cases of adult pneumonia are not severe; however, particular subsets of patients and certain pathogens are more likely to be associated with serious complications when pneumonia occurs.

The diagnosis of serious pulmonary infection in the adult is complex because of the emergence of "new" infectious agents, patient syndromes, and types of antibiotics. *Legionella pneumophila,* a now commonly recognized cause of community pneumonia, also is responsible for outbreaks of pneumonia in numerous hospitals. The acquired immunodeficiency syndrome (AIDS) has been the harbinger of devastating pulmonary infections due to cytomegalovirus (CMV), *Mycobacterium avium-intracellulare* (MAI), and *Pneumocystis carinii.* Use of third-generation cephalosporins is implicated as a cause of enterococcal pneumonia.

DIAGNOSIS

SPUTUM SAMPLES

Examination of sputum samples is the time-honored method to identify bacterial pathogens in the lower airway. Gram-stained sputum smears, unfortunately, are among the least sensitive microbiologic methods for making a specific etiologic identification. The sensitivity of sputum Gram stains is only 40% to 60%. If stringent criteria are used to determine the quality of the sample (greater than 25 leukocytes, less than 10 squamous cells per × 100 field), 75% of obtained samples will be judged as inadequate. Sputum cultures may also be misleading. Specimens obtained during antibiotic therapy may yield organisms resistant to the agent given.

PROTECTED BRUSH

Specimens collected by brushings or suction aspiration through the inner channel of a bronchoscope are probably no more effective in establishing an etiologic agent than Gram stain and culture of expectorated sputa. The bronchoscopic protected catheter brush has been recommended for use in intubated and ventilated patients. Seven of ten patients with suspected infection had positive cultures using the protected brush technique; in each case, the organism matched cultures obtained by reference methods (*i.e.*, blood or pleural fluid). Many of the patients would have been managed appropriately with antibiotic selection based on the culture of tracheal secretions obtained by aspiration through the suction channel of the bronchoscope.

TRANSTRACHEAL ASPIRATION

Transtracheal aspiration (TA) is an invasive technique which requires an experienced physician and patients who have no contraindications. It is most useful in diagnosing acute bacterial, mycoplasmal, anaerobic, and viral infections but may also be useful as a diagnostic technique in patients with unusual infections such as aspergillus and pneumocystis. The procedure has been shown to be more sensitive and specific than sputum culture or culture obtained by transbronchoscopic swabs. Transtracheal aspiration is associated with several complications including bleeding, violent coughing, and cervical and mediastinal emphysema. Suggested patient requirements are the ability to cooperate, a platelet count exceeding 100,000/ml, no other bleeding disorder, and a Pa_{O_2} greater than 60 mm Hg with supplemental oxygen.

TRANSTHORACIC NEEDLE ASPIRATION

Transthoracic needle aspiration is performed with an 18- to 25-gauge needle and may be done with fluoroscopic guidance to permit the sampling of localized lesions. Recently, this technique has been used to identify the etiology of pulmonary infiltrates in immunocompromised patients. Using this method, Bandt was able to identify the causative organism in 16 of 21 immunosuppressed patients with pulmonary infiltrates undiagnosed by TTA and other less invasive methods. Complications include hemoptysis and pneumothorax.

TRANSBRONCHIAL/OPEN LUNG BIOPSY

Transbronchial and open lung biopsy are techniques used almost exclusively for the compromised host in whom the differential diagnosis of diffuse and localized pulmonary infiltrates often includes noninfectious diseases such as radiation pneumonitis, lung injury caused by cytotoxic drugs, pulmonary hemorrhage, and tumor invasion. Infectious agents commonly detected include *Legionella* species, *P. carinii,* cytomegalovirus, nocardia, mycobacteria, and fungi. Transbronchial biopsy is best reserved for normal hosts with infiltrative processes suspected to be malignant or granulomatous in nature; the diagnostic yield in the immunocompromised host may be as low as 5%. On the other hand, open lung biopsy may provide specific diagnostic information even in patients with nondiagnostic transbronchial biopsies.

TREATMENT

NORMAL HOST

Antibiotic therapy may be justified for patients with pneumonia in whom a precise etiologic agent is unknown. For example, normal hosts who develop pneumonia in the community can be treated with penicillin or erythromycin since the usual etiology will be virus, *Pneumococcus, Mycoplasma,* or *Legionella.* Patients with a productive cough and a sputum smear suggestive of gram-positive diplococci should be treated with penicillin. Patients with "atypical" pneumonia will frequently present with a milder illness characterized by an upper respiratory tract prodrome and a nonproductive cough. The distinction between this presentation and that due to viral infection (no specific treatment) may be difficult during the initial management period; erythromycin or tetracycline is suitable for this group of patients. A primary consideration in selecting dosage should be whether or not *Legionella* infection is strongly suspected.

COMPROMISED HOST

The "abnormal host, that is, the patient with diabetes or COPD, the alcoholic, the immunocompromised, and the stressed hospital patient is at risk for developing pneumonia with unusual organisms acquired both in the community and during hospitalization. A major difficulty in the diagnosis of pneumonia in these patients is in differentiating between colonizing bacteria and pathogenic bacteria in sputum or endotracheal aspirate cultures. Empiric antibiotic therapy may be necessary early in the management strategy pending results of reliable cultures such as blood and pleural fluid, particularly for immunocompromised patients. Several issues must be addressed before therapy is selected for the abnormal host with pneumonia. Has the patient recently received antibiotics? Does the patient have an underlying disease process that might affect the immunologic response to infection (*i.e.*, leukemia, lymphoma, acquired immune deficiency)? Has the patient received steroids or other types of chemotherapy? Does the patient have underlying chronic lung disease, diabetes, an alcoholic history? The chest radiograph appearance and the rate of progression may provide useful clues to the cause of pulmonary infiltrates in the abnormal host. Evidence of consolidation and lobar, nodular, or patchy involvement suggests bacterial or fungal infection or noninfectious causes such as hemorrhage, tumor, thromboembolic disease,

TABLE 41-1 CAUSES OF SERIOUS ADULT PNEUMONIA

	Normal Host	Abnormal Host
Usual Organisms	Pneumococcus *M. pneumoniae* *H. influenza* Viruses	Pneumococcus Gram-negative bacilli Anaerobic bacteria *S. aureus*
Unusual Organisms	Legionella Mycobacterium *F. tularensis* *Y. pestis* Group A streptococcus Meningococcus *B. anthracis*	Enterococcus Group B streptococcus *L. micdadei* Aspergillus Nocardia *P. carinii* Cytomegalovirus Mycobacteria

(Modified from Bradsher, RW: Overwhelming pneumonia. *Med Clin North Am* 1983; 67:1233)

and pulmonary edema. Diffuse bilateral interstitial infiltrates suggest viral, mycobacterial, fungal, or *P. carinii* infection, lymphangitic spread of tumor, or drug-induced pulmonary disease. An acute process that evolves during a 24-hour period or less is also suggestive of bacterial pneumonia or pulmonary emboli, edema, or hemorrhage. A chronic course that evolves over one or more weeks, particularly during antibiotic therapy, suggests mycobacterial, fungal, nocardial, or parasitic infection.

The recommended empiric antimicrobial regimen then should be tailored to treat the most likely offending pathogens for a given patient scenario. A cephalosporin, aminoglycoside, antipseudomonal penicillin, and erythromycin in appropriate combination will adequately treat most gram-positive and gram-negative coccal and bacillary bacteria, *Legionella* and *Chlamydia*. The addition of trimethoprim-sulfamethoxazole, which is effective against *Pneumocystis* and *Nocardia*, may be indicated for the deteriorating patient who has received steroids or other chemotherapeutic agents. It is important to remember that empiric antibiotic therapy in the abnormal host with pneumonia may obscure potential information derived from open lung biopsy; the choice between these two approaches rests largely, as usual, on clinical judgment.

As medical technology evolves and new patient populations emerge in the hospital and community, clinicians will face an expansive array of complicated pulmonary infections. Bradsher reviewed the topic of overwhelming pneumonias and divided patients and organisms into several groups: normal host infected with usual and unusual organisms and abnormal host infected with usual and unusual organisms (Table 41-1). This grouping acknowledges the weathering of the once well-defined boundary between community- and hospital-acquired infections and has obvious implication for empiric antibiotic therapy.

For further information, please see Chapter 87 in Civetta JM, Taylor RW, Kirby RR: Critical Care. *Philadelphia: J. B. Lippincott, 1988*

BIBLIOGRAPHY

Abraham SN, Beachey EH, Simpson WA: Adherence of *Streptococcus pyogenes, Escherichia coli,* and *Pseudomonas aeruginosa* to fibronectin-coated and uncoated epithelial cells. *Infect Immunol* 1983; 41:1261

Aisner J, Murillo J, Schimpff SC, et al: Invasive aspergillosis in acute leukemia: Correlation with nose cultures and antibiotic use. *Ann Intern Med* 1979; 90:4

Anderson LJ, Patriarca PA, Hierholzer JC, et al: Viral respiratory illnesses. *Med Clin North Am* 1983; 67:1009

Austrian R, Gold J: Pneumococcal bacteremia with special reference to bacteremic pneumococal pneumonia. *Ann Intern Med* 1964; 60:759

Bandt PD, Costellino RA: Needle diagnosis of pneumonitis. Value in high risk patients. *JAMA* 1972; 220:1578

Bartlett JG, Finegold SM: Anaerobic infections of the lung and pleural space. *Am Rev Respir Dis* 1974; 110:56

Berk SL, Holtsclaw SA, Smith JK, et al: Nontypable *Hemophilus influenzae* in the elderly. *Arch Intern Med* 1982; 142:537

Bradsher RW: Overwhelming pneumonia. *Med Clin North Am* 1983; 67:1233

Brewin A, Arangol L, Hudley WK, et al: High-dose penicillin therapy and pneumococcal pneumonia *JAMA* 1974; 230:409

Chester A: Mycoplasma pneumonia with bilateral pleural effusions. *Am Rev Respir Dis* 1975; 112:451

Dingle JH, Badger GF, Feller AE, et al: A study of illness in a group of Cleveland familes: A plan of study and certain general observations. *Am J Hyg* 1953; 58:16

Dorff GJ, Rytel MW, Farmer SG, et al: Etiologies and characteristic features of pneumonias in a municipal hospital. *Am J Med Sci* 1973; 266:349

Douglas RG Jr: Viral respiratory diseases. In Galasso GJ, Merigan JC, Buchanan RA (eds): *Antiviral Agents and Viral Diseases of Man,* pp 385–459. New York, Raven Press, 1979

Douglas RG Jr, Betts RF: Influenza viruses. In Mandell GL Douglas RG Jr, Bennett JE (eds): *Principles and Practice of Infectious Diseases,* pp 1135–1167. New York, John Wiley & Sons, 1979

Drew WL, Mintz L, Miner RC, et al: Prevalence of cytomegalovirus infection in homosexual men. *J Infect Dis* 1981; 143:188

Fanta CH, Pennington JE: Fever and new lung infiltrates in the immunocompromised host. *Clin Chest Med* 1981; 2:19

Fekety FR, Caldwell J, Gump D, et al: Bacteria, viruses and mycoplasmas in acute pneumonia in adults. *Am Rev Respir Dis* 1971; 104:499

Follansbee SE, Busch DF, Wofsy CB, et al: An outbreak of *Pneumocystis carinii* pneumonia in homosexual men. *Ann Intern Med* 1982; 96:705

George RB, Mogabgab WJ: Atypical pneumonia in young men with rhinovirus infections. *Ann Intern Med* 1969; 71:1703

George WL, Finegold SM: Bacterial infections of the lung. *Chest* 1982; 81:502

Gerson SL, Talbot GH, Hurwitz S, et al: Prolonged granulocytopenia: The major risk factor for invasive pulmonary aspergillosis in patients with acute leukemia. *Ann Intern Med* 1984; 100:345

Gleen GM, Jakub GJ, Low RB: Defense mechanisms of the respiratory membrane. *Am Rev Respir Dis* 1977; 115:479

Gump DW, Frank RO, Winn WC, et al: Legionnaires' disease in patients with associated serious disease. *Ann Intern Med* 1979; 90:538

Haley CE, Cohen ML, Halter J, et al: Nosocomial Legionnaires' disease. *Ann Intern Med* 1979; 90:583

Harris AA, Levin S, Trenholme GM: Selected aspects of nosocomial infections in the 1980's. *Am J Med* 1984; 77:3

Higuchi JH, Johanson WG: The relationship between adherence of *Pseudomonas aeruginosa* to upper respiratory cells in vitro and susceptibility to colonization in vivo. *J Lab Clin Med* 1980; 95:698

Jacobs MR, Koornhof HJ, Robins–Browner M: Emergence of multiply resistant pneumococci, *N Engl J Med* 1978; 299:735

Johanson WG, Higuchi JH, Chaudhuri TR, et al: Bacterial adherence to epithelial cells in bacillary colonization of the respiratory tract. *Am Rev Respir Dis* 1980; 121:55

Johanson WG Jr, Pierce AK, Sanford JP, et al: Nosocomial respiratory infections with gram-negative bacilli. *Ann Intern Med* 1972; 77:701

Johanson WG, Pierce AK, Sanford JP: Changing pharyngeal bacterial flora of hospitalized patients. *N Engl J Med* 1969; 281:1137

Johanson WG, Woods DE, Chaudhuri T: Association of respiratory tract colonization with adherence of gram-negative bacilli to epithelial cells. *J Infect Dis* 1979; 139:667

Kalinske RW, Parker RH, Brandt D, et al: Diagnostic usefulness and safety of transtracheal aspiration. *N Engl J Med* 1967; 276:604

Kim TC, Arora HS, Aldrich TK, et al: Atypical mycobacterial infections. *South Med J* 1981; 74:1304

Kovacs JA, Hiemenz JW, Macher AM: *Pneumocystis carinii* pneumonia: A comparison between patients with the acquired immunodeficiency syndrome and patients with other immunodeficiencies. *Ann Intern Med* 1984; 100:663

Leach RP, Coonrod JD: Detection of pneumococcal antigens in the sputum in pneumococcal pneumonia. *Am Rev Respir Dis* 1977; 116:847

Levin DP: The clinical spectrum of *Mycoplasma pneumoniae* infections. *Med Clin North Am* 1978; 62:961

Louria DB, Kaminski T: The effects of four anti-microbial drug regimens on sputum superinfection in hospitalized patients. *Am Rev Respir Dis* 1962; 85:649

McCauley DI, Naidich DP, Leitman BS: Radiographic patterns of opportunistic lung infections and Kaposi sarcoma in homosexual men. *Am J Radiol* 1982; 139:653

MacFarlane JT, Fitch RG, Ward MJ: Hospital study of adult community-acquired pneumonia. *Lancet* 1982; 2:225

Mackowiak PA, Martin RM, Jones SR, et al: Pharyngeal colonization by gram-negative bacilli in aspiration prone persons. *Arch Intern Med* 1978; 298:1224

Meyer RD: Legionella infections: A review of five years of research. *Rev Infect Dis* 1983; 6:258

Miller RP, Bates JH: Pleuropulmonary tularemia. *Am Rev Respir Dis* 1969; 99:31

Muder RR, Yu VL, Zuravleff J: Pneumonia due to the Pittsburg pneumonia agent: New clinical perspective with a review of the literature. *Medicine* 1983; 62:120

Mufson MA, Chang V, Gill V: The role of viruses, mycoplasma and bacteria in acute pneumonia in adults. *Am J Epidemiol* 1970; 91:192

Mufson MA, Chang V, Gill V, et al: The role of viruses, mycoplasmas and bacteria in acute pneumonia in civilian adults. *Am J Epidemiol* 1967; 86:526

Murray JF, Felton CP, Garay SM, et al: Pulmonary complications of the acquired immunodeficiency syndrome. *N Engl J Med* 1984; 310:1082

National Nosocomial Infections Study Report, Annual Summary 1983. *MMWR* 1985; 33:1SS

Pagani J, Libshitz HI: Opportunistic fungal pneumonia in cancer patients. *Am J Radiol* 1981; 137:1033

Palmer DL, Schmidt–Nowara WW, Wagner D: Pulmonary plague: Pneumonic and

ARDS forms. Program Abstract no. 83. Washington, DC, 22nd Interscience Conference on Antimicrobial Agents and Chemotherapy, 1982

Pasculle AW, Myerowitz RL, Rinaldo CR: New bacterial agent of pneumonia isolated from renal transplant recipients. *Lancet* 1979; 2:58

Pecora DV, Brook R: A comparison of transtracheal aspiration with other methods of determining the bacterial flora of the lower respiratory tract. *N Engl J Med* 1963; 269:664

Pennington JE: Nosocomial respiratory infection. In Mandell GL, Dougllas RG, Bennett JE (eds): *Principles and Practice of Infectious Disease,* 2nd ed, p 1620. New York, John Wiley & Sons, 1984

Perman HH, Maclachlan WWG: Tularemic pneumonia. *Ann Intern Med* 1931; 5:687

Phair JP, Bassaris HP, Williams JE, et al: Bacteremic pneumonia due to gram-negative bacilli. *Arch Intern Med* 1983; 143:2147

Plotkin SA, Brachman PS, Utell M: An epidemic of anthrax, the first in the 20th century. *Am J Med* 1960; 29:992

Rein MF, Gwaltney JM, O'Brien WM, et al: Accuracy of Gram's stain in identifying pneumococci in sputum. *JAMA* 1978; 239:2671

Rubin RH: Pneumonia in the immunocompromised host. In Fishman AP (ed): *Update: Pulmonary Diseases and Disorders,* pp 1–25. New York, McGraw-Hill, 1982

Rubin RH: The cancer patient with fever and pulmonary infiltrates: Etiology and diagnostic approach. In Remington JS, Swartz MN (eds): *Current Clinical Topics in Infectious Diseases,* pp 288–303. New York, McGraw-Hill, 1980

Rubin RH, Russell PS, Levin M, et al: Summary of a workshop on cytomegalovirus infections during organ transplantation. *J Infect Dis* 1979; 139:728

Rumbaugh IF, Prior JA: Lung abscess: A review of 41 cases. *Ann Intern Med* 1961; 55:223

Sackner MA, Hirsch J, Epstein S: Effect of cuffed endotracheal tubes on tracheal mucous velocity. Chest 1975; 68:774

Sackner MA, Landa JF, Greeneltch N: Pathogenesis and prevention of tracheobronchial damage with suction procedures. *Chest* 1973; 64:284

Sanders E: Bacterial interference. I. Its occurrence among the respiratory tract flora and characterization of inhibition of group A streptococci by viridans streptococci. *J Infect Dis* 1969; 120:698

Sanford JP: Pneumonia caused by gram-positive bacteria. In Fishman AP (ed): *Pulmonary Diseases and Disorders,* pp 1130–1140. New York, McGraw-Hill, 1980

Sanford JP, Pierce AK: Lower respiratory tract infections. In Bennett JV, Brachman PS (eds): *Hospital Infections,* pp 255–286. Boston, Little, Brown & Co, 1979

Silva JJ, Nealon TJ, Reinarz JA: A selective phagocytic defect for killing of *N. meningitidis* during adenoviral infection. *Clin Res* 1972; 20:55

Slavin ER, Walsh JJ, Pollack AD: Late generalized tuberculosis: A clinical pathologic analysis and comparison of 100 cases in the pre-antibiotic and antibiotic era. *Medicine* 1980; 59:552

Sprunt K, Redman W: Evidence suggesting importance of role of interbacterial inhibition in maintaining balance of normal flora. *Ann Intern Med* 1968; 68:578

Stamm WE: Gram-negative pneumonias: Diagnosis and management, *Drug Ther* 1979; 9:69

Stamm WE, Martin SM, Bennett JV: Epidemiology of nosocomial infections due to gram-negative bacilli: Aspects relevant to development and use of vaccines. *J Infect Dis* 1977; 136:S151

Stevens RM, Teres D, Stillman JJ, et al: Pneumonia in an intensive care unit. *Arch Intern Med* 1974; 134:106

Stover DE, White DA, Romano PA, et al: Diagnosis of pulmonary disease in acquired immunodeficiency syndrome. *Am Rev Respir Dis* 1984; 130:659

Sullivan RJ, Dowdle WR, Marine WM, et al: Adult pneumonia in a general hospital ward. *Arch Intern Med* 1972; 129:935

Tarpay M: Importance of antimicrobial susceptibility testing of *Streptococcus pneumoniae. Antimicrob Agents Chemother* 1979; 14:628

Tobin MJ, Grenvik A: Nosocomial infection and its diagnosis. *Crit Care Med* 1984; 12:191

Toledo–Pereyra LH, DeMeester TR, Kinealey A, et al: The benefits of open lung biopsy in patients with previous non-diagnostic transbronchial lung biopsy. *Chest* 1980; 77:647

Valenti WM, Trudell RG, Bentley DW: Factors predisposing to oropharyngeal colonization with gram-negative bacilli in the aged. *N Engl J Med* 1978; 298:1108

Verghese A, Berk SL: Bacterial pneumonia in the elderly. *Medicine* 1983; 62:271

Verghese AC, Berk SL, Boelen LJ, et al: Group B streptococcal pneumonia in the elderly. *Arch Intern Med* 1982; 142:1642

Villers D, Derriennic M, Raffi F, et al: Reliability of bronchoscopic protected brush catheter in intubated and ventilated patients. *Chest* 1985; 88(4):527

Wallace JM, Batra P, Gong H, et al: Percutaneous needle lung aspiration for diagnosing pneumonitis in the patient with acquired immunodeficiency syndrome. *Am Rev Respir Dis* 1985; 131:389

Wallace RJ Jr, Musher DM, Martin RR: *Hemophilus influenzae* pneumonia in adults. *Am J Med* 1978; 64:87

Weg J: Chronic respiratory infections. In Guenter CA, Welch MH (eds): *Pulmonary Medicine,* pp 432–452. Philadelphia, JB Lippincott, 1982

Wilson WR, Cockerill FR, Rosenow EC: Pulmonary disease in the immunocompromised host. *Mayo Clinic Proc* 1985; 60:610

Winterbauer RH, Hutchinson JF, Reinhardt GN, et al: The use of quantitative cultures and antibody coating of bacterial to diagnose bacterial pneumonia by fiberoptic bronchoscopy. *Am Rev Respir Dis* 1983; 128:98

Wolinsky E: Non-tuberculous mycobacteria and associated diseases. *Am Rev Respir Dis* 1979; 119:107

Woods DE, Bass JA, Johanson WG, et al: Role of adherence in the pathogenesis of *Pseudomonas aeruginosa* lung infection in cystic fibrosis patients. *Infect Immunol* 1980; 30:694

Woods DE, Straus DC, Johanson WG, et al: Role of fibronectin in the prevention of adherence of *Pseudomonas aeruginosa* to buccal cells. *J Infect Dis* 1981; 143; 784

Yu VL: Enterococcal superinfection and colonization after therapy with Moxalactam, a new broad-spectrum antibiotic. *Ann Intern Med* 1981; 94:784

Yu VL, Kroboth FJ, Shonnard J: Legionnaires' disease: New clinical perspective from a prospective pneumonia study. *Am J Med* 1982; 73:357

42

Acute Respiratory Failure in Chronic Obstructive Pulmonary Disease

DEFINITIONS

Chronic obstructive pulmonary disease (COPD) is a generic term that encompasses a variety of disease processes, the most common of which are chronic bronchitis, emphysema, asthma, bronchiectasis, and cystic fibrosis. The emphasis in this chapter will be on the diagnosis and management of adult patients with chronic bronchitis or emphysema; however, many of the principles also apply to patients with other types of obstructive lung disease.

Chronic bronchitis is defined clinically as a chronic productive cough, present on most days for at least 3 months of the year, for at least 2 consecutive years. Pathophysiologically, it is defined as excessive mucus secretion and mucous gland hypertrophy within the tracheobronchial tree. Emphysema is defined as the anatomic alteration of the lung characterized by an abnormal enlargement of the air spaces distal to the terminal and respiratory bronchioles. Additionally, this anatomic alteration is associated with destructive changes of the alveolar walls and alveolar capillary membranes. Most patients with COPD have features of both.

By definition, acute respiratory failure occurs when the respiratory system is unable to maintain alveolar ventilation sufficient to eliminate carbon dioxide produced by the body. Therefore, acute respiratory failure is associated with alveolar hypoventilation and elevation of the arterial partial pressure of carbon dioxide (Pa_{CO_2}). At the level of the alveolar capillary membrane, the amount of oxygen added and carbon dioxide eliminated is reduced, resulting in the development of both hypoxemia and hypercapnia.

Patients with acute respiratory failure superimposed on COPD generally have dyspnea and worsening of their chronic cough, productive of thick mucoid or purulent sputum, for several days. These symptoms are associated with a deterioration in the arterial oxygen tension (Pa_{O_2}) and often with elevation of the Pa_{CO_2}. Acute respiratory failure with alveolar hypoventilation and elevated Pa_{CO_2} in a previously normal patient is associated with a proportionately decreased *p*H but only slightly higher than normal serum bicarbonate level. This situation is in contrast to patients with chronic respiratory failure and alveolar hypoventilation with elevated Pa_{CO_2}. The kidneys retain bicarbonate to compensate for the elevated Pa_{CO_2}, resulting in a low-normal arterial *p*H, an increased serum bicarbonate concentration, and a proportionately decreased serum chloride level. Therefore, patients with acute respiratory failure superimposed on COPD usually can be distinguished from patients with chronic respiratory failure by arterial blood gas analysis.

DIAGNOSIS

The first step in the acute setting is to establish a prior diagnosis of chronic bronchitis or emphysema by history, physical examination, chest radiograph, electrocardiogram (EKG), arterial blood gas analysis, and previously performed pulmonary function tests. Patients with COPD generally have a long history of regular tobacco use. Those with chronic bronchitis typically manifest a chronic productive cough, progressive dyspnea on exertion, and occasionally wheezing. The predominant symptom in patients with emphysema is chronic and progressive exertional dyspnea; a productive cough and wheezing are usually absent.

Physical examination of patients with COPD reveals prolonged expiration and diffusely reduced breath sounds. Chronic bronchitic patients may appear cyanotic, with rhonchi and wheezing; emphysematous patients are characterized by asthenia and a barrel-shaped chest and may have dry crackles.

Patients with moderate to severe COPD often have associated hypoxemia. Chronic hypoxemia, either intermittent or continuous, results in secondary erythrocytosis, pulmonary hypertension, and cor pulmonale. Physical and laboratory manifestations of cor pulmonale include a loud pulmonary component of the second heart sound, a right ventricular heave, jugular venous distention, lower extremity edema, and EKG evidence of right ventricular hypertrophy and P-pulmonale.

The chest radiograph usually shows evidence of hyperinflation. Characteristically, in a posteroanterior radiograph, the dome of the diaphragm is below the 10th interspace posteriorly. In addition, specifically in patients with chronic bronchitis, increased peribronchial and bronchial marking may be noticed. Patchy areas of hyperlucency and fibrosis, a flat diaphragm, and attenuated pulmonary vasculature are frequently seen in emphysematous patients.

Routine pulmonary function testing is useful in diagnosing and characterizing patients with COPD. The pathophysiologic hallmark is a decrease in the ratio of the force expiratory volume in 1 second (FEV_1) to forced vital capacity (FVC). In addition to decreased expiratory flow rates, patients with chronic bronchitis often manifest an elevated residual volume, hypoxemia, and, in moderately severe disease, hypercapnia. Significant improvement in spirometric testing often occurs after they inhale bronchodilators. Patients with emphysema have an increase in both residual volume and total lung capacity; a decrease in the diffusing capacity for carbon monoxide, and relatively well-preserved Pa_{O_2} and Pa_{CO_2} until very late stages of disease. They have minimal improvement in spirometry after inhaling bronchodilators.

These historical, physical, and laboratory features are useful in identifying patients with COPD. However, the clinical distinction between chronic bronchitis and emphysema is largely artificial because most patients have features of both disease processes.

When acute respiratory failure complicates underlying COPD, cough and dyspnea are exacerbated. Clinical signs of acute hypoxemia and hypercapnia, although often present, are nonspecific. Disturbances of consciousness, headache, and abnormal muscle movements may be noted. A bounding pulse, tachycardia, and initial hypertension are followed in severe cases by hypotension with associated vasodilatation and diaphoresis. Definitive assessment of the adequacy of oxygenation and ventilation depends on arterial blood gas analysis.

TREATMENT

Arterial P_{CO_2} is related to carbon dioxide production ($\dot{V}_{CO_2}$) and to the amount of carbon dioxide eliminated by alveolar ventilation ($\dot{V}_A$):

$$Pa_{CO_2} = \frac{\dot{V}_{CO_2}}{\dot{V}_A} \times 0.863 \qquad (1)$$

Treatment of an acute exacerbation of COPD is designed to provide adequate oxygenation, to decrease carbon dioxide production by decreasing the work of breathing, and to increase alveolar ventilation, thus decreasing Pa_{CO_2}. Management should be directed toward identifying and treating the specific factor(s) precipitating acute respiratory failure. If acute bacterial infection is suspected, sputum Gram stain and cultures of sputum and blood should be obtained, and the patient placed on appropriate antibiotic coverage. In similar fashion, CHF must be treated with digitalis and diuretics; inappropriate oxygen therapy corrected by careful and controlled oxygen administration; the injudicious use of sedatives eliminated; a pulmonary thromboembolus treated by heparin or streptokinase infusion; and a pneumothorax relieved by tube thoracostomy.

CONSERVATIVE THERAPY

In the vast majority of patients, a specific precipitating cause may not be identified, although an acute viral upper respiratory tract infection often is responsible. Most of these patients respond favorably to conservative treatment, including continuous supplemental oxygen administration, inhaled and intravenous bronchodilators, intravenous steroids and antibiotics, vigorous hydration, aggressive chest physical therapy and tracheal suctioning, avoidance of sedatives, physical stimulation to keep them awake, and diuretics as needed to control pulmonary congestion. In one study of 91 consecutive hospitalized patients, 81 were managed successfully on this regime. Acute mortality for this group was 13%.

Oxygen

The low Pa_{O_2} often seen with acute exacerbations of COPD responds well to administered oxygen in terms of increased arterial oxygen saturation (Sa_{O_2}), arterial oxygen content (Ca_{O_2}), and tissue oxygenation (Fig. 42-1). The overall improvement is effected without raising the Pa_{O_2} to normal levels which may, in this subgroup of patients, depress respiratory drive. Traditionally, the rise in Pa_{CO_2} seen after the administration of supplemental oxygen is ascribed to elimination of the hypoxic stimulus to breathe. Other causes such as the effect of oxygen on the carbon dioxide dissociation curve of blood (Haldane effect) are also implicated. The problem was evaluated by Aubier in 22 patients with COPD and acute airway infection. After 15 minutes of oxygen administration, minute ventilation decreased slightly to 93% of the control value, and Pa_{CO_2} increased by an average of 23 mm Hg. Presumably, if no other changes occurred, the decrease in minute ventilation should have resulted in only a 5 mm Hg incrase in Pa_{CO_2}. An additional 7 mm Hg increase

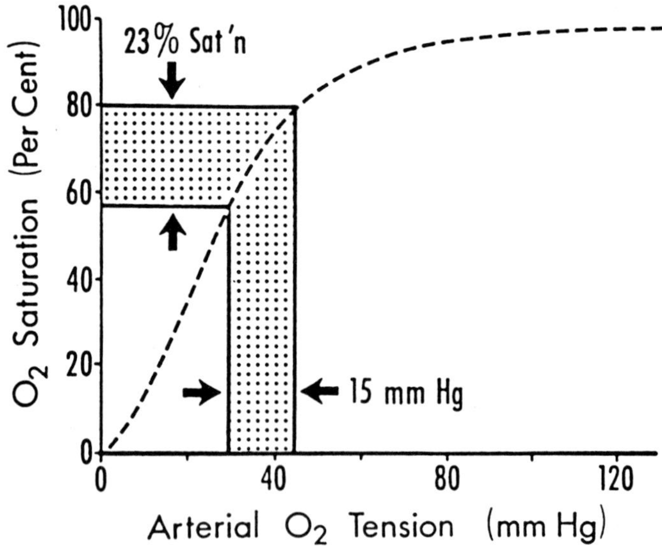

Figure 42-1 Oxyhemoglobin dissociation curve illustrates the effect of a 15-mm Hg increase in Pa_{O_2} occurring on the steep portion of the curve on percent oxygen saturation. (Block AJ: Practical management of pulmonary insufficiency. In Eliot RS [ed]: *The Acute Cardiac Emergency, Diagnosis and Management*, p 194. Mount Kisco, NY, Futura Publishing Co, 1972)

in Pa_{CO_2} might be explained by the Haldane effect, leaving almost half of the increase due to increased carbon dioxide production or dead space ventilation (*i.e.*, an inhomogeneity of $\dot{V}/\dot{Q}$ ratios throughout the lungs).

Oxygen can be safely administered by a venturi mask or nasal cannula. The safest technique for hypoxemic and hypercapnic COPD patients uses a 28% venturi mask. A 5 liter/min of flow of oxygen through the jet entrains 50 liters of air to produce an accurate 28% inspired oxygen concentration. The total flow of 55 liter/min ensures adequate carbon dioxide removal.

Bronchodilators

The relief of bronchial obstruction is desirable to decrease the work of breathing, carbon dioxide production, and alveolar hypoventilation. Various inhaled β_2-selective sympathomimetics are available, several of which have been introduced during the last 5 years. Most have an onset of action between 5 and 15 minutes and a duration between 3 and 6 hours.

Metaproterenol is administered by either a metered-dose inhaler or a gas-powered nebulizer. The usual dose is 0.3 ml of a 5% solution diluted with 2.5 ml of normal saline. Albuterol has a slightly longer duration of action than metaproterenol and is administered by a metered-dose inhaler. Like metaproterenol, terbutaline can be administered by either a metered-dose inhaler or nebulizer. The dose for nebulization is 5 ml of a 0.1% solution administered every 4 hours.

In general, these agents should be administered by metered-dose inhaler. However, with uncooperative patients or those who are unable to use a metered-dose inhaler correctly, a gas-powered nebulizer can be used. The dosage schedule is every 4 hours regardless of the variable half-lives of the different drugs. Oral preparations of all the β_2-sympathomimetics are available; however, the inhalation route is the preferred delivery method and is better tolerated with fewer side-effects by most patients.

Aminophylline is also useful. In addition to its pharmacologic relaxation of bronchial and vascular smooth muscle, it augments cardiac rate and contractility and acts as a respiratory stimulant. Murciano believes diaphragm strength is improved and fatigue decreased in patients with stable COPD. An increase in FVC, FEV_1, and maximum transdiaphragmatic pressure can be demonstrated, thus indicating an increase in the maximal inspiratory diaphragmatic force. These effects are noted 7 days after therapy is initiated and persist for 30 days, suggesting that aminophylline has a potent and long-lasting effect on diaphragmatic strength in patients with fixed airway obstruction.

Oral theophylline and intravenous aminophylline preparations are available. In acutely ill patients, aminophylline is preferable. In patients who have not taken methylxanthines regularly, aminophylline should be given as a 6 mg/kg loading dose over approximately 30 minutes, followed by a continuous intravenous maintenance dose of approximately 0.5 mg/kg/hr. When patients have taken theophylline preparations chronically, but do not have evidence of toxicity, one half the loading dose should be administered. Patients who routinely take theophylline preparations and have symptoms or signs of toxicity on hospital admission should not receive any methylxanthines until the serum theophylline level is known.

The usual therapeutic theophylline range is between 10 and 20 μg/ml. For patients receiving oral theophylline preparations, measurement should be performed at the time of peak absorption to avoid toxicity. Measurement just before administration of a slow-release, sustained-action preparation indicates a trough level which may be useful in maximizing theophylline effectiveness.

Corticosteroids

Corticosteroids are an important component of conservative treatment. They should be reserved for those individuals with acute exacerbations that do not appear to be due to bacterial infections, and commonly are used in cases of acute, probably viral, tracheobronchitis. Their mechanisms of action in this population is to decrease inflammation and thereby relieve bronchospasm.

Intravenous corticosteroids, generally are used for more than 3 days. After patients demonstrate subjective and objective evidence of improvement in air flow obstruction, a tapering course of prednisone is employed over several weeks. Inhaled beclomethasone dipropionate does not have any role in the management of acute respiratory failure complicating COPD.

Antibiotics

Acute bacterial pneumonia should be suspected in patients who present with fever, a cough productive of purulent sputum, localized crackles or consolidation, leukocytosis, and radiographically demonstrated pulmonary infiltrate(s). Initial antibiotic therapy should be guided by the sputum Gram stain and modified according to sputum, pleural fluid, or blood culture results. Antibiotics are also indicated in those patients with a change in their sputum production, but without clear evidence of bacterial infection.

Initial parenteral therapy with a broad-spectrum antibiotic such as ampicillin, erythromycin, or cefazolin is recommended. In toxic patients, antibiotic coverage should be extended with an aminoglycoside to cover gram-negative infections until the results of sputum, pleural fluid, and blood cultures return. In less ill patients, antibiotic therapy can be initiated orally with either ampicillin, tetracycline, erythromycin, cephalexin, or trimethoprim/sulfamethoxazole.

Many patients become severely hypoxemic, hypercapnic, and acidotic when they fall asleep. Therefore, when they are initially admitted to the hospital, they should receive continuous physical stimulation so that they do not sleep. The goal is to improve their condition sufficiently during the first 24 to 48 hours of hospitalization so that they can then take short naps. Hypnotics, minor tranquilizers, or other drugs with sedative properties should not be administered.

The majority of patients with acute exacerbations of COPD initially are placed at "bed rest." During this period, heparin should be administered in a subcutaneous dose of 5000 U, twice daily, to prevent deep venous thrombosis and subsequent pulmonary thromboembolism. Few studies actually document the effectiveness of this regimen. However, because very few side-effects occur, and because a number of studies confirm the effectiveness of low-dose subcutaneous heparin in other bedridden patients, its use in COPD patients seems indicated.

AGGRESSIVE THERAPY

When conservative medical therapy is unsuccessful, tracheal intubation and mechanical positive-pressure ventilation are indicated. The timing of intubation and assisted ventilation cannot be predicted on specific arterial blood gas values or tests of lung function. However, stupor and coma due to carbon dioxide retention or severe respiratory acidemia are indications for intubation. Other indications include the necessity to protect the airway in comatose patients and to aid in the control of profuse and viscous secretions in debilitated patients who are unable to cough effectively.

Intubation

Choices are 7.5- to 8.0-mm internal diameter (ID) endotracheal tubes for nasotracheal intubation and 8.0- to 8.5-mm ID tubes for orotracheal insertion.

Currently available endotracheal tubes have large-volume, low-pressure cuffs to decrease the incidence of pressure necrosis of the trachea. Immediately after intubation, the endotracheal tube cuff should be inflated to allow a minimal leak around the tube. Tube location within the tracheobronchial tree should be confirmed by both physical examination and a portable chest radiograph.

Mechanical Ventilation

When it is used, mechanical ventilation should incorporate a time-cycled, volume-limited, positive-pressure ventilator. The techniques most commonly used are intermittent mandatory ventilation/synchronized intermittent ventilation (IMV/SIMV) and assist-control ventilation (AV).

Too much controversy has been generated in an attempt to define the superiority of one ventilatory mode over the other. Extensive clinical experience proves that both techniques are capable of achieving adequate oxygenation and ventilation in patients with acute respiratory failure.

Initial tidal volume should be adjusted between 10 and 15 ml/kg. Inspired oxygen should be adjusted to maintain a Pa_{O_2} between 75 and 90 mm Hg. When IMV is used, the initial ventilator rate should be set between four and eight breaths per minute, and adjusted to maintain a normal pH. With AV, the initial control ventilator rate also should be set between eight and ten breaths per minute. Adequate humidification is essential in intubated COPD patients.

Continuous positive airway pressure (CPAP) can be combined with both IMV and AV in treating refractory hypoxemia associated with diffuse alveolar infiltrative diseases. Functional residual capacity is increased, and more normal $\dot{V}/\dot{Q}$ ratios and oxygenation often result. Hypoxemia in patients with acute exacerbations of COPD usually responds to relatively low concentrations of supplemental oxygen. However, in those patients with cardiogenic and noncardiogenic pulmonary edema and hypoxemia that are poorly responsive to the administration of a F_{IO_2} of 0.5, CPAP may be beneficial. The major complications associated with CPAP are pulmonary barotrauma and hypotension with resultant decreased tissue oxygenation. Because of these potentially serious complications, and because most patients do not have refractory hypoxemia, CPAP plays a minor role in this patient population.

For further information, please see Chapter 90 in Civetta JM, Taylor RW, Kirby RR: Critical Care. *Philadelphia: J. B. Lippincott, 1988*

BIBLIOGRAPHY

American Thoracic Society (A Statement by the Committee on Diagnostic Standards for Nontuberculous Respiratory Diseases). Definitions and Classifications of Chronic Bronchitis, Asthma, and Pulmonary Emphysema. *Am Rev Respir Dis* 1962; 85:762

Aubier M, Murciano D, Milic–Emili J, et al: Effects of the administration of O_2 on ventilation and blood gases in patients with chronic obstructive pulmonary disease during acute respiratory failure. *Am Rev Respir Dis* 1980; 122:747

Block AJ: Practical management of pulmonary insufficiency. In Eliot RS (ed): *The Acute Cardiac Emergency, Diagnosis and Management,* p 189. Mount Kisco NY, Futura Publishing Co, 1972

Campbell EJM: The J Burns Lecture—The management of acute respiratory failure in chronic bronchitis and emphysema. *Am Rev Respir Dis* 1967; 96:626

Cherniack RM: The management of acute respiratory failure. *Chest* 1970; 58:427

Matthay RA, Depew CC: Obstructive airway disease: Rational therapy with theophylline agents. *Geriatrics* 1980; 35:65

Murciano D, Aubier M, Lecocguic Y, et al: Effects of theophylline on diaphragmatic strength and fatigue in patients with chronic obstructive pulmonary disease. *N Engl J Med* 1984; 311:349

Smith JP, Stone RW, Muschenheim C: Acute respiratory failure in chronic lung disease. *Am Rev Respir Dis* 1968; 97:791

43 Status Asthmaticus

Critically ill asthmatic patients are often encountered in the emergency room (ER), hospital ward and intensive care unit (ICU). The term "status asthmaticus" implies that the patient is refractory to traditional beta-agonist and theophylline therapy. This condition is usually associated with a prolonged asthma attack and inflammatory changes that have occurred are not easily reversed by standard bronchodilator therapy. The *initial* management of severe life-threatening bronchospasm is similar for patients with new-onset severe bronchospasm and for patients with status asthmaticus. Therapies may diverge, however, because patients with status asthmaticus may be unresponsive to initial therapeutic intervention and require prolonged, aggressive, and sometimes controversial therapy. Pathologic lung changes are shown in Figures 43-1 to 43-5.

DIAGNOSIS

The differential diagnosis of patients with wheezing includes asthma, COPD, "cardiac asthma" (acute congestive heart failure), upper airway obstruction, endobronchial obstruction, organophosphate poisoning, pulmonary embolism, anaphylaxis, and toxic fume exposure (Table 43-1). A wheezing patient with a long smoking history and no history of childhood asthma is less likely to respond briskly to therapy and probably has predominantly fixed disease. Treatment is similar to that for acute asthma but the patient's response is often delayed.

Upper airway obstruction is characterized by stridor (inspiratory wheezing) heard loudest over the upper airway. Risk factors are usually evident and include foreign body aspiration, previous tracheal intubation, upper respiratory tract infection, or neck mass. Endobronchial obstruction does not usually produce respiratory distress in adults unless it is of acute onset (*i.e.*, foreign body aspiration superimposed on poor respiratory reserve).

The absence of wheezing is an ominous finding in the severely distressed asthmatic because it implies minimal air movement and is a harbinger of respiratory arrest. The presence of inspiratory wheezing implies that proximal

TABLE 43-1 DIFFERENTIAL DIAGNOSIS—ASTHMA

Entity	Clue
COPD	Smoking history, less responsive to bronchodilators
CHF	History, cardiomegaly, rales, wheezes
Upper airway obstruction	History, wheezing heard loudest over neck and upper chest
Endobronchial obstruction	History, localized wheezing
Organophosphate poisoning	History, wheezing, bronchorrhea, sialorrhea
Pulmonary embolism	Rare, risk factors, chest pain
Anaphylaxis	Insect sting, recent medication history, urticaria
Toxic fume exposure	History, poorly responsive to bronchodilators

airway mucosal edema or bronchospasm is probably present, causing impairment of both inspiratory and expiratory flow.

Hyperinflation of the lungs and large swings in intrathoracic pressure lead to an accentuated pulsus paradoxus. The paradoxical pulse is often appreciated during routine blood pressure measurement as the systolic blood pressure falls during inspiration. Normally this is not greater than 10 mm Hg.

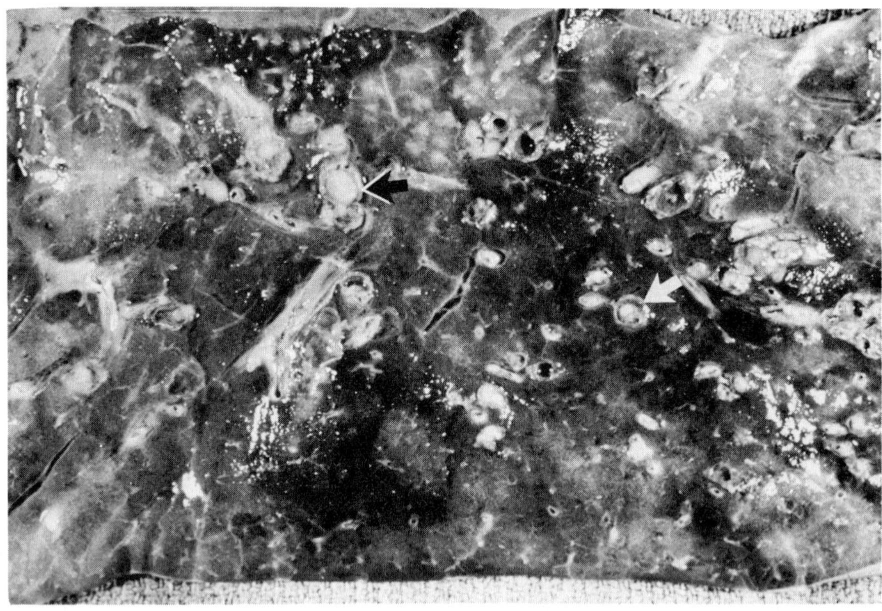

Figure 43-1 Gross necroscopy material from a patient dying of asthma. The patient had been seen 3 times over 8 days and was on maximum outpatient medication with unknown compliance. On the third visit to the hospital the patient arrested and could not be resuscitated. Profound mucous plugging of segmental and subsegmental bronchi is seen (*arrows*).

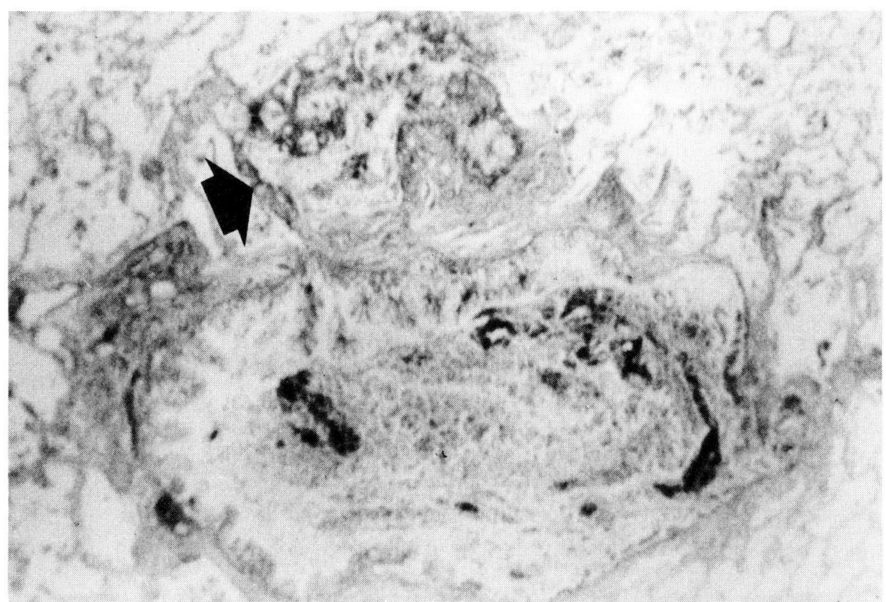

Figure 43-2 Same patient. This scanning low-power photomicrograph demonstrates two bronchioles. The smaller of the two bronchioles (*arrow*) is depicted at the top. Both are occluded with mucus and debris.

A value greater than 15 mm Hg in an acute asthmatic is usually associated with an FEV_1 of < 0.9 liter. Pulsus paradoxus is nonspecific and occurs in other disease states such as pericardial tamponade, cardiomyopathy, severe COPD, and acute hemorrhage.

History and physical examination alone do not reliably predict the severity of airway obstruction in the acute asthmatic. Although spirometry is the best objective measure of airway obstruction, the severely ill asthmatic is rarely able to perform a full forced vital capacity (FVC) maneuver. Curiously, this is the very patient in whom it is needed most. The patient's inability to maximally inspire or to maintain a full maximum expiratory effort usually prohibits use of routine spirometry. After the patient improves, however, spirometry may be important in making disposition decisions.

An objective assessment of airway obstruction in the severe asthmatic can usually be made by measuring the PEFR. This test requires patient cooperation only in the early part of the FVC maneuver. Because the greatest expiratory flow rates exist in early expiration, the majority of severe asthmatics are able to perform this maneuver. Normal expiratory flow rates vary considerably with age, sex, and height. In adults a PEFR less than 100 liters/min implies severe obstruction to air flow. Adults with PEFR of 300 liters/min or greater usually do not require hospitalization.

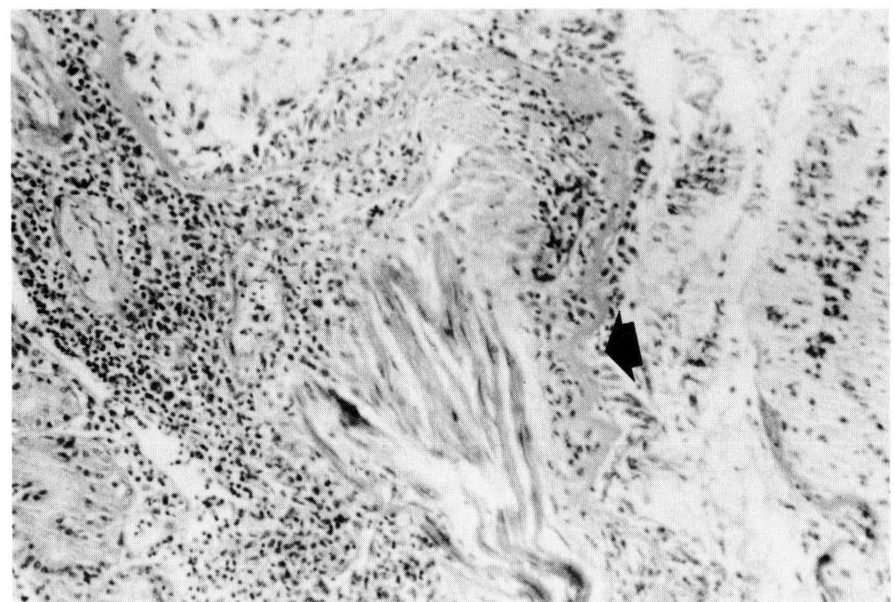

Figure 43-3 Same patient. This higher magnification view depicts, on the right side, mucus and debris within an airway lumen. The wall of the lumen, depicted on the left (*arrow*), demonstrates hyperplasia of the smooth muscle and eosinophilic infiltration.

Although arterial blood gases (ABGs) are useful for decisions regarding hospital admission or tracheal intubation, they add little in the early management of acute asthma. Most asthmatics respond dramatically to initial therapy so that ABGs obtained on presentation are rarely predictive of outcome. Often the patient is improved with aggressive therapy before the blood gas result is returned. Therefore, early attention should center around aggressive therapeutic intervention.

Arterial blood gases may be used to stage asthma. Stage I is characterized by normal values. Patients in stage II have a decreased Pa_{CO_2} and a normal Pa_{O_2} (hyperventilation has led to normalization of Pa_{O_2}). Stage III is associated with a decrease in both Pa_{CO_2} (hyperventilation is now unable to totally compensate for a widened $P(A-a)O_2$). Stage IV is characterized by a normal Pa_{CO_2} and a further decrease in Pa_{O_2} (inspiratory fatigue is now prominent). Patients in stage V have respiratory failure with an increased Pa_{CO_2} and a marked decrease in Pa_{O_2}. These findings indicate an impending respiratory arrest. A normal Pa_{CO_2} should alert the physician to respiratory fatigue and the danger of respiratory arrest. This classification system is best applied after initial aggressive treatment of asthmatic patients and may be inappropriate if applied before initial therapy. In contrast to asthma, this classification has little utility in patients with COPD.

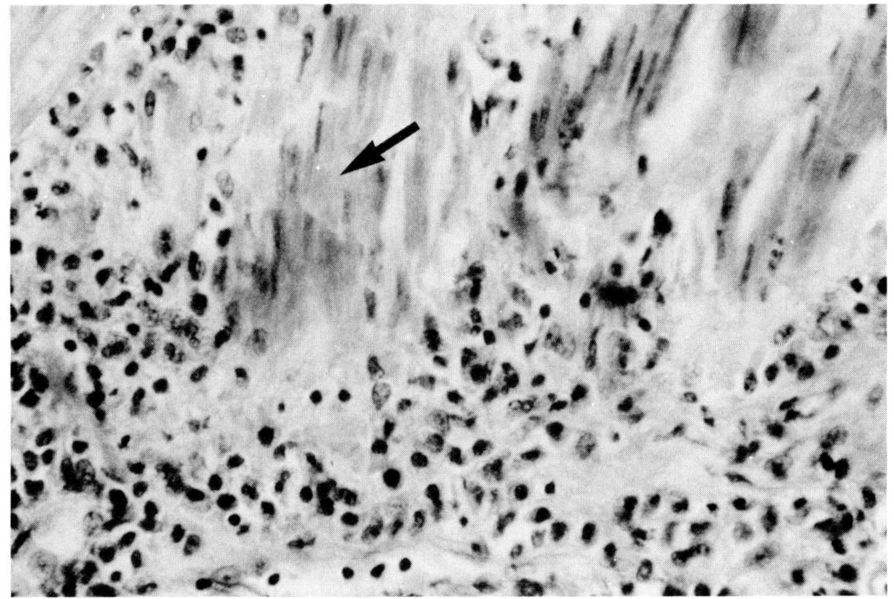

Figure 43-4 Same patient. An even higher magnification demonstrates smooth muscle proliferation (*arrow*) and massive pulmonary infiltration of eosinophils.

TREATMENT

DRUGS

Beta-Adrenergic Therapy (Table 43-2)

Metaproterenol, albuterol, and terbutaline are highly β_2-selective agents and should be delivered by inhalation as the preferred agents in treating acutely ill asthmatic patients. Clinical differences between these three agents, when inhaled, are minimal. Begin initial therapy in the acutely ill asthmatic with a β_2-selective agonist, every 15 minutes three or four times or until the patient shows significant improvement.

When these agents are delivered parenterally or orally, they lose much of their β_2 selectivity. When subcutaneous terbutaline is compared with subcutaneous epinephrine, equal cardiac side-effects are seen. Oral β_2-selective agents should not be used as primary treatment for patients with acute asthma because the therapeutic:toxicity ratio is less than with inhaled agents. Subcutaneous beta-agonist therapy (epinephrine, terbutaline) also has a disadvantageous therapeutic:toxicity ratio when compared with inhaled β_2-selective agonists. Subcutaneous epinephrine or terbutaline might, however, be useful in several situations. Inhaled agents are often difficult to administer to children. In addition, the pediatric population has a reduced susceptibility

TABLE 43-2 BETA-ADRENERGIC AGONISTS

Agent	Relative Potency	Route of Administration	Mechanism of Action	Duration (hr)	Dosage
Metaproterenol	3	Oral	$\beta_2 > \beta_1$	3–5	0.3–0.5 mg/kg t.i.d. to q.i.d.
		Aerosol, 5% solution	$\beta_2 > \beta_1$	3–5	0.01–0.3 ml/kg q.i.d.*
Albuterol	4	Oral	$\beta_2 >> \beta_1$	4–6	0.10–0.15 mg/kg t.i.d. to q.i.d.
		Aerosol, 0.5% solution	$\beta_2 >> \beta_1$	4–6	0.01 ml/kg up to 1 ml q.i.d.*
Fenoterol	4	Oral	$\beta_2 >> \beta_1$	4–6	0.01 mg/kg t.i.d. to q.i.d.
	4	Aerosol, 0.5% solution	$\beta_2 >> \beta_1$	4–6	0.01 ml/kg up to 1 ml q.i.d.*
Terbutaline	4	Oral	$\beta_2 >> \beta_1$	4–6	0.075 mg/kg t.i.d. to q.i.d.
	4	Parenteral, 0.1% solution (s.q.)	$\beta_2 >> \beta_1$	4–6	0.01 ml/kg, maximum of 0.25 ml every 15 min × 2
Epinephrine	3	Parenteral, 0.1% solution (s.q.)	α, β_1 β_2	1–2	0.01 ml/kg maximum of 0.3–0.5 ml every 15 min × 3
Isoproterenol	4	Aerosol, 0.5% solution	$\beta_1 = \beta_2$	1–2	0.02 ml/kg, up to 0.5 ml q.i.d.
Isoetharine	2	Aerosol, 1% solution	$\beta_2 \geq \beta_1$	2–3	0.02 ml/kg up to 0.5 ml q.i.d.

(Modified from Myers DL: Pharmacologic therapy of respiratory failure. In Kirby RR, Taylor RW [eds]: *Respiratory Failure*, p. 484. Chicago, Year Book Medical Publishers, 1986)

s.q., subcutaneous; t.i.d., three times daily; q.i.d., four times daily.

*More frequent dosing is often required initially; see text.

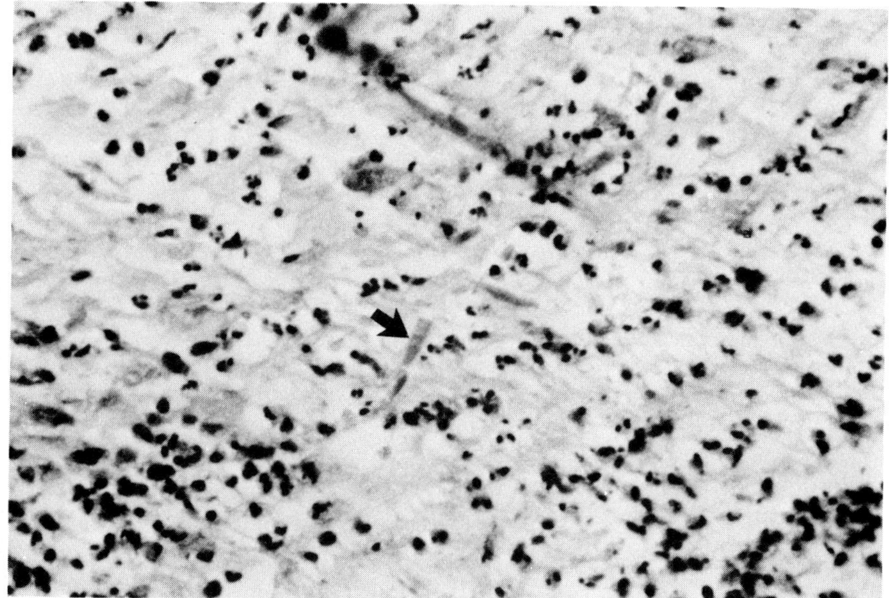

Figure 43-5 Same patient. This high magnification view vividly shows mucosal debris with an admixture of exfoliated respiratory epithelium and eosinophils. A Charcot-Leyden crystal is noted in the center of the field (*arrow*). These elongated amorphous structures are thought to be produced from excretions of eosinphils.

to β_1 toxicity making subcutaneous administration a useful route of drug delivery. Rapid delivery of beta-agonists to the airway is desirable in seriously ill asthmatic patients with impending respiratory arrest. The combination of inhaled and subcutaneously administered beta-agonists has been useful. It has been argued that bronchodilation is enhanced when drug is delivered by the airway and by the circulation. No clear data support this concept. Although the subcutaneous administration of beta-agonists induces greater peripheral airway bronchodilation than an equal amount of inhaled agent the difference is not clinically significant.

Two types of nebulizer systems are available for inhalation therapy, the face mask and the hand-held nebulizer with a mouthpiece. The mouthpiece is preferred because it delivers more drug. However, more patient cooperation is required with the hand-held system because a good seal must be maintained around the mouthpiece. In the severely ill asthmatic the face-mask system may be necessary. The hand-held mouthpiece nebulizer system must be used if anticholinergic medication is used. Contamination of the ocular area may occur if a face mask is used for delivery of an anticholinergic agent. Pupillary dilatation and precipitation of glaucoma may occur. Patients with known glaucoma or bladder neck obstruction should not receive atropine.

If subcutaneous adrenergic therapy is chosen, the epinephrine dose for adults is 0.3 to 0.5 ml of a 1:1000 dilution depending on age and weight. This may be repeated in the initial management every 15 minutes as many as three times. An alternative agent is subcutaneous terbutaline, 0.25 mg (Table 43-2).

Theophylline

Patients who fail to respond to beta-agonist therapy or patients who present with a severe asthma attack (PEFR < 100 liters/min) should receive intravenous aminophylline. If the patient has not been receiving a theophylline preparation, a loading dose of aminophylline, 6 mg/kg in the moderate attack and 7.5 mg/kg in the severe attack, should be given over 15 to 30 minutes. After the loading dose is given, aminophylline should be administered by continuous infusion with an infusion pump at a rate of 0.7 mg/kg/hr. This dosage must be modified depending on the patient's underlying condition (Table 43-3).

Steroids

Corticosteroids are an essential part of asthma therapy, especially when mucosal edema and mucus plugging have important pathologic roles. Methylprednisolone given in a dose of 60 to 125 mg every 4 to 6 hours has become accepted therapy in the early management of the asthmatic patient. The benefit derived by the asthmatic is probably due to a combination of enhancement of β_2-receptor responsiveness, interruption of arachidonic acid inflammatory pathways, decrease in capillary basement membrane permeability, decreased leukocyte attachment, modulation of calcium migration intracellularly, reduction in airway mucus production, and suppression of IgE receptor binding.

Anticholingergics

Although atropine was recognized as one of the earliest effective drugs for treatment of asthma, it was largely abandoned when beta-adrenergic ago-

TABLE 43-3 MAINTENANCE DOSES OF AMINOPHYLLINE IN ACUTE ASTHMA

Condition	Continuous Infusion Dose (mg/kg/hr)
Otherwise healthy adult	0.7
Teenager	0.9
Older than age 50	0.5
History of cardiac or liver dysfunction	0.2–0.3
Smoking adult	0.9

nists were developed, due to fewer side-effects and a perceived better efficacy of the beta-agonists. An intense interest in anticholinergic therapy has resurfaced. Inhaled atropine is effective in treating bronchospasm in patients with asthma and COPD. Although anticholinergic agents may offer significant benefit to the asthmatic, they are probably more useful in patients with COPD. The dose of atropine in patients with COPD is 0.025 mg/kg in a total volume of 3 to 5 ml. This dose is probably appropriate for the asthmatic as well. It should be given by a hand-held nebulizer with a mouthpiece and not by face mask to avoid atropine deposition in the eyes and the associated problems of glaucoma exacerbation or pupillary dilation. Few systemic side-effects occur at the recommended dose. Earlier concerns regarding drying or inspissation of airway secretions are unfounded.

TRACHEAL INTUBATION/MECHANICAL VENTILATION

Indications for early tracheal intubation include apnea or near apnea, central cyanosis, mental status changes, or depressed level of consciousness. Inability to adequately oxygenate or ventilate an asthmatic mandates tracheal intubation. A sustained respiratory rate in excess of 40 breaths per minute implies impending respiratory fatigue and may mandate tracheal intubation. The awake and alert asthmatic tolerates nasotracheal better than orotracheal intubation.

Mechanical ventilation in the asthmatic is often feared by the clinician because of published reports of a significant increase in morbidity and mortality with its use. How much of this morbidity and mortality is related to the severity of the disease and how much is due to the intervention itself is not clear. Significant complications do occur in the mechanically ventilated asthmatic including barotrauma, machine failure, endotracheal tube malfunction, and pneumonia.

For further information, please see Chapter 91 in Civetta JM, Taylor RW, Kirby RR: Critical Care. *Philadelphia: J. B. Lippincott, 1988*

BIBLIOGRAPHY

Amory DW, Burnham SC, Cheney FW: Comparison of the cardiopulmonary effects of subcutaneously administered epinephrine and terbutaline in patients with reversible airway obstruction. *Chest* 1975; 67:279

Bone RC, Hiller C: Modern treatment of bronchial asthma. *JACEP* 1978; 7:269

Brandstetter RD, Gotz VP, Mar DD: Identifying the acutely ill patient with asthma. *South Med J* 1981; 74:713

Brenner BE: Bronchial asthma in adults: Presentation to the emergency department: Part I. Pathogensis, clinical manifestations, diagnostic evaluation, and differential diagnosis. *Am J Emerg Med* 1983; 1:50

Brenner BE: Bronchial asthma in adults: Presentation to the emergency department:

Part II. Sympathomimetics, respiratory failure, recommendations for initial treatment, indications for admission, and summary. *Am J Emerg Med* 1983; 3:306

Bryant DH: Nebulized ipratropium bromide in the treatment of acute asthma. *Chest* 1985; 88:24

Chodosh S: Rational management of bronchial asthma. *Arch Intern Med* 1978; 138:1394

Fanta CH, Rossing TH, McFadden ER: Emergency room treatment of asthma. *Am J Med* 1982; 72:416

Franklin W. Treatment of severe asthma. *N Engl J Med* 1974; 290:1469

George RB: Some recent advances in the management of asthma. *Arch Intern Med* 1982; 142:933

Gross NJ, Skorodin MS: The place of anticholinergic agents in the treatment of airways obstruction. *Immunol Allergy Pract* 1986; 8:224

Haskell RJ, Wong BM, Hansen JE: A double-blind, randomized clinical trial of methylprednisolone in status asthmaticus. *Arch Intern Med* 1983; 143:1324

Hiller FC, Wilson FJ: Evaluation and management of acute asthma. *Med Clin North Am* 1983; 67:669

Hopewell PC, Miller RT: Pathophysiology and management of severe asthma. *Clin Chest Med* 1984; 5:623

Marney SR: Asthma: Recent developments in treatment. *South Med J* 1985; 78:1084

Martin TG, Elenbaas RM, Pingleton SH: Use of peak expiratory flow rates to eliminate unnecessary arterial blood gases in acute asthma. *Ann Emerg Med* 1982; 11:70

Nowak RM, Pensler MI, Sarkar DD, et al: Comparison of peak expiratory flow and FEV_1 admission criteria for acute bronchial asthma. *Ann Emerg Med* 1982; 11:64

Pak CCF, Kradjan WA, Lakshminarayan S, Marini JJ: Inhaled atropine sulfate. *Am Rev Respir Dis* 1982; 125:331

Scoggin CH, Sahn SA, Petty TL: Status asthmaticus—A nine-year experience. *JAMA* 1977; 238:1158

Shim C, Williams J: Bronchial response to oral versus aerosol metaproterenol in asthma. *Ann Intern Med* 1980; 93:428

Smith CS, Williams MH: Relationship of wheezing to the severity of obstruction in asthma. *Arch Intern Med* 1983; 143:890

Storms WW: Ipratropium bromide (Atrovent): A new anticholinergic bronchodilator for the treatment of asthma. *Immunol Allergy Pract* 1986; 8:32

Tashkin DP, Trevor E, Chopra SK, Taplin GV: Sites of airway dilatation in asthma following inhaled versus subcutaneous terbutaline. *Am J Med* 1980; 68:14

44
Hemoptysis

Massive hemoptysis is an uncommon pulmonary condition that mandates rapid stabilization and treatment. It has been defined by various authors as 100 to 600 ml of blood loss daily into the tracheobronchial tree. Mortality is directly proportional to three factors: rate and volume of blood loss, and the patient's underlying medical condition. Massive hemoptysis is most often associated with inflammatory lung disease of which active and inactive tuberculosis make up a large proportion of the cases. The source of the bleeding is usually from the bronchial circulation.

Optimal management involves a team approach which includes the intensivist, pulmonologist, radiologist, anesthesiologist, and thoracic surgeon. The greatest immediate risk to the patient is asphyxia. Successful temporizing measures to control bleeding in the airway include selective intubation of the main stem bronchi, endobronchial tamponade, intravenous pitressin, and bronchial artery embolization. If the site of bleeding can be localized by bronchoscopy and if the patient has adequate pulmonary reserve, surgical resection should be accomplished.

DIAGNOSIS

A directed, abbreviated history can provide valuable information regarding the cause of hemorrhage and may result in the expeditious institution of lifesaving therapy. The interviewer should attempt to localize the source, estimate the quantity, and determine the onset, duration, and character of the hemoptysis. In addition, conditions *associated* with hemoptysis should be identified. (Table 44-1).

Although bronchogenic carcinoma is an infrequent cause of massive hemoptysis, the diagnosis must be entertained in patients over age 40 who are cigarette smokers. In reality many patients have multiple risk factors. They may have a history of a positive purified protein derivative (PPD) skin test for tuberculosis or an exposure to tuberculosis coexistent with chronic obstructive pulmonary disease (COPD) and chronic bronchitis. The duration of hemop-

TABLE 44-1 KEY HISTORICAL POINTS

Present illness
- Patient age
- Onset and duration of hemoptysis
- Source of bleeding
  - Upper respiratory tract
  - Lower respiratory tract
  - Gastrointestinal tract
- Amount of blood
- Characteristics of sputum
- Associated chest pain/trauma
- Smoking
- Medications
- Tuberculosis exposure

Medical history
- Cardiopulmonary disease
- Autoimmune disease
- Blood dyscrasia

Review of systems
- Nasal symptoms
- Oropharyngeal symptoms
- Laryngeal symptoms
- Gastrointestinal symptoms
- Hematuria

tysis may be helpful with long-standing minor hemoptysis favoring bronchiectasis or bronchogenic carcinoma.

Some patients may be able to localize the site of bleeding to a particular side of the chest. This may be helpful in positioning the patient to minimize aspiration. One study by Kinasewitz demonstrated that 51 to 67 patients were unable to correctly identify the site of a cough stimulus by the bronchoscope. Thus, information obtained from the patient regarding the site of bleeding should be kept in its proper perspective.

Many patients find it difficult to identify the organ system responsible for bleeding, let alone the hemithorax. Careful questioning regarding nausea, hematemesis, melena, or prior gastrointestinal disease may be helpful. The appearance of the specimen may aid in diagnosing the site of hemorrhage. In hemoptysis, bright red blood is mixed with frothy sputum, and the specimen should be devoid of food particles. The suctioning of blood or hemoccult positive material from the stomach by a nasogastric tube may not reliably differentiate hematemesis from hemoptysis. Some patients, particularly women with hemoptysis, swallow coughed up blood which makes quantification of hemoptysis inaccurate.

The presence of purulent material in the sputum suggests bronchiectasis or lung abscess. A history of valvular heart disease suggests a diagnosis of mitral stenosis. The report of tearing chest pain prompts consideration of a ruptured aortic aneurysm. The presence of hematuria may indicate a medication overdose or interaction or the presence of an alveolar hemorrhage syndrome.

Important physical findings possibly present in the patient with massive hemoptysis are listed in Table 44-2. As mentioned previously, the more debilitated the patient the higher the risk of death, primarily from aspiration. Obtunded patients with an inadequate cough reflex may suffer dire consequences after aspirating small amounts of blood. Although it is unusual for patients to be hypovolemic as a result of hemopthysis, if the airway is adequately maintained a small percentage of patients risk exsanguination. Also, chronically ill patients with hemoptysis may be hypovolemic secondary to decreased fluid intake. It is therefore prudent to assess these patients' volume status. Routine preoperative laboratory studies (Table 44-3) should be obtained in anticipation of thoracotomy.

A chest radiograph should be obtained on all patients, preferably a posteroanterior and lateral film. The radiograph may yield specific information such as a new alveolar infiltrate representing pulmonary hemorrhage, a pulmonary mass or cavity, evidence of lung abscess, an enlarged left atrium with Kerley B lines suggesting mitral stenosis, or a lobulated mass suggestive of an arteriovenous malformation. The abnormality on chest radiograph may not correspond to the site of bleeding.

TREATMENT

Maintenance of the patient's airway is of prime importance. The task may be considerable if the rate of bleeding is brisk. Supplemental oxygen should be given to all patients with massive hemoptysis because blood fills the trach-

TABLE 44-2 IMPORTANT PHYSICAL FINDINGS

General
Level of consciousness
Orthostatic changes
Head and neck
Ulceration of nasal septum
Telangiectasia
Oropharyngeal lesion
Laryngeal lesion
Adenopathy
Chest
Chest trauma/rib fracture
Localized wheezes, rales, rhonchi
Diastolic rumble/opening snap
Extremities
Clubbing
Petechiae/ecchymosis

TABLE 44-3 LABORATORY STUDIES

Complete blood count
PT/PTT
Electrolytes, BUN creatinine
Urinalysis
Sputum
Smear and culture for bacteria, acid-fast bacilli, and fungus
Sputum cytology
PPD (intermediate strength)
Chest radiograph

eobronchial tree and ventilation/perfusion mismatch worsens. Two large bore intravenous cannulae should be placed to allow access for fluid and medication administration, and to prepare the patient for possible surgery. Six units of blood should be typed and cross-matched. Cough should be suppressed but not abolished with 30 to 60 mg of codeine intramuscularly every 6 hours. Excessive chest manipulation, such as percussion and spirometry, should be avoided. The risk of spirometry provoking bleeding is probably small, but in the presence of massive hemoptysis, ventilatory reserve may be significantly underestimated, therefore making the test of questionable value. The patient should be positioned with the presumed bleeding side down in the lateral decubitus and slight Trendelenburg position. This will lessen spill over into the "good lung" and promote drainage of the airway. If bronchospasm or purulent sputum has been identified, appropriate intravenous antibiotics or bronchodilators should be started. Adequate suction and a large endotracheal tube (8.0-9.0 mm) and a laryngoscope should be present at the bedside.

If, prior to bronchoscopy, the bleeding becomes so rapid that respiratory arrest is imminent, the following measures may be attempted. The endotracheal tube can be advanced until breath sounds are no longer heard over the left side of the chest (normally the right main stem bronchus lies in the same axis as the trachea). If the patient is not bleeding from this side the cuff can be inflated and the patient ventilated with the airway protected. If the patient is bleeding from the side that is selectively intubated, a Foley catheter or Fogarty catheter can be placed in the airway and inflated. The endotracheal tube can then be slowly withdrawn until bilateral breath sounds are once again present. Tube placement should be verified by a chest radiograph. Intravenous vasopressin (0.2–0.3 u/min) may be given. This has been reported as an effective temporizing measure.

A Carlens or Robertshaw double-lumen tube offers no significant advantage over selective intubation. Placement of these tubes requires experienced personnel. In addition, the small lumen of the Carlens tube makes suctioning difficult. If mechanical ventilation is needed, some authors have suggested that positive end-expiratory pressure (PEEP) may be therapeutic by providing a measure of tamponade to the site of hemorrhage by the increase in intrathoracic pressure. This therapy should be used with caution. because PEEP may increase the risk of hypotension and barotrauma associated with mechanical ventilation, particularly in patients with COPD. Once the patient has been stabilized, attempts to identify the site of bleeding and institute definitive therapy must be made. Figure 44-1 illustrates in algorithmic fashion how this may be approached.

Bronchoscopy is the procedure of choice for the diagnosis of the site of bleeding. Both rigid bronchoscopy and flexible fiberoptic bronchoscopy have been used successfully with similar diagnostic yields. The choice of which scope to use depends on the rate of bleeding and the personal experience of the pulmonary and thoracic surgery consultants. If bleeding is considerable and on-going, the patient is best handled in the operating room with rigid bronchoscopy. The rigid bronchoscope provides better suction and the capability to ventilate the patient. If bleeding is less severe, a large-channel flexible bronchoscope may be used, such as the Olympus T1. This bronchoscope will pass freely through an endotracheal tube that is 8.0 mm or larger. The flexible scope offers the advantage of direct visualization of the upper lobes and opportunity to place a Fogarty catheter in a segmental or subsegmental bronchus if the bleeding site is identified. Segmental lavage with iced isotonic saline may aid in identifying and controlling the hemorrhage. This method has been used successfully with both rigid and flexible bronchoscopy. Topical epinephrine, in a 1:20,000 dilution, may be helpful if an endobronchial lesion such as an adenoma is the source of hemorrhage.

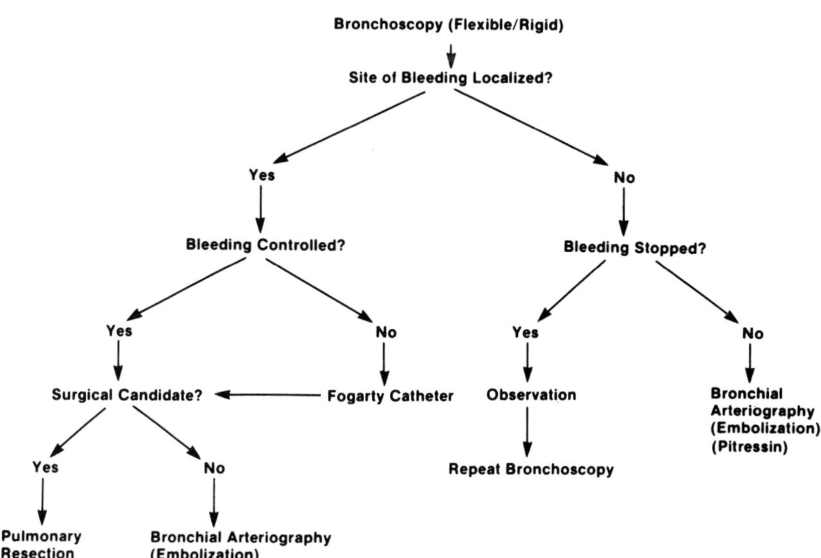

Figure 44-1 Management of massive hemoptysis.

Once the site of bleeding has been localized and controlled, a decision regarding definitive therapy must be made. If the patient is an operative candidate, pulmonary resection should be performed. Criteria for inoperability include forced vital capacity or forced expired volume in 1 second of less than 40% predicted, unresectable carcinoma, and bilateral pulmonary disease with inability to localize the site of bleeding by bronchoscopy.

If the site of bleeding cannot be localized by bronchoscopy and the patient is still actively bleeding, bronchial arteriography may be attempted. Angiographic findings that implicate a particular site as the source of bleeding are localized hyperemia, massive systemic-to-pulmonary artery or vein shunt, pericavity vascularity, and extravasation of contrast medium (a rare finding). The role of chest computed tomography (CT) and nuclear medicine studies (Tc-sulfur colloid and Tc-labeled red blood cells) in localizing bleeding is uncertain at the present time. If the site of bleeding cannot be localized and the bleeding has stopped at the time of bronchoscopy, observation with serial hematocrits, chest radiography and arterial blood gases in conjunction with repeat bronchoscopy may be most prudent.

In patients who are not surgical candidates and who continue to bleed, bronchial artery embolization should be attempted. If Gelfoam is used as the material for embolization and care is taken not to embolize the spinal artery, complications are minimal. Uflacker's series of 75 patients reported immediate control of hemoptysis in 64 patients (76.6%) and a recurrence rate of 21.7% during the follow-up period ranging from 1 to 47 months. If no abnormalities are identified on the bronchial arteriogram, the nonbronchial systemic vessels should be investigated to identify the source of bleeding. If bleeding persists after a thorough investigation of the bronchial and nonbronchial systemic arteries with embolization where appropriate, the pulmonary circulation should be studied.

For further information, please see Chapter 92 in Civetta JM, Taylor RW, Kirby RR: Critical Care. *Philadelphia: J. B. Lippincott, 1988*

BIBLIOGRAPHY

Barth DH, Mertens MA: Interventional radiology. *Med Clin North Am* 1984; 68:1647

Bobrowitz ID, Ramakrishna S, Shim YS, et al: Comparison of medical vs surgical treatment of major hemoptysis. *Arch Intern Med* 1983; 143:1343

Brenner B: *Comprehensive Management of Respiratory Emergencies.* Rockville Aspen Systems Corp, 1985

Conlan AA, Hurwitz SS: Management of massive hemoptysis with the rigid bronchoscope and cold saline lavage. *Thorax* 1980; 35:901

Crocco JA, Rooney JJ, Fankushen DS, et al: Massive hemoptysis. *Arch Intern Med* 1968; 121:495

Garzon AA, Cerruti MM, Golding ME, et al: Exsanguinating hemoptysis. *J Thorac Cardiovasc Surg* 1982; 84:829

Garzon AA, Gourin A: Surgical management of massive hemoptysis. A ten-year experience. *Ann Surg* 1978; 187:267
Gourin A, Garzon AA: Control of hemorrhage in emergency pulmonary resection for massive hemoptysis. *Chest* 1975; 68:120
Gourin A, Garzon AA: Operative treatment of massive hemoptysis. *Ann Thorac Surg* 1974; 18:52
Haponik EF, Britt EJ, Smith PL, et al. Computed chest tomography in the evaluation of hemoptysis. *Chest* 1987; 91:80
Haponik EF, Rothfeld B, Britt EJ, et al: Radionuclide localization of massive pulmonary hemorrhage. *Chest* 1984; 86:208
Holsclaw DS, Grand RJ, Shwachman H, et al: Massive hemoptysis in cystic fibrosis. *J Pediatr* 1970; 76:829
Imgrund SP, Goldberg SK, Walkenstein MD, et al: Clinical diagnosis of massive hemoptysis using the fiberoptic bronchoscope. *Crit Care Med* 1985; 13:438
Kinasewitz GT, Long RJ, George RB, et al: Inability of awake patients to correctly locate a cough stimulus. *South Med J* 1985; 78:970
Magee G, Williams MH Jr: Treatment of massive hemoptysis with intravenous pitressin. *Lung* 1982; 160:165
Noseworthy TW, Anderson BJ: Massive hemoptysis. *Can Med Assoc J* 1986; 135:1097
Pursel SE, Lindskag GE: Hemoptysis. A clinical evaluation of 105 patients examined consecutively on a thoracic surgical service. *Am Rev Respir Dis* 1961; 84:329
Uflacker R, Kaemmerer A, Picon PD, et al: Bronchial artery embolization in the management of hemoptysis: Technical aspects and long term results. *Radiology* 1985; 157:637
Vujic I, Pyle R, Hungerford GD, et al: Angiography and therapeutic blockade in the control of hemoptysis. The importance of nonbronchial systemic arteries. *Radiology* 1982; 143:19
Winzelberg GG, Wholey MH, Jarmolowski, CA, et al: Patients with hemoptysis examined by Tc-99m sulfur colloid and Tc-99m-labeled red blood cells: A preliminary appraisal. *Radiology* 1984; 153:523
Wolfe JD, Simmons DH: Hemoptysis: Diagnosis and management. *West J Med* 1977; 127:383

45
Pleural Effusions

Fluid moves from the parietal pleura to the pleural space and then to the visceral pleura. This movement is caused by pressure differentials in the thoracic cavity. The lung exhibits recoil (wants to collapse when inflated), much like a child's balloon. The chest wall also has recoil, but its recoil is more like that of a compressed stiff spring (similar to an automotive suspension spring). At normal lung volumes a negative pleural surface pressure results when the outward pull of the chest wall is counterbalanced by the inward pull of the lung. The hydrostatic pressure in the parietal pleura is positive, and the resultant gradient favors the (normal) movement of fluid from the chest wall lining into the pleural space. This movement is opposed somewhat by the higher oncotic pressure of fluid in the parietal pleura compared with pleural fluid. The net pressure gradient from parietal pleura to pleural space remains positive, however. The hydrostatic pressure of the visceral pleura is also positive, opposing fluid movement from the pleural space into the visceral pleura. However, the oncotic pressure of fluid in the visceral pleura counteracts the hydrostatic pressure, and the resultant driving pressure favors fluid movement from pleural space to visceral pleura. The magnitude of forces favoring fluid movement from the parietal pleura to the pleural space is less than that of the forces favoring movement from the pleural space to the visceral pleura, and fluid normally does not accumulate in the pleural space.

It has been estimated that under normal conditions up to 100 ml of fluid enters the pleural space per hour. Since the lung can theoretically absorb up to 300 ml/hr, no fluid accumulates. These numbers apply only to protein-free fluid. The lung also has a large lymphatic drainage system speculated to be capable of removing 500 ml of fluid daily from the pleural space.

Pleural effusions are thought to occur from several mechanisms that alter the homeostatic physiology described above. They are often missed in a critically ill patient, especially in the first few days of illness.

DIAGNOSIS

In the absence of hypotension or indwelling femoral devices, most patients can be briefly supported and examined in the sitting position. Areas of decreased breath sounds should be searched for by auscultation, as should regions of increased dullness to percussion. This position also allows examination of the skin of the back and buttocks—areas that commonly never see the light of day during the patient's ICU stay, but can yield significant findings about fluid status (presacral edema), infection (decubiti), drug reactions or fever (rashes), and patient comfort (foreign bodies such as plastic catheter sheaths, suction tips, and other items can be found under patients who cannot complain).

The radiographic manifestations of pleural fluid when viewed from various projections are well described. Pleural fluid is always more dense than air and thus causes an area of increased opacification on the film. A key to correct diagnosis of pleural fluid on chest radiograph lies in recognizing the projection used when the film was taken. Unless the fluid is loculated, it moves to the most dependent portion of the thoracic space. If the film is taken supine, the fluid may only form a diffuse "haziness" through which lung markings will still be seen (distinguishing it somewhat from a large pulmonary infiltrate, which should obscure lung markings and perhaps contain air bronchograms). No air–fluid level exists, and effusions viewed in a supine projection may be missed altogether or diagnosed as another process. Due to the positive pressure fluid exerts in the pleural space, most large effusions cause some shift of the mediastinum to the contralateral side. Atelectasis or total lung collapse can be associated with an effusion, but simple radiographic separation of effusion from collapse (and more importantly, quantification of amount of fluid present) is usually impossible. For these reasons "blind" aspiration of a radiographically opacified hemithorax on the assumption that all the abnormality is due to fluid is inadvisable. Radiographs in Figures 45-1 through 45-5 demonstrate these principles. Differences in transudative and exudative effusions are summarized in Table 45-1.

TREATMENT

Once an effusion has been confirmed as present, the decision must be made whether or not to attempt thoracentesis. A prerequisite for any invasive procedure is knowledge of the "current anatomy" of the patient—not just where structures are *supposed* to be in relation to anatomic landmarks, but where they really *are* at the time of the procedure. For thoracentesis to be performed safely, one must know *exactly* the fluid and diaphragm locations. Normally a standard set of radiographs (posteroanterior, lateral, lateral decubitus) provides the information, but these views may be unavailable or suboptimal in the ICU patient. If discussion with the radiologist and repeat views do not

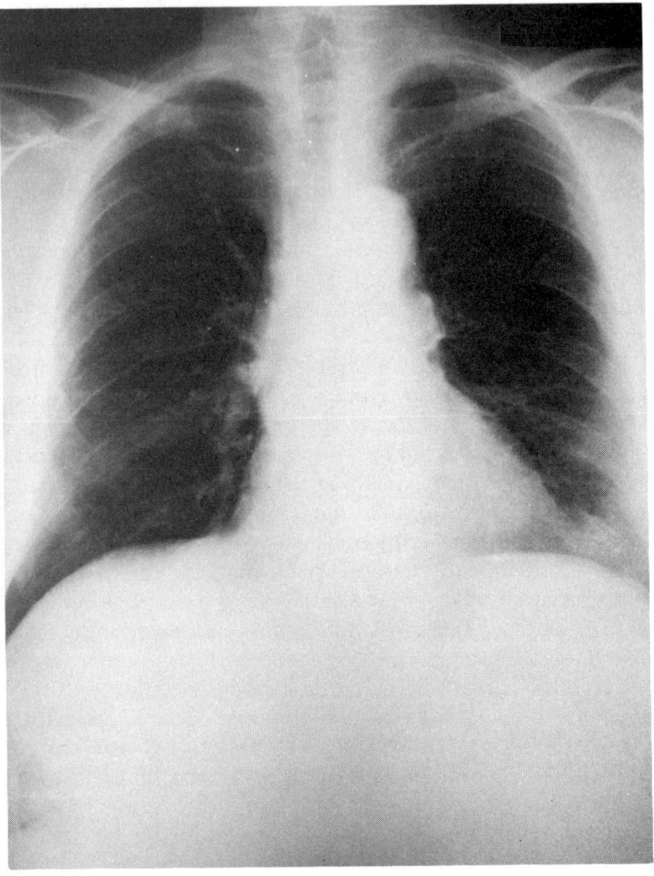

A

Figure 45-1 A. Normal upright posterior-anterior chest radiograph. This standard view is most familiar to physicians. Unfortunately, this view is hard to obtain in critically ill patients, because it requires an upright posture with the film plate in front of the patient and the beam source 6 feet from the plate. **B**. Same patient as in A, but film taken as semirecumbent portable view several days later after surgery. Note the apparent enlargement of the heart and mediastinum produced by this view. Also note the "field of view" of this film—the top of the thorax is not seen. It is most helpful to tell the radiographic technician the area of greatest interest to ensure that it will be seen on the film. Intensive care patients may act as "moving targets," and often require personnel to support them if they cannot comply with requests to "hold still and take a deep breath." This film has an area of increased density in the left lung base that may represent either consolidation of lung parenchyma or pleural fluid (or both). The right

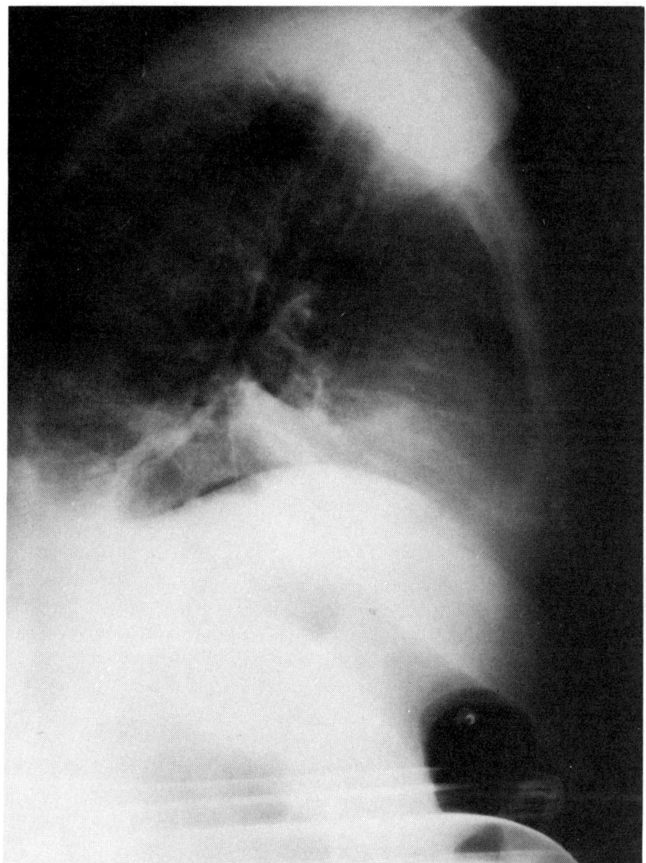

B

Figure 45-1 *(continued)*

hemidiaphragm is also elevated which may represent a right subpulmonic effusion or volume loss from lobectomy. One should never assume that a homogeneous density below a lung is fluid; it may be abdominal contents below an abnormally elevated diaphragm. **C.** Upright lateral view of same patient obtained the same day as in B. This view confirms both an increase in lower lobe lung density due to atelectasis and the presence of fluid in the posterior gutter. What is *NOT* confirmed is the hemithorax in which the fluid is located. Figure 1, B suggests that fluid could be present on either side. (A subsequent left lateral decubitus film confirmed the fluid to be left-sided.)

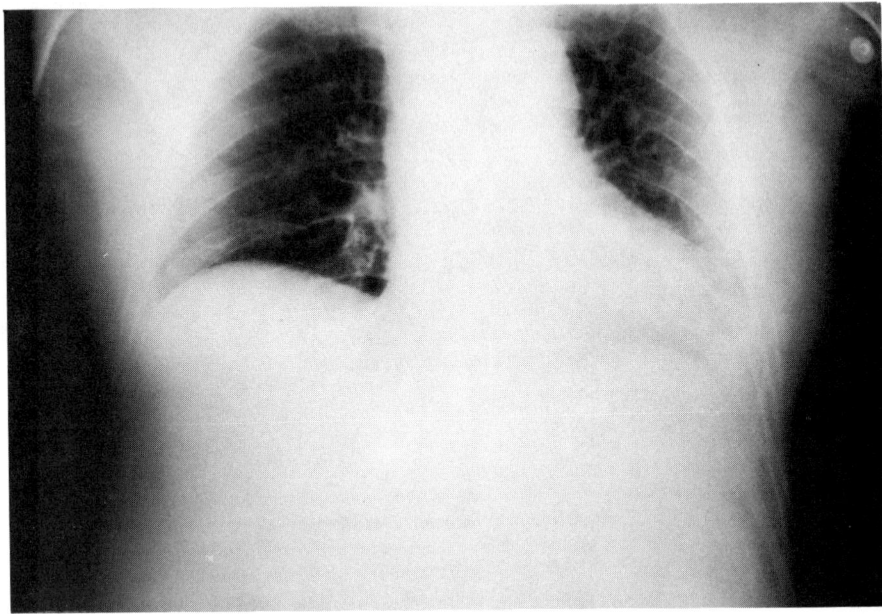

C

Figure 45-1 *(continued)*

→

Figure 45-2 A. Supine portable view of a patient recovering from coronary artery bypass surgery. Note the homogeneous opacification of the left hemithorax, without air bronchograms. The vasculature of the left lung can be seen "through" the increased density. These findings suggest a left-sided pleural effusion. **B.** Same patient as in A, but this view was obtained with the patient in the sitting position. The left upper lung field has cleared remarkably. There is persistent opacification of the left lower lung field, strongly suggesting a left pleural effusion. *(continued)*

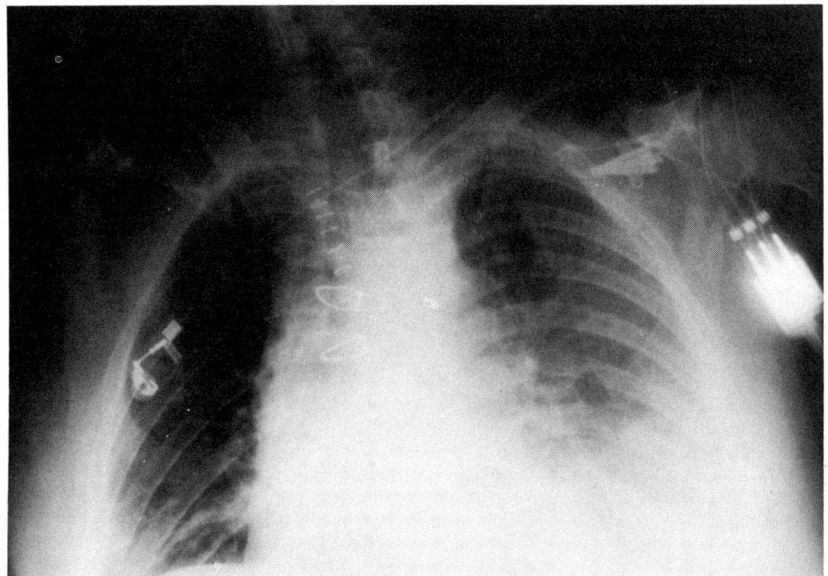

A

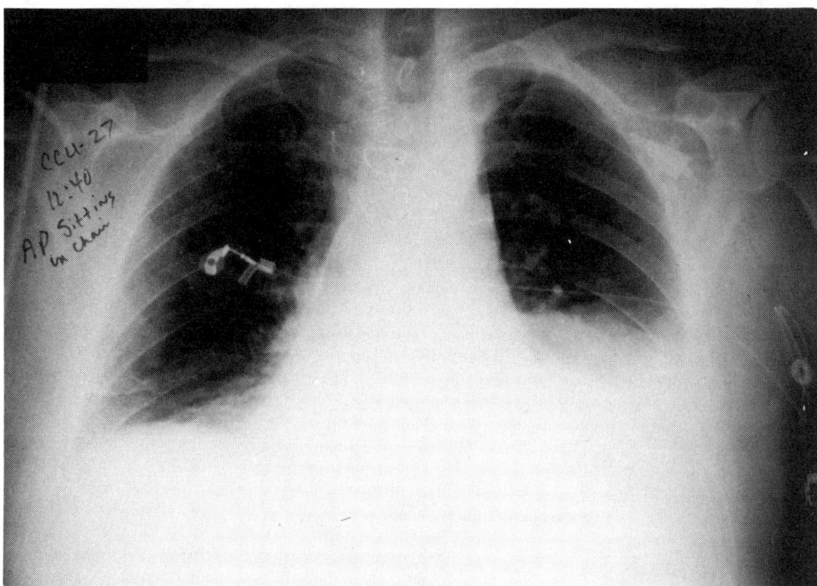

B

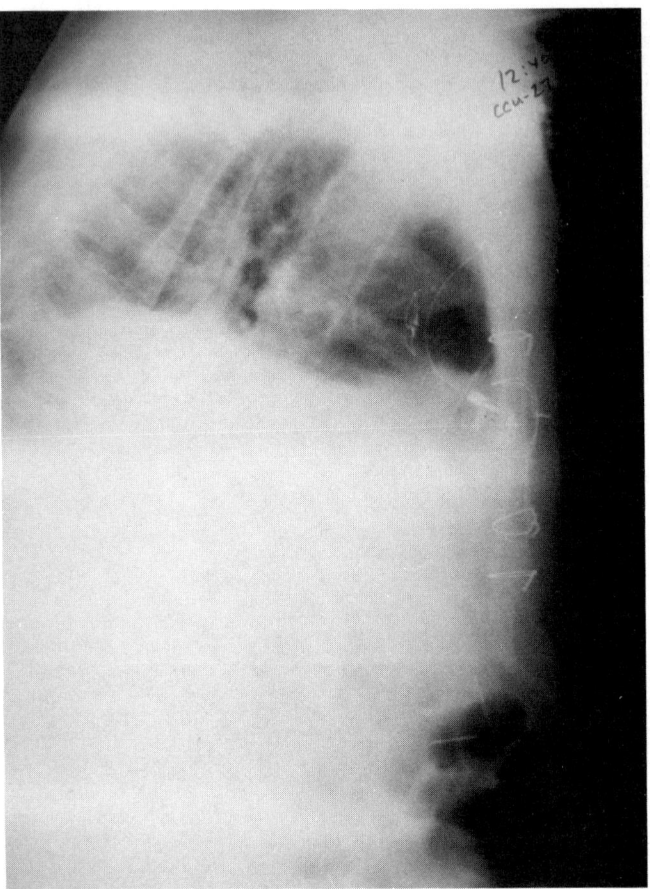

C

Figure 45-2 *(continued)* C. Same patient. This portable upright lateral view confirms the presence of a large pleural effusion. Review Figures 45-2A and 45-2B. Is there evidence for a similar, but smaller, right-sided effusion? This patient had congestive heart failure, and a left thorocentesis yielded a transudative fluid.

Figure 45-4 Semirecumbent view of a patient with ARDS after a right lobectomy. Note the density in the right lower lung field that could represent fluid. The region did not move on lateral decubitus views, suggesting loculation if fluid was present. A chest CT did not document significant amounts of fluid. The abnormality was due to right diaphragmatic elevation secondary to loss of lung volume from lobectomy, along with atelectasis.

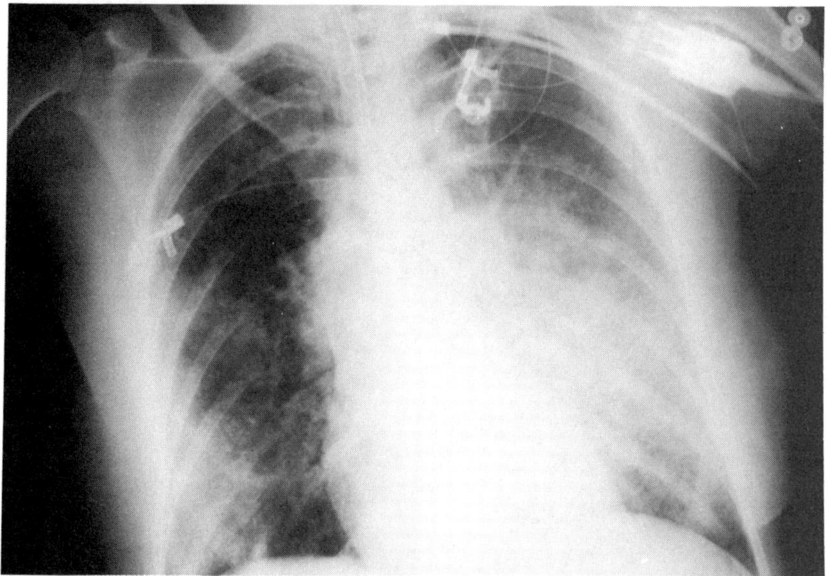

Figure 45-3 Portable supine radiograph of a patient with aspiration pneumonia and ARDS following a drug overdose. The left hemithorax has increased density, but it is not homogeneous. The pulmonary vessels of the left lung are obscured, and air bronchograms are present. The left costophrenic angle is preserved. A similar process involves the right lung to a lesser degree. A film taken only hours previously showed significantly fewer abnormalities. No pleural effusion is present.

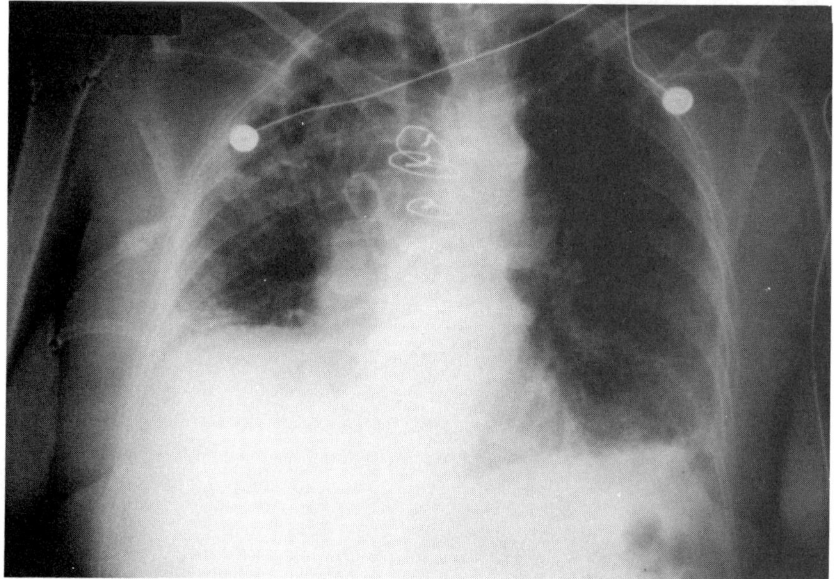

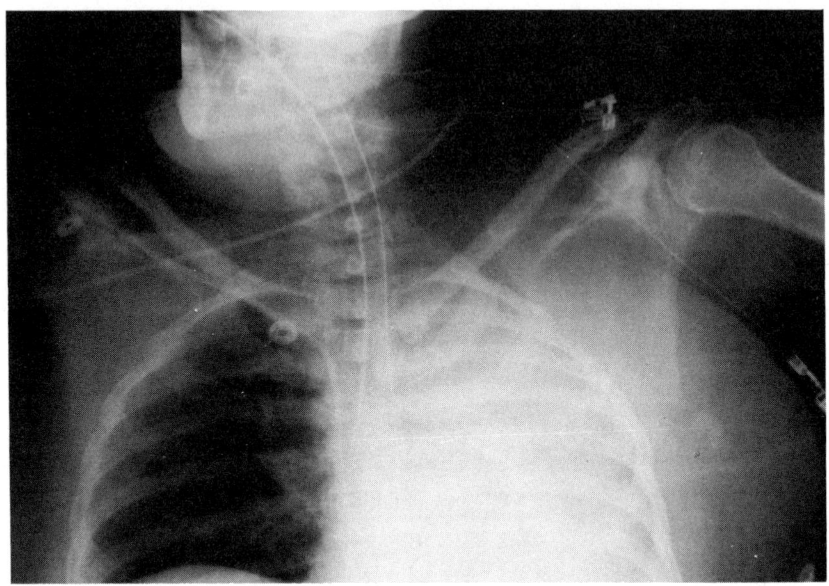

A

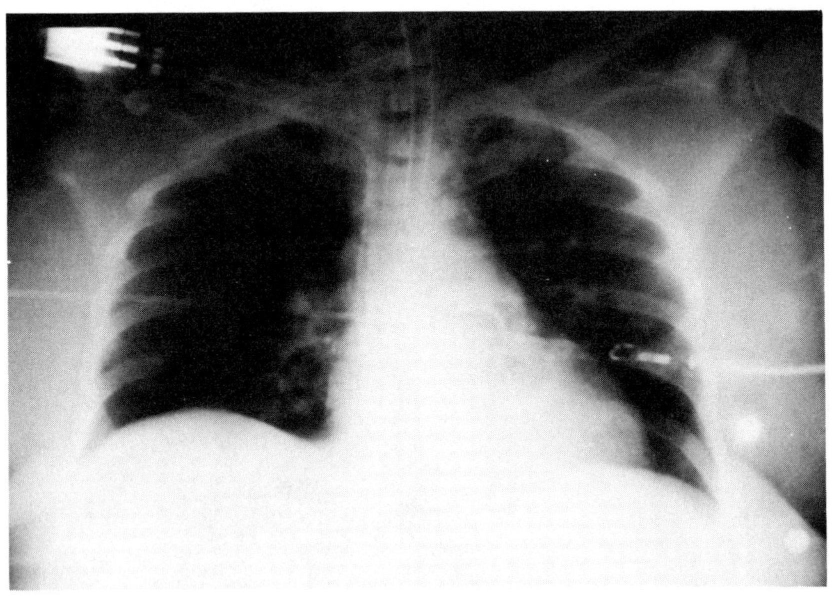

B

Figure 45-5 A. Portable supine view of a ventilator-dependent patient. Note the opacification of the entire left hemithorax. The patient was febrile when this film was taken. Should immediate thorocentesis be performed to rule out empyema? **B.** Portable supine film of same patient, but obtained 8 hours later. The left lung is now normal. Note the right main stem intubation present in figure 5, A. If the opacification in A was due solely to massive pleural effusion, there should be contralateral shift of the heart and mediastinum. Figure 5, A demonstrates complete atelectasis of the left lung, with shift of the heart and mediastinum to the ipsilateral side. Although massive atelectasis can produce an associated effusion, the quantity and location of the fluid cannot be determined from the routine film, and thorocentesis (especially in a ventilator-dependent patient) can be hazardous.

←

clearly demonstrate and locate fluid in the pleural space, ultrasound of the chest may be useful. Chest computerized tomography (CT) can also help to confirm the presence and location of an effusion, but it requires transporting the patient to the scan suite.

If fluid cannot be reasonably identified and localized, thoracentesis should not be attempted. Failure to confirm that an initial physical or radiographic finding is due to pleural fluid usually means the amount of fluid, if present at all, is small. The risk involved in thoracentesis increases for small amounts of fluid. The likelihood that small amounts of fluid represent a significant disease process is also small. It has been recommended that thoracentesis *not* be attempted unless greater than 1 cm of fluid "layers out" in the lateral decubitus position.

Even when clearly present in significant volume, pleural effusions in critically ill patients require *expedient* thoracentesis in only three settings: if the fluid is suspected to be infected, if the fluid is suspected to be blood, or if it is strongly suspected that the effusion is causing ventilatory compromised by reducing lung and thoracic volume in the affected hemithorax. For all other processes, analysis of the fluid may provide useful information, but such data are not mandatory and urgent thoracentesis is not necessary.

TABLE 45-1 CHARACTERISTICS OF TRANSUDATIVE VERSUS EXUDATIVE EFFUSIONS

	Transudates	**Exudates**
Fluid/serum lactate dehydrogenase (LDH)	< 0.6	> 0.6
Fluid/serum protein	< 0.5	> 0.5
Fluid/normal serum LDH	$< 2/3$	$> 2/3$

(Modified from Light RW: *Pleural Diseases.* Philadelphia, Lea &Febiger, 1983)
Notes: (1) Fluid and serum values should be obtained simultaneously; (2) exudative fluids need meet only *one* of the EXUDATE criteria; (3) transudative fluids must meet *all* of the TRANSUDATE criteria; (4) this scheme will properly classify 99% of pleural effusions.

For further information, please see Chapter 93 in Civetta JM, Taylor RW, Kirby RR: Critical Care. *Philadelphia: J. B. Lippincott, 1988*

BIBLIOGRAPHY

Forsberg L, Tylen U: Ultrasound examination of lesions in the thorax. *Acta Radiol Diagn* 1980; 21:375

Health and Public Policy Committee, American College of Physicians: Diagnostic thoracentesis and pleural biopsy in pleural effusions. *Ann Intern Med* 1985; 103:799

Jay SJ: Pleural effusions. *Postgrad Med* 1986; 80(pt 1):164

Jay SJ: Pleural effusions. *Postgrad Med* 1986; 80(pt 2):181

Jay SJ: Diagnostic procedures for pleural disease. *Clin Chest Med* 1985; 6:33

Light RW: *Pleural Diseases.* Philadelphia, Lea & Febiger, 1983

Moller A: Pleural effusion: Use of the semi-supine position for radiographic detection. *Radiology* 1984; 150:245

Pugatch RD, Spirn PW: Radiology of the pleura. *Clin Chest Med* 1985; 6:17

Raasch BN, Carsky EW, Lane EJ, O'Callaghan JP, Heitzman ER: Pleural effusion: Explanation of some typical appearances. *AJR* 1982; 139:899

Rosa UW: Pleural effusion: How to avoid a diagnostic stalemate. *Postgrad Med* 1984; 75:253

Rudikoff JC: Early detection of pleural fluid. *Chest* 1980; 77:109

Sahn SA: Pleural manifestations of pulmonary disease. *Hosp Pract* 1981; (Mar):73

Woodring JH: Recognition of pleural effusion on supine radiographs: How much fluid is required? *AJR* 1984; 142:59

46
Airway Pressure Support

The care of patients with acute lung injury has changed significantly since Avery and colleagues suggested in 1956 that "alkalotic apnea" be employed for the treatment of patients with flail chest injuries. Ashbaugh and associates described in 1967 the use of positive end-expiratory pressure (PEEP) in conjunction with controlled mechanical ventilation to improve lung function in such patients, and in 1973 Downs introduced the notion that such patients could breathe spontaneously between mechanical breaths. Later it was found that very high levels of PEEP and continuous positive airway pressure (CPAP) could be applied, and that morbidity and mortality were improved with such treatment. Subsequently, a variety of airway pressure patterns have been employed to treat patients with acute lung injury, and a great deal of controversy has been generated.

A rational approach to the successful treatment of these patients necessitates a detailed understanding of the pathophysiologic processes that occur, a comprehensive appreciation of the equipment required to generate various airway pressure patterns, and an understanding of the patient–machine interface. The latter area has been complicated by confusing terminology, fallacious claims by manufacturers, and a contention by some that technical considerations are of minimal relevance in the treatment of critically ill patients. The following paragraphs outline a physiological basis for the application of positive airway pressure therapy and support.

PRACTICAL CONSIDERATIONS

Continuous positive airway pressure is applied in a variety of clinical situations. Controversy surrounds the efficacy of CPAP therapy and prophylaxis. Determination of efficacy requires objective and relevant criteria. The use of CPAP does not increase the Pa_{O_2} of patients who have little derangement in pulmonary function. Postoperatively, a patient with atelectasis may have a marked reduction in lung volume, but because hypoxic pulmonary vasoconstriction (HPV) diverts pulmonary blood flow away from the collapsed lung tissue, Pa_{O_2} is relatively normal. Even if CPAP reverses the atelectasis, arterial blood gas analysis probably will not reveal any significant effect.

Continuous positive airway pressure may increase the respiratory distress of a postoperative patient with obstructive lung disease whose functional residual capacity (FRC) is greater than normal because of gas trapping. Obviously, the criteria for applying CPAP must be precise and the measures of efficacy direct. Because CPAP increases lung volume, it should be used when an increase in FRC is desirable, not when a patient is merely at risk for decreased lung volume and arterial hypoxemia, or has hypoxemia secondary to obstructive lung disease with gas trapping. Prophylactic CPAP probably has no role. The patient with postoperative atelectasis but normal arterial oxygenation may be a candidate for therapeutic CPAP. Criteria for efficacy in this situation should be an increase in FRC and resolution of atelectasis, not an increase in Pa_{O_2}.

Following some operative procedures, especially those involving the upper abdomen, CPAP increases FRC to a greater extent than any other therapeutic maneuver, including incentive spirometry and intermittent positive-pressure breathing. The level of CPAP used depends on the decrement in FRC and lung–thorax compliance. After major abdominal procedures, lung–thorax compliance is reduced slightly by postoperative pain and splinting. Functional residual capacity may be reduced by up to 1 liter in adult patients. Theoretically, if lung–thorax compliance is 75 ml/cm H_2O (normal = 100 ml/cm H_2O) and FRC is reduced to 750 ml, 10 cm H_2O, CPAP will return expiratory lung volume to normal. Five to 10 cm H_2O is sufficient in nearly all postoperative patients with little or no coexisting lung disease.

The most effective way to supply CPAP is in conjunction with tracheal intubation. However, the intubation is fraught with complications, discomfort, and an increased risk of pulmonary infection. Ambulation is impaired, effective coughing is inhibited, and sedation often is required. Therefore, application of CPAP with a mask is desirable in many clinical settings. Patients must be sufficiently alert and unrestrained to remove the mask should regurgitation occur, since the airway is not protected. Gastric drainage is unnecessary in the majority of patients, as long as CPAP is less than 15 to 20 cm H_2O. Standard anesthesia masks are not acceptable for CPAP. The mask must be soft and nonirritating. It must be loosely strapped to the face to prevent pressure necrosis, especially on the bridge of the nose. A sufficient flow of gas must be provided to allow substantial leaks in the system, while maintaining an effective level of CPAP. Considerations of flow resistance, increased work of breathing created by the equipment, and inspiratory flow requirements are of major importance. When mask CPAP is used, inspired gas should be at room temperature and 80 to 100% relative humidity. Heated humidification is uncomfortable and unnecessary.

Patients with acute lung injury have marked decreases in lung volume and lung compliance. They often require higher levels of CPAP to achieve an acceptable FRC and to improve arterial oxygenation. Work of breathing is increased with acute lung injury, so equipment design is critical. A variety of criteria are employed to determine optimum CPAP in such patients. A Pa_{O_2} of 65 to 70 mm Hg achieved with an inspired oxygen fraction (FI_{O_2}) of 0.25 to 0.30 is desirable. Occasionally, this goal is impossible, even when obviously excessive CPAP is applied. Regardless of the Pa_{O_2}, apply CPAP to a level that minimizes work of breathing as assessed by spontaneous respiratory rate and depth of breathing.

When CPAP is initiated or changed, lung volume is rapidly altered. The change in FRC appears nearly complete within seconds. Similary rapid changes in Pa_{O_2} occur. Therefore evaluate the patient's response to therapy almost immediately. In this manner, an optimum level is selected within a short time of initiation of therapy. Since Pa_{O_2} is influenced by mixed venous blood oxyhemoglobin saturation, both mixed venous and arterial blood may have to be sampled on occasion to accurately assess gas exchange efficiency.

How often the CPAP level should be reassessed once an optimum level is reached is unclear. However, up to 80% of patients in a surgical ICU receive a higher level of CPAP than is necessary because their improvement goes undetected. Although work of breathing can be assessed frequently, arterial and mixed venous blood sampling is limited to several times daily for both physiological and economic considerations. In all probability, continuous oximetric measurement of arterial and mixed venous oxyhemoglobin saturation will enhance the assessment of pulmonary gas exchange and allow more frequent and appropriate alteration in CPAP therapy.

If the above approach to CPAP adjustment is adopted, "weaning" will be unnecessary. Adjustment will occur continuously until ambient airway pressure is appropriate. Any sign of deterioration in pulmonary function, such as increased arterial hypoxemia or apparent work of breathing, is an indication for reapplication of the previous level of CPAP. Clinical experience indicates that tracheal extubation may be performed safely once 5 cm H_2O CPAP is attained. Intermittent mask CPAP is often useful once continuous CPAP is discontinued.

EQUIPMENT CONSIDERATIONS

A myriad of devices to produce positive airway pressure have been introduced during the past two decades. Advances in respiratory therapy have occurred, but the complexity of equipment and therapy has greatly increased the clinician's responsibility and knowledge requirements. The uninformed practitioner charged with the care of patients with compromised pulmonary function can no longer use disdain for technology as an acceptable excuse for ignorance.

Currently available systems provide CPAP by a number of mechanisms, none of which is ideal. In order to prevent significant fluctuation in Paw, measures must be taken to ensure that inspiratory flow is equivalent to patient demand at all times. Early attempts supplied a continuous flow of gas to the inspiratory side of the breathing circuit. Peak inspiratory flow demand may be as high as 100 to 200 liters/min. Providing such flow continuously is impractical, so a compliant reservoir often is placed in the inspiratory circuit. Compliance of the reservoir shold be such that small decrements in reservoir volume produce negligible change in pressure. Thus, rather large, distensible rubber bags are suggested. Less compliant bags result in significant decreases in Paw.

Humidifier resistance causes a decrease in Paw during spontaneous inspiration and must be avoided. Similarly, high-resistance valves should not be placed in the inspiratory side of the breathing circuit. Exhalation valve flow resistance is potentially detrimental and may precipitate barotrauma (pneumomediastinum, subcutaneous emphysema, and pneumothorax). Flow resistance of the PEEP valve also causes marked increase in expiratory work of breathing (Fig. 46-1).

Less widely appreciated is the increase in inspiratory work of breathing that may be imposed by PEEP valve flow resistance. Whenever flow resistance exists, a continuous gas flow through the circuit elevates Paw. For example, if 10 cm H_2O CPAP is desired and a gas flow of 50 liters/min continuously flows through the circuit, an exhalation valve with flow resistance of 0.1 cm H_2O/liter/min will produce a circuit pressure of 5 cm H_2O. To obtain 10 cm

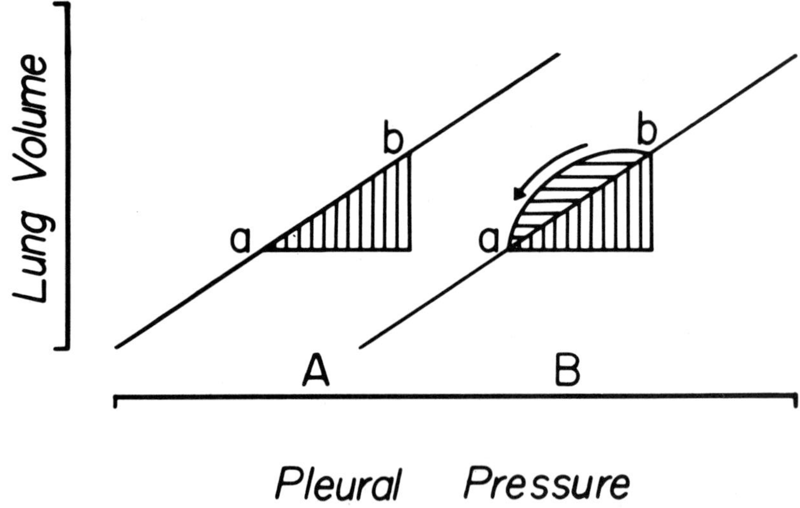

Figure 46-1 The shaded area *(A)* represents works expended to increase lung volume from point a to b when an ideal, nonflow-resistive circuit is used to provide CPAP. When exhalation valve resistance is significant *(B)*, an expiratory gas flow increases airway pressure and creates a resistive work depicted by the shaded area above the pressure-volume curve.

H_2O CPAP, a threshold resistance of 5 cm H_2O will have to be added. During peak inspiration, if the patient's inspiratory flow is 60 liters/min, no flow through the PEEP valve occurs at peak inspiration (it all goes to the patient) and Paw will decrease to 5 cm H_2O. Thus, inspiratory work of breathing is increased. During exhalation, if expiratory flow from the patient is 50 liters/min, total flow through the valve is 100 liters/min, and expiratory Paw rises transiently to 15 cm H_2O (Fig. 46-2). Such a fluctuation in Paw increases both inspiratory and expiratory work of breathing (Fig. 46-3B), compared to the ideal situation (Fig. 46-3A).

Many ventilators provide CPAP with little or no continuous gas flow, in which case the previous discussion has limited relevance. Inspiratory gas flow is provided on demand and optimally should match the flow-rate desired by the patient. To date, no ventilator accomplishes this task. For a variety of reasons, an inspiratory pressure drop is common, and inspiratory work of breathing is increased, often to intolerable levels. To decrease the work of breathing, some devices overshoot the flow demand of the patient and provide positive-pressure ventilation. Although the work of breathing by the patient and the ventilator may appear to balance, patient discomfort and tachypnea are observed frequently.

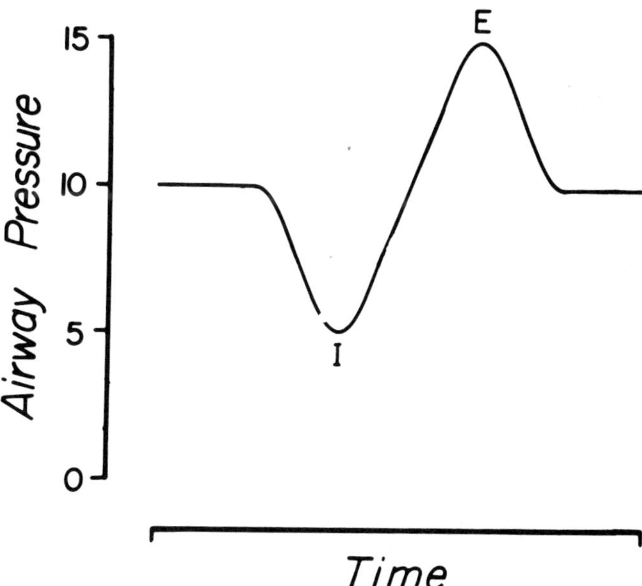

Figure 46-2 With a continuous flow of gas through the circuit, exhalation valve flow resistance results in a drop in airway pressure during inspiration and an increase in airway pressure during exhalation. Both deviations in airway pressure represent increased work of breathing.

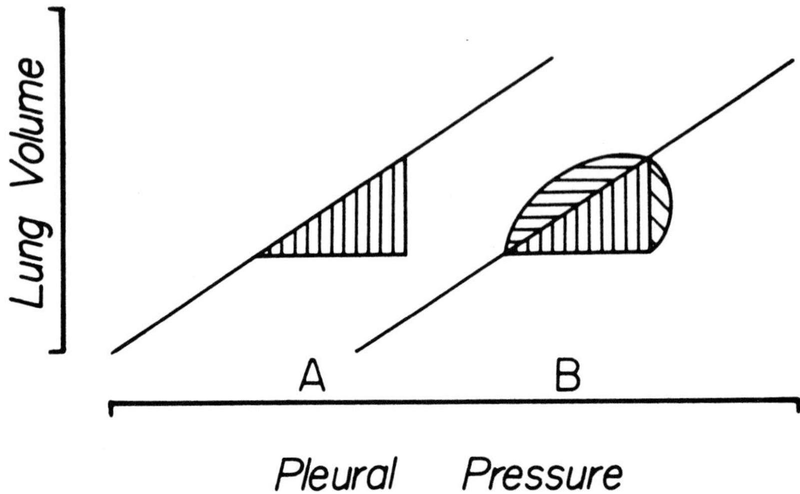

Figure 46-3 The added work of breathing resulting from exhalation valve flow resistance is depicted by the shaded areas above the pressure–volume curve and to the right of the normal elastic work diagram.

For further information, please see Chapter 95 in Civetta JM, Taylor RW, Kirby RR: Critical Care. *Philadelphia: J. B. Lippincott, 1988*

BIBLIOGRAPHY

Ashbaugh DB, Bigelow DB, Petty TL, et al: Acute respiratory distress in adults. *Lancet* 1967; 2:319

Avery AE, Mörch ET, Benson DW: Critically crushed chests: A new method of treatment with continuous hyperventilation to produce alkalotic apnea and internal pneumatic stabilization. *J Thorac Surg* 1956; 32:291

Banner MJ, Lampotang S, Boysen PG, et al: Flow resistance of expiratory positive-pressure valve systems. *Chest* 1986; 90:212

Douglas ME, Downs JB: Pulmonary function following severe acute respiratory failure and high levels of positive end-expiratory pressures. *Chest* 1977; 71:18

Downs JB, Klein EF Jr, Desautels D, et al: Intermittent mandatory ventilation: A new approach to weaning patients from mechanical ventilators. *Chest* 1973; 64:331

Gibney RTN, Wilson RS, Pontoppidan H: Comparison of work of breathing on high gas flow and demand valve continuous positive airway pressure systems. *Chest* 1982; 82:692

Katz JA, Kraemer RW, Gjerde GE: Inspiratory work and airway pressure with continuous positive airway pressure delivery systems. *Chest* 1985; 88:519

Kirby RR, Downs JB, Civetta JM, et al: High level positive end-expiratory pressure (PEEP) in acute respiratory insufficiency. *Chest* 1975; 67:156

Poulton TJ, Downs JB: Humidification of rapidly flowing gas. *Crit Care Med* 1981; 9:59

Rose DM, Downs JB, Heenan TJ: Temporal responses of functional residual capacity and oxygen tension to changes in positive end-expiratory pressure. *Crit Care Med* 1981; 9:79

Stock MC, Downs JB, Gauer PK, et al: Prevention of postoperative pulmonary complications with CPAP, incentive spirometry, and conservative therapy. *Chest* 1985; 87:151

47
Pulmonary Barotrauma

Pulmonary barotrauma (PBT) is considered by many physicians to be a limiting feature of ventilator therapy. Reluctance to use the full capability of ventilatory support for fear of causing a pneumothorax or other life-threatening complications may lead to the patient's death from hypoxemia. In fact, extra-alveolar air is infrequently an immediate threat to life, and time is usually available to care for the patient. When a patient develops ventilator-related pulmonary barotrauma, the most pressing goal is to minimize the impact of the extra-alveolar air on pulmonary and cardiovascular function.

PNEUMOTHORAX

The development of pneumothorax during positive-pressure ventilation demands efficient evaluation and decompression if barotrauma morbidity is to be minimized. If the patient is experiencing pulmonary or cardiovascular compromise, an intravenous cannula (16 gauge, 2½ inches long) with attached syringe can be placed in the second anterior intercostal space on the side of the suspected pneumothorax. In the presence of a tension pneumothorax, the plunger will be forced out of the syringe barrel if the pressure is sufficiently high, and the pneumothorax will be temporarily relieved.

When a pneumothorax is present or suspicion of pneumothorax is sufficiently high, a chest tube should be placed. If the patient is not severely compromised and time is available for evaluation, a chest radiograph should be obtained before placement. Tube thoracostomy should be performed using a 30 Fr or larger tube placed in the midaxillary line through the fifth intercostal space. This location avoids the pectoralis major and latissimus dorsi muscles, and the catheter may be easily directed to the superior aspect of the pleural space, allowing efficient drainage of the pleural air. Although radiography-assisted chest tube placement is seldom used in patients requiring long-term ventilatory therapy, radiographic guidance, including computerized tomography, may be necessary to decompress the air collection adequately (Fig. 47-1). Patients who require tube thoracostomy for pneu-

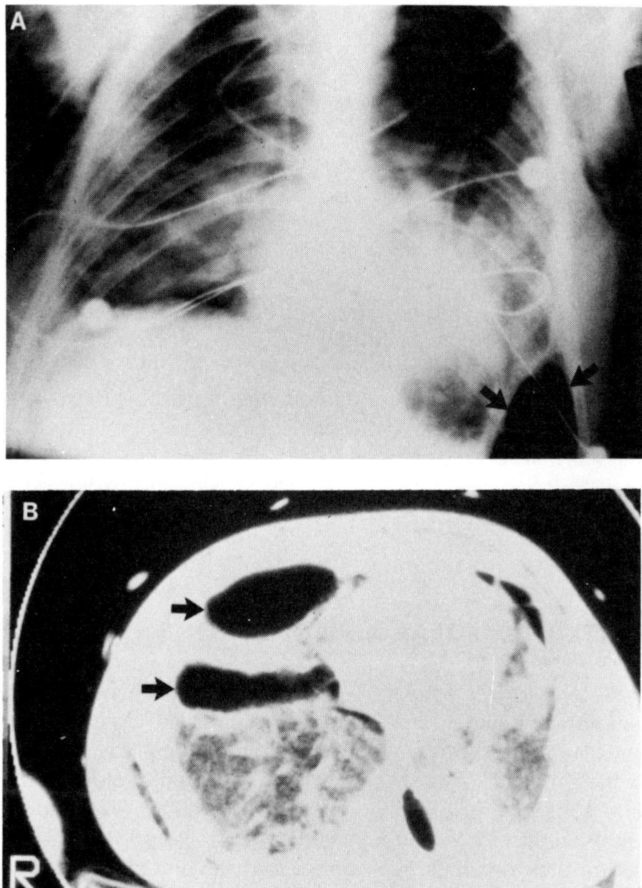

Figure 47-1 Radiographs from a 22-year-old with ARDS after 30 days of mechanical ventilation. **A.** AP radiograph illustrates only one pleural air collection (*arrows*), at the left costophrenic angle. **B.** A CT scan demonstrates two unrecognized right lung extra-parenchymal air collections (*arrows*) which necessitated CT scan-guided decompressions.

mothorax during a period of positive-pressure ventilation often require pleural drainage for a longer period than the usual 2 to 4 days when they are breathing spontaneously.

Timely treatment of pneumothorax is supported by data from Steier and colleagues, who showed that a delay of longer than 30 minutes in chest tube insertion in patients with a ventilator-related pneumothorax was associated with 31% mortality (9 deaths in 29 patients). When immediate decompression was carried out (less than 30 minutes after recognition of pneumothorax), mortality was only 7% (3 of 45 patients). In contrast, Zwillich and associates prospectively analyzed complications of assisted ventilation and found no correlation between the occurrence of pneumothorax and mechanical-ventilation-related mortality.

The presence of an ipsilateral chest tube should not lull one into thinking a tension pneumothorax cannot also be present. Gobein and colleagues determined that tension pneumothorax can and does occur in mechanically ventilated patients with adult respiratory distress syndrome (ARDS) with a functioning ipsilateral chest tube in place. In 15 of the 16 patients reviewed, a loculated tension pneumothorax was present in the subpulmonic or paracardiac region, although no shift of the mediastinum was clinically detectable. Reines reported a second pneumothorax in 11 of 16 patients (78%) with acute respiratory failure who were treated with more than 15 cm H_2O positive end-expiratory pressure (PEEP) despite a functioning ipsilateral chest tube. Six of 11 (54%) were loculated and under tension. Pollack and associates described similar findings in six infants with pneumothorax following cardiac surgical procedures. Five of the 6 (83%) had a second pneumothorax while an ipsilateral chest tube was in place.

OTHER EXTRA-ALVEOLAR AIR CONDITIONS

Other extra-alveolar air conditions that may require immediate therapy include pneumomediastinum, pneumopericardium, and, occasionally, intravascular air if a nonlethal dose is entrained. Pneumomediastinum infrequently occurs as the only sign of serious PBT, since mediastinal air is usually decompressed by subsequent formation of subcutaneous emphysema, pneumothorax, or pneumoretroperitoneum. If an anatomic anomaly such as prior pleural scarring or previous neck operation prevents decompression of the mediastinal air, the excessive pressure (tension mediastinum) may compromise venous return and produce cardiovascular collapse. Patients may complain of chest pain, and a classic Hamman's sign ("mediastinal crunch") is present in up to 50%. Electrocardiographic changes sometimes are present and can confuse the diagnosis, especially if the patient develops chest pain. If cardiovascular compromise is present and tension mediastinum is diagnosed, decompression is required. In infants, relief can be provided by insertion of a small catheter into the anterior mediastinum. In adults, the most efficient method of mediastinal decompression is by incision 2 to 3 cm cephalad to the suprasternal notch, followed by opening of the deep fascia beneath the sternum. The infrequency of this complication makes this a rarely needed technique.

Pneumopericardium can also require immediate therapy. Isolated signs of cardiac tamponade may be present if the mediastinal air selectively decompresses into the pericardium. Therapy may include pericardiocentesis, using a technique similar to that for decompressing a pericardial effusion.

If entrainment of intravascular air appears to have occurred, a head down, left lateral decubitus position (Durant's position) is often recommended. Unlike venous air embolism, however, barotrauma-induced intravascular air may also be found in the left side of the heart, making the choice of a decubitus position a problem. If air entrainment is nonlethal and the patient is stabilized, hyperbaric oxygen therapy may be indicated; this is an unusual clinical problem.

PREVENTION

A central problem in the management of patients with PBT is providing the required ventilatory assistance without contributing to additional morbidity or mortality. Mortality from acute respiratory failure ranges from 20% to 80%, whereas barotrauma-related mortality during mechnical ventilation is less than 1%. Thus, every effort should be made to maintain oxygenation through increased expiratory pressure (PEEP and continuous positive airway pressure, or CPAP) and FI_{O_2}, while the number of mechanically administered positive-pressure breaths is reduced. Such alterations of ventilator therapy may decrease the incidence and progression of PBT, although the incidence appears primarily related to the patient's underlying pulmonary pathology. A treatment plan may be modeled after the guidelines in Table 47-1.

FREQUENCY OF MECHANICAL BREATHS

Mechanical ventilation of the neonate with respiratory distress syndrome (RDS) provides much of our understanding of PBT. In 1976, Mannino and colleagues reported that lowering the number of mechanically delivered breaths with intermittent mandatory ventilation (IMV) compared to controlled ventilation, decreased the incidence of neonatal PBT from 69% to 18%. Similar findings were reported by Mathru and associates in adults. They found the incidence of PBT was 22% in patients treated with controlled ventilation and PEEP, versus 7% in a similar IMV and PEEP group (Table 47-2).

PEAK INSPIRATORY PRESSURE

In addition to decreasing the number of mechanically delivered breaths, the peak inspiratory pressure (PIP) also should be reduced whenever possible.

TABLE 47-1 DECREASING THE INCIDENCE OF PULMONARY BAROTRAUMA

Minimize the number of mechanically delivered breaths.
Minimize peak inspiratory pressures (flow rates, sedation, relaxants).
Maintain intravascular volume.
Use selective (independent) lung ventilation if indicated.
(Do not allow respiratory death to occur by avoiding high PEEP/CPAP.)

TABLE 47-2 INCIDENCE OF PULMONARY BAROTRAUMA IN ADULTS WITH ALTERATION OF VENTILATION MODE

	CMV	**IMV**
MV rate	12/min	6/min (initially)
PIP (cm H_2O)	34 ± 9	51 ± 14
PEEP/CPAP (cm H_2O)	15 ± 4	27 ± 5
PBT	22%	7%
PA artery catheterization	5%	48%

(Mathru M, Rao TLK, Venus B: Ventilator-induced barotrauma in controlled mechanical ventilation versus intermittent mandatory ventilation. *Crit Care Med* 1983; 11:359. Used with permission of Williams & Wilkins.)

Early data supporting this concept also came from neonatal studies. Moylan and colleagues noted a change in the incidence of PBT following an alteration in ventilatory management technique in neonates with RDS at the Massachusetts General Hospital. From 1971 until 1974, ventilatory pressures were maintained while the F_{IO_2} was decreased to 0.4 during the weaning of mechanically ventilated neonates. From 1974 until 1975, the F_{IO_2} was reduced only to 0.6, whereupon the ventilatory pressures were decreased. The results of this study show significant differences in the two periods and clarify the relationship of PIP to PBT (Table 47-3).

This association also has been found in adults. Petersen and Baier noted stratification of PBT incidence in patients requiring increased PIP (Table 47-4). Because of the relationship of high PIP to PBT in many reports, high-frequency ventilation (HFV) is suggested as a method to decrease the incidence. Carlon and coworkers reported 309 patients with acute respiratory failure at Memorial Sloan-Kettering Cancer Institute who were selected randomly to receive either conventional volume-controlled IMV or HFV. Mechanical ventilation in all cases lasted more than 12 hours. Pulmonary barotrauma occurred in 6 of 157 conventionally ventilated patients (3.8%) and in

TABLE 47-3 INCIDENCE OF ALVEOLAR RUPTURE IN INFANTS WITH RDS

Ventilatory Pressures Maintained Until F_{IO_2} Reduced to 0.4		**Ventilatory Pressures Maintained Until F_{IO_2} Reduced to 0.6**
60 ± 18 hr	PIP > 40 cm H_2O	8 ± 2 hr
17 ± 7 hr	PIP > 50 cm H_2O	1 ± 0.7 hr
90 ± 14 hr	PEEP > 5 cm H_2O	71 ± 7 hr
51%	ALVEOLAR RUPTURE	24%

(Moylan FMB, Walker AAA, Kramer SS, et al: The relationship of bronchopulmonary dysplasia to the occurrence of alveolar rupture during positive pressure ventilation. *Crit Care Med* 1978; 6:140. Used with permission of Williams & Wilkins.)

TABLE 47-4 PEAK INSPIRATORY PRESSURES DURING POSITIVE-PRESSURE VENTILATION AND INCIDENCE OF PULMONARY BAROTRAUMA

PIP (CM H_2O)	Incidence PBT
>70	43% (10/23)
50–70	8% (4/53)
< 50	0% (0/157)

(Peterson GW, Baier H: Incidence of pulmonary barotrauma in a medical ICU. *Crit Care Med* 1983; 11:67. Used with permission of Williams & Wilkins.)

4 of 152 HFV patients (2.6%). These differences were clinically and statistically nonsignificant. Mean airway pressures were 12 cm H_2O in the HFV patients and 37 cm H_2O in the conventionally ventilated patients, suggesting that the relationship between PIP and PBT may not be causal and may instead reflect only the noncompliance of the patient's lungs.

INTRAVASCULAR VOLUME

The aforementioned recommendations for reducing the incidence of PBT are reasonably well supported. Less clear is the connection between hypovolemia and PBT. In 1969 Lenaghan and associates reported a study of expansion rupture of the lung in normovolemic and hypovolemic dogs. Normovolemic dogs did not experience PBT until airway pressures of 62 ± 9 cm H_2O were reached, whereas dogs rendered hypovolemic by hemorrhage sustained PBT at 33 ± 7 cm H_2O. Thus, prevention of hypovolemia may be important in decreasing the risk of PBT. Mathru and colleagues documented a difference in the incidence of PBT in two groups of patients receiving different ventilatory management. Hypovolemia, as a contributing factor to PBT, was not directly addressed. However, only 5% of the patients in the group with a 22% incidence of PBT underwent pulmonary artery (PA) catheterization, while in the group with a 7% incidence of PBT, almost 50% had PA catheters inserted, presumably with more attention to maintenance of intravascular volume. Since the question of hypovolemia was not central to this study, no definitive statements can be made in this regard. Nevertheless, hypovolemia is a likely contributor to an increased incidence of PBT.

SELECTIVE VENTILATION

Asynchronous independent lung ventilation also is an option for patients with unilateral lung disease as a cause of PBT or those with primarily unilateral PBT. If the air leak can be lateralized, ventilation to that lung can be altered to provide decreased frequency and PIP of mechanical breaths.

For further information, please see Chapter 97 in Civetta JM, Taylor RW, Kirby RR: Critical Care. *Philadelphia: J. B. Lippincott, 1988*

BIBLIOGRAPHY

Brown DL: Pulmonary barotrauma. In Kirby RR, Taylor RW (eds): *Respiratory Failure,* pp 602–611. Chicago, Year Book Medical Publishers, 1986

Carlon GC, Howland WS, Ray C, et al: High frequency jet ventilation: A prospective randomized evaluation. *Chest* 1983; 84:551

Gobein RP, Reines HD, Schabel SI: Localized tension pneumothorax: Unrecognized form of barotrauma in adult respiratory distress syndrome. *Radiology* 1982; 142:15

Hillman KM: Pulmonary barotrauma. *Clin Anaesthesiol* 1985; 3:877

Hillman KM, Barber JD: Asynchronous independent lung ventilation (AILV). *Crit Care Med* 1980; 8:390

Hurd TE, Novak R, Gallagher TJ: Tension pneumopericardium: A complication of mechanical ventilation. *Crit Care Med* 1984; 12:200

Lenaghan R, Silva YJ, Walt AJ: Hemodynamic alterations associated with expansion rupture of the lung. *Arch Surg* 1969; 99:339

Mannino FL, Feldman BH, Heldt GP, et al: Early mechanical ventilation in RDS with a prolonged inspiration. *Pediatr Res* 1976; 10:464

Mathru M, Rao TLK, Venus B: Ventilator-induced barotrauma in controlled mechanical ventilation versus intermittent mandatory ventilation. *Crit Care Med* 1983; 11:359

Moylan FMB, Walker AM, Kramer SS, et al: The relationship of bronchopulmonary dysplasia to the occurrence of alveolar rupture during positive pressure ventilation. *Crit Care Med* 1978; 6:140

Petersen GW, Baier H: Incidence of pulmonary barotrauma in a medical ICU. *Crit Care Med* 1983; 11:67

Pollack MM, Fields AL, Holbrook PR: Pneumothorax and pneumomediastinum during pediatric mechanical ventilation. *Crit Care Med* 1979; 7:536

Reines HD: Manifestations of barotrauma in acute respiratory failure. *Am Surg* 1981; 47:421

Steier M, Ching N, Roberts EB, et al: Pneumothorax complicating continuous ventilatory support. *J Thorac Cardiovasc Surg* 1974; 67:17

Van Stiegmann G, Brantigan CO, Hopeman AR: Tension pneumomediastinum. *Arch Surg* 1977; 112:1212

Zwillich W, Pierson DJ, Creagh CE, et al: Complications of assisted ventilation: A prospective study of 354 consecutive episodes. *Am J Med* 1974; 57:161

48

Extracorporeal Circulation for Respiratory Failure

This chapter reviews the history of extracorporeal circulation for cardiac and respiratory support and describes the techniques of extracorporeal membrane oxygenation (ECMO) in some detail. Most of the description relates to ECMO for newborn respiratory failure, since the technique is established as a standard treatment in that group of patients. The principles described in the discussion of infant ECMO relate to the use of the technique for children and adults also. Commentary is added where appropriate for adult patients. The use of extracorporeal circulation for cardiac failure is summarized briefly.

ECMO CONSULTATION

Should ECMO be considered for your patient with severe respiratory failure unresponsive to optimal management? Definitely *yes* if the patient is a newborn infant over 34 weeks' gestational age. *Possibly,* if the patient is a child or adult with treatable and reversible pulmonary disease of only a few days' duration. Definitely *not* if the patient has extensive pulmonary fibrosis, or other incurable disease, necrotizing pneumonitis, or has been treated with a ventilator with high pressure and high oxygen concentration for a week or more.

If the patient is a candidate of ECMO, how do you do it? *If you have to ask, do not do it!* Send the patient to a center where ECMO is routinely practiced. Although the necessary equipment is fairly simple, this is not a procedure that can be done on the spur of the moment. As of this writing, many centers throughout the world are capable of treating neonates and children. Very few accept adult patients.

What is ECMO? Extracorporeal membrane oxygenation is the term used to describe prolonged extracorporeal cardiopulmonary bypass achieved by extrathoracic vascular cannulation. A modified heart-lung machine is used, consisting of a venous blood drainage reservoir, a servoregulated roller pump, a membrane lung to exchange oxygen and carbon dioxide, and a heat exchanger to maintain temperature (Fig. 48-1). The patient must be

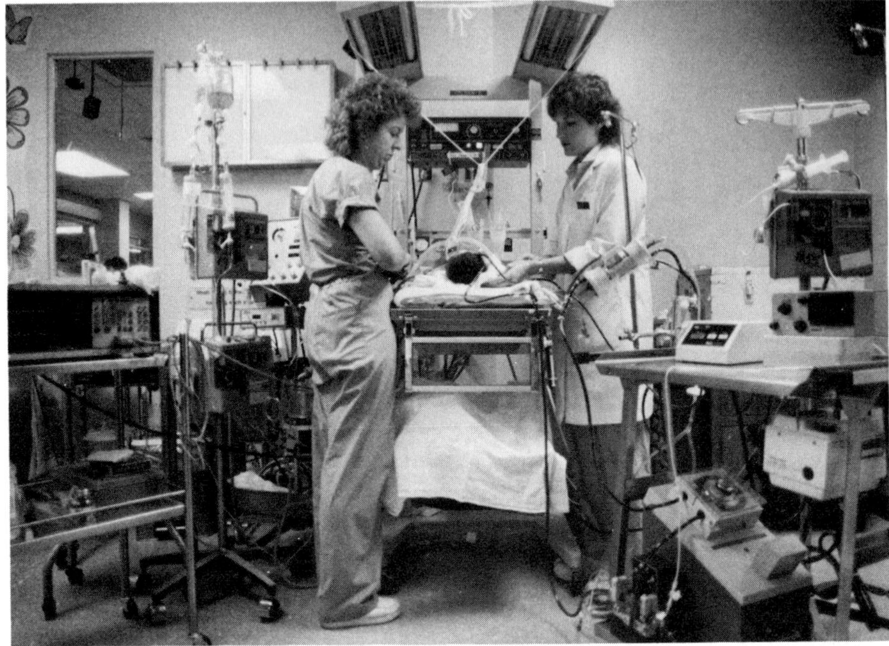

Figure 48-1 The ECMO system in use for neonatal respiratory failure (Bartlett RH: In Welch et al: *Pediatric Surgery.* Chicago, Year Book Medical Publishers, 1986)

maintained with continuous heparin anticoagulation to prevent thrombosis within the circuit.

Is extracorporeal circulation helpful for cardiac failure? Yes, in all age groups and disease categories, but only if there is reason to think that the cardiac disease will recover in a few days. Moderate left ventricular failure is better treated by intra-aortic balloon pumping. Severe left ventricular failure may be better managed by left-atrial-aortic extracorporeal circulation. Total venoarterial ECMO is reserved for patients with right ventricular or biventricular failure, unresponsive to other modes of therapy, in which heart recovery or replacement is anticipated within a few days.

PATIENT SELECTION

The indication for ECMO support is acute reversible respiratory or cardiac failure unresponsive to optimal ventilator and pharmacologic management, but from which recovery can be expected within a reasonable period (10 days) of extracorporeal support. The requirement for systemic heparinization limits the population for whom ECMO is appropriate to patients without bleeding complications, thereby excluding premature infants (<35 weeks' gestation), and patients with active bleeding.

NEONATES

As noted, ECMO has been applied to infants with a mortality risk of 80% or greater as determined by retrospective analysis of local patient populations. Included were neonates who, despite optimum medical management, demonstrated acute deterioration ($Pa_{O_2} < 40$ mm Hg or pH < 7.15 for 2 hr), failure to improve ($Pa_{O_2} < 55$ mm Hg and hypotension requiring inotropic support), uncontrolled tension pneumothoraces or pneumomediastinum, or deterioration following diaphragmatic hernia repair. Excessive alveolar-to-arterial oxygen gradients, $P(A{-}a)O_2$, also have been proposed as a qualification for ECMO. In a retrospective review by Krummel, a $P(A{-}a)O_2$ greater than 620 mm Hg for 12 consecutive hours correlated with over 90% mortality. The oxygenation index: mean airway pressure $\times$ FI_{O_2} $\times$ 100 divided by postductal Pa_{O_2} is useful. After optimal conventional therapy, an oxygenation index consistently over 25 defines 50% mortality and over 40 defines 80% mortality.

Contraindications to ECMO include any evidence of intracerebral hemorrhage or other brain damage, multiple congenital anomalies, and irreversible lung damage. Mechanical ventilation over 7 days is a relative contraindication and over 10 days an absolute contraindication, although exceptions have been noted. In congenital diaphragmatic hernia, the absence of a "honeymoon period" (Pa_{O_2} greater than 70 mm Hg) is evidence of hypoplasia incompatible with normal growth and development, and hence is a contraindication. Possible ECMO candidates are evaluated with cranial ultrasound to rule out intraventricular hemorrhage, and cardiac ultrasound to rule out congenital cardiac anomalies. Entry criteria should be evaluated at each hospital before ECMO therapy is begun because of regional differences in patient populations and treatment protocols.

ADULTS

Very few centers consider adult patients as candidates for ECMO at the present time. However, when adult ECMO centers are established, the indications should be severe ARF of few days' duration with a predicted mortality rate of 80% or greater. Reversible ARF in adults is difficult to define, so adult entry criteria for ECMO are controversial. Care must be taken to avoid patients with established pulmonary fibrosis. Lung biopsy is often necessary to determine the diagnosis and to measure the extent of fibrosis. Patients with the potential for bleeding or those with major destruction of lung tissue are not candidates for ECMO.

TECHNIQUES AND MANAGEMENT

NEONATES

After the medical decision to begin ECMO is made, the necessary parental consent is obtained while the circuit is prepared and primed with approximately 350 ml of heparinized blood. Because the blood volume in the circuit is as much as twice the blood volume of the neonate, the appropriate hematocrit, pH, and electrolyte concentration must be adjusted before cardiopulmonary bypass is instituted. A surgical and operating room support team performs the dissection and cannulation under local anesthesia in the neonatal intensive care unit (NICU). An oblique incision in the right side of the neck above the clavicle anterior to the sternocleidomastoid muscle exposes the internal jugular vein and common carotid artery. The infant is given a 150-U/kg bolus of heparin as a loading dose. The vessels are ligated distally, and cannulas are inserted in a proximal direction from the ligation site. The venous cannula is threaded through the right internal jugular vein into the right atrium, and the arterial cannula is threaded into the common carotid so that its tip rests at the entrance to the aortic arch. The largest catheters that fit "comfortably" inside the artery and vein are used. Catheter positions are confirmed by chest radiograph or ultrasound. Positioning and flow resistance of the venous drainage catheter determine the maximum blood flow; the catheter should be capable of delivering total cardiac support of 120 ml/kg/min. The common carotid artery has been successfully ligated without complications, presumably because of abundant collateral flow.

Once cannulation is accomplished and bypass initiated, blood drains by gravity through the venous catheter to a servoregulated roller pump. The pump then perfuses the blood through a 0.4 or 0.8 m^2 membrane lung (SciMed, Minneapolis, Minnesota). Gas exchange occurs in the membrane lung as oxygen is added to the blood, while water vapor and carbon dioxide are removed. Because carbon dioxide removal is much more efficient than oxygen transfer, exogenous carbon dioxide often must be added to the oxygen inflow to avoid hypocapnic alkalosis. The blood then passes through a small heat exchanger and returns to the patient. Blood flow is gradually increased during the initial 15 to 20 minutes of bypass until approximately 80% of the infant's cardiac output flows through the circuit. Oxygenated blood from the circuit then mixes in the aortic arch with poorly oxygenated blood from the left ventricle and ductus arteriosus to yield an oxygen content adequate for the infant's metabolic requirements.

Once extracorporeal support is established, and appropriate pH, Pa_{O_2} and Pa_{CO_2} are obtained, ventilator settings are reduced to minimize barotrauma and oxygen toxicity (PIP, 20 cm H_2O; PEEP, 3 cm H_20; rate 10/min; FI_{O_2}, 0.3). Flow is maintained at a level that achieves full respiratory support until lung improvement occurs. The usual flow for full support is 80 to 120 ml/kg/min (usually 300–400 ml/min) and is set to maintain Pa_{O_2} between 70 and 90 mm Hg. Adequate support is defined as that level of extracorporeal flow that results in normal arterial and mixed venous oxygenation, mean arterial pressure, and organ function. During ECMO, chest physiotherapy continues, and suctioning is accomplished through the endotracheal tube. Paralyzing agents and vasoactive drugs are discontinued, and patients are maintained alert and awake.

Anticoagulation must be maintained during the entire course of treatment.

Heparin is administered into the circuit with a loading dose (150 U/kg) followed by a constant infusion of approximately 30 U/kg/hr. Whole blood activated clotting time (ACT) measured each hour is maintained at two to three times normal values. Platelets, which may be destroyed by the membrane lung, are administered when thrombocytopenia of 80,000 or less is observed. Hematocrit is maintained between 40% and 45% with packed red blood cell transfusions. Maintenance intravenous fluids are delivered directly into the bypass circuit as is total parenteral nutrition, which is begun on the third day of life. Antibiotics (ampicillin and gentamicin) are administered until ECMO is completed. A chest radiograph and cranial ultrasound study are obtained daily.

As the lungs begin to recover, extracorporeal blood flow is reduced in a stepwise fashion until only 10% to 20% of the infant's cardiac output (usually 40–50 ml/min) is diverted through the circuit. Arterial P_{O_2} is maintained between 70 and 90 mm Hg. After an idling period of 8 to 12 hours to ensure continued lung function, the circuit is disconnected, the cannulas removed, and the vessels ligated proximally. Initially following decannulation, the infant is maintained with mechanical ventilation but is usually weaned to an oxygen hood within 48 to 72 hours. During the first 3 to 4 days off ECMO, the platelet count must be monitored closely for a precipitous drop as damaged platelets are removed from the circulation.

The ductus arteriosus actually closes spontaneously during the course of ECMO. If it does not, surgical closure is indicated while the patient is still on bypass. Termination of ECMO is indicated when there are signs of irreversible brain damage, uncontrollable bleeding, or irreversible lung damage (when the patient is dependent on ECMO for more than 10 days).

ADULTS

The general principles described for infants also apply to adult patients. Vascular access is achieved under local anesthesia using the right internal jugular vein and the right axillary artery. Since it is essential to deliver the oxygenated blood into the aortic arch, the femoral artery is not a suitable access site unless a very long catheter is used. The common carotid artery is acceptable if adequate right-sided brain blood flow can be demonstrated (by clamping of the carotid artery under local anesthesia). In adults, 80 ml/kg/min is adequate blood flow. As in the neonate, the extracorporeal flow is increased until satisfactory gas exchange is achieved with low ventilator settings. Management and weaning of adults is similar to neonates, and survivors require bypass an average of 5 days. Complications are related to bleeding and circuit component failure.

The technique of venovenous ECMO as performed by Gattinoni and Kolobow is somewhat different from that of the venoarterial ECMO just described. The rationale of this technique is to prevent damage to diseased lungs by reducing their motion (pulmonary rest), although three to five "sighs" with low-frequency positive-pressure ventilation (LFPPV) are provided each minute to "preserve" the functional residual capacity (FRC). With this method, oxygen uptake and carbon dioxide removal are dissociated: oxygenation is accomplished primarily through apneic oxygenation, whereas carbon dioxide is cleared through extracorporeal removal ($ECCO_2R$). The combination LFPPV–$ECCO_2R$ is performed at an extracorporeal blood flow of 20% to 30% of cardiac output. Vascular access may be jugulofemoral, femoral–femoral, or saphenosaphenous. Venovenous access emphasizing carbon dioxide removal is promising in adults, although most patients go through a phase of diminished lung function that may require systemic oxygenation as well.

COMPLICATIONS

NEONATES

The average duration of ECMO is 4 days. Technical complications include tubing rupture, air in the circuit/air embolism, oxygenator or heat exchanger malfunction, power failure, malposition of the venous or arterial cannulas requiring repositioning, and unintentional decannulation. The overall incidence of technical complications is approximately 20%. Although none of the technical complications has been a direct cause of mortality, stopping ECMO to change an oxygenator or ruptured tubing often causes physiological instability. Patient complications in descending order of frequency include intracranial hemorrhage, seizures, other significant bleeding, patent ductus arteriosus (which may require surgical ligation), hypertension, cardiac arrest, cannulation problems, pericardial tamponade, cardiac failure, renal failure, pneumothorax, and sepsis.

Because of systemic heparinization, bleeding complications are common. Intracranial bleeding occurs primarily in premature infants less than 2 kg birth weight or less than 35 weeks' gestation. Some oozing at the cannulation site is present in almost all patients. Major life-threatening bleeding from other sites, however, occurs in approximately 11%. Significant bleeding is managed by lowering the heparin dose to allow the ACT to be approximately 200 seconds, and by increasing the platelet count to greater than 100,000. Discontinuation of the heparin for 1 to 2 hours may be considered. These measures may, of course, lead to clotting in the circuit, particularly the membrane lung.

When pulmonary vasospasm relaxes, recovery of lung function begins; flow through the ductus reverses (becomes left-to-right), and the ductus usually closes within 24 hours. The ductus may remain patent with major left-to-right shunting occurring in approximately 20% of patients. When persistent for more than 24 to 48 hours, ductus ligation should be performed during ECMO.

Cardiovascular complications include hypoxic cardiac arrest requiring cardiopulmonary resuscitation during cannulation, systemic hypertension requiring vasoactive drugs, hemopericardium with tamponade, and global myocardial dysfunction. Major complications related to decannulation or vessel ligation are rare, but brief paralysis is induced to minimize the chance of air embolism. Renal failure may be treated with dialysis or continuous hemofiltration through the ECMO circuit. This procedure is successful in removing extracellular fluid, and hemofiltration is used freely for symptomatic fluid overload. After 10 days of support, the complication rate may exceed the potential benefit, although the absolute limits of ECMO have yet to be determined.

Intracranial hemorrhage, active gastrointestinal bleeding, or a gestational age under 35 weeks are contraindications to ECMO. The frequent use of whole blood ACT (the Bason method) is essential to monitor heparin effect and titrate the continuous infusion. Methods using other activators can be misleading. If accessible bleeding persists when the ACT is under 200 seconds and the platelet count is greater than 100,000, aggressive operative management is appropriate.

ADULTS

Bleeding and mechanical circuit problems occur in the adult also. Intracranial bleeding is unlikely except in patients with recent cranial trauma. Gastrointestinal and nasopharyngeal bleeding are more common. Platelet transfusion is rarely necessary.

For further information, please see Chapter 48 in Civetta JM, Taylor RW, Kirby RR: Critical Care. *Philadelphia: J. B. Lippincott, 1988*

BIBLIOGRAPHY

Bone RC: Extracorporeal membrane oxygenation for acute respiratory failure (editorial). *JAMA* 1986; 256:910

Cilley RE, Zwischenberger JB, Andrews AF, et al: Intracranial hemorrhage during extracorporeal membrane oxygenation in neonates. *Pediatrics* 1986; 78:699

Gattinoni L, Pesenti A, Mascheroni D, et al: Low-frequency positive-pressure ventilation with extracorporeal CO_2 removal in severe acute respiratory failure. *JAMA* 1986; 256:881

Kirkpatrick BV, Krummel TM, Mueller DG, et al: Use of extracorporeal membrane oxygenator for respiratory failure in term infants. *Pediatrics* 1983; 72:872

Kolobow T, Bowman RL: Construction and evaluation of an alveolar membrane artifical heart-lung. *Trans Am Soc Artif Intern Organs* 1963; 9:238

Krummel TM, Greenfield LJ, Kirkpatrick BV, et al: Alveolar-arterial oxygen gradients versus the neonatal pulmonary insufficiency index for prediction of mortality in ECMO candidates. *J Pediatr Surg* 1984; 19:380

Zapol WM, Snider MT, Hill JD: Extracorporeal membrane oxygenation in severe acute respiratory failure: A randomized prospective study. *JAMA* 1979; 242:2193

49
Pulmonary Function Testing in the Critical Care Unit

Measurement of pulmonary function in the intensive care unit (ICU) is quite different from testing performed in the pulmonary function laboratory. In the ICU, pulmonary function analysis may help determine the need for mechanical ventilation, or it may monitor ventilator safety, determine disease progression, or help decide when to wean the patient from mechanical ventilation. Test selection is important; some tests performed in the pulmonary function laboratory have little significance in the ventilated or acutely ill patient; a different set of normals is necessary (Table 49-1).

ACUTE ASTHMA

During an acute asthmatic event, resistance in the large and small airways progressively increases. Hyperinflation and air trapping occur, causing a reduction in vital capacity (VC). The diaphragm is placed at a mechanical disadvantage, decreasing respiratory muscle efficiency. As the respiratory muscles fatigue, ventilatory failure occurs; progressive respiratory acidosis and hypoxia result. Careful, repeated physical examination and arterial blood gases historically have been most useful in following asthma. Repeated determinations of peak expiratory flow rate (PEFR) and VC are less invasive and provide more objective measurements of disease progression. After four hours of treatment, improvement in PEFR greater than 50% of the admission peak flow rate predicts a rapid response to maximal therapy. Carbon dioxide tension (P_{CO_2}), forced expiratory volume in 1 second (FEV_1), and VC differences do not always provide a reliable predictor to the speed of recovery. Those patients who have a 50% improvement in the presenting value of PEFR will obtain maximum improvement within 1 week of admission, whereas those who do not may take considerably longer.

Patients with asthma and a PEFR 25% less than that predicted are particularly at risk for respiratory failure. During treatment, bronchodilator response may be monitored with PEFR and VC; a comparison of the postbronchodilator value of the previous treatment with the prebronchodilator value of the current

TABLE 49-1 SELECTED FORMULAS TO CALCULATE PULMONARY FUNCTION VARIABLES

Variables	Formulas	Normal Values
Lung volumes		
Tidal volume	$V_T = \dot{V}insp \times T_I$	10–15 ml/kg (lean body weight)
Minute ventilation	$\dot{V}_E = V_T \times f$	6–10 liters/min
Alveolar ventilation	$\dot{V}_A = V_E - V_D \times f$	4.2–6.2 liters/min
Deadspace	$V_D = V_T(Pa_{CO_2} - PE_{CO_2}/Pa_{CO_2})$	$V_D/V_T = 0.30–0.40$ $V_D = 150$ ml
Mechanics		
Dynamic compliance	$Cdyn = V_T/Ppeak$	0.028 liters/ml H_2O ($V_T = 0.81$)*
Static compliance	$Cstat = V_T/Pplat$	0.045 liters ml H_2O ($V_T = 0.81$)*
Airway resistance	$Raw = Ppeak - Pplat/\dot{V}$	2.5 ml H_2O/(liters/sec)
Respiratory system resistance	$Rresp = Ppeak/\dot{V}$	10 ml H_2O/liters/sec†
Work		
Mechanical	$W = \int P \times dV_T$	0.85 kg-m/min or 0.08 kg-m/liter

* Bone RC: Diagnosis of causes for acute respiratory distress by pressure-volume curves. *Chest* 1976; 70:740.
† Peters RM, Hilberman M, Hogan JS, Crawford DA: Objective indications for respiratory therapy in post-trauma and postoperative patients. *Am J Surg* 1972; 124:262.

treatment may indicate the need for a shorter, more frequent treatment schedule.

CHRONIC OBSTRUCTIVE PULMONARY DISEASE

Chronic obstructive pulmonary disease (COPD) is a broad disease category encompassing a number of distinct pathological processes, but in this discussion, it is limited to bronchitis and emphysema.

Bronchitis is characterized by mucus secretion, increased airways resistance, ventilation perfusion ($\dot{V}/\dot{Q}$) mismatch, and an increase in work of breathing. Hypoxemia and respiratory acidosis during exacerbation are common. For this reason, determination of arterial blood gases (ABGs) is important in the acute setting. PEFR and VC are useful for the same reasons as in asthma. Postoperatively, the bronchitic may experience increased secretions and decreased cough due to pain leading to atelectasis, increased $\dot{V}/\dot{Q}$ mismatch, and possibly, respiratory failure. Arterial blood gas determinations, serial physical examination, repeated PEFR, and VC facilitate management in these patients.

Emphysema is characterized by alveolar wall destruction and reduction in alveolar capillary units; an increase in compliance and deadspace ventilation results. Airways collapse and sputum production in some individuals result in air-flow obstruction. VC is often reduced because of air trapping, which produces an increased residual volume (RV). The increased compliance promotes hyperinflation and places the diaphragm at a mechanical disadvantage, decreasing efficiency. ABGs are usually preserved due to good $\dot{V}/\dot{Q}$ matching in the remaining alveolar capillary units and correlate poorly with the degree of dyspnea during an acute exacerbation. The deadspace to tidal volume ratio (V_D/V_T) increases slowly with disease progression and so is not particularly useful during an acute exacerbation. Some exacerbations are accompanied by increase in sputum production and $\dot{V}/\dot{Q}$ mismatching; there is considerable overlap between individuals with predominant emphysema or bronchitis. In this setting, initial determination of ABGs is important and measures of air flow (PEFR and VC) may be of help in determining treatment response.

RESTRICTIVE DISEASES

A reduction in respiratory system compliance due to increased lung or chest wall stiffness results in reduced total lung capacity (TLC) and VC. Expiratory flow rates are usually normal. Reduced TLC and lung compliance may be seen in several conditions, including diffuse pulmonary fibrosis, pulmonary parenchymal infiltrative diseases such as bronchopneumonia or extensive carcinoma, and conditions which increase lung water, including cardiogenic and noncardiogenic pulmonary edema. ABGs, lung compliance, and V_D/V_T

are reasonable parameters to follow in the ventilated patient. A reduced chest wall compliance and relatively normal lung parenchyma characterize chest wall restriction. Resulting decreases in respiratory system compliance occur in high cord transection, scleroderma, burns, and kyphoscoliosis. Displacement or compression of the lungs by morbid obesity, effusion, large tumors, or ascites may also reduce TLC and produce restriction, usually without affecting lung compliance. If reducing TLC and VC leads to significant atelectasis, reduction in lung compliance may occur. With spinal cord transection, respiratory system compliance may be followed to determine when ventilator weaning may begin, as there is usually improvement with time.

Adult respiratory distress syndrome (ARDS), although defined by a clinical constellation of findings, is characterized by interstitial edema progressing to alveolar filling and destruction of alveolar capillary units with fibrosis. Increases in deadspace and V_D/V_T, reduction in VC, progressive hypoxemia, and a decrease in lung compliance result. Serial ABGs should be followed as the process worsens, and V_D/V_T, minute ventilation, and venous admixture ($\dot{Q}s/\dot{Q}t$) are very helpful during the recovery phase in determining when to wean from the ventilator.

NEUROMUSCULAR DISEASES

Myasthenia gravis, Guillain-Barré syndrome, motor neuron diseases, and spinal cord interruption may all lead to respiratory failure. In general, decreased muscular ability leads to reduced ventilation or an inability to respond to respiratory stress. Characteristically, VC is reduced and respiratory rate increased. Cough is weak, and thus the ability to clear secretions is compromised, leading to atelectasis, decreased compliance, $\dot{V}/\dot{Q}$ mismatch, and hypoxemia. Hypoventilation with respiratory acidosis may occur precipitously. In myasthenia gravis, the maximum minute ventilation and peak inspiratory pressure (PIP) or VC may be helpful in diagnosis and following response to anticholinergic medication. Serial VC and PIP determinations predict respiratory failure better than serial ABGs in progressive neuromuscular diseases like Guillain-Barré syndrome. A VC less than 1 liter or a PIP above -30 ml of water is a criterion for intubation. Difficulty with secretion clearance may become manifest when the mean maximal expiratory pressure is below $+40$ ml of water; this may also be an indicator for intubation.

REDUCED DRIVE

Reduced central ventilatory drive is responsible for hypoxemia and respiratory acidosis of varying degrees in several situations, including drug overdoses, central nervous system accidents, sleep apnea, the obesity hypoventilation syndrome, and central hypoventilation. Reduced minute ventilation, poor secretion clearance, atelectasis, and respiratory acidosis result. With extreme obesity, there may be an additional chest wall restrictive abnormality, reducing functional residual capacity (FRC). Serial ABGs and specifically the arterial carbon dioxide tension (Pa_{CO_2}) must be followed in these patients. Spontaneous minute ventilation and VC during the recovery phase of drug overdose will help determine the time to wean. Actual measurement of respiratory drive is not commonly done in the intensive care setting.

EXTUBATION VERSUS WEANING

Indications to discontinue mechanical ventilation must not be confused with indications to remove an artificial airway. Patients with altered states of consciousness, recurrent aspiration, or copious secretions may achieve ventilator independence, yet require continued airway protection.

There is little justification for pursuing tests of weaning readiness in unstable, critically ill patients. Withdrawal of mechanical ventilation should not be considered until the underlying problem that necessitated mechanical support improves. Correction of nonpulmonary factors affecting the ability to breathe spontaneously are important prior to weaning attempts.

Various tests have been proposed to evaluate the need for continued ventilatory support. Such criteria seek to minimize premature weaning attempts, while decreasing unnecessary time spent on the ventilator. Generally, these tests can be separated into three areas of assessment: ability to oxygenate, resting ventilatory needs, and respiratory mechanical capability. They are based on three basic physiologic parameters: a $\dot{Q}s/\dot{Q}t$ of less than .15 to .20, a V_D/V_T of less than 0.6, and an adequate "respiratory reserve" to enable a doubling of the resting work of breathing. Most other criteria listed are derivations of these three factors.

VENTILATION NEEDS

Carbon dioxide tension and blood *p*H are dependent on alveolar ventilation. Increased carbon dioxide production must be matched with increased alveolar ventilation to maintain a steady-state Pa_{CO_2} and *p*H. Fever, sepsis, shivering and high glucose loads during total parenteral nutrition may increase carbon dioxide production and ventilatory demands.

Three physical findings seen during spontaneous ventilation tests may predict weaning failure: rapid shallow respirations, respiratory alternans (alternating between abdominal and rib cage breathing), and abdominal paradox (the inward movement of the abdominal wall during inspiration in the supine position). These clinical signs, if present, may predict those patients still in need of ventilatory support; prospective confirmation is pending.

For further information, please see Chapter 33 in Civetta JM, Taylor RW, Kirby RR: Critical Care. *Philadelphia: J. B. Lippincott, 1988*

BIBLIOGRAPHY

Cohen CA, Zagelbaum G, Gross D, et al: Clinical manifestations of inspiratory muscle fatigue. *Am J Med* 1982; 73:308

DeHaven CB, Hurst JM, Branson RD: Evaluation of two different extubation criteria: Attributes contributing to success. *Crit Care Med* 1986; 14:92

Fleury B, Murciano D, Talamo C, et al: Work of breathing in patients with chronic obstructive disease in acute respiratory failure. *Am Rev Respir Dis* 1985; 131:822

Martin TG, Elenbass RM, Pingleton SH: Use of peak expiratory flow rates to eliminate unnecessary arterial blood gases in acute asthma. *Ann Emerg Med* 1982; 11:70

Morganroth ML, Morganroth JL, Nett LM, Petty TL: Criteria for weaning from prolonged mechanical ventilation. *Arch Intern Med* 1984; 144:1012

Peters RM, Hilberman M, Hogan JS, Crawford DA: Objective indications for respiratory therapy in post-trauma and postoperative patients. *Am J Surg* 1972; 124:262

Petheram IS, Jones OA, Collins JV: Patterns of recovery of airflow obstruction in severe acute asthma. *Postgrad Med J* 1979; 55:877

Prakish O, Meij S, Borden B, Saxena PR: Cardiorespiratory monitoring during open heart surgery. *Crit Care Med* 1981; 9:530

Sahn SA, Lakshminarayan MB: Bedside criteria for discontinuation of mechanical ventilation. *Chest* 1973; 63:1002

Seleky PA, Wasserman K, Klein M, Ziment I: A graphic approach to assessing interrelationships among minute ventilation, arterial carbon dioxide tension, and ratio of physiologic dead space to tidal volume in patients on respirators. *Am Rev Respir Dis* 1978; 117:181

Sivak ED: Prolonged mechanical ventilation, an approach to weaning. *Cleve Clin Q* 1980; 47:89

50 Practical Application of Blood Gas Measurements

DETERMINANTS OF Pa_{CO_2}

The normal arterial partial pressure of carbon dioxide (Pa_{CO_2}) is 40 mm Hg (range, 36–44 mm Hg). Hypoventilation is defined as a Pa_{CO_2} above 44 mm Hg, and hyperventilation is a Pa_{CO_2} below 36 mm Hg.

Production of carbon dioxide is often ignored because it is relatively constant in most settings. However, in catabolic and hypermetabolic states, carbon dioxide production may increase significantly and affect Pa_{CO_2}. In the absence of shivering, production is decreased by hypothermia.

Total ventilation ($\dot{V}_E$) is partitioned between gas distributed to the alveoli and that passing to the non-gas-exchange (deadspace) areas of the lungs. Thus,

$$\dot{V}_E = \dot{V}_D + \dot{V}_A \quad (1)$$

where $\dot{V}_D$ is deadspace ventilation and $\dot{V}_A$ is alveolar ventilation. The conducting airways are termed anatomic deadspace. Alveoli that are ventilated but not perfused make up the alveolar deadspace.

If volume is related to time, then

$$\dot{V}_E = V_T \times f/min \quad (2)$$

$$\dot{V}_A = V_A \times f/min \quad (3)$$

where V_T is tidal volume (including deadspace volume) and V_A is alveolar volume. The elimination of carbon dioxide is proportional to alveolar ventilation and the alveolar partial pressure of carbon dioxide (PA_{CO_2}):

$$\dot{V}_{CO_2} \propto \dot{V}_A \times PA_{CO_2} \quad (4)$$

Because measurement of PA_{CO_2} is not always possible, PA_{CO_2} is assumed = Pa_{CO_2}. This relationship holds reasonably well in normal situations but can be quite aberrant in some clinical settings (*i.e.*, pulmonary embolism, profound pulmonary hypotension). Everything else being equal, however, increased $\dot{V}_A$ should be associated with decreased Pa_{CO_2}, whereas a decrease of $\dot{V}_A$ is associated with an elevation of Pa_{CO_2}.

DETERMINANTS OF Pa_{O_2}

When you measure the Pa_{O_2} from a sample of arterial blood, you need information on the alveolar gas composition to which the blood was exposed. First, estimate the alveolar P_{O_2} (PA_{O_2}); next, assume that both alveolar and arterial gas equilibration have occurred; finally, compare the estimated PA_{O_2} and the measured Pa_{O_2}. The initial step entails calculation of the partial pressure of humidified, inspired oxyen (PI_{O_2}):

$$PI_{O_2} = (PB - P_{H_2O}) \times FI_{O_2} \tag{5}$$

At sea level, PB = 760 mm Hg, PH_2O = 47 mm Hg (37°C body temperature) and, in this example, $FI_{O_2} = 0.21$. Thus,

$$PI_{O_2} = (760 - 47) \times 0.21 = 150 \text{ mm Hg}$$

Dead space gas maintains the same partial pressure. At the alveolar level, however, oxygen is removed and carbon dioxide added to the gas mixture. Total alveolar and atmospheric pressures are equal, but the composition and partial pressures of gases in the two phases differ. The total pressure in each phase is equal to the sum of its partial pressures:

$$PA = PA_{O_2} + PA_{CO_2} + PA_{N_2} + PA_{H_2O} \tag{6}$$

where PA = the total alveolar gas pressure (equal to PB).

Since PA_{N_2} and PA_{H_2O} remain essentially constant when ambient air is breathed, an *increase* in PA_{CO_2} implies a *decrease* in PA_{O_2}. Thus, pulmonary capillary blood exposed to a lower PA_{O_2} enters the systemic circulation with a lower than normal PA_{O_2}. The overall relationship defining these variables is described by the ideal alveolar air equation:

$$PA_{O_2} = PI_{O_2} - \frac{PA_{CO_2}}{R} + \left[PA_{CO_2} \times FI_{O_2} \times \frac{1 - R}{R}\right] \tag{7}$$

where R = the respiratory quotient, $\dot{V}_{CO_2}/\dot{V}_{O_2}$ (normally 0.8). This expression can be simplified to

$$PA_{O_2} = PI_{O_2} - (Pa_{CO_2} \times 1.25) \tag{8}$$

ABNORMALITIES OF OXYGENATION

If the lung functioned as a perfect gas exchange organ, PA_{O_2} and Pa_{O_2} would be equal. To the extent that perfect ventilation and perfusion matching ($\dot{V}/\dot{Q}$) do not occur, a gradient between PA_{O_2} and Pa_{O_2} ($P(A-a)O_2$ is established. An increase of $P(A-a)O_2$ implies a deterioration in lung function. Alveolar

TABLE 50-1 CAUSES OF INCREASED $P(A\text{-}a)O_2$ GRADIENT

Post-traumatic pulmonary insufficiency
Aspiration of gastric contents
Sepsis
Viral pneumonia
Smoke inhalation/respiratory burns
Inhalation of toxic chemicals
Oxygen toxicity
Near-drowning
Fat embolism
Uremia
Pancreatitis
Neurogenic pulmonary edema
Altitiude pulmonary edema

hypoventilation also results in hypoxemia when *air* is breathed but is *not* associated with an increase of $P(A-a)O_2$. A number of abnormalities increase this gradient and produce hypoxemia (Table 50-1).

Although it is theoretically possible that substances lie between the alveoli and the pulmonary capillaries and inhibit oxygen diffusion, this abnormality is of little clinical importance in the etiology of *acute* hypoxemia.

A relative shunt results from reduced but finite ventilation that is less than the corresponding perfusion. Thus, some oxygenation of mixed venous blood occurs, but to a level far less than normal. This abnormality is the most common cause of hypoxemia in acute and chronic respiratory insufficiency. Diffusion block and relative shunt are corrected when patients inspire 100% oxygen.

When mixed venous blood passing through the lungs does not come into contact with the alveoli, it is "shunted" past the gas-exchange surface. Venous admixture results when this shunted blood mixes with oxygenated blood from other normal lung areas. Absolute shunt is minimally improved by the administration of 100% oxygen.

A decrease in arterial oxygenation usually is thought to reflect increases of absolute or relative shunt and an overall deterioration of lung function. However, changes in cardiac output, by virtue of their effect on the content of oxygen in mixed venous blood, also ultimately affect Pa_{O_2}. Increases in cardiac output tend to minimize hypoxemia and the $P(A-a)O_2$ gradient that results from any right-to-left absolute and relative shunting. Conversely, decreases in cardiac output tend to accentuate this hypoxemia and to increase the $P(A-a)O_2$. Mechanical ventilation and positive end-expiratory pressure (PEEP) are used to improve lung function. However, by virtue of their potentially adverse effects on cardiac output, such therapy can be associated with a decreased Pa_{O_2}. Thus, pulmonary *and* cardiac function must be assessed to evaluate any given set of arterial blood gases accurately.

For more information, please see Chapter 29 in Civetta JM, Taylor RW, Kirby RR: Critical Care. *Philadelphia: J. B. Lippincott, 1988*

BIBLIOGRAPHY

Bendixen HH, Egbert LD, Hedley–Whyte J, et al: *Respiratory Care*. St. Louis, CV Mosby, 1965

Comroe JH: *Physiology of Respiration*. Chicago, Year Book Medical Publishers, 1962

Comroe JH, Forster RE, Dubois AB, et al: *The Lung*, 2nd ed. Chicago, Year Book Medical Publishers, 1962

Egan DF: *Fundamentals of Inhalation Therapy*. St. Louis, CV Mosby, 1969

Hodgkin JE, Collier CA: Blood gas analysis and acid–base physiology. In Burton GG, Hodgkin JE (eds): *Respiratory Care: A Guide to Clinical Practice*, 2nd ed, pp 258–266. Philadelphia, JB Lippincott, 1984

Nunn JF: *Applied Respiratory Physiology*, pp 140–183. London, Butterworths, 1987

VI. Neurologic/ Psychiatric Disorders

51
Altered Mental Status and Coma

A rapid, effective, and orderly evaluation of the patient in coma is critical in the first minutes after arrival in the emergency room. Once this initial evaluation is completed and the patient is stabilized, a more comprehensive evaluation is necessary first to determine the anatomy of the lesion producing coma and then to establish the etiology of the coma. The outcome may rest on therapy initiated within minutes of the patient's arrival. This chapter first outlines the necessary initial steps to be taken in the emergency evaluation of coma. A more detailed evaluation of the comatose patient is then described, to help define the anatomy of the lesion and guide subsequent evaluation. The three processes that cause coma—bilateral hemispheric lesions, brain-stem lesions, and diffuse metabolic/toxic lesions—are discussed. Finally, the assessment and treatment of the deteriorating comatose patient, including patterns of brain herniation, are described.

EMERGENCY EVALUATION

When the comatose patient is brought into the emergency room, a rapid, simple, and methodic evaluation must be conducted. This 5-minute evaluation is designed to reveal any problems that may lead to death or prolonged morbidity if left untreated.

AIRWAY/BREATHING

First, check the airway and respiratory excursions. If in doubt, intubate the trachea. Elective intubation in an unrushed, controlled setting is far preferable to emergency intubation after the patient develops acute respiratory distress. Check arterial blood gases to ensure adequate ventilation. If the patient is suspected to have a neck injury, radiologic assessment must be done first to prevent injury to the spinal cord. If time does not permit radiologic assessment, a cricothyroidotomy or emergency tracheostomy is indicated.

The patient may require mechanical ventilation, based on the arterial blood gases and the physician's clinical judgment. Keep in mind that a comatose patient who initially presents with adequate ventilation may subsequently deteriorate, particularly if the coma is caused by acute intoxication or trauma.

CIRCULATION

Remember that cardiac dysfunction (*i.e.*, myocardial infarction or dysrhythmia) or hypotension (due to blood loss or septic shock) may cause coma. Acute brain dysfunction during herniation may secondarily alter cardiac rate, rhythm, and blood pressure. Whatever the etiology, maintenance of adequate cardiac output and blood pressure is essential to survival. Cardiac rate and rhythm must be continuously monitored, and abnormalities treated aggressively.

METABOLIC

The laboratory evaluation is sometimes critical in diagnosing the cause of coma. Blood should be drawn for determination of serum electrolytes, glucose, urea nitrogen, complete blood count, Chem-20, and prothrombin and partial thromboplastin times. Additional blood is drawn in serum tubes for studies indicated from the later evaluation (*e.g.*, drug screen, liver function tests, and serum ammonia). Glucose should be administered intravenously as early as possible to *all* patients in coma, without waiting for laboratory results. Hypoglycemia is unfortunately often neglected as a cause of coma, or recognized too late. Hypoglycemia can produce all degrees of alteration of consciousness, from lethargy to coma, and can cause focal neurologic signs.

Seizures may cause additional brain damage. The most widely recommended treatment is intravenous diazepam (approximately 10 mg) to stop the seizure, followed by intravenous phenytoin (500 mg–1 g at a rate less than 50 mg/min). These drugs are not benign in this setting. Diazepam may cause respiratory depression or arrest, and phenytoin may cause hypotension or bradycardia. Adequate respiratory support, including artificial ventilation if necessary, and frequent monitoring of vital signs are critical. A more detailed discussion of treating status epilepticus is found in Chapter 53.

Metabolic acidosis or alkalosis may cause or worsen coma. Abnormalities of acid–base balance and blood chemistry should be corrected. Similarly, hypo- or hyperthermia can contribute to the patient's altered mental state and must be treated.

Wernicke's encephalopathy is a rare but potentially treatable cause of coma. The administration of glucose may precipitate Wernicke's disease in a patient who is alcoholic or malnourished. Thiamine, 50 mg to 100 mg, should be administered.

A common cause of coma is abuse of legal or illegal drugs. The primary treatment of drug overdose is supportive, particularly in maintaining ventilation. More specific therapy is available for narcotic ovedose and for anticholinergic sedative overdose. Narcotic overdose is treated with naloxone hydrochloride, 0.4 mg IV every 5 minutes until the patient is conscious. The duration of action is 2 to 3 hours. Since many narcotics, including methadone, have a longer half-life, the patient may relapse and need to be treated again. Sedatives with anticholinergic effects, such as the tricyclic antidepressants, can produce coma.

Increased intracranial pressure (ICP) may result from some causes of coma and can cause morbidity or death if not aggressively treated.

Infection of the central nervous system may produce an altered mental state. Infection elsewhere in the body may also alter the level of consciousness. Blood cultures and lumbar puncture may need to be obtained quickly in the emergency room.

All points previously outlined must be evaluated in every patient in coma, and evaluation must be initiated within minutes after arrival in the emergency room. A patient brought in comatose after an automobile accident, for example, may have had the accident because of hypoglycemia.

BEDSIDE EVALUATION OF COMA

Once the initial evaluation is completed and the patient has been stabilized, a comprehensive evaluation is conducted to determine the anatomic lesion causing coma. The simple, brief bedside evaluation of the comatose patient outlined below usually reveals the level of the neuraxis responsible for the altered mental state.

The descriptions of acutely altered mental state are easier to label than to define. The spectrum of states between "alert" and "comatose" is difficult to quantitate. Decreasing levels of consciousness are commonly described by the following terms: clouding of consciousness, delirium, obtundation, stupor, and coma. A stuporous patient is unresponsive except to vigorous stimuli, while a comatose patient is unresponsive to all external stimuli.

Lesions in either of two anatomic sites can impair consciousness. Stupor or coma is produced by bilateral hemispheric lesions affecting the ascending retricular activating system, or by a brain-stem lesion affecting the reticular core. The bedside neurologic examination helps determine the site of the lesion.

The reticular activating system occupies the central core of the brain-stem. This dense population of neurons receives collaterals from every major somatic and spinal sensory pathway. Experimental lesions in animals and neuropathologic studies in man demonstrate that a lesion in the brain-stem reticular core can cause coma. Specifically, lesions in the midbrain and pons, extending anywhere from the posterior hypothalamus to the lower third of pons, produce coma. Brain-stem lesions causing coma are paramedian, and ventral to the ventricular system, involving both sides of the midline and most of the dorsal-ventral axis of the tegmentum. Brain-stem lesions exclusively localized to the medulla do not impair consciousness.

The brain stem reticular core communicates with the cerebral hemispheres through a diffuse fiber pathway, the ascending reticular activating system, which passes primarily through the central tegmental fasciculus. Three major ascending pathways arise from the reticular formation. One pathway ascends to the thalamic reticular nucleus and then to the cortex. The second ascends through the hypothalamus to the basal forebrain. The third pathway originates in the midbrain raphe and locus ceruleus and projects to the neocortex. Lesions in the cerebral hemispheres that produce coma must be large and bilateral. A lesion involving exclusively one hemisphere does not produce coma unless it secondarily affects the function of the other hemisphere.

The bedside neurologic examination of the comatose patient determines whether the lesion is in the brain stem, involving the reticular core, or is in both hemispheres, involving the ascending reticular activating system. This evaluation consists of examining spontaneous and induced movements, the pattern of respiration, pupils and ocular movements.

SPONTANEOUS AND INDUCED MOVEMENTS

Simple observation of the patient at the bedside reveals much about the depth of stupor or coma and about the anatomic lesion. The patient may have semipurposeful movements (e.g., arm flailing) or may have no movements. There may be more spontaneous or evoked movement on one side, indicating a lesion involving one corticospinal tract more than the other. The patient may have tonic or clonic movements that can be either massive or subtle and focal (indicating seizure activity). Movement evoked by a mildly painful stimulus is examined next. Noxious stimuli include rubbing the sternum with a closed fist or pressing the nasal bridge. The pattern of motor response elicited by pain may reveal the anatomic level producing the altered mental state. Purposeful movement (e.g., withdrawing the examiner's hand) indicates a higher level of function than no movement. Painful stimuli may also produce posturing, which has great localizing value. Decerebrate rigidity is induced by painful stimuli, and involves extension, adduction, and pronation of the arms, and extension of the legs with plantar flexion of the feet. Decerebrate posturing almost always signifies a brain-stem lesion, from the mesencephalon to the vestibular nuclei. Decorticate posturing produces flexion of the arms with extension of the legs. Lesions of the cerebral hemispheres produce decorticate posturing.

RESPIRATION

Examination of the respiratory pattern may facilitate anatomic localization. Figure 51-1 diagrams the various respiratory patterns commonly encountered in the comatose patient and their anatomic localization. Cheyne–Stokes respiration is a regular crescendo–decrescendo pattern in the depth of respiration; there may be a brief apneic spell between cycles. Cheyne–Stokes respirations are seen commonly in deep bilateral subcortical lesions. Hyperventilation, a sustained hyperpnea, can result from lesions in the brain stem, but most commonly is a compensatory mechanism for primary pulmonary dysfunction. True central neurogenic hyperventilation is present when the

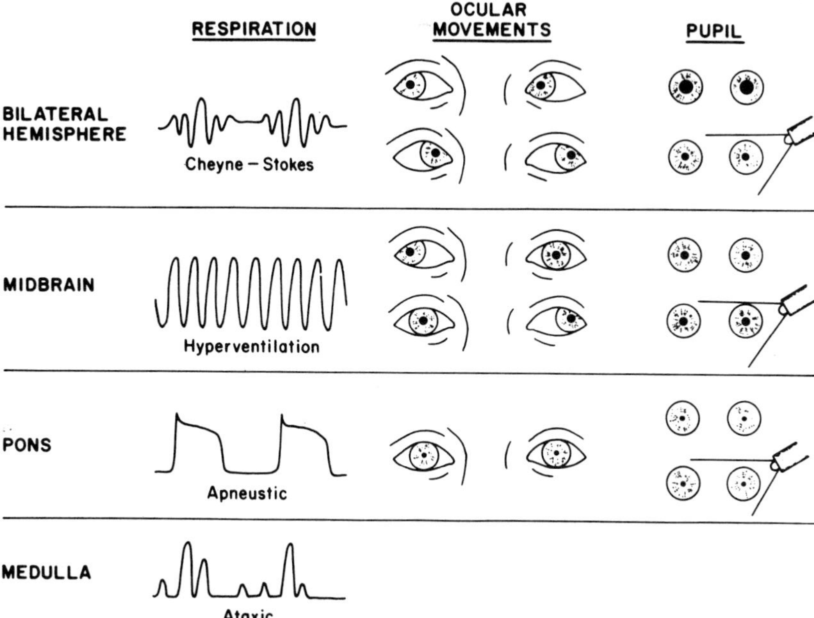

Figure 51-1 Respiratory patterns, extraocular movements, and pupillary findings in comatose patients with lesions in different locations of the central nervous system.

patient is breathing room air and arterial blood gases reveal an elevated Po_2, lowered Pco_2, and an elevated *p*H. Patients meeting these strict criteria are rare, and usually have lesions in the low midbrain and middle third of the pons. Most commonly, comatose patients who are hyperventilating are attempting to compensate for pulmonary dysfunction and are mildly hypoxic. Apneustic breathing is characterized by a long inspiratory pause at full inspiration. This respiratory pattern indicates a lesion at the midpontine level, involving the dorsolateral tegmentum. Ataxic breathing is characterized by chaotic respiration of random depth and rate. Lesions of the dorsomedial medulla, compromising the primary respiratory centers, produce this respiratory pattern. Cluster breathing consists of clusters of breaths with irregular pauses, and is produced by lesions in the lower pons or upper medulla.

OCULAR MOVEMENTS

Examination of eye movements elicited by stimulation of the vestibular mechanism often reveals important localizing information. Two tests of ocular function are easily conducted at the bedside, and are important components of the initial neurologic assessment. Both the oculocephalic maneuver and the ice water caloric test rely on the same anatomic pathways to produce eye movements.

To perform the oculocephalic test, the patient's head is rapidly rotated from side to side, which stimulates both the vestibular apparatus and proprioceptors in the neck. A normal response in the comatose patient is conjugate deviation of the eyes in the direction opposite the head turning. Conjugate deviation of the eyes implies that the pathways between the vestibular nuclei, the abducens nuclei, and the oculomotor nuclei are all intact, and therefore indicates that the brain stem is functional. A patient with an intact oculocephalic response usually has a bilateral hemispheric lesion causing coma. If no eye deviation is produced by the oculocephalic maneuver, no anatomic conclusions can be drawn, and the ice water caloric test, which uses a more effective stimulus, must be employed. An oculocephalic test producing disconjugate eye movements suggests a brain-stem lesion preventing effective communication between the vestibular and occular nuclei, as shown in Figure 51-1.

To conduct the ice water caloric test, the ears are first examined to determine that the tympanic membrane is intact, and the patient's head is elevated 30° above the horizontal plane, thereby placing the lateral semicircular canal in the vertical plane. Up to 120 ml of ice water is instilled into the external canal by a catheter attached to a syringe. The eye movements are then observed. In the conscious patient, cold water stimulation of the semicircular canal produces tonic conjugate deviation of the eyes toward the side of the stimulus with superimposed nystagmus, the fast component away from the side of the stimulus. The tonic eye movements are mediated by information arising in the vestibular nuclei, traveling to the paramedian pontine reticular formation, then to the abducens and oculomotor nuclei. The fast saccadic nystagmus is mediated by impulses traveling from the posterior portion of the frontal lobes, descending through the genu of the internal capsule. In the comatose patient with bilateral hemispheric lesions, ice water vestibular stimulation will therefore produce tonic conjugate eye deviation and no nystagmus, because the tonic deviation is mediated by the brain stem and the nystagmus results from fibers originating in the frontal lobes. The comatose patient with a brain-stem lesion will usually demonstrate either of two abnormalities. The lesion may be in the middle or upper brain stem, involving the medial longitudinal fasciculus, which transmits information from the abducens nuclei to the oculomotor nucleus. In this case, the eye opposite the side of stimulation will not adduct across the midline (due to failure of the oculomotor nucleus), while the eye on the side of stimulation will fully abduct (due to the normal function of the abducens nucleus). If the lesion is in the lower brain stem, the patient may have no response to ice water stimulation due to destruction of the vestibular nuclei or of the paramedian pontine reticular formation (the "lateral gaze centers") near the abducens nuclei.

PUPILS

The size of the pupil represents a balance between parasympathetic input, which constricts the pupil, and sympathetic input, which dilates the pupil. The pupillary examination is critical because it often reveals important anatomic information and can be quantitatively assessed to help evaluate the patient over time. Therefore, a careful measure of the pupils, recorded in the hospital chart, is essential. A table displaying pupillary diameters recorded in millimeters in ambient light and with direct and consensual stimuli must be a part of the initial and follow-up evaluations. A "large pupil" recorded by a physician in the emergency room may or may not be the same "large pupil" seen later by the ICU physician.

The pupils in a comatose patient with bilateral cortical lesions are usually small and reactive. Three drug types may produce coma by depressing bilateral cortical function and can also produce pupillary disturbances directly. Atropine and scopolamine are muscarinic receptor antagonists that directly inhibit the parasympathetic input to the eye and therefore produce fixed and dilated pupils. Glutethimide overdose can produce coma and frequently produces unequal pupils that are 4 to 8 mm. Opiates (such as heroin and morphine) can also produce coma by depressing cortical function and produce pinpoint pupils.

Brain-stem lesions causing coma may produce pupillary abnormalities with localizing value. Lesions in the midbrain, involving the tectum, interrupt the pupillary light reflex and produce midposition pupils that do not respond to light. Lesions of the midbrain tegmentum interrupt both parasympathetic and sympathetic pathways to produce midposition, fixed, and nonreactive pupils. A lesion involving the third nerve, or oculomotor nucleus in the midbrain, may produce a dilated pupil that is sluggishly reactive to light, and may also produce oculomotor paresis.

A pontine lesion producing coma destroys the descending sympathetic fibers and stimulates the parasympathetic input, producing pinpoint pupils. The light reflex is still intact, although it is often difficult to see without a magnifying glass.

Lesions of the medulla, by themselves, do not produce coma, as noted previously. However, if a lesion producing coma extends to the lateral medulla, Horner's syndrome may result from interruption of the sympathetic pathway, producing pupillary constriction and ptosis (see Figure 51-1).

The orderly bedside examination of the comatose patient for spontaneous and evoked motor movement, respirations, ocular movements, and pupillary size and response is an invaluable aid in assessing whether the patient is comatose from a bilateral hemispheric lesion or a brain-stem lesion. These observations, in addition to the routine history and physical examination, help direct the subsequent evaluation.

For more information, please see Chapter 99 in Civetta JM, Taylor RW, Kirby RR: Critical Care. *Philadelphia: J. B. Lippincott, 1988*

BIBLIOGRAPHY

Edwards RH, Simon RP: Coma. In Baker AB, Joynt RJ (eds): *Clinical Neurology.* Philadelphia, Harper & Row, 1986

Feldman MH: The decerebrate state in the primate. I. Studies in monkeys. *Arch Neurol* 1971; 25:501

Glaser J: *Neuroophthalmology,* p 247. Hagerstown, MD, Harper & Row, 1978

Kinkel W: Computerized tomography in clinical neurology. In Baker AB, Joynt RJ (eds): *Clinical Neurology.* Philadelphia, Harper & Row, 1986

McKissock W, Richarson A, Walsh L: Spontaneous cerebellar hemorrhage: A study of 34 consecutive cases treated surgically. *Brain* 1960; 83:1

Peele TL: *The Neuroanatomic Basis for Clinical Neurology,* 3rd ed, p 248. New York, McGraw Hill, 1977

Plum F, Posner JB: *The Diagnosis of Stupor and Coma.* Philadelphia, FA Davis, 1980

Prensky AL, Coben LA: Electroencephalography. In Baker AB, Joynt RJ (eds): *Clinical Neurology.* Philadelphia, Harper & Row, 1986

Romer FK: Bacterial meningitis: A 15 year review of bacterial meningitis from departments of internal medicine. *Dan Med Bull* 1977; 24:35

Smith BH: Infections of the dura and its venous sinus. In Banker AB, Joynt RJ (eds): *Clinical Neurology.* Philadelphia, Harper & Row, 1986

52
Cerebrovascular Disease/Stroke

Stroke is a term for a variety of disorders characterized by the sudden onset of a neurologic deficit caused by ischemia or hemorrhage in a localized region of the brain. It is the clinical manifestation of a complex process that can involve the cerebrovasculature directly (as from atherosclerosis) or indirectly (as from cardiac emboli). Stroke is a serious condition, representing the third leading cause of death in American adults, and patients often present to a critical care setting. The acute management of such patients revolves around three key questions:

1 Is the diagnosis of stroke correct?

2 Is the stroke in the distribution of the carotid arteries (cerebral hemispheres) or the vertebral–basilar system (brain stem)?

3 Is the stroke due to an embolus, thrombus, lacune, or hemorrhage?

Answers to these questions determine the appropriate diagnostic work-up and therapeutic interventions, as well as the patient's prognosis.

DIFFERENTIAL DIAGNOSIS

Most patients who suddenly develop a localized neurologic problem have, in fact, had a stroke. Stroke is by far the most common acute, focal, non-traumatic brain disease. The differential diagnosis of stroke thus is not extensive, but there is nevertheless an unfortunate tendency to assume that any neurologic symptom that appears abruptly must be due to vascular disease.

As shown in Table 52-1, many symptoms that can occur as a feature of stroke, especially brain-stem stroke, are seldom due to vascular disease when they occur alone, unaccompanied by other evidence of neurologic damage. Thus, a patient with a sudden attack of vertigo is unlikely to have had a brain-stem stroke. Similarly, dysarthria, headache, and double vision have multiple etiologies, in which vascular disease appears far down the list. It is particularly important that changes in mental status not be attributed to cerebrovascular disease until other, more likely, metabolic, toxic, and infec-

TABLE 52-1 SYMPTOMS SELDOM RESULTING FROM CEREBROVASCULAR DISEASE

Vertigo alone	Confusion
Dysarthria alone	Memory loss
Dysphagia alone	Delirium
Diplopia alone	Coma
Headache	Syncope
Tremor	Incontinence
Tonic-clonic motor activity	Tinnitus

tious etiologies have been excluded. Confusion, delirium, memory loss, and coma are rarely caused by stroke. Most of the confusion about the diagnosis of stroke occurs in patients with altered mental status. Table 52-2 lists the diseases most commonly mistaken for stroke.

EVALUATION OF STROKE

The history, focusing on the characteristic features of each type of stroke discussed above, is the most reliable, reproducible, and cost-effective way of evaluating cerebrovascular disease. Often other conditions can be eliminated, and the anatomy and etiology of the stroke can be determined from the history alone.

The physical examination complements the history, but examination of the vascular system is surprisingly unrewarding. Atherosclerosis may present few outward signs, but the physical examination may still be valuable (see Table 52-3).

Measurement of blood pressure in both arms while the patient is supine and sitting gives clues to the state of the circulation, and may reveal hypertension, orthostatic hypotension, and proximal subclavian stenosis. Palpation of carotid and temporal arteries may reveal insufficient circulation, but palpation of the carotid arteries is actually a poor measure of their patency, and even severe carotid stenosis may cause little change in the pulse. The value of palpation is also limited because atherosclerosis usually involves the internal carotid artery, but only the common carotid artery can be felt. Disease in other arteries, such as the femorals, correlates poorly with the condition of

TABLE 52-2 CONDITIONS MOST FREQUENTLY MISTAKEN FOR STROKE

Seizures	Peripheral neuropathy and Bell's palsy
Metabolic encephalopathy	Multiple sclerosis
Cerebral tumor	Hypoglycemia
Subdural hematoma	Encephalitis
Cerebral abscess	Migraine
Vertigo, Ménière's disease	Psychogenic illness

TABLE 52-3 BEDSIDE AIDS IN EVALUATING CEREBROVASCULAR DISEASE

History
Activity—thrombosis on awakening, bleed during activity
Onset—sudden or stepwise
Recovery—rapid for emboli
Anatomy—multiple vascular territories for emboli
Mental status—diminished, with headache and nausea, in bleeds
Predisposing factors—diabetes, hypertension, heart disease, dysrhythmia, angina, coagulopathy, migraine, oral contraceptives

Physical Examination
Vascular evaluation
- Carotid circulation
  - Abnormal carotid or temporal artery pulses
  - Carotid bruits
  - Retinal microemboli and ischemic retinopathy
- Vertebral-basilar circulation
  - Bruits at the subclavian–vertebral junction
  - Unequal blood pressures in the arms

Cardiac evaluation
- Myocardial infarction
- Dysrhythmias
- Prosthetic valves
- Endocarditis

Neurologic evaluation
- Carotid circulation
- Vertebral basilar circulation

the carotids and is seldom a useful guide to the management of stroke patients.

Carotid bruits are vexatious physical findings. Although various authors have attempted to correlate certain features of bruits with internal carotid artery stenosis, most such reports have not been reproduced. No characteristic feature, including the volume, pitch, or duration of the bruit, reliably indicates the degree or the nature of constriction of the vascular lumen. Many bruits reflect benign conditions. The clinical significance of carotid bruits is minimized because they are audible in many asymptomatic individuals without atherosclerosis who never suffer from cerebrovascular disease, but may be absent in severely diseased vessels. Thus, carotid artery bruits may or may not reflect underlying atherosclerosis, and while carotid bruits may be a general marker of atherosclerosis, there are many false-positives and false-negatives when evaluating stroke patients. Therefore, even if a carotid bruit is detected, it may be difficult to decide whether it is relevant to the patient's symptoms, and it should not be given undue emphasis in the overall evaluation.

Retinal vessels mirror the brain vasculature and ophthalmoscopy allows direct observation of arterial narrowing, as from hypertension or diabetes. Also, embolic strokes may be suspected because of the presence of embolic material in the retinal arteries. Cholesterol particles that embolize to the eye often lodge in bifurcations and are visible as shiny, refractile, orange-yellow crystals called Hollenhorst plaques. Retinal emboli composed of platelets and fibrin are grayish-white in color. Both kinds of emboli usually indicate the presence of carotid stenosis and ulceration, but emboli from the heart may also find their way to the retinal vessels.

Examination of the heart should focus on detecting thrombogenic diseases, including myocardial infarction, dysrhythmias, prosthetic valves, and bacterial endocarditis. The presence of heart disease is important because of the high morbidity and mortality from coronary artery disease after stroke, and because the determination that a stroke is embolic may rest on finding a cardiac source of embolus. As many as 9% of patients with a stroke have had a concomitant myocardial infarction, which is often silent. The history must therefore address chest pain, diaphoresis, nausea, dyspnea, and other symptoms of cardiac ischemia. Palpitations, dizziness, and light-headedness are clues to dysrhythmias.

The physician should inquire about intravenous drug use and search for needle tracks, especially in younger patients. A fourth heart sound may indicate a recent myocardial infarction, while murmurs may reflect underlying valvular heart disease. Computed tomographic (CT) scanning, magnetic resonance imaging (MRI), lumbar puncture, and electroencephalography are invaluable diagnostic aids in the evaluation of cerebrovascular disease.

MANAGEMENT

GENERAL PRINCIPLES

Following a completed stroke, care of the patient should emphasize supportive measures. The patient should be admitted to the hospital and a diagnostic work-up initiated, as outlined above. The airway, breathing, and circulation should be supported if the patient is comatose or unstable. It is usually preferable to err on the side of hypertension in patients with ischemic stroke; lowering the blood pressure too quickly may further enlarge the area of ischemia. Most patients have a transient blood pressure elevation after a stroke, and this can usually be monitored without intervention. Other support includes maintenance of hydration and normal blood glucose, as well as proper electrolyte balance.

The leading causes of death after a stroke are not neurologic, and critical care of the stroke patient usually centers around management of medical problems.

The leading cause of morbidity and mortality after a stroke (Table 52-4) is pneumonia, which is usually due to aspiration, since the stroke often causes weakness of facial and pharyngeal muscles and disturbance of the swallowing reflexes. Patients should have their oral intake restricted until it is clear that they can swallow well. Fever after a stroke is almost always due to an infection and should prompt a search for pneumonia.

TABLE 52-4 LEADING CAUSES OF DEATH IN THE FIRST FEW DAYS AFTER A STROKE

Pneumonia
Pulmonary embolism
Cardiac ischemia and dysrhythmias
The stroke itself

Stroke patients who are either bedridden or have lost mobility in their limbs are at high risk for a deep venous thrombosis, and pulmonary embolism is another common cause of complications following stroke. Prophylaxis for pulmonary embolism is a controversial subject, but a case can be made for low-dose heparin therapy (e.g., 5000 units sc b.i.d.).

There is a definite correlation between atherosclerosis in the coronary and cerebral arteries, and most patients admitted with a stroke have underlying coronary artery disease. Many patients with a stroke have had a concomitant myocardial infarction or will suffer one within a few days. The myocardial ischemia is often "silent" or unrecognized, and the patient must be questioned and examined diligently for any symtoms that could indicate cardiac ischemia. Because patients are often aphasic, confused, or unresponsive after a stroke, their EKG (and possibly serum creatine kinase level) should always be examined so that a myocardial infarction is not overlooked. Preexisting heart disease, combined with the catecholamine release that often accompanies a stroke, accounts for a high incidence of cardiac dysrhythmias in stroke patients. Although these are occasionally serious or even fatal, studies have not shown the benefit of continuous cardiac monitoring or aggressive antidysrhythmic therapy as a routine part of stroke care. Rather, each patient must be observed carefully and treatment individualized.

TREATMENT

It seems certain that a great potential for recovery exists after a stroke, since many affected neurons are merely damaged rather than destroyed. Therapy to salvage these reversibly injured cells could have a major impact on improving the stroke outcome. Similarly, our scientific knowledge of atherosclerosis, platelet function, microcirculation, and biochemical mechanisms of hypoxia and cell injury, as well as the pharmacology of drugs that affect these processes, has expanded enormously in recent years. The nihilistic view that stroke will forever remain an untreatable condition is thus not warranted. Nevertheless, these advances have not yet been translated into real clinical benefits, and the situation today is one in which a wide variety of medical and surgical treatments are applied to stroke victims, often aggressively and dogmatically, despite the lack of any solid evidence that they are truly effective. In fact, despite the vast increase in our understanding of cerebrovascular diseases, the clinician today has little more to offer than did his or her mentor a generation ago. There is no treatment, medical or surgical, that has been proven to alter the natural history of a completed stroke.

Thrombotic Stroke

Symptoms of a cerebral thrombosis may present in a gradual or stuttering fashion. If deficits are worsening before the clinician's eyes, the situation is usually referred to as a stroke in evolution. To stop the progressive ischemia, such patients are usually treated with anticoagulants. Well-controlled trials assessing the efficacy of anticoagulation in minimizing the severity of evolving strokes have proven difficult to design, and the available data are inconclusive regarding whether anticoagulation (*e.g.*, with heparin or warfarin compounds) is actually effective. Nevertheless, the standard of practice among most neurologists is to treat such patients with heparin. Anticoagulation is clearly not of benefit to patients who have already completed their stroke.

If anticoagulation is to be given, a CT scan is first obtained to exclude any intracerebral hemorrhage. If the scan is negative, the patient is then begun on intravenous heparin, administered at the rate of approximately 1000 units/hour, with close monitoring of the prothrombin time (PT) and partial thromboplastin time (PTT). Many authorities advocate that the patient not be given a bolus or loading dose of heparin, since this may increase the likelihood of intracerebral hemorrhage. The PTT should be maintained at 1½ times normal, and over the next few days the patient is usually switched to warfarin to maintain the PT at the same level. Oral anticoagulation is then continued for several weeks, although the exact duration is rather arbitrary.

The contraindications to anticoagulation include very advanced age or pronounced medical frailty, a large cerebral infarction (which would contain a great deal of necrotic brain tissue), uncontrolled hypertension, or the presence of active bleeding (either within the head or at another site, such as a gastrointestinal hemorrhage).

The other mechanism by which patients with a thrombotic stroke may become critically ill is the development of increased intracranial pressure (ICP). Cytotoxic edema is common after a stroke, as the ischemic brain tissue breaks down and dies. This process usually reaches a peak within 3 to 5 days after the initial insult—a crucial time in the management of stroke patients. As the brain tissue becomes edematous and swells, the pressure within the confined cranial vault increases, leading to a worsening of the focal neurologic deficit and a progressive global decline in other neurologic functions. The first evidence of increased ICP is usually a gradually worsening mental status, with the patient becoming increasingly lethargic and finally stuporous and comatose. If severe, the increased ICP can lead to herniation of the brain and death.

Intervention must be rapid to reverse the rising ICP. Intubation and subsequent hyperventilation leads to vasoconstriction, which in turn provides more room within the skull for the expanding brain. The mainstay of treatment is diuretics (such as 40–80 mg of intravenous furosemide) and osmolar agents such as mannitol or glycerol. A dose of 150 to 200 mg of mannitol can be administered intravenously as a bolus, and then 50 to 100 mg can be given every few hours as needed to decrease the edema. High doses of steroids, such as 6 mg of dexamethasone every 4 hours, may be of some value, although the onset of action is delayed (hence, they are not effective within the first few hours).

The question may be raised of whether it is feasible to surgically correct a stenotic or newly thrombosed artery in a patient who has just suffered a thrombotic stroke. This should be discouraged. Immediate angiography and surgery for an acute stroke has an unacceptably high morbidity and mortality rate, and restoration of brain function has been disappointing. There are no firm indications for angiography or surgery in the critical care management of stroke patients.

Embolic Stroke

As with all ischemic strokes, there is no adequate therapy for a completed embolic stroke. However, embolic cerebral infarction often occurs in the setting of active, ongoing embolization from a cardiac source. Emboli from the heart may arise from a prosthetic valve, a mural thrombus or aneurysm from a recent myocardial infarction, a fibrillating atrium, or valvular heart disease. A decision must often be made whether or not to immediately administer anticoagulants to a patient who presents with an embolic stroke from one of these cardiac sources. Although reliable controlled data are again scarce, it is probably best to begin anticoagulation immediately in most patients. This should be done as outlined above, after obtaining a CT scan that excludes intracerebral hemorrhage, using a dose of intravenous heparin of about 1000 units/hour. Anticoagulation via the oral route with warfarin can be initiated quickly, always maintaining the clotting studies about 1½ to 2 times normal, but no more than that.

Anticoagulation carries some risk of converting a bland ischemic cerebral infarction into a hemorrhagic one, with concomitant clinical worsening. On the other hand, a delay in initiating anticoagulation, even of only a few days, poses the risk of subsequent embolization and further strokes. On balance, the risk of clinical deterioration following immediate anticoagulation is very small and does not outweigh the definite benefit of preventing further embolization by administering heparin. Table 52-5 reviews the key points in anticoagulation for the treatment of stroke.

Lacunar Stroke

There is usually little in the way of emergency intervention or critical care required in the management of lacunar stroke, other than general medical and supportive measures. Occasionally, lacunar strokes can also evolve or progress, but many authorities recommend against anticoagulating a lacunar stroke in evolution, since the risk of bleeding from one of the small perforating vessels may be much greater than any benefit accrued. These strokes are so small that edema is seldom a significant problem, and patients with lacunar strokes usually recover very well, regardless of the severity of the initial deficit.

TABLE 52-5 ANTICOAGULATION AFTER A STROKE

I. Indications/Contraindications
   A. May be useful
      1. Stroke in evolution
      2. Nonseptic emboli from the heart
   B. Usually not useful
      1. Completed stroke of any type
      2. Transient ischemic attacks
      3. Lacunae
II. Technique
   A. CT scan to rule out hemorrhage
   B. Intravenous heparin at 1000 units/hour, without a prior loading dose
   C. Maintain PTT at 1½ times normal
   D. Duration of treatment is controversial—may switch to oral warfarin compounds if chronic therapy is needed

Intracerebral Hemorrhage

The main danger from intracerebral hemorrhage again lies in increased ICP due to the mass of blood within the brain. This is the one setting after a stroke in which acute lowering of the blood pressure may be indicated, in order to lower ICP. Observation for and management of increased ICP should then proceed as discussed earlier.

Subarachnoid Hemorrhage

A ruptured intracranial aneurysm, the most common cause of subarachnoid hemorrhage, is a catastrophic event. Half of all patients die during the initial hospital period. Subarachnoid hemorrhage may occur at any age, with the peak incidence in the sixth decade, and there is a slight female predominance. It may also occur at any time, and the relationship between the ruptured aneurysm and hypertension, exercise, or other precipitating events is controversial.

Clinically, sudden rupture of an aneurysm causes abrupt, excruciating headache, usually diffuse and generalized, and often described as the worst headache the patient has ever experienced. The intracranial blood may also cause a stiff neck and increased ICP with nausea and vomiting. Focal neurologic signs such as hemiparesis or cranial nerve palsies may occur, arising from the territory of the ruptured blood vessel. Usually, there is at least some decrease in the level of consciousness, and as many as 50% of patients may become comatose or die immediately following subarachnoid hemorrhage. Patients thus usually present to a critical care setting as a diagnostic problem of stupor or coma. The stiff neck and history of preceding severe headache are the main clues distinguishing a subarachnoid hemorrhage from the many metabolic causes of coma.

An EKG with rhythm strip is mandatory because the catecholamine surge and hypertension after subarachnoid hemorrhage often precipitate cardiac dysrhythmias. Bleeding parameters should also be measured, including PT,

PTT, and platelet count. The syndrome of inappropriate antidiuretic hormone secretion (SIADH) may follow an intracranial bleed, so serum electrolytes must be checked.

Neurologic investigation of the patient with suspected subarachnoid hemorrhage begins with CT scanning, which should be the initial imaging study. A CT scan without contrast enhancement detects subarachnoid hemorrhage in approximately 75% of patients. Sometimes the CT scan localizes the site of the bleeding, and the aneurysm itself may be visualized. The CT scan may also rule out other causes of coma and focal neurologic deficits, or may show a large hematoma that would preclude a lumbar puncture.

The definitive test for subarachnoid hemorrhage is a lumbar puncture that reveals blood within the cerebrospinal fluid (CSF). If the CT scan is equivocal or negative, examination of the spinal fluid is confirmatory. Lumbar puncture is safe provided the CT scan does not show a focal mass of blood. If there is any question that blood in the CSF is due to a traumatic tap rather than a subarachnoid hemorrhage, the spinal fluid should be spun down in a centrifuge; blood that is more than 2 hours old leaves a xanthochromic supernatant, confirming that blood was present before the lumbar puncture.

Although CT scanning and lumbar puncture can demonstrate blood in the subarachnoid space, angiography is necessary for precise characterization of bleeding intracranial lesions such as aneurysm or arteriovenous malformations. Usually, this is deferred until just before surgery, so that any vasospasm present can be evaluated in close temporal relation to the operation.

Patients with subarachnoid hemorrhage are prone to deterioration in the days following their initial bleed, often because of arterial spasm; hence, surgical mortality in this period is high. The constant delicate adjustments needed to balance the many complications of subarachnoid hemorrhage demand an intensive care setting. The patient must be guided through a mine field of potentially disastrous problems until he is stable enough for definitive treatment—surgical obliteration of the aneurysm.

Most patients are so ill after subarachnoid hemorrhage (grades 3 through 5; Table 52-6) that surgery poses an unacceptable risk of morbidity and mortality. Surgery must therefore be delayed until the patient has improved and the medical problems have resolved. During this time, the patient is subject to a host of complications. Some authorities advocate expeditious angiography and definitive surgery within the first day or so following subarachnoid hemorrhage if the patient is stable (grade 1 or 2), so that subse-

TABLE 52-6 GRADING OF PATIENTS WITH SUBARACHNOID HEMORRHAGE

Grade 1: Fully conscious, no neurologic deficits
Grade 2: Mild drowsiness, no neurologic deficits
Grade 3: Drowsiness and confusion, focal neurologic deficits
Grade 4: Stupor, moderate or severe neurologic defects
Grade 5: Coma

quent difficulties can be managed without fear of rebleeding. The timing of aneurysm surgery remains controversial, however, and is best guided by the experience of the surgeons at a given medical center.

Continued bleeding from the aneurysm, which is often fatal, is one of the most serious complications of subarachnoid hemorrhage and tends to occur early: 20% of patients will rebleed, half of them within the first few days. Precautions include bed rest in a calm environment, often with sedatives. Stool softeners are usually given as well. Antihypertensive medication, such as hydralazine or propranolol, may be administered to prevent an elevated blood pressure from bursting the aneurysm. If the pressure is lowered too much, however, cerebral vasospasm may be induced or worsened. As a compromise, a pressure of about 140/90 is usually considered adequate. Treatment with antifibrinolytic agents to prevent rebleeding, such as ϵ-aminocaproic acid, is not clearly beneficial and has fallen into disfavor.

Vasospasm begins about 3 days after the bleed and may persist for 3 weeks, rendering surgery impossible. The spasm is often sufficiently severe to cause a cerebral infarction, which should be suspected if the patient develops new focal deficits during this time. Angiography may be necessary to confirm vasospasm. The specific substances within blood or the factors induced by the bleeding that are responsible for the cerebral vasospasm are not known. It is difficult to prevent vasospasm, but maintenance of blood pressure and intravascular volume appears helpful. Some studies suggest that calcium channel blockers, such as nimodipine or nifedipine in doses of 20 mg *q.i.d.*, may minimize vasospasm.

Other complications include hydrocephalus caused by blood blocking the reabsorptive pathways of the spinal fluid. Ventricular drainage by a shunt may also be required. Seizures are usually best managed with phenytoin, which can be given at a loading dose of 15 mg/kg (usually, about 1 g for the normal-sized person) and maintained at 300 mg/day.

The neurosurgical service should be involved as soon as possible after the subarachnoid hemorrhage to assist in the patient's management.

For more information, please see Chapter 101 in Civetta JM, Taylor RW, Kirby RR: Critical Care. *Philadelphia: J. B. Lippincott, 1988*

BIBLIOGRAPHY

American-Canadian Cooperative Study Group: Persantine-aspirin trial in cerebral ischemia, part II: Endpoint results. *Stroke* 1985; 16:406

Bousser MG, Eschwege E, Haguenau M, et al: AICLA controlled trial of aspirin and dipyridamole in the secondary prevention of atherothrombotic cerebral ischemia. *Stroke* 1983; 14:5

Brust JCM: Transient ischemic atacks: Natural history and anticoagulation. *Neurology* 1977; 27:701

Canadian Cooperative Study Group: A randomized trial of aspirin and sulfinpyrazone in threatened stroke. *N Engl J Med* 1978; 299:53

Cerebral Embolism Task Force: Cardiogenic brain embolism. *Arch Neurol* 1986; 43:71
Crowell RM, Zervas NT: Management of intracranial aneurysm. *Med Clin North Am* 1979; 63:695
Dimant J, Grob D: Electrocardiographic changes and myocardial damage in patients with acute cerebrovascular accidents. *Stroke* 1977; 8:448
Fields WS, Lemak NA, Frankowski RF, et al: Controlled trial of aspirin in cerebral ischemia. *Stroke* 1977; 8:301
Fisher CM, Roberson GH, Ojemann RG: Cerebral vasospasm with ruptured saccular aneurysm—The clinical manifestations.
Hart RG, Easton JD: Management of cervical bruits and carotid stenosis in preoperative patients. Stroke 1983; 14:290
Hier DB, Davis KR, Richardson EP, et al: Hypertensive putaminal hemorrhage. *Ann Neurol* 1977; 1:152
McCarthy ST: Low dose heparin as a prophylaxis against deep-vein thrombosis after acute stroke. *Lancet* 1977; 2:800
Mohr JP: Lacunes. *Stroke* 1982; 13:3
Mohr JP, Caplan LR, Melski JW, et al: The Harvard cooperative stroke registry. *Neurology* 1978; 28:754
Norris JW, Hachinksi VC: Misdiagnosis of stroke. *Lancet* 1982; 1:328
Przelomski MM, Roth RM, Gleckman RA, et al: Fever in the wake of a stroke. *Neurology* 1986; 36:427
Rokey R, Rolak LA, Harati Y, et al: Coronary artery disease in patients with cerebrovascular disease: A prospective study. *Ann Neurol* 1984; 16:50
Sorensen PS, Pedersen H, Marguardsen J, et al: Acetylsalicylic acid in the prevention of stroke in patients with reversible cerebral ischemic attacks. *Stroke* 1983; 14:15
Strittmatter W, Gilmer W, Rolak L: Low yield in the diagnostic workup of transient ischemic attacks. *Ann Neurol* 1986; 36:178
Weir B: Antifibrinolytics in subarachnoid hemorrhage. *Arch Neurol* 1987; 44:116
Weksler BB, Lewin M: Anticoagulation in cerebral ischemia. *Strok* 1983; 14:658

53 Status Epilepticus

In the most general terms, status epilepticus is defined as epileptic seizures that are so frequently repeated or so prolonged as to create a fixed and lasting epileptic condition. In most cases status consists of recurrent seizures without an intervening return to normal consciousness. Any of the classified seizures can develop into status epilepticus; however, generalized tonic–clonic (convulsive) status epilepticus is a medical emergency and is the focus of most of this chapter. Mortality and morbidity of generalized tonic–clonic status increase with duration of the status. It is critical that convulsive status be stopped within 60 minutes to prevent both systemic and neurologic complications (See Table 53-1).

DEFINITIONS AND CLASSIFICATION

Seizures are usually classified as generalized or partial. Generalized seizures are accompanied electrically by synchronous epileptiform activity in both cerebral hemispheres. In primary generalized seizures, bilaterally synchronous epileptiform activity occurs in both cerebral hemispheres from onset; secondary generalized seizures begin as partial seizures that spread and result in epileptiform activity in both cerebral hemispheres. Primary generalized seizures include tonic–clonic (grand mal), tonic, clonic, myoclonic, atonic, and absence (petit mal) seizures. Partial seizures, those which begin with epileptiform activity in one brain region, are defined as "simple partial" if consciousness is not impaired during the seizure and as "complex partial" if consciousness is impaired. The initial clinical manifestation of partial seizures depends on the function of the brain region involved in the seizure onset. If the motor strip is the site of origin, the initial manifestation is abnormal motor activity, usually clonic, of the contralateral limbs.

Although this classification scheme is helpful in addressing the clinical and EEG characteristics of the seizures, a more useful classification with regard to the management and treatment of status epilepticus divides the status into convulsive, nonconvulsive, and simple partial. Convulsive status includes gen-

TABLE 53-1 PROTOCOL FOR TREATMENT OF GENERALIZED TONIC–CLONIC STATUS

1. Provide for maintenance of vital signs. Maintain airway, give oxygen. Observe and examine the patient.
2. Obtain 50 ml of blood for glucose, calcium, electrolytes, BUN, liver function, and anticonvulsant drug level analysis; CBC; and toxicology screen. Begin normal saline IV and give 50 ml of 50% glucose and 100 mg thiamine. Monitor EKG, blood pressure, and, if possible, EEG.
3. Use intravenous diazepam to stop seizures, 5 mg in 1–2 minutes; may repeat every 5–10 minutes if seizures recur, up to a total dose of 30 mg. An alternative approach is to use lorazepam, 2–4 mg IV every 5 minutes, up to a total dose of 10 mg.
4. Give phenytoin, 18 mg/kg IV, at a rate of less than 50 mg/min. If cardiac dysrhythmias or hypotension occur, slow the infusion rate.
5. If seizures persist after administration of phenytoin, intubate the patient and then give phenobarbital intravenously at a rate of 50–100 mg/min until the seizures stop or a total of 20 mg/kg has been given.
6. If seizures continue, arrange for anesthesia. While waiting, review the laboratory results and correct any abnormalities. Paraldehyde mixed in normal saline to produce a 4% solution may be given intravenously, using a glass syringe. Titrate until seizures stop. An alternative therapy is intravenous lidocaine, 1–3 mg/kg as a loading dose and then 2–10 mg/kg/hr. At these dosages, lidocaine may cause seizures.
7. If seizures continue after 60 minutes, general anesthesia, neuromuscular blockade, and EEG monitoring are required. Either inhalation anesthetic (isoflurane) or barbiturate anesthetic (sodium pentobarbital, 5 mg/kg as a loading dose and then 1–3 mg/kg/hr) may be used.

eralized tonic–clonic seizures with either a partial or generalized onset. Tonic, clonic, or myoclonic seizures may also occur with sufficient frequency to constitute a convulsive status; however, these seizure types (discussed later) rarely develop into status in adults. Nonconvulsive status includes absence and complex partial seizures; it is not accompanied by major motor signs but is associated with various degrees of impaired consciousness and automatic behavior. Simple partial status is usually characterized by unilateral, restricted motor seizures that are continuous and do not impair consciousness (epilepsia partialis continua). Because generalized tonic–clonic status (also referred to as convulsive status) is the most common form of status epilepticus in adults, it is the main focus of this chapter. The diagnosis and treatment of nonconvulsive status and simple partial status are addressed at the end of the chapter.

ETIOLOGY

About half of adult patients with convulsive status epilepticus have a preexisting diagnosis of epilepsy. Convulsive status is rarely the presenting symptom of primary generalized epilepsy. About 25% of patients have cryptogenic or idiopathic seizures (*i.e.*, seizures without a definite etiology). The other 75% have symptomatic seizures caused by a brain lesion or metabolic abnormality. Only about 1% to 2% of patients with cryptogenic seizures develop status, whereas about 9% of those with symptomatic epilepsy develop convulsive status.

In a series of adult patients presenting with convulsive status to a metropolitan public hospital emergency room, Aminoff and Simon found that the most common cause was anticonvulsant drug noncompliance (28% of all patients; 50% of patients with preexisting epilepsy). Other causes included association with alcohol withdrawal (15%), cerebrovascular lesions (10%), drug intoxication (10%), and acute metabolic derangement (8%). In other series, 5% to 25% of patients with convulsive status had brain tumors (usually in the frontal lobes), 10% to 25% had an acute or chronic traumatic lesion, 10% to 15% had an acute or old cerebrovascular lesion, and 5% to 10% had a central nervous system (CNS) infection. Seizures may occur in association with acute cerebrovascular lesions (infarction, intracerebral hemorrhage, subarachnoid hemorrhage) or as the result of a previous cerebrovascular accident. Metabolic etiologies include hyponatremia, hypoglycemia, hypocalcemia, uremia, hepatic encephalopathy, anoxic-hypoxic encephalopathy, and hyperosmolar states. Commonly used drugs that may produce seizures and status include theophylline and its derivatives, isoniazid, lidocaine, tricyclic antidepressants, phenothiazines, and the penicillins.

In most series, the seizures of more than half of the patients had focal features. These included asymmetric tonic or clonic motor activity and eye deviation. The presence of focal CNS lesions was not a prerequisite for the seizures to have focal features. Even metabolic etiologies can be accompanied by seizures with focal features, and in such situations the focus of seizure origin may shift or alternate between sides.

In summary, convulsive status manifested by generalized tonic–clonic seizures is usually associated with a precipitating etiology. An etiology or precipitating factor is not found in only 15% to 25% of the patients. In patients with previously diagnosed epilepsy, the most common precipitating causes are anticonvulsant medication noncompliance or alcohol withdrawal. Other considerations include systemic infections, sleep deprivation, metabolic alterations, or drug intoxication. In patients without a previous seizure history, convulsive status is usually associated with a CNS lesion or acute metabolic derangement. In this group of patients, neoplasm, trauma, and cerebrovascular insults must be considered, as well as any acute metabolic insult. During the course of treatment, these considerations must be kept in mind and appropriate laboratory studies ordered.

INITIAL THERAPY AND MANAGEMENT

The first step in management is to determine whether the patient is in status. Convulsive status can be defined as successive generalized tonic–clonic seizures without an intervening return to normal consciousness. If a patient presents with a single convulsion, he is not in status unless he has a second convulsion before regaining consciousness. Most patients with generalized convulsive status do not have continuous generalized seizures but have four or five generalized tonic–clonic seizures per hour. Between seizures, the patient is comatose or markedly obtunded.

The initial therapy for a patient who has a history of a recent seizure and has not regained consciousness consists of maintaining adequate ventilation and circulation. An airway should be inserted and oxygen given by mask. If the patient is having a tonic–clonic seizure, no attempt should be made to open his mouth with a tongue depressor or other device; doing so might damage the gums or tongue, or could dislodge teeth that the patient might then aspirate. Instead, oxygen should be administered, and the patient's head should be turned to one side to prevent aspiration. The seizure usually terminates within a few minutes, and an airway can then be inserted. Airways aid in suctioning secretions that accompany tonic–clonic seizures. The tonic component of generalized seizures is associated with cyanosis and hypoxia; however, intubation is usually not necessary unless there is evidence of respiratory depression following the seizure.

An intravenous catheter should be inserted, and at least 50 ml of blood should be obtained for laboratory studies. Studies should include determinations of serum electrolytes, blood urea nitrogen (BUN), liver function, calcium, glucose, anticonvulsant drug levels, a complete blood count, alcohol level, and toxicology screen. Arterial blood gas determinations may be useful but must be interpreted in light of the consequences of a generalized convulsion (see above). Once the blood is drawn, an infusion of normal saline should be started and 50 ml of 50% glucose given. Because a carbohydrate load in a patient deficient in thiamine may precipitate Wernicke's encephalopathy, 100 mg of thiamine should also be administered. Normal saline should be used because phenytoin precipitates in glucose-containing solutions.

During this initial period, the physician should observe and be able to describe the patient's seizure activity. A brief physical examination is done for signs of systemic disease, trauma, and any focal neurologic signs. If the patient presents without a history, he should be examined for an identification tag stating that he has epilepsy or for medications he might have with him. If the patient is already hospitalized, his diagnosis and the medications that he is receiving should be reviewed. The next step in treatment depends on whether the patient is in convulsive status epilepticus or is merely in a postictal state. If the patient has a second generalized seizure before regaining consciousness, appropriate pharmacologic therapy should be instituted, as outlined in Table 53-1. Intravenous diazepam or derivatives should not be given to a patient who has had a single seizure and is postictal. This initial pharmacologic therapy should be given only if the patient is in convulsive status (*i.e.*, is having successive generalized tonic–clonic seizures without an intervening return to consciousness).

LABORATORY EVALUATION OF ETIOLOGY

Laboratory data obtained during the initial management of a patient in status epilepticus often reveal the etiology. Further evaluation depends on the clinical setting and whether the patient has been diagnosed previously as being epileptic. An EEG is helpful in determining whether the patient has a generalized epileptiform abnormality, a focal epileptiform abnormality, or an underlying metabolic abnormality. If a patient presents with convulsive status as a first seizure and without an obvious metabolic etiology, a complete evaluation should be performed to determine whether there is an underlying lesion. Unenhanced computerized tomography (CT) of the brain should be performed to detect the presence of acute hemorrhage, and an enhanced CT should be done to detect neoplasms, abscesses, or vascular malformations. Magnetic resonance imaging (MRI) may detect lesions (especially low-grade neoplasms) not seen with CT scan and is an appropriate alternative in some cases.

Lumbar puncture is indicated whenever an infectious etiology or a subarachnoid hemorrhage not seen on CT scan is suspected. When focal features or papilledema are detected on examination or there is a clinical picture of transtentorial herniation, a CT or MRI scan should be performed before the lumbar puncture. Patients with convulsive status may have elevated temperatures and increased white blood cell counts that are not accompanied by underlying infection. Nonetheless, these findings require that a CNS infection be ruled out by lumbar puncture. As many as 18% of patients with recent convulsive status may have a pleocytosis without CNS infection. Usually, the total cell count is below 100 and may consist of either polymorphonuclear or mononuclear cells. The protein is often elevated, but the glucose is usually normal or higher than normal. These abnormalities are believed to be a consequence of a blood–brain barrier breakdown during status. Patients with pleocytosis and fever should be treated as if they had meningitis until cultures are negative.

PROGNOSIS

The prognosis for patients with convulsive status depends on the duration of the status and the underlying etiology. Mortality has decreased recently but is still approximately 10%. In most cases, death results from the underlying pathology responsible for the patient's seizures. In adults, the neurologic sequelae of status have not been well studied. Intellectual impairment may occur as a consequence of the patient's status rather than the underlying pathology. The morbidity of status is higher in children than in adults. Most studies have found that the longer convulsive status remains uncontrolled, the greater the associated morbidity and mortality.

For more information, please see Chapter 100 in Civetta JM, Taylor RW, Kirby RR: Critical Care. *Philadelphia: J. B. Lippincott, 1988*

BIBLIOGRAPHY

Aminoff MJ, Simon RP: Status epilepticus: Causes, clinical features and consequences in 98 patients. *Am J Med* 1980; 69:657

Browne TR: Paraldehyde, chlormethiazole, and lidocaine for treatment of status epilepticus. *Adv Neurol* 1983; 34:509

Delgado-Escueta AV, Enrile-Bacsal F: Combination therapy for status epilepticus: Intravenous diazepam and phenytoin. *Adv Neurol* 1983; 34:477

Gastaut H: Classification of status epilepticus. *Adv Neurol* 1983; 34:15

Goldberg MA, McIntyre HB: Barbiturates in the treatment of status epilepticus. *Adv Neurol* 1983; 34:499

Janz D: Etiology of convulsive status epilepticus. *Adv Neurol* 1983; 34:47

Kofke WA, Snider MT, Young RSK, et al: Prolonged low flow isoflurance anesthesia for status epilepticus. *Anesthesiology* 1985; 62:653

Leppik IE, Derivan AT, Homan RW, et al: Double-blind study of lorazepam and diazepam in status epilepticus. *JAMA* 1983; 249:1452

Meldrum BS, Vigouroux RA, Brierley JB: Systemic factors and epileptic brain damage. Prolonged seizures in paralyzed, artificially ventilated baboons. *Arch Neurol* 1973; 29:82

Simon RP: Physiologic consequences of status epilepticus. *Epilepsia* 1985; 26:S58

54
Neurologic Infections

Infections of the central nervous system (CNS) are often rapidly fatal or debilitating when undiagnosed but almost invariably treatable when suspected and diagnosed early. This presents the clinician with a challenge for rapid diagnosis and treatment. Recently developed diagnostic techniques, such as computerized tomography (CT) and cerebrospinal fluid (CSF) antigen assays, have supplemented the traditional CSF examination. The possibility of safely arriving at an accurate diagnosis has improved dramatically. Similary, the introduction of new therapeutic agents directed at bacteria, viruses, and fungi has greatly improved our opportunity for effecting a cure with minimal complications.

CLINICAL PRESENTATION AND INITIAL DIAGNOSTIC MEASURES

SUSPECTED CNS INFECTION WITH NO FOCAL NEUROLOGIC SIGNS

The absence of focal neurologic signs is reassuring but not absolute in ruling out mass lesions or dangerous cerebral edema. Even though mass lesions may be present without focal signs, the absence of such signs reduces the risk of lumbar puncture. In general, proceeding directly to CSF examination is justified in the setting of suspected CNS infection with no focal signs.

Bacterial Meningitis

Neurologic infection may be difficult to recognize at the extremes of life. In very young infants and occasionally in the aged, the typical signs of meningeal irritation may be attenuated or absent. Subtle clues, such as irritability and poor feeding, may be the only indications of infection in infants. In elderly patients, clinical signs of bacterial meningitis may be limited to confusion, lethargy, and fever. Lumbar puncture is therefore performed earlier in such patients. In normal hosts, signs of meningitis are more typical. Meningeal irritation and altered mental status are most frequent, with headache, nausea, vomiting, and photophobia often present. Involuntary rigidity of the neck muscles resulting from meningeal irritation is a classic clinical clue to bacterial meningitis. Brudzinski's sign is positive when flexion of the neck results in involuntary knee and hip flexion. Pain and difficulty extending the knee in a supine patient in 90° thigh flexion at the hip is the classic Kernig's sign and is a strong clinical clue to meningeal irritation. Nuchal rigidity may be difficult to elicit in comatose or immunosuppressed patients and in those with diffuse neurologic impairment. Meningism may occur in patients without meningeal irritation in the presence of lobar pneumonia, septicemia, mastoiditis, cervical adenitis, cervical osteoarthritis, and peritonsillar abscess. Similarly, cervical osteoarthritis may manifest pain and suggestive neck stiffness in the elderly in the absence of meningeal irritation. Convulsions or coma occur on presentation in as many as one third of patients with bacterial meningitis. Cranial neuropathies may occur and do not necessarily reflect increased intracranial pressure (ICP) or poor prognosis, particularly when they are present early.

Non-neurologic signs may be useful during the examination of patients with suspected neurologic infection. Patients with meningococcal meningitis commonly have pleomorphic petechial lesions and large purpuric or echymotic lesions. Erythema nodosum and bullous disease as well as an evanescent morbilliform rash may also be seen in meningococcal disease but are less specific. In addition to a careful examination of the skin, the clinician should direct attention to potential primary sites of non-neurologic infections, such as pneumonia, endocarditis, otitis media, suppurative sinusitis, pyoderma, or joint infections. These foci of infection may be secondary or predisposing to bacterial meningitis and occur in as many as one third of patients with bacterial meningitis.

Epidemiologic and Clinical Clues to Specific Pathogens. Rapid institution of antimicrobials may be life- or function-sparing when managing neurologic infections. Unfortunately, Gram stain and cultures of the CSF are not always successful in the presumptive identification of pathogens. A careful assessment of epidemiologic and clinical clues may help to narrow the field of potential pathogens to a workable few and allow a rational selection of antimicrobials.

HAEMOPHILUS INFLUENZAE, which accounts for 10,000 cases in the United States each year, is the most frequent cause of bacterial meningitis. Passively acquired maternal antibodies protect the neonate until immunity begins to wane at approximately 3 months of age. This risk persists until approximately age 6, when active immunity begins to provide some protection. Exceptions may exist when additional risk factors are superimposed upon the age factor. *H. influenzae* meningitis may occur in adults, but is rarely in epidemic form and usually preceded by a defect in humoral immunity, asplenia, or suppurative sinus disease. Higher incidence has been reported in Eskimos, Navajo Indians, and blacks. Crowding and low socioeconomic status may result in higher risk, but have yet to be established. Peak incidence of the disease follows a spring and fall distribution except in the southern states, where winter is the predominant season.

NEISSERIA MENINGITIDIS infection is most common in the very young and decreases in frequency through young adulthood; by age 45, it causes less than 10% of meningitis. Although large epidemics continue to occur in other parts of the world, only sporadic and small clusters have been reported in the United States over the past four decades. The majority of cases are caused by serogroup B, which is not well covered by available vaccines. Each serogroup has characteristic although loosely overlapping clinical patterns, with serogroups A and C associated with epidemic disease and meningococcemia, serogroup B with sporadic disease, and serogroup Y with pulmonary disease. Studies in military recruit populations have proven that crowding and pharyngeal carriage rates are not related to epidemics. The presence of petechiae should alert the clinician to the possibility of *N. meningitidis,* since these lesions are present in half of such cases but are unusual with other pathogens. Similiar rashes occur uncommonly with enteroviral disease, and if meningism is present may lead to antibiotic therapy while awaiting cultures. Approximately 5% of cases present with fulminant meningococcemia, often progressing to shock and death before CSF abnormalities are detected. Although uncommon, an unusual alteration of mental status may occur during *N. meningitidis* meningitis, characterized by stimulated, manic behavior. A high frequency of joint involvement is reported, and serositis is frequent with articular, pericardial, and tendon sheath inflammation appearing after the first week of disease. Recurrent disease due to this pathogen is extremely uncommon, in contrast to the pneumococcus, which is often associated with recurrences. Patients with a deficiency of the terminal components of complement (C5-8) and immunoglobulin A are susceptible to fulminant meningococcemia.

STREPTOCOCCUS PNEUMONIAE (pneumococcus) usually causes meningitis in the normal host only at the extremes of life. The peak incidence is under age 1 and over age 50. Over half of cases have an antecedent suppurative focus of infection of the sinuses, ear, or lung. Risk factors include asplenia, humoral immunity deficit, and dural tears, particularly when contiguous to a sinus. Recurrence in such patients is not uncommon. Because of the intense inflammation and dense exudative process associated with infections caused by this organism, coma, seizure, and focal neurologic signs are more common early in the disease and may result in a higher rate of morbid sequelae.

GRAM-NEGATIVE ROD (GNR) meningitis is often hospital acquired and may occur in the setting of head trauma, recent neurosurgery, or other procedures involving breach of the dura. Neonates and granulocytopenic patients are at particular risk of GNR meningitis, as are patients with ventricular shunts and other remote sites of GNR infection such as pyelonephritis. Other risk factors are parameningeal foci of infection, trauma, chronic debilitated status, and advanced age. The clinical presentation of GNR meningitis is different from that associated with other pathogens. Meningeal signs may be minimal in the debilitated, chronically ill, and elderly or very young patients who are more frequently affected. Cervical arthritis in the elderly may obscure the presence of meningism. These factors have led to an aggressive approach to lumbar puncture in patients with neurologic signs and the above risk factors.

Aseptic Meningitis

Presenting symptoms and signs of nonbacterial meningitis may be indistinguishable from those of bacterial meningitis. In general, however, patients are less ill, with lower fever and a less toxic appearance. Headache is often severe in adults, whereas confusion, lethargy, and lassitude may dominate the clinical picture in children. Many infectious and noninfectious diseases may present with the aseptic meningitis syndrome. Notable among these are partially treated bacterial meningitis, leptospirosis, Lyme disease, lymphogranuloma venereum, syphilis, tuberculosis, fungal disease, and collagen vascular diseases.

Viral meningitis occurs throughout the year but is more common during the summer and fall months, thus mimicking the seasonality of the enteroviruses, which are the most common cause. Bacterial meningitis is more common during the winter and spring months. Either may occur throughout the year, however. Viral prodrome often precedes the aseptic meningitis complication and may provide valuable clues to the specific cause. Antecedent parotitis may suggest mumps, or a morbilliform rash during a measles epidemic may presage a complicating meningitis or encephalitis. In the final analysis, even the best clinical and epidemiologic clues are insufficient to distinguish bacterial meningitis from septic meningitis, and the clinician must resort to CSF examination and culture.

SUSPECTED CNS INFECTION WITH FOCAL NEUROLOGIC SIGNS

The presence of focal neurologic signs or papilledema suggests that an intracranial mass lesion is present. In such cases, the clinician should consider delaying lumbar puncture until a CT scan can be performed to rule out cerebral edema or mass effect and thus eliminate the possibility of uncal herniation. Rapid neurologic deterioration and even death may occur following lumbar puncture in 25% of patients with intracranial abscess. When meningeal signs are present and neurodiagnostic studies are judged necessary, therapy should not be delayed for the performance of CT scans or lumbar punctures. A single dose of a well-selected antibiotic may be lifesaving and should not be delayed beyond the first hour after presentation. Cultures of the CSF are not substantially affected by a single dose of intravenous antibiotic. Careful examination should be performed to detect remote foci of infection that may have seeded a brain abscess or subdural empyema. Examination of the sinuses and ear canals may disclose infection contiguous to intracranial suppuration.

Spinal Epidural Abscess

Epidural abscess is an uncommon problem, and the diagnosis is often delayed or missed entirely. A high index of suspicion is essential because fewer than one fourth of cases are suspected on admission. Typical presenting findings are fever, malaise, and back pain. The vague and non-specific nature of these early clues often leads the clinician to consider a viral or self-limited process. Progression of the infection is followed by persistent spinal pain, nerve root pain, and eventually weakness and anesthesia, with sphincter control deficits. The duration of back pain before diagnosis is highly variable but averages 16 days (range, 2–42 days). Nerve root pain is present in more than 90% of patients and, although it may be a presenting finding, it usually follows the onset of persistent spinal ache by 2 to 3 days.

Spread may occur from local contiguous foci such as decubiti or vertebral osteomyelitis, or may be a local consequence of recent spinal surgery. In such cases, gram-negative pathogens are somewhat more common. The mode of spread in 25% to 50% of cases is hematogenous from a remote suppurative focus. Cutaneous infections are most common, followed by urinary tract infections, sepsis, pneumonia, and infected intravenous catheters. Approximately three fourths of patients have clinical or historical evidence of an antecedent infection when spinal epidural abscess is diagnosed. *Staphylococcus aureus* is overwhelmingly the most common cause of spinal epidural abscess, accounting for 69% to 90% of cases. Gram-negative pathogens and a variety of opportunistic pathogens occur but are much less likely. In some parts of the world, *Mycobacterium tuberculosis* is very common, but it accounts for less than 25% of epidural abscesses in the United States. The indolent nature of tuberculous disease renders it less of a surgical emergency, and medical cures are the rule. Alternate diagnostic possibilities to be considered include disc herniation, acute transverse myelitis, inflammatory joint disease, and neoplasm.

When the typical clinical picture suggests the diagnosis, immediate evaluation is necessary. Plain radiographs of the affected area may show evidence of vertebral osteomyelitis, which is accompanied by epidural abscess in approximately 20% of cases. A negative study is not helpful in that delayed evidence of osteomyelitis is characteristic and paravertebral mass is often not apparent. Myelography is almost always abnormal and is the procedure of choice to document the process. The role of CT scanning and magnetic resonance imaging (MRI) is increasing but has yet to be established. Cerebrospinal fluid typically shows an increased protein, a mild polymorphonuclear pleocytosis (often less than 150), and a normal glucose.

Once documented, a spinal epidural abscess is a neurosurgical emergency. Antibiotic therapy without drainage is ineffective. Presumptive antistaphylococcal therapy should be initiated preoperatively with nafcillin and maintained for 3 to 4 weeks or longer, if appropriate to the management of any associated infection. When vertebral osteomyelitis or bacterial endocarditis is present, 6 to 8 weeks of parenteral therapy should be given. Antibiotics should be altered for optimal coverage when the definitive microbiologic diagnosis is made.

Cranial Epidural Abscess

This process is similar to spinal epidural abscess but is much less common. Spread from infected sinuses or orbital infection is the usual cause, but abscess may follow trauma, neurosurgery, or other CNS infection. Subdural empyema is commonly present and usually accounts for any observed neurologic deficits. The role of CT scanning is better documented in cranial epidural abscess and has replaced cerebral angiography as the diagnostic procedure of choice.

Subdural Empyema

Accumulation of pus in the space between the dura and the arachnoid often arises by direct extension from infections of the paranasal sinuses or middle ear or from osteomyelitis. Frontal sinusitis with or without cranial osteomyelitis is a predisposing factor in as many as three fourths of cases of nontraumatic subdural empyema. Presenting signs and symptoms result from increased intracranial pressure, meningeal irritation, or surrounding cortical inflammation at the site of the empyema. Meningeal signs are present in 80% of patients and focal neurologic findings in 80% to 90%. The clinical presentation may be dominated by complications, such as brain abscess or cortical vein thrombosis. The technique of choice for documenting subdural empyema is CT scanning, but multiple case reports and small series have documented a small proportion of false-negative CT scans in subdural empyema. The microbiology is similar to that of chronic sinusitis or brain abscess, with streptococci, staphylococci, anaerobic streptococci, and gram-negative rods commonly present. A combination of medical and surgical therapy is required for a successful outcome. A recent large series documents that craniotomy results in a higher success rate than drainage through burr holes. Empirical antibiotic coverage may be instituted with penicillin G or, alternatively, with chloramphenicol, but is adjusted to specific therapy based on culture and sensitivity reports when available.

Brain Abscess

Brain abscess is an uncommon infection that occurs about one fifth as often as bacterial meningitis. Diagnosis can be challenging because many patients are afebrile and have an indolent clinical course that may not suggest the presence of infection or brain abscess. Mortality from brain abscess was once high, and even into the antibiotic era death rates of 40% to 60% were reported. Dramatic reductions in mortality, however, have resulted since the introduction of better imaging techniques for intracranial disease. Drainage procedures guided by CT have provided earlier microbiologic diagnosis and more effective drainage of intracranial suppuration.

Brain abscess may arise from direct contiguous spread from nearby infection or from hematogenous spread from a remote site of infection. Direct spread is often from a nearby extracerebral site of infection, such as frontal sinusitis or mastoiditis, and these lesions are commonly located in the frontal or temporal lobes. In contrast, brain abscess arising from hematogenous spread is often in the distribution of the middle cerebral artery. Typical underlying infections for hematogenous spread include bacterial endocarditis, pneumonia, or skin and soft tissue infections. Patients with congenital heart disease and right-to-left shunting or pulmonary arteriovenous fistulae are more likely to have brain abscesses from hematogenous spread because the pulmonary vascular bed is bypassed. Abdominal or pelvic infections seldom lead to brain abscesses. Increased recognition of brain abscess in the immunocompromised host over the past two decades is a result of better imaging techniques and higher prevalence resulting from immunosuppression. In these patients, *Nocardia asteroides,* phycomycoses, *Cryptococcus neoformans, Toxoplasma gondii, Candida* species, and other opportunistic pathogens should be considered in addition to usual brain abscess pathogens. Because of an increased likelihood of brain abscess in immunocompromised patients with meningitis, these patients should receive early consideration for brain imaging studies.

Patients with brain abscess will often have a short duration of symptoms. The most common presentation is severe headache, alterations of mood or consciousness, irritability, confusion, and nausea and vomiting of less than 2 weeks duration. Fever is present in approximately half of patients with brain abscess and is less common in adults and the elderly. In about two thirds of patients, a clue to the origin will be apparent at the time of initial diagnosis.

Once the diagnosis of brain abscess is suspected, a brain imaging technique, such as radionuclide scan or CT scans should be performed to determine the extent of cerebral edema and the size and position of the lesion. Cerebrospinal fluid examination by lumbar puncture should not be done because of an enhanced risk of complications with increased ICP. Further, CSF is not generally helpful in the diagnosis of brain abscess because it merely reflects changes characteristic of a parameningeal focus of infection and often will not contain the causative pathogens. Only after midline shifts, large lesions, and cerebral edema have been excluded by CT scanning should a lumbar puncture be performed. The CT scan may become positive early in the course of brain abscess, before the development of encapsulated suppuration. This "cerebritis" stage of brain abscess may be amenable to antibiotic therapy and may not require surgical drainage.

Surgical or CT-guided drainage of the necrotic and purulent material is essential for an effective cure. Better imaging techniques have produced earlier diagnoses, and some literature reflects adequate management with antibiotics alone in the cerebritis stage. In carefully selected patients who pose a high surgical risk, antibiotics alone may be curative when given in high doses over long periods. These cases are an exception to the rule that drainage of purulent material is required. Antibiotic therapy should include coverage for anaerobes as well as aerobes, since anaerobes are present in approximately half of cases of brain abscess. Intravenous penicillin and chloramphenicol should be administered in divided doses when brain abscess is documented. If *S. aureus* is suspected because of penetrating head injury or occurrence of brain abscess following craniotomy, a penicillinase-resistant penicillin, such as oxacillin or nafcillin, should be substituted for penicillin G. Antibiotic therapy should be maintained for a minimum of 3 to 4 weeks unless management of an underlying infection, such as endocarditis or osteomyelitis, requires longer treatment.

Prognosis is determined partly by the extent of underlying disease, delay in diagnosis and drainage, and age of the patient. Mortality has declined dramatically from 60% in the 1960s and earlier to under 20% during the present era of high suspicion and early diagnosis.

Herpes Encephalitis

Herpes encephalitis in the adult is caused by herpesvirus hominis (HVH) type I and occasionally type II, and is the most common fatal encephalitis in the United States. Neonatal encephalitis is most often caused by type II HVH acquired during passage through an infected birth canal. Adults typically present with a subacute febrile syndrome characterized by headache and altered mentation. Focal neurologic findings and seizure are present in 70% of cases.

Presumptive diagnosis can be made with a combination of CT scan, EEG, and CSF examinations, but definitive diagnosis requires biopsy of affected brain tissue. Typically, CSF shows elevated opening pressures, moderate pleocytosis (50–500 lymphocytes), normal glucose, and elevated protein. Some reports have suggested that the presence of red cells in the CSF, in the right clinical setting, indicates herpes encephalitis, but this has not borne up under careful scrutiny. Completely normal CSF is seen in a small minority of cases. Serology for herpes antibodies in CSF is too insensitive and results are too long delayed to be clinically useful. The EEG and CT scan are abnormal in 80% and 60% of cases, respectively, but alone are insufficient to establish a definitive diagnosis. The combination of clinical findings and neurodiagnostic studies was correct in only 57% of cases entered into a large cooperative study, emphasizing the need for biopsy. Brain biopsy has proven a safe and effective method of establishing the diagnosis. Much debate has focused on the need for biopsy in the current era of safe and relatively effective therapy. The need to exclude other potentially treatable diseases is the most compelling reason to proceed with a diagnostic biopsy.

Dramatic improvement in therapy of herpes encephalitis has reduced morbidity and mortality. Recent trials have proven acyclovir to be superior to adenine-arabinoside; acyclovir in a dose of 10 mg/kg every 8 hours for 10 days is now the treatment of choice. Mortality of less than 20% and morbid sequelae of less than 50% can now be expected in a disease that was once fatal in 70% of cases, with high survivor morbidity.

For more information, please see Chapter 102 in Civetta JM, Taylor RW, Kirby RR: Critical Care. *Philadelphia: J. B. Lippincott, 1988*

BIBLIOGRAPHY

Boor V, Paulson OB, Rasmussen N: Pneumococcal Meningitis: Late neurologic sequelae and features of prognostic impact. *Arch Neurol* 1984; 41:1045

Cherubin CE, Eng RHK: Experience with the use of cefotaxime in the treatment of bacterial meningitis. *Am J Med* 1986; 80:398

Cherubin CE, Mar JS, Sierra MF, et al: Listeria and gram negative bacillary meningitis in New York City; 1972–1979: Frequent cases of meningitis in adults. *Am J Med* 1981; 71:199

Hodges GR, Perkins RL: Hospital associated bacterial meningitis. *Am J Med Sci* 1976; 271:335

Kaplan K: Brain abscess. *Med Clin North Am* 1985; 69:345

Kennedy DH, Fallon RJ: Tuberculous meningitis. *JAMA* 1979; 241:264

Spagnuolo PJ, Elnor JJ, Lerner PI, et al: Hemophilus influenzae meningitis: The spectrum of disease in adults. *Medicine* 1982; 61:74

Tauber MG, Sande MA: Principles in the treatment of bacterial meningitis. *Am J Med* 1984; 76:224

Whitley RJ, Alfred CA, Hirsch MS, et al: Herpes simplex encephalitis: Adenine arabinoside versus acyclovir therapy. *N Engl J Med* 1986; 314:144

Whitley RJ, Soong SJ, Linnemann C, et al: Herpes simplex encephalitis: Clinical assessment. *JAMA* 1982; 274:317

55 Guillain–Barré Syndrome

Guillain–Barré syndrome is one of the most common neurologic disorders that can cause a previously healthy person to develop, over a course of several days to weeks, complete muscle paralysis and respiratory failure. The syndrome became a household word following the National Influenza Immunization Program of 1976 when over 1000 cases were reported. Persons who received the A/New Jersey/76 (swine) influenza vaccine had an increased incidence of Guillain–Barré syndrome—approximately 5 to 6 times that of unvaccinated people. An estimated 10 cases for every 1 million persons vaccinated occurred in the 10 to 12 weeks following vaccination. Younger patients (<25 years) appeared to have a lower relative risk and a lower case fatality rate. Subsequent national influenza vaccination programs have not been associated with an increased risk of developing Guillain–Barré syndrome.

PATHOGENESIS

The cause of Guillain–Barré syndrome is unknown. However, a growing body of evidence has implicated both humoral and cellular immune factors. Most patients have a history of a recent viral prodrome or some other event in the several weeks preceding onset of paralysis, although the relationship between the antecedent events and the pathogenesis of Guillain–Barré syndrome remains unclear. Examination of biopsied and postmortem neural tissue typically shows inflammatory lesions throughout the peripheral nervous system, consisting of lymphocyte and macrophage invasion of the myelin sheaths with segmental demyelination. Although cranial nerve lesions are common, central nervous system demyelination has not been noted. Support for humorally mediated demyelination comes from the observation that injection of cell-free serum from patients into rat sciatic nerve produces demyelinated lesions similar to those seen in Guillain–Barré syndrome. Antibodies to peripheral nerve tissue and myelin have been isolated from patients with Guillain–Barré syndrome, although their specificity and correlation with disease activity remain uncertain. Circulating immune complexes have been identified in some patients.

Although myelin destruction predominates, severe cases are associated with axonal disruption and wallerian degeneration. Electrodiagnostic studies which disclose evidence of primarily axonal destruction (*i.e.*, fibrillations, positive sharp waves) predict a prolonged course with residual neurologic impairment.

Similar pathologic lesions have been noted in the autonomic nervous system and seem to correlate with the autonomic derangements that may complicate the clinical course.

EPIDEMIOLOGY

Since the epidemic of Guillain–Barré syndrome following the National Influenza Immunization Program of 1976, the annual reported incidence in the United States and Europe has been 0.6 to 1.9 per 100,000 population. The disorder may occur at any age, with no discernible geographic or seasonal distributions. Most cases are sporadic, although infrequent clusters have been identified. A usually minor respiratory or gastrointestinal infection within the previous 8 weeks is present in approximately 65% of affected patients. Approximately 25% of patients ultimately require mechanical ventilation for periods ranging from several weeks to over 1 year. With meticulous intensive supportive care, the case fatality rate has been reduced to approximately 5%. Full recovery is the rule, although up to 15% of patients experience residual neurologic deficit and 5% of survivors are severely disabled.

CLINICAL FEATURES

The clinical presentation may be variable and patients may not always fit the "typical case" description. The presence of a preceding viral syndrome is common, but is not essential to the diagnosis. Initial symptoms are often sensory, consisting of paresthesias, dysesthesias, and neuritic-type pain. Patients may initially be misdiagnosed as having conversion symptoms, somatization disorder, or hysteria. The onset of objective weakness and areflexia within hours to days should alert the clinician that he or she is not dealing with functional weakness. Symmetric weakness usually begins in the lower extremities and progresses to involve muscles of the trunk, diaphragm, arms, and facial muscles. Bilateral facial paresis eventually develops in more than 50% of patients. Proximal muscle weakness is typically more prominent than distal weakness. Involvement of bulbar muscles may impair swallowing and the ability to handle secretions. Autonomic demyelination results in marked lability of the blood pressure, with rapid and unpredictable swings between hypertension and hypotension. Other autonomic manifestations include persistent facial flushing, urinary retention, tachydysrhythmias and bradydysrhythmias. Neuropathic lesions in the afferent limb of the baroreceptor system may lead to the syndrome of inappropriate antidiuretic hormone secretion (SIADH) and resulting hyponatremia. Extreme elevations in CSF protein (> 1500 mg/dl) have been associated with symptoms of increased intracranial pressure (ICP) and clinical papilledema. Occasional patients have evidence of mild glomerulonephritis manifested as transient proteinuria—sometimes in the nephrotic range. In the usual case, maximum neurologic deficit is reached within 2 to 3 weeks, followed by stabilization and gradual recovery over weeks to months.

Several clinical variants of the syndrome have been identified, including opthalmoplegia, ataxia, and areflexia (Miller Fisher syndrome); "descending paralysis," with ocular, facial, and pharyngeal paresis occurring before limb paresis; instances of almost pure respiratory muscle failure; and pure dysautonomic syndromes.

Occasional patients seemingly recover from the acute paralysis but then suffer a relapse of paresis with a subsequent protracted course. Other patients may have a progressive course following the initial attack of Guillain–Barré syndrome. These syndromes are referred to as chronic relapsing polyneuropathy and differ from acute demyelinating polyneuropathy in that the chronic form appears more responsive to prednisone therapy. The chronic relapsing syndrome has been associated with neurofibromatosis and HLA-Aw30 and HLA-Aw31.

TREATMENT

The most immediate threat to life of the patient with Guillain–Barré syndrome is respiratory failure from intercostal and diaphragmatic muscle paralysis. Patients may often "look good," only to suffer precipitous respiratory arrest because the extent of weakness has not been appreciated. Arterial blood gas monitoring is worthwhile, but it should be emphasized that hypoxemia and hypercapnia are late findings and indicate that respiratory arrest is imminent. Tracheal intubation should not be delayed until there is evidence of deteriorating blood gases. Respiratory reserve is best monitored by serial determinations of forced vital capacity and negative inspiratory pressure at least every 2 hours until stabilization. Elective intubation should be performed when the vital capacity approaches 15 ml/kg (approximately 1 liter in the average adult) or sooner if there is associated pharyngeal paresis and difficulty handling secretions. As the vital capacity drops further, the ability to effectively cough and clear secretions is impaired, resulting in atelectasis and ventilation–perfusion mismatch producing hypoxemia. Hypercapnia usually occurs after the appearance of hypoxemia when the bellows function of the diaphragm and intercostal muscles is lost. Failure to intubate early in the course may result in the need for emergency intubation under suboptimal conditions, thereby causing unnecessary risk to the patient. Once the patient is intubated, it is unnecessary to proceed to immediate tracheotomy. Some patients may recover within several days to 2 weeks, obviating the need for tracheotomy. If after 10 to 14 days the patient shows no signs of imminent recovery, tracheotomy should be considered. On the other hand, if the patient has been steadily gaining strength, one might choose to wait several more days before proceeding with tracheotomy.

Meticulous attention to monitoring the patient and the ventilator is essential to avoiding mechanical mishaps that can result in death. The ventilator must be equipped with monitors for volume and pressure changes, and should have audible alarms to detect disconnection from the patient. The alarms should be checked daily to ensure they are working. Remember, a paralyzed patient with a tube through the vocal cords cannot call for help.

Frequent chest physiotherapy, tracheal suction, and turning help reduce the risk of nosocomial pneumonia. However, the incidence of acquired pneumonia in Guillain–Barré syndrome patients remains high and should be anticipated. Prophylactic antibiotics are not advised; when pulmonary infiltrates and fever develop, empirical antibiotic therapy should be started pending the results of Gram stains, cultures, and sensitivities. The initial choice of antibiotics should be based on the likely pathogens and sensitivity patterns unique to the particular hospital.

Frequent turning (every 2 hours) decreases the risk of skin breakdown and decubitus formation. Attention should be paid to limb positioning to avoid compressive neuropathies—particularly around the ulnar and peroneal nerves. Physical therapy should be initiated to prevent contractures, foot drop, and muscle atrophy.

Autonomic dysfunction usually responds to the appropriate pharmacologic agents (*i.e.*, α-blockers and β-blockers for severe hypertension). The development of asystole or advanced degrees of heart block may require emergency insertion of a temporary transvenous pacemaker.

Neuritic pain in the limbs and back is common and may respond to quinine or tricyclic antidepressants. Small doses of codeine may occasionally be required to obtain adequate analgesia.

Adequate nutrition must be maintained to avoid a catabolic state and help reduce the risk of infection. Sufficient calories can usually be given through the enteral route (a small silastic feeding tube or gastrostomy). Occasionally, autonomic derangements are of sufficient severity to result in ileus and inability to effectively use the gastrointestinal tract for feeding. Parenteral nutrition may initially be started through a peripheral vein; if gastrointestinal dysfunction is persistent, long term central hyperalimentation should be utilized.

Lower extremity thromboembolism and pulmonary embolism are significant risks in the bedridden paralyzed patient. In addition, anticardiolipin antibody has been reported in patients with Guillain–Barré syndrome which may further increase the risk of thrombosis. Compressive pneumatic boots have been advocated but may result in pressure neuropathy of the peroneal nerve as it crosses the fibular head. Since pulmonary emboli have occurred in some patients treated with fixed-dose subcutaneous heparin, it may be preferable to use adjusted-dose subcutaneous heparin (adjusting the dose to maintain a 6-hour postdose PTT in the upper 5 seconds of control). Alternatively, warfarin may be employed to maintain a prothrombin time in the range of 1.25 to 1.5 times control.

The use of plasmapheresis in acute Guillain–Barré syndrome has generally shown favorable results, although its exact role is still somewhat controversial. At the present time, plasmapheresis should probably be reserved for patients with acute-onset progressively worsening weakness. There is little evidence that patients with mild weakness or those in whom the clinical state has improved or plateaued for more than 1 week will benefit from plasmapheresis.

Corticosteroid therapy (*i.e.*, prednisone) has not been convincingly shown to alter the course and may even by detrimental. Certain patients with the chronic relapsing variant of polyneuropathy may, however, benefit from steroids or other immunosuppressive therapy.

Depression and psychological aberrations related to the "locked-in" syndrome are common. Patients should be frequently reassured that the outlook for full recovery is good. An optimistic and emphatic attitude on the part of the physician and nursing staff is of inestimable value in this regard.

For more information, please see Chapter 104 in Civetta JM, Taylor RW, Kirby RR: Critical Care. *Philadelphia: J. B. Lippincott, 1988*

BIBLIOGRAPHY

Harrison BM, Hansen LA, Pollard JD, et al: Demyelination induced by serum from patients with Guillain–Barré syndrome. *Ann Neurol* 1984; 15:163

Mendell JR, Kissel JT, Kennedy MS, et al: Plasma exchange and prednisone in Guillain–Barré syndrome: A controlled randomized trial. *Neurol* 1985; 35:1551

Moore P, James O: Guillain–Barré syndrome: Incidence, management and outcome of major complications. *Crit Care Med* 1981; 9:549

O'Donohue WJ, Baker JP, Bell GM, et al: Respiratory failure in neuromuscular disease—Management in a respiratory intensive care unit. *JAMA* 1976; 235:733

Ropper AH: Severe acute Guillain–Barré syndrome. *Neurol* 1986; 36:429

Ropper AH, Keline SM: Guillain–Barré syndrome: Management of respiratory failure. *Neurol* 1985; 35:1662

56 Myasthenia Gravis

Myasthenia gravis is an autoimmune neuromuscular disorder characterized by fatigability and weakness of skeletal muscles resulting from decreased availability of acetylcholine receptors in the postsynaptic membrane. It is an uncommon disease with an estimated prevalence of approximately 1 per 20,000 population. Neither race nor geographic area appears related to the incidence of the disorder. Although myasthenia gravis is rare before the second decade of life, it may occur at any age. There is a markedly different age of peak onset between the sexes. Women appear to have a peak age of onset in young adulthood (third or fourth decade), whereas among men the onset tends to be later in life (sixth and seventh decades). Among young adults with myasthenia gravis there is a female preponderance of approximately 2:1, whereas there is a slight male preponderance among elderly patients.

As yet undetermined genetic factors may play a predisposing role in the pathogenesis of myasthenia gravis. There is an increased incidence of HLA-B8 in young female patients who have thymic hyperplasia. In elderly males with thymoma, there is no increased incidence of HLA-B8 but the incidence of HLA-A2, HLA-A3, and HLA-A7 is increased. Transient neonatal weakness has been noted in 10% to 20% of infants born to mothers who have myasthenia gravis. The occurrence of neonatal weakness has not been shown to correlate with the severity of the mother's illness or with her titer of antibody to acetylcholine receptors.

PATHOGENESIS

The essential feature that leads to the skeletal muscle weakness of myasthenia gravis is decreased transmission across the neuromuscular junction because of a decreased number of acetylcholine receptors (AChRs) on the postsynaptic membrane.

Three fourths of patients with myasthenia gravis have abnormalities of the thymus gland. Of these, approximately 85% have germinal cell hyperplasia (typically, young female patients) and the remaining 15% have gross or microscopic thymomas (typically, elderly male patients). Although the relationship of thymic abnormalities to the etiology of the disease is uncertain, thymectomy has become an accepted form of therapy for adolescents and young adults with generalized disease and for all patients with thymoma. Patients with ocular myasthenia gravis, children, and elderly patients represent more controversial treatment groups. Thymectomy may be expected to produce clinical remission or significant improvement in up to 70% of patients, although benefits may not be apparent for a year or more. Initiating factors that trigger B lymphocytes to produce anti-AChRabs and the precise role of the thymus gland in the pathogenesis of the disease remain to be elucidated.

A number of other autoimmune diseases have been associated with myasthenia gravis, particularly thyroid disease, which may be present in up to 10% of patients. The incidences of rheumatoid arthritis, systemic lupus erythematosus, and pernicious anemia also appear to be increased. Numerous autoantibodies, including antinuclear antibodies, antiparietal cell antibodies, and antithyroglobulin antibodies, may be found in the serum of patients with myasthenia gravis. Antibodies to striated muscle have been particularly associated with thymoma.

The autoimmune nature of chronic graft-versus-host disease, which develops in up to 30% of long-term survivors following allogeneic bone marrow transplant, may predispose to the formation of antibodies to acetylcholine receptors and subsequent development of clinical myasthenia gravis.

Penicillamine, a drug commonly used to treat rheumatoid arthritis and Wilson's disease, has been associated with the development of clinical myasthenia and the formation of anti-AChR antibody. Withdrawal of the drug results in clinical improvement of weakness and decreased titers of anti-ACh antibody.

CLINICAL FEATURES

The dominant feature of myasthenia gravis is progressive weakness of certain muscles when used repetitively, with partial recovery following a period of rest. The disease usually develops insidiously over a period of weeks to months, although explosive onset with rapid generalized weakness is occasionally seen. At first, the attacks of weakness are transient and may resolve with a good night's rest. Unilateral or bilateral ptosis and diplopia are the usual initial complaints, reflecting predominant involvement of the extraocular muscles. Up to 20% of patients have disease confined to the eye muscles and are said to have "ocular myasthenia." Any weakness of muscle groups in addition to the extraocular muscles is referred to as "generalized myasthenia." If generalized progression does not occur within several years, it is unlikely to occur at all. Involvement of bulbar muscles may manifest as weakness of the jaw muscles while chewing food, with inability to retract the corners of the mouth leading to a peculiar transverse, snarling smile ("myasthenic facies"). Weakness of the pharyngeal and laryngeal muscles may cause a nasal, garbled-sounding voice with reduced volume on prolonged talking. Regurgitation of swallowed liquids through the nose may be reported. Involvement of the arm, leg, and trunk muscles may occur asymmetrically in any combination. Typically, proximal muscle weakness is more prominent than distal weakness. Weakness may not be apparent in the well-rested patient, but can usually be elicited with repetitive exercise (e.g., ptosis following sustained upward gaze). Patients with extensive involvement may be weak even at rest. Muscle atrophy is rare but is occasionally seen in older patients. The remainder of the physical examination is usually normal.

DIAGNOSIS

Confirmation of the clinical diagnosis of myasthenia gravis is aided by use of the edrophonium test and EMG. Edrophonium is a short-acting acetylcholinesterase inhibitor that allows a build-up of acetylcholine in the neuromuscular junction, thereby improving motor strength in the myasthenic patient. Before administering edrophonium, baseline testing of muscle strength is performed. Edrophonium (10 mg per 1-ml ampule) is withdrawn into a syringe and 2 mg is administered through a previously established intravenous catheter. Muscle strength is retested after approximately 30 seconds, with particular attention to respiratory function (measuring vital capacity or negative inspiratory pressure), swallowing, extremity strength, and oculomotor function. If no improvement has occurred, the remaining 8 mg of edrophonium is injected. A definite improvement in strength that occurs within 1 minute and lasts several minutes strongly supports a diagnosis of myasthenia gravis. If functional weakness is a possibility, the test should also be performed using an injectable saline control. Pretreatment with atropine (0.5–1.0 mg) may help block distressing muscarinic side-effects. Occasional patients with myasthenia may show an ambiguous response to edrophonium—particuarly those with limited ocular myasthenia. If the diagnosis remains uncertain, a low-dose curare test may be considered.

TREATMENT

Patients with myasthenia gravis who complain of dyspnea or difficulty swallowing should be admitted to the hospital immediately. Rapid asessment of respiratory function should be carried out: if vital capacity is less than 1.0 to 1.5 liters, the patient should be transferred to an intensive care unit for close observation and possible elective intubation. Weakened facial muscles may hinder use of the spirometer, in which case a negative inspiratory pressure measurement is a good parameter to follow. One should not delay intubation if the patient has marginal respiratory compensation; it is better to perform a timely elective intubation because patients can abruptly fatigue and suffer respiratory arrest or mucus plugging from voluminous secretions. A careful search for infection is mandatory because these patients are frequently receiving immunosuppressive therapy, which increases the risk of infection. Even those patients who are not taking immunosuppressive drugs appear to be at increased risk for infection because of difficulty handling secretions and poor pulmonary toilet from weakened respiratory muscles. A frequent mistake is to delay initiation of antibiotics too long or to miss a seemingly trivial infection that may have precipitated the crisis. Although aminoglycosides may produce mild neuromuscular blockade and weakness, they can be used if indicated based on the likely source of infection (or on sensitivity reports).

Patients with respiratory failure should have a clear airway maintained with repeated gentle suction, postural drainage, and periodic inflations with intermittent positive-pressure breathing to prevent segmental atelectasis and hypostatic pneumonia. Incentive spirometry may cause respiratory muscle fatigue and should be avoided. If mechanical ventilation is required, anticholinesterase drugs should be withdrawn for 72 to 96 hours. A "drug holiday" may restore the effectiveness of anticholinesterases when they are restarted. Plasmapheresis should be considered for patients in myasthenic crisis—especially in conjunction with the initiation of immunosuppressive therapy with corticosteroids or azathioprine. Plasmapheresis may also be useful in preparing patients for thymectomy and as an adjunct to initiating immunosuppressive therapy to effect more rapid improvement. Refractory cases have also been treated with high-dose intravenous immunoglobulin (400 mg/kg/day for 5 days) with favorable outcome, although confirmation of these results must await completion of a randomized, double-blind, placebo-controlled trial. The use of pulse therapy with high-dose methylprednisolone (2 g infused intravenously over 12 hours, repeated at 5-day intervals for a total of two or three doses) may also be of benefit for severely ill patients in myasthenic crisis. Pulse therapy appears to produce less initial worsening and more rapid improvement in severely affected patients than conventional doses of prednisone. Further studies should be awaited before widespread use is adopted in myasthenic crises.

If elective surgery is required in a patient with myasthenia gravis, oral anticholinesterase medication may be stopped and the equivalent dose given by intravenous infusion (*e.g.*, 1 mg neostigmine IV is equivalent to 60 mg pyridostigmine PO). The amount of neostigmine required should be infused over a period that approximates the oral dosing interval (*e.g.*, pyridostigmine 60 mg PO every 4 hours may be given as neostigmine 1 mg IV infusion over each 4 hours). Intravenous methylprednisolone may be substituted for oral prednisone in a dose equivalent to the "on" day if the patient has been on alternate-day steroids. Curare-like muscle relaxants should not be used.

For more information, please see Chapter 105 in Civetta JM, Taylor RW, Kirby RR: Critical Care. *Philadelphia: J. B. Lippincott, 1988*

BIBLIOGRAPHY

Arsura EL, Bick A, Brunner NG, et al: High-dose intravenous immunoglobulin in the management of myasthenia gravis. *Arch Intern Med* 1986; 146:1365

Arsura EL, Brunner NG, Namba T, et al: High-dose intravenous methylprednisolone in myasthenia gravis. *Arch Neurol* 1985; 42:1149

Drachman DB: Myasthenia gravis (two-part series). *N Engl J Med* 1978; 298:136, 193

Drachman DB, Adams RN, Josifek LF, et al: Functional activities of autoantibodies to acetylcholine receptors and the clinical severity of myasthenia gravis. *N Engl J Med* 1982; 307:760

Mann JD, Johns TR, Campa JF: Long-term administration of corticosteroids in myasthenia gravis. *Neurology* 1976; 26:729

Rowland LP: Controversies about the treatment of myasthenia gravis. *J Neurol Neurosurg Psychiatry* 1980; 43:644

Seybold ME: Myasthenia gravis—A clinical and basic science review. *JAMA* 1983; 250:2516

57 Monitoring of Neurologic Function

Unlike hemodynamic or respiratory function monitoring in the intensive care unit (ICU), no objective method for continuously monitoring the brain's electrical activity is widely accepted. The neurologic examination, Glasgow Coma Score (GCS), and standard electroencephalogram (EEG) assess the patient's neurologic status intermittently and have major limitations. Newer techniques including processed EEGs, somatosensory evoked responses (SERs), and auditory brain stem evoked responses (ABRs), popularized in the operating theater, have not yet been integrated on a regular basis in the ICU.

Prevention of secondary damage due to ischemia and hypoxia is essential. Critical threshold levels for blood pressure/flow which maintain cerebral function in a normal individual may not be appropriate for the progressively failing brain in a patient with cerebral vasospasm following a subarachnoid hemorrhage.

Maintenance of normal cerebral perfusion pressure (CPP), which is mean arterial blood pressure (MAP) minus mean intracranial pressure (ICP), over a wide range of blood pressure (autoregulation) is lost in a variety of pathologic states. Autoregulation may be disrupted in the damaged areas and in areas remote from the injury site. Moderate hypotension of little consequence in normal patients can lead to cerebral ischemia, while sudden hypertension predisposes to an abnormal increase in cerebral blood flow (CBF) and cerebral edema.

Twenty percent of the cardiac output is directed to the brain, which comprises only 2% of the adult body weight. When CBF falls below 23 ml/100 g/min, a neurologic deficit results in awake monkeys. If it decreases below 18 to 21 ml/100 g/min in anesthetized animals, EEG recordings are altered, while below 15 ml/100 g/min, SERs are reduced. Nevertheless, an evoked response can still be obtained when CBF is reduced by 80%. Synaptic failure may be reflected by subtle changes such as a decrease in the amplitude of the cortical SER or loss of fast EEG activity. As CBF decreases below 10 ml/100 g/min, effluxes of cellular potassium and edema formation are common. At even lower CBF levels, these abnormalities increase. If prompt action is not taken, infarction and cellular death occur, depending on the degree and duration of ischemia. Total ischemia at normal body temperature of more than 15 minutes' duration is usually associated with brain cell death. However, at least experimentally, cellular survival may be possible after as much as 2 hours of incomplete focal ischemia. Thus, absence of the EEG or cortical SERs indicates that severe ischemia is present but does not mean necessarily that cellular death has occurred. Prompt reversal of ischemia and the associated electrophysiologic abnormalities usually can be achieved by improvement of CPP. Nevertheless, an estimate of CBF based on the CPP, which generally is adequate for the normal brain, is of little help in a damaged brain with loss of autoregulation.

Irreversible brain damage may be prevented by aggressive intervention. Successful intraoperative neurologic monitoring suggests a natural extension of such techniques to the ICU for the early detection of cerebral failure due to hypotension, hypoxia, increased ICP, or mass lesions.

Direct monitoring techniques test the function of central nervous system (CNS) structures and pathways and include the neurologic examination, ABRs, SERs, and standard or processed EEG recordings. The computed tomographic (CT) scan, conversely, provides anatomic information (although functional changes often can be inferred from observed structural alterations). Blood pressure, pulse, serum electrolytes and glucose, arterial blood gas values and *p*Ha indirectly reflect the metabolic environment of the brain. Clinicians who use electrophysiologic monitoring must keep these factors, other physiologic variables, and the patient's medications in mind. A flat EEG obtained from a patient in barbiturate coma or one who is profoundly hypothermic is not indicative of brain death, but absent evoked responses strongly support such a diagnosis.

NEUROLOGIC EXAMINATION

The neurologic examination is always available for precise and frequent monitoring. However, patients' responses to verbal commands are compromised by muscle relaxants, tranquilizers, barbiturates, narcotics, and other medications, making its use unsatisfactory in many clinical circumstances. Numerous drugs given routinely in most ICUs impair cognitive function.

In trauma patients, alcoholic intoxication is a frequent predisposing factor further complicating neurologic examination. Nevertheless, a decreased level of consciousness should not be attributed to alcohol alone unless other drugs and intracranial pathology have been ruled out. A CT scan should be performed as soon as possible if the effects of alcohol obscure the neurologic examination.

"Classical" physical findings may not be present to ascertain the presence or absence of increased ICP. Cushing's triad, the association of increased ICP with systemic hypertension and bradycardia, is present less than 25% of the time even when ICP is greater than 30 mm Hg. If a value greater than 15 mm Hg is accepted as abnormal, the detection rate of under 25% is clearly unsatisfactory and has resulted in increased utilization of direct ICP monitoring.

GLASGOW COMA SCORE (SCALE)

The Glasgow Coma Score (Table 57-1) is a clinical grading system commonly used for determining severity of brain injury. Coma is defined as an inability to obey commands, speak, or open the eyes. The accepted value for severe brain injury is a GCS of 8 or less. Patients with a score of 7 or less require immediate tracheal intubation and possibly hyperventilation. A GCS of 3 is assigned to ventilator-dependent patients with no response to verbal or painful stimulation. The GCS reflects the patient's ability to process and act on information presented, and is a useful tool for assessing depth of coma and predicting outcome.

Because of the widespread use of tracheal intubation, pharmacologically induced neuromuscular paralysis, and mechanical ventilator-induced hyperventilation, the GCS can only be accurately ascertained before and after but not during such therapy.

STANDARD ELECTROENCEPHALOGRAM

The EEG reflects spontaneous and on-going electrical acitivity recorded on the surface of the scalp. Changes in the EEG are closely linked to critical thresholds in CBF but also result from altered Pa_{O_2}, temperature, and external stimulation (Table 57-2). However, standard EEG recording is not routinely

TABLE 57-1 MODIFIED GLASGOW COMA SCORE

Sign	Evaluation	Score
Eye opening	Spontaneous	4
	To speech	3
	To pain	2
	None	1
Best verbal response	Oriented	5
	Confused	4
	Inappropriate	3
	Incomprehensible	2
	None	1
Best motor response	Obeys commands	6
	Localizes pain	5
	Withdrawal to pain	4
	Flexion to pain	3
	Extension to pain	2
	None	1

TABLE 57-2 EEG ALTERATIONS

Depression	Activation
Hypoxia (Sa_{O_2} < 65%; Pa_{O_2} < 40 mm Hg)	Hyperoxia
Hypocapnia	Hypercapnia
Anesthetics	Anesthetics (*i.e.*, enflurane)
Postseizure	Stimulation
Hypotension	Seizure
Hypoglycemia	
Hypothermia	

performed in the ICU due to insufficient technical personnel, the difficulty of on-line EEG interpretation, numerous electrically induced artifacts, and drug-induced suppression of cortical activity.

COMPUTED TOMOGRAPHY

An increase of ICP or decrease of intracranial compliance is suggested when a CT scan reveals a mass lesion with a 0.5-cm or greater midline shift or encroachment on the major cerebrospinal fluid (CSF) cisterns. Absence of the basal cisterns on a CT scan is associated with high mortality, particularly when the GCS is 3 or 4. Initial CT visualization of the basal cisterns does not guarantee a good outcome, since later ischemia and hypoxia can rapidly change the prognosis. Mass lesions demonstrated in the posterior, frontal, and temporal lobes frequently are associated with brain stem compression.

INTRACRANIAL PRESSURE

The only direct assessment of ICP is obtained by measurement. Accurate monitoring of ICP depends on the type of monitor placed and the criteria used for determining abnormal values. The Richmond subarachnoid bolt is popular since it does not require brain tissue penetration or knowledge of ventricular positions. However, it requires constant attention to maintain an unobstructed pathway to the subarachnoid space. Ventriculostomy catheters may be impossible to place when cerebral edema causes shifting or collapse of the lateral ventricle system. Subdural or epidural catheters placed through a burrhole can also be used, as can implanted ICP transducers. The latter are beset by numerous technical difficulties related to calibration and stability, however, and are not widely used.

Normal ICP is less than 15 mm Hg. Prolonged uncontrollable ICP above

29 mm Hg is associated with a poor outcome. Patients may exhibit increases in ICP due to pain, suctioning, laryngoscopy, tracheal intubation, and venous obstruction related to head positioning rather than because of intracranial pathology.

In patients with an intracranial mass effect and a shift of the ventricular system, small fluctuations in ICP can produce considerable deterioration in neurologic function. Intracranial pressure reaches the phase of rapid rise prior to clinical signs of pupillary dilatation. Thus a normal ICP does not exclude a mass lesion. Monitoring of patients during the acute phase of injury when the ICP is normal is as important as later monitoring when it is uncontrollable. A high ICP suggests decreased CPP and the possibility of regional or global ischemia. As cerebral edema increases, the microvascular network around the neurons collapses and ischemia results. Intracranial compliance determinations are felt by some investigators to have greater prognostic value than the mean ICP.

EVOKED RESPONSES

Unlike EEG recordings which reflect on-going cerebral activity, evoked responses are associated with specific external stimuli. Somatosensory evoked responses commonly use median, peroneal, and posterior tibial nerve stimulation and, ideally, recordings from the peripheral nerve, dorsal spinal cord, and sensory cortex (Fig. 57-1). Auditory brain stem evoked responses use cochlear nerve stimulation and recording of brain stem transmission.

Auditory evoked responses are particularly useful to predict an unfavorable outcome in head trauma patients as well as in other patients being assessed for brain death. Otologic pathology occurring with bilateral basilar skull fracture may account for absence of a response despite intact brain stem function.

If the ABRs demonstrate brain stem function, a nuclear cerebral perfusion scan will document CBF. In the late stages of cerebral failure, blood flow may be present only in the saggital sinus, but this finding does not establish brain death. A well-formed ABR is strong evidence for brain stem function, even in the absence of brain stem reflexes.

In the SER pathway (see Figure 57-1), a recordable Erb's point following median nerve stimulation reflects intact peripheral nerve conduction. A more central SER recorded over the cervical area (CII) demonstrates intact cervical conduction (spinal cord dorsal columns). Finally, a normal cortical SER indicates that conduction through the brain stem to the cortex is present. A recordable Erb's point in a patient without demonstrable cervical pathology and with no brain stem and cortical SERs supports a diagnosis of absent brain stem and cortical function. Lack of EEG activity, except in the setting of pharmacologic sedation or hypothermia, further substantiates the diagnosis of brain death.

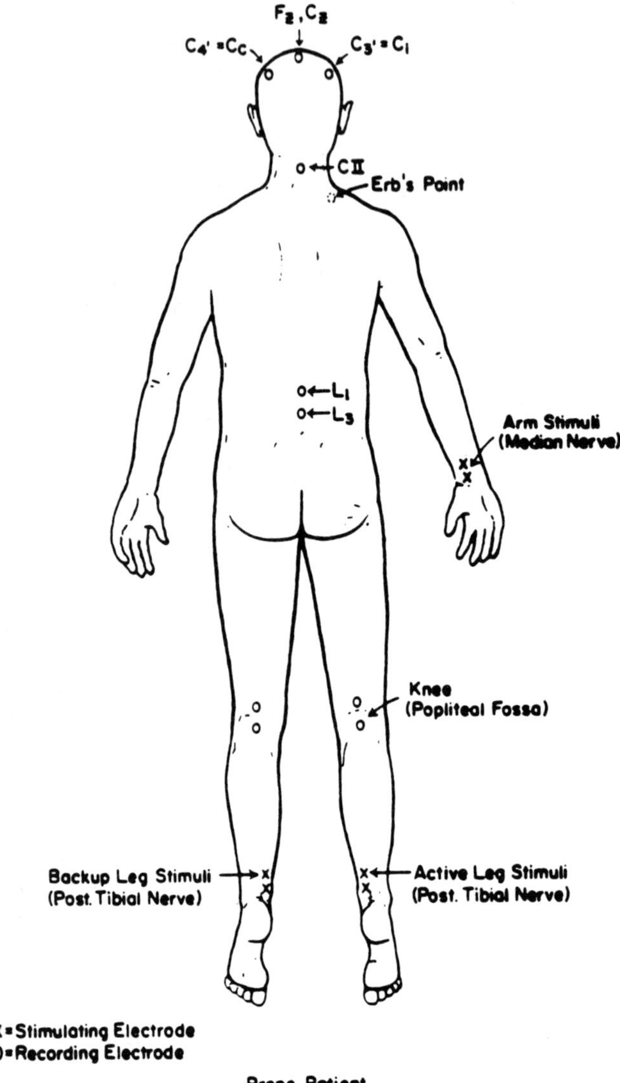

Figure 57-1 Recording of SERs. At least two channels are used, each consisting of a pair of electrodes. One electrode is placed along the anatomic pathway; the other serves as a reference. Following median or posterior tibial stimulation, recordings of interest include Erb's point, CII (cervical cord) and cortical areas: C3′, Cz, C4′ C3′ is contralateral to the stimulation site, 3 cm posterior to C3 (not shown); C4′ is ipsilateral to the stimulation site, 3 cm posterior to C4 (not shown). Cz is recorded at the cortex. (Gravenstein JS, Paulus DA: *Clinical Monitoring Practice,* 2nd ed, p 27. Philadelphia, JB Lippincott, 1987)

OTHER ORGAN SYSTEMS

The emphasis in this chapter is on neurologic monitoring, *per se*. However, other organ system functions can be important and may play a major role in the patient's ultimate outcome. This fact is easily recognized in cases of multisystem trauma or failure (shock, sepsis, and so forth), but is just as true in many episodes of primary CNS dysfunction.

An excellent example involves subarachnoid hemorrhage from a ruptured cerebral aneurysm. In an attempt to prevent secondary cerebral vasospasm and a worsening of the ischemic insult, many neurosurgeons favor vigorous fluid administration with colloids and crystalloids to augment cardiac output and presumably CBF, particularly to the involved areas. Although the efficacy of this treatment is not fully documented, its use appears to be increasing. Patients with otherwise normal cardiopulmonary function tolerate this regimen reasonably well. Those with marginal function may not. Episodes of pulmonary edema resulting from overly zealous fluid therapy necessitate vigorous diuretic therapy and positive-pressure ventilatory support. Rather than awaiting the rather insensitive endpoint of fluffy pulmonary infiltrates appearing on a chest radiograph, one might consider the selective use of pulmonary artery catheterization to evaluate cardiovascular and pulmonary integrity more precisely.

For more information, please see Chapter 34 in Civetta JM, Taylor JW, Kirby RR: Critical Care. *Philadelphia: J. B. Lippincott, 1988*

BIBLIOGRAPHY

Astrup J, Symon L, Branston NM, et al: Cortical evoked potential and extracellular potassium and hydrogen at critical levels of brain ischemia. *Stroke* 1977; 8:51

Goldie WB, Chiappa KH, Young RR, et al: Brainstem auditory and short latency somatosensory evoked responses in brain death. *Neurology* 1981; 31:248

Javes TH, Morowitz RB, Krowell RM, et al: Thresholds of cerebral ischemia in awake monkeys. *J Neurosurg* 1981; 54:773

Jennett B: Assessment of the severity of head injury. *J Neurol Neurosurg Psychiatry* 1976; 39:647

Jennett B, Teasdale G, Galbraith S, et al: Severe head injuries in three countries. *J Neurol Neurosurg Psychiatry* 1977; 49:291

Lassen NA: Cerebral blood flow and oxygen consumption in man. *Physiol Rev* 1959; 39:183

Lorenzo AV, Bresnan MJ, Barlow CF: Cerebrospinal fluid absorption deficit in normal pressure hydrocephalus. *Arch Neurol* 1974; 30:387

Marshall LF, Smith RW, Shapiro HM: The influence of diurnal rhythms in patients with intracranial hypertension: Implications for management. *Neurosurg* 1978; 2:100

Pashayan AG: Monitoring the neurosurgical patient. In Gravenstein N (ed): *Problems in Anesthesia: Monitoring,* pp 104–120. Philadelphia, JB Lippincott, 1987

Sharpiro HM: Neurosurgical anesthesia and intracranial hypertension. In Miller RD (ed): *Anesthesia,* p 1563. Philadelphia, JB Lippincott, 1986

Siesjo BK: Cerebral circulation and metabolism. *J Neurosurg* 1984; 60:883

Starr A: Auditory brainstem responses and brain death. *Brain* 1976; 99:543

Sullivan HG, Becker DP: Intracranial pressure monitoring and interpretation. In *Anesthesia and Neurosurgery,* p. 58. St. Louis, CV Mosby, 1980

Sundt TM Jr, Sharbrough FW, Piepgras DG, et al: Correlation of cerebral blood flow and electroencephalographic changes during carotid endarterectomy. With results of surgery and hemodynamics of cerebral ischemia. *Mayo Clin Proc* 1981; 56:533

Tabaddor K, Danziger A, Whisoff HS: Estimation of intracranial pressure by CT scan in closed head trauma. *Surg Neurol* 1982; 18:212

Teasdale G, Jennett B: Assessment of coma and impaired consciousness. A practical scale. *Lancet* 1974; 2:81

58
Behavioral Disturbances

Behavioral disturbances are common in the ICU. 10% to 15% of the patients on acute medical and surgical wards suffer from delirium or confusional states during hospitalization. The incidence of confusional states increases greatly in hospitalized patients over 60 years of age, and delirium occurs in almost all patients who have been burned over greater than 40% of the body surface area. Other behavioral disorders resulting from a critically ill patient's fear, anxiety, denial, anger, depression, dependency, and personality are encountered daily by physicians and critical care nurses (Table 58-1). Regardless of your expertise, there are times when a psychiatric consultation is needed.

WHAT TO DO FIRST

When faced with a patient who has a behavioral disturbance, the first question must be: "Is the patient delirious?" This is a crucial decision point in the evaluation. If a delirium or confusional state is present, the focus of the differential diagnosis must become the etiologic agent(s) causing the problem. The importance of discovering and correcting the underlying cause of a delirium cannot be over-emphasized. Unfortunately, terms like "ICU psychosis," which infer a cause-and-effect relationship between the ICU setting and delirium, result in diagnostic apathy. Intensive care unit psychosis implies that the problem is somehow natural or expected when a patient is critically ill; therefore, delirium can be ignored. The evidence for such an etiology is flimsy. How many patients have been diagnosed as having "ICU fever" or "ICU dysrhythmia?" The brain's highly complex, multifactorial reaction to metabolic, anoxic, toxic, and infectious insults is delirium. Delirium is the tangible sign of cerebral insufficiency, just as angina is the ordinary warning sign of heart ischemia. The appearance of a delirium, which is often referred to as acute brain failure, should promote martialing of the same medical forces as failure of any other vital organ. Mortality associated with delirium is not trivial. From 20% to 76% of acutely ill patients diagnosed as delirious die within a few months. Far from being a natural phenomenon or "disease

TABLE 58-1 PSYCHIATRIC DISTURBANCES IN THE ICU

Agitation	Depression
Anxiety	Despondency
Apathy	Fear
Confusion	Hostility
Denial	Personality
Dependency	Psychosis

of medical progress," brain failure is ominous, signaling a need for renewed concern and prompt attention.

CLINICAL FEATURES OF A DELIRIUM

A delirium has certain characteristics (Table 58-2). The patient often manifests prodromal symptoms such as restlessness, anxiety, irritability, or sleep disruption prior to the onset. One of the hallmark findings is rapid fluctuation in the degree of confusion. Patients may be grossly confused and hallucinating during the night and have brief lucid intervals interspersed with confusional periods during the day. They also have difficulty sustaining attention. During the interview, they typically are distracted by environmental events, such as a loud noise or a nurse checking the intravenous infusion, and forget the question asked. Their inability to sustain attention and preoccupation with internal events undoubtedly play a key role in the severe memory impairment and orientation difficulties found in delirium.

Delirious patients, except for lucid intervals, are usually disoriented to time, often disoriented to place, but very rarely, if ever, disoriented to person. Following recovery from a delirium, some patients will be amnesic for the entire episode, others will have islands of memory, and a few will recall the

TABLE 58-2 CLINICAL FEATURES OF DELIRIUM

Prodrome
Rapidly fluctuating course, reversible, lucid intervals
Altered arousal and psychomotor abnormality
Attention decreased
Sleep–wake disturbance
Impaired memory
Thinking and speech disorganized
Perceptions altered
Disorientation
Emotional lability
Dysgraphia/constructional apraxia/dysomic aphasia
Motor abnormalities

entire period. Those patients who experience paranoid delusions with a relatively clear sensorium usually recall the ICU experience.

Another clinical feature of delirium deserves particular emphasis. Though usually aroused, the reticular activating system (RAS) of the brain stem may be hypoactive in delirium, in which case a patient appears apathetic, somnolent, and quietly confused. In most patients, RAS hyperactivity induces agitation, hypervigilance, and psychomotor hyperactivity. Some patients have a mixed picture that swings back and forth between hypoactive and hyperactive states. The medical staff often "diagnoses" the patient with a retarded (hypoactive) delirium as depressed. This diagnosis in an apathetic, quietly confused patient sometimes leads to inappropriate treatment with antidepressant medications.

The sleep–wake cycle of delirious patients is often reversed. They may be somnolent during the day and active during the night when the nursing staff is sparse. Restoration of the normal diurnal sleep cycle is an important part of treatment. In addition, delirious patients' thought patterns are disorganized and their reasoning defective. They often experience misperceptions involving illusions, delusions, and hallucinations. These misperceptions often are woven into a loosely knit delusional, and frequently, paranoid system. Visual hallucinations are common and can involve simple visual distortions or complex scenes. During a delirium, they occur more frequently than auditory hallucinations. Tactile hallucinations are the least frequent. As the severity of the delirium increases, spontaneous speech becomes incoherent and rambling.

Motor system abnormalities such as tremor, myoclonus, asterixis ("liver flap"), or reflex and muscle tone changes can also be present. The tremor associated with delirium, particularly when toxic–metabolic in origin, is absent at rest but apparent during movement. Myoclonus and asterixis occur in many toxic and metabolic conditions. Symmetric reflex and muscle tone changes also are seen.

IS DELIRIUM PRESENT?

The bedside mental status examination for cognitive dysfunction is not difficult. Folstein's Mini-Mental State (MMS) examination provides a good screening tool for organicity and is also used to follow the patient's clinical course serially. The MMS examination tests for orientation, memory, attention, dysgraphia, and constructional apraxia. A score of 15 or less out of a total of 30 on the MMS signals the presence of delirium or dementia.

The electroencephalogram (EEG) is diagnostically helpful in difficult cases. Delirium is a clinical manifestation of global cerebral dysfunction. As mentioned earlier, one of the interchangeable terms for delirium is acute brain failure. The EEG characteristically, but not always, shows global cerebral slowing. A low-voltage, fast-activity pattern as in delirium tremens also can be present. Remember that the EEG appears worse than the mental status examination in the delirious patient; conversely, the mental status examination of the demented patient is usually much worse than predicted from simple review of the EEG (*i.e.*, the EEG is usually normal in dementia until the later stages).

IF DELIRIUM IS PRESENT, WHAT IS NEXT?

The differential diagnosis of delirium is extensive. Confusional states, particularly in the elderly, may have multiple contributory causes. An elderly, delirious patient can have a low hematocrit, multiorgan system disease (e.g., pulmonary insufficiency, cardiac failure, or preexisting brain damage) and be taking multiple medications. Each potential contribution to the delirium needs to be pursued and, to whatever degree possible, reversed. A method for organizing the differential diagnosis of a delirious patient is helpful. This diagnositic system is found in Table 58-3 and is represented by the mnemonic WHHHHIMP.

In hospital and emergency room patients, prescribed medications are common causes of delirium (Table 58-4). A thorough medication history and review of the patient's medication records are essential. The doctor's order sheets can be misleading since drugs may have been ordered but not given. Correlation of changes in behavior with medication administration or discontinuation can be helpful in sorting through a difficult case.

A more comprehensive list of diagnoses that can cause delirium is summarized in Table 58-5. The mnemonic used, I WATCH DEATH, may seem melodramatic, but the mortality rate within the first 3 months following the diagnosis of delirium is approximately 30%.

TREATMENT

The goal of evaluation is to discover specific reversible causes for delirium. A delirious patient with a blood pressure of 260/150 and papilledema must immediately receive antihypertensive medications. The alcoholic patient having withdrawal symptoms must receive appropriate pharmacologic intervention with drugs such as thiamine and a benzodiazepine. If a specific cause

TABLE 58-3 DELIRIUM—DIFFERENTIAL DIAGNOSIS OF URGENT ITEMS

Wernicke's encephalopathy/withdrawal
Hypertensive encephalopathy
Hypoglycemia
Hypoperfusion of CNS
Hypoxemia
Intracranial bleed
Meningitis/encephalitis
Poisons/medications

TABLE 58-4 DRUGS THAT CAUSE DELIRIUM (REVERSIBLE DEMENTIA)

Analgesics
- Meperidine (Normeperidine)
- Opiates
- Pentazocine
- Salicylates

Antibiotics
- Acyclovir (antiviral)
- Aminoglycosides
- Amodiaquine
- Amphotericin B (antifungal)
- Cephalosporins
- Chloramphenicol
- Chloroquine (antimalarial)
- Ethambutol
- Gentamicin
- Interferon (antiviral)
- Isoniazid
- Rifampin
- Sulfonamides
- Tetracyclines
- Ticarcillin
- Vancomycin

Anticholinergics
- Antihistamines
  - Chlorpheniramine (Ornade, Teldine)
- Antiparkinson drugs
  - Benzotropine (Cogentin)
  - Biperidine (Akineton)
- Antispasmodics
- Belladonna alkaloids

Anticholinergics *(continued)*
- Diphenhydramine (Benadryl)
- Phenothiazines (especially Thioridizide)
- Promethazine (Phenergan)
- Tricyclic antidepressants (especially amitriptyline)
- Trihexyphenidyl (Artane, Pipanol, Tremin)

Anticonvulsants
- Phenobarbital
- Phenytoin (Dilantin)
- Sodium valproate (Depakene)

Anti-inflammatory
- ACTH
- Corticosteroids
- Ibuprofen (Motrin, Advil)
- Indomethacin (Indocin)
- Naproxen (Naprosyn)
- Phenylbutazone (Butazolidin, Azolid)
- Steroids

Antineoplastics
- Aminoglutethimide
- DTIC
- 5-Fluoruracil
- Hexamethylenamine
- L-Asparaginase
- Methotrexate (high dose)

Antineoplastics *(continued)*
- Tamoxifen
- Vinblastine
- Vincristine

Antiparkinsons
- Amantadine (Symmetrel)
- Bromocriptine
- Carbidopa (Sinemet)
- Levodopa (Larodopa)

Cardiac
- Beta-blockers
- Captopril
- Clonidine (Catapres)
- Digitalis (Digoxin, Lanox)
- Disopyramide (Norpace)
- Lidocaine (Xylocaine)
- Mexilitene
- Methyldopa (Aldomet)
- Quinidine (Quinidine Quiaglute, Duraquine)
- Procainamide (Pronestyl)
- Tocainide

Drug withdrawal
- Alcohol
- Barbiturates
- Benzodiazepines

Sedative–hypnotics
- Barbiturates (Miltown, Equanil)

Sedative–hypnotics *(continued)*
- *Benzodiazepines*
- *Glutethimide*

Sympathomimetics
- Aminophylline
- Amphetamines
- Cocaine
- Ephedrine
- Phenylephrine
- Phenylpropanolamine
- Theophylline

Miscellaneous drugs
- Baclofen
- Bromides
- Chlorpropamide (Diabinese)
- Cimetidine (Tagamet)
- Disulfiram (Antabuse)
- Ergotamines
- Lithium
- Metrizamide (Amipaque)
- Metronidazole (Flagyl)
- Phenelzine
- Podophyllin (by absorption)
- Procarbazine
- Propylthiouracil
- Quinacrine
- Ranitidine
- Timolol Ophthalmic

TABLE 58-5 CAUSES OF DELIRIUM (I WATCH DEATH)

Infectious	Encephalitis, meningitis, syphilis
Withdrawal	Alcohol, barbiturates, sedatives–hypnotics, benzodiazepine
Acute metabolic	Acidosis, alkalosis, electrolyte disturbance, hepatic failure, renal failure
Trauma	Heat stroke, postoperative severe burns, closed head
CNS pathology	Abscesses, hemorrhage, normal pressure hydrocephalus, seizures, stroke, tumors, vasculitis
Hypoxia	Anemia, carbon monoxide poisoning, hypotension, pulmonary/cardiac failure
Deficiencies	B_{12}, hypovitaminosis, niacin, thiamine
Endocrinopathies	Hyper(hypo)adrenalcorticism, hyper(hypo)glycemia, parathyroid
Acute vascular	Hypertensive encephalopathy, shock
Toxins/drugs	Medications, pesticides, solvents
Heavy metals	Lead, manganese, mercury

for the confusional state cannot be found, a number of interventions are helpful in controlling unacceptable behavior.

Haloperidol is the drug of choice when you must treat a delirium of unknown etiology. It is a potent antipsychotic, with virtually no anticholinergic or hypotensive properties, is not a respiratory depressant, and can be given parenterally. Intravenous haloperidol is the safest drug for control of agitation in the critically ill patient. Recommended dosages of haloperidol for the agitated patient are summarized in Table 58-6.

Other useful antipsychotic medications include thiothixene (Navane) and droperidol (Inapsine). Droperidol is used as a preanesthetic agent and for control of nausea and vomiting. It is a butyrophenone like haloperidol and has comparable antipsychotic potency. Droperidol is approved for intrave-

TABLE 58-6 GUIDELINES FOR INTRAVENOUS HALOPERIDOL

Level of Agitation	Starting Dose
Mild	0.5–2.0 mg
Moderate	2.0–5.0 mg
Severe	5.0–10.0 mg

Note:
(1) Clear IV tubing with normal saline.
(2) For elderly, use starting dose in the low range
(3) Allow 30 min between doses.
(4) For continued agitation, double previous dose.
(5) After 3 doses, give 0.5–1.0 mg of lorazepam IV concurrently or alternate lorazepam with haloperidol every 30 min.
(6) Once patient is calm, add the total mg of haloperidol and administer same number of mg over the next 24 hr.
(7) Assuming the patient remains calm, reduce dose 50% every 24 hr.
(8) Oral dose is twice the IV dose.

nous use but has the disadvantage of having a higher potential than haloperidol for causing hypotension. Less potent antipsychotic medications are thioridazine (Mellaril) and chlorpromazine (Thorazine). Because higher milligram doses are required, they are more likely to cause hypotension, have more anticholinergic side-effects, and should be used with caution in the unstable patient with cardiovascular disease. Obtain psychiatric consultation before using thioridazine or chlorpromazine in critically ill patients.

Having a calm family member remain with a paranoid, agitated patient is reassuring and can prevent mishaps. In lieu of a family member, close supervision by reassuring staff is important. Both nurses and family members can frequently reorient the disoriented patient to date and surroundings. Placing a clock, calendar, and familiar objects in the room may be helpful. Adequate light in the room decreases frightening illusions at night. Despite recommendations to the contrary, a private room for the delirious patient is appropriate only if adequate supervision can be assured. A room with a window is helpful to orient the patient to normal diurnal cues.

If the patient normally wears eyeglasses or a hearing aid, improving the quality of sensory input by returning these devices is useful. A common error on medical and surgical wards is to group delirious patients in the same room. This process slows recovery and makes reorientation of confused patients virtually impossible.

WHEN DELIRIUM IS NOT PRESENT

What should you do if the patient has a behavior disorder, but the MMS examination and recent clinical history indicate that no cognitive dysfunction is present? The next step is to continue the examination with the goal of uncovering the concerns, realistic or not, that the patient has about his medical condition. Some patients can easily identify fears, anxiety, and depressive ideas concerning their medical condition, but this task is not always easy. Certain characteristic emotional responses are encountered in different intensive care settings (Table 58-7).

TABLE 58-7 FREQUENCY OF CONSULTATION REQUESTS ACCORDING TO TYPE OF ICU

CCU	Surgical ICU	Respiratory ICU	Medical ICU
Anxiety Depression Management (AMA sign-out, dependency) Hostility Delirium	Delirium Depression Anxiety weaning from ventilator	Depression Anxiety weaning from ventilator Management (drug dependency, dependency)	Delirium Management (suicide attempt) Depression Anxiety

When the critical care physician is called regarding a patient with a behavioral problem, the first concern is whether a change in medical status prompted the behavior (e.g., shortness of breath prompts agitation). Concern of the physician for the patient's medical condition not only rules out problems but also helps to establish rapport. Once medical problems are discounted and rapport is established, the interviewer can ask open-ended questions about the current situation. The basic approach used is to uncover and correct the critically ill patient's unrealistic or distorted expectations. For example, "What is worrying you most right now?" If you cannot establish sufficient rapport, or if the patient is unable or unwilling to talk, request a psychiatric consultation.

AGITATION

Agitation is excessive motor activity resulting from a patient's internal discomfort. This discomfort may result from physical pain, anxiety, fear, or akathisia (an internal sense of discomfort often with motor restlessness that occurs as a side-effect of neuroleptic medications). If a delirium is not present, other sources for the agitation must be explored.

For many critically ill patients, the cause of their anxiety and fear is the threat of death. In your conversations with the patient, if fears of dying are not mentioned, ask, "You look scared. How are you doing," or ask directly, "Are you worried that you may die?" If the patient answers that he/she believes he/she is dying, your response depends on the reality of those fears. If dying is an unrealistic possibility, reassurance and realistic explanations about the current situation markedly decrease the level of anxiety and fear. If dying is a likely or definite outcome of the illness, ask the patient, "What frightens you most about dying?" The patient may reply, "I'm afraid of the pain I will have" or "I have never been religious and don't know what to expect." In the former case, you can reassure the patient that he/she will be kept comfortable and free of moderate or severe pain. In the latter case, you can offer to arrange a consultation visit from a chaplain who can offer reassurance and advice.

Medications are helpful in treating anxiety and fear. Benzodiazepines reduce anxiety in most patients. When you prescribe benzodiazepines for critically ill patients, considerations of the half-life of the drug, onset of action, drug interactions, and the route of metabolism are important. Diazepam produces a rapid, high level in the central nervous system (CNS) and is clinically useful when rapid tranquilization is desired. Drug interactions can result in behavioral changes. Cimetidine increases the half-life of longer-acting benzodiazepines, resulting sometimes in confusion or lethargy. Short-acting benzodiazepines, such as oxazepam or lorazepam, are recommended in patients with liver damage to prevent build-up of drugs and their metabolites.

When anxiety is severe and is manifested as fear or panic, major tranquilizers (neuroleptics) are more efficacious. For example, a young man is admitted to the CCU to rule out myocardial infarction. He is noted to be extremely anxious with agitation, and oxazepam, 15 mg orally four times a day, is ordered. Despite the medication, he continues to be agitated, hypervigilant, and resists sleep. Inquiry into the patient's concerns reveals a strong family history of deaths associated with heart attacks. The patient is afraid to sleep "because I might not wake up," and he is "watching the monitors in case the alarms don't work." The patient, on a 0 (no anxiety) to 10 (terror) scale of anxiety, reports a 9.5 (*with* benzodiazepine treatment). He is then given perphenazine (Trilifon), 2 mg orally three times a day. His anxiety promptly drops to a self-rating 3 out of 10, and all objective signs of emotional discomfort disappear. When panic emerges, as it did in this patient, low-dose major tranquilizers such as haloperidol 1 or 2 mg twice each day; perphenazine, 2 mg orally three times each day; thiothixene, 1 or 2 mg three times per day; or trifluoperazine (Stelazine) 2 mg three times per day, can markedly reduce the level of anxiety.

Neuroleptic drugs, including droperidol, prochlorperazine (Compazine) and metoclopramide (Reglan), are associated with extrapyramidal side-effects such as akathisia. Patients usually report a sense of inner restlessness and sometimes manifest agitation. Akathisia is difficult to treat, and may or may not be improved by giving the patient diphenhydramine (Benadryl), benzodiazepines (usually diazepam), or anticholinergic drugs such as trihexyphenidyl (Artane) or benztropine mesylate (Cogentin). Propranolol may also reduce akathisia. If symptoms do not remit, neuroleptics may have to be discontinued.

DEPRESSION OR APATHY

Clinical depression consists of a depressed mood with a symptom constellation that includes sleep disturbance, decreased interests, increased sense of guilt, decreased energy, decreased ability to concentrate, decreased (or more rarely increased) appetite, altered psychomotor state (either decreased or increased), and suicidal ideation or preoccupation with death. Many of these symptoms are difficult to interpret, since almost all seriously ill patients have problems with sleep, energy, and appetite, and some have difficulty with concentration. How, then, does one decide if a patient is depressed? The following characteristics help to identify critically ill patients who are also clinically depressed. These are sustained depressed mood, either increased (agitation) or decreased psychomotor movements, suicidal ideation, and, very importantly, a sense of helplessness and hopelessness about the current situation. The depressed patient also feels worthless. If the latter two symptoms are present, the patient requires treatment for depression. Failure to treat depression increases the mortality and morbidity of all medical illness.

Apathy and depression do coexist in certain patients (*i.e.*, depressed patients often are apathetic about the future). Apathy, however, also exists as a separate entity. These patients are indifferent about the current medical condition and do not feel sad, hopeless, or worthless. They are not clinically depressed, although they may be misdiagnosed as depressed. One might say they are pseudodepressed. Apathy in this group of patients is a product of brain dysfunction, probably in the frontal lobe. It occurs in hypoaroused, delirious patients, demented patients, and in some poststroke and brain-damaged patients. Nondepressed apathetic patients are not likely to respond to antidepressant medications. In fact, their mental status may worsen secondary to the anticholinergic side-effects of these drugs. A nondelirious subgroup may respond to stimulants. Methylphenidate (Ritalin) in doses of 10 mg twice per day, or dextroamphetamine 10 mg once per day, may energize the patient and improve rehabilitation. The afternoon dose of stimulants should be given before 3 PM so that the patient's ability to fall asleep is not impaired.

Certain medications are depressogenic. Thus, review of the depressed patient's medication regimen is necessary. Frequent offenders are reserpine, methyldopa, propranolol, guanethidine, hydralazine, and clonidine.

REFUSAL TO COOPERATE

This problem can manifest itself as denial of serious illness, such as a threatened AMA sign-out, or refusal to follow a treatment plan, such as sneaking cigarettes or failure to remain in bed while on strict bed rest. As Hackett and Cassem suggest, "Although the threat to sign out can mean that the individual does not take the illness seriously (*e.g.*, is not frightened enough), the threat to sign out issued by an acutely ill patient should be assumed to be a reaction to panic unless proven otherwise." Basically, when faced with flight or fight response to the severe stress of acute illness, the patient opts for flight.

If the patient seems incompetent (*i.e.*, is incapable of understanding the situation because of mental dysfunction), get a psychiatric consultation to document mental status. If the patient is competent and is demanding to leave against medical advice, try the following approach. Remain calm. Anger is a tempting response to this situation, but taking an adversarial stance rarely changes the patient's decision. In a calm, direct way, inform the patient about the medical difficulties, stressing the fact that the illness is manageable. Mobilize the patient's family. If certain members of the family can help to calm the patient, they are invaluable assets in this situation. If the family is as panicky as the patient, which is very rarely the case, keep the family and patient separated. As soon as possible, medicate the patient with a low-dose antipsychotic medication such as haloperidol, 1 or 2 mg, or perphenazine, 2 to 5 mg orally.

Many patients who refuse to comply with medical treatment are rebelling against dependency. The natural response of the staff to this rebellious behavior is to demand complete compliance. To do so is to fight a losing battle, with the staff attempting to function as the police and the patient feeling like a misunderstood criminal. The patient believes that his/her body has forsaken him/her by becoming ill, and now the medical staff is demanding total surrender. Certainly a fertile setting for rebellion! When faced with this situation, the staff should review the treatment plan and decide where flexibility can be allowed and where it is contraindicated. Use statements such as, "Would you like your sponge bath this morning or in the evening?" or "Your digitalis should be taken on schedule to keep your heart rhythm regular, but you can refuse your Valium. If you want the Valium later, just let us know." This gives the patient some sense of control in a situation where he/she is feeling totally powerless.

HOSTILITY

Anger in the critically ill springs from many roots. Patients may be frightened or feel threatened. They commonly ask, "What did I do to deserve this?" The nursing and physician staff may be the recipients of the resultant anger. If patients have complaints, hear them out, and correct the problem if appropriate. Empathize with the situation, "I know you are having a difficult time." For most patients, anger is a temporary state of affairs and will pass as they and the staff become adjusted to each other and to the situation. However, a few patients who exhibit chronic hostility have life-long difficulties with interpersonal relationships. A psychiatric consultation is indicated. These are difficult even for the psychiatrist to treat, and marginal control of the anger may be as much as can be achieved.

DEPENDENCY

Critically ill patients who regress to an infantile state during hospitalization (helpless behavior and unrealistic demands) irritate the medical staff. The latter may become so intent on controlling their own anger that they overcompensate and give in to the patients' demands. Unfortunately, acquiescence to unreasonable demands results in further regression and more demands. When dealing with a regressed patient, the staff must enforce reasonable limits and guide the patient towards rehabilitation. Firm demands for self-care and increased independence are recommended.

Transfer of the patient out of the ICU with a consequent reduced level of medical vigilance has both good and bad aspects. The patient is improving (good news), and the level of medical observation and monitoring are about to be reduced (bad news). The patient should be told in advance when transfer will occur and should be assured that less monitoring is appropriate because medical improvement has occurred. In some cases, a transitional status, such as a stepdown unit, offers reassurance before transfer to a general medical ward.

For more information, please see Chapter 141 in Civetta JM, Taylor RW, Kirby RR: Critical Care. *Philadelphia: J. B. Lippincott, 1988*

BIBLIOGRAPHY

Avery D, Winokur G: Mortality in depressed patients with electroconvulsive therapy and antidepressants. *Arch Gen Psychiatry* 1976; 33:1029

Cassem NH: Psychiatric and ethical issues in the critical care unit. In Parrillo JE (ed): *Current Therapy in Critical Care Medicine,* p 331. Philadelphia, BC Decker, 1987

Cassem NH, Hackett TP: The setting of intensive care. In Hackett TP, Cassem NH (eds): *Massachusetts General Hospital Handbook of General Psychiatry,* p 319. St. Louis, CV Mosby, 1978

Desmond PV, Patwardhan RV, Schenker S, et al: Cimetidine impairs elimination of chlordiazepoxide (librium) in man. *Ann Intern Med* 1980; 93:266

Engel GL: Delirium. In Freedman AM, Kaplan HI (eds): *Comprehensive Textbook of Psychiatry.* Baltimore, Williams & Wilkins, 1967

Epstein LJ, Simon A: Organic brain syndromes in the elderly. *Geriatrics* 1967; 22:145

Flint FJ, Richards SM: Organic basis of confusional states in the elderly. *Br Med J* 1956; 2:1537

Katons W, Raskind M: Treatment of depression in the medically ill with methylphenidate. *Am J Psychiatry* 1980; 137:963

Kaufmann MW, Murray GB, Cassem NH: Use of psychostimulants in medically ill depressed patients. *Psychosomatics* 1982; 23:817

Kennard MA, Bueding E, Wortis WB: Some biochemical and electroencephalographic changes in delirium tremens. *Q J Stud Alcohol* 1945; 6:4

Klerman GL: Depression in the medically ill. *Psychiatr Clin North Am* 1981; 4:301

Lipowski ZJ: *Delirium (Acute Brain Failure in Man),* p 515. Springfield, IL, Charles C. Thomas Publishers, 1980

Lipowski ZJ: Delirium updated. *Compr Psychiatry* 1980; 21:190

McKegney FB: Intensive care syndrome: Definition, treatment and prevention of new "disease of medical progress." *Conn Med* 1966; 30:633

Murray: Personal communication, Massachusetts General Hospital

Wilson LM: Intensive care delirium. *Arch Intern Med* 1972; 130:225

VII. Gastrointestinal Disorders

59 Gastrointestinal Bleeding

Gastrointestinal hemorrhage remains a frequent cause of emergency hospitalization, resulting in 50 to 100 patients per 100,000 population per annum being admitted. Although reported mortality rates range from 9% to 29%, the average mortality figure remains at approximately 10%. Disappointingly, the mortality rate from this disease process has remained unchanged over the past 30 years. Although improvements in technology have enhanced diagnostic accuracy, few studies have documented decreased mortality based on better diagnosis or improved therapy.

Patients may be admitted from the emergency room with gastrointestinal hemorrhage of various etiologies, including acid peptic disease, Mallory–Weiss tears, or esophageal varices. These patients are in contrast to critically ill patients often with multiple organ system failure (MOSF) who present with non-gastrointestinal disease such as acute respiratory failure, sepsis, multisystem trauma, head injury, or burns. This group has gastrointestinal disease as a common manifestation of systemic illness, resulting in "stress ulceration," probably more aptly described as acute mucosal erosions. Such lesions are notoriously difficult to manage. Prophylaxis markedly enhances this group's chances of survival, whereas the need for surgery has resulted in dismal mortality rates.

INITIAL MANAGEMENT

Most patients with gastrointestinal bleeding are admitted after initial evaluation and resuscitation directly to intensive care units. Although not all patients warrant admission, the following criteria may be used to select those patients benefiting from such intensive therapy:

1 Greater than 500 ml blood loss;

2 History of hypotension; and

3 Presence of hypovolemic shock.

HISTORY

A brief history to establish the differential diagnosis should be obtained and should include the pain patterns, which may suggest peptic ulcer disease, biliary tract disease, or pancreatitis. For example, the onset of gastrointestinal bleeding after prolonged retching and vomiting suggests the possibility of a Mallory–Weiss tear. Stigmata of alcoholic liver disease should also be sought, since these raise the possibility of bleeding esophageal varices. Attention should be paid to the surgical history, particularly to the presence of an aortic reconstruction. Gastrointestinal bleeding after such procedures must be considered as aorto–duodenal fistulas until proven otherwise. History of drug ingestion should be solicited, especially the use of salicylates, alcohol, nonsteroidal anti-inflammatory drugs, steroids, and anticoagulants.

INFUSIONS/CATHETERIZATION

Since the initial aim is to stabilize the patient, one or more large-bore peripheral intravenous infusions should be started promptly. Resuscitation should begin with the administration of physiologic crystalloid solutions. Blood products may be needed, depending on the estimated amount of hemorrhage. An orthostatic drop of 10 mm Hg in the systolic pressure or an increase of 20 or more beats per minute in the pulse rate suggests the loss of 10% to 15% of circulating blood volume (approximately 750–1000 ml), which may be replaced by crystalloid solutions alone. The loss of 20% to 25% of circulating blood volume (1500–2000 ml) necessitates the immediate replacement of shed blood plus crystalloid solution. Red blood cell mass should be replaced milliliter for milliliter. In addition, isotonic crystalloid losses should be replaced at a rate of 3 ml for each milliliter of estimated blood loss.

A Foley catheter should be placed to monitor urinary output as a measure of adequate volume repletion. Patients with suspected upper gastrointestinal hemorrhage require a large-bore nasogastric tube. Less than 1% of all cases of gastrointestinal hemorrhage will occur in the absence of guaiac-positive nasogastric aspirate. Therefore, the absence of guaiac-positive material from the nasogastric tube fairly rules out the presence of upper gastrointestinal hemorrhage. Patients who require rapid volume replacement or who have multisystem disease may well require central venous catheters. More appropriately, such patients may require the placement of a balloon-tipped, flow-directed pulmonary artery (PA) catheter to allow adequate volume replacement as well as to measure other physiologic parameters.

DIAGNOSIS

LABORATORY STUDIES/SYSTEMIC EVALUATION

Initial laboratory studies should include routine hemograms and stool and gastric aspirates to be tested for blood. Electrolytes, amylase, liver and renal functions, and a coagulation profile should be assessed early in the resuscitation effort. With the widespread use of nonsteroid anti-inflammatory drugs, particular attention must be paid to qualitative defects in platelet function. In these cases, platelet transfusion may be indicated even with a "normal" platelet count. Every effort should be made to correct any underlying coagulation defect early in treatment.

Patients hospitalized for MOSF or for protracted illness are candidates at high risk for gastrointestinal bleeding, frequently from acute mucosal erosions (discussed later). Obvious sources of bleeding should be sought immediately. For example, in patients recently having upper gastrointestinal surgery for peptic ulcer disease, technical problems are the most common cause of early postoperative hemorrhage. In patients with upper gastrointestinal bleeding after portosystemic decompressive procedures, the vascular anastomosis must be examined (angiographically) to ensure its patency.

After surgically correctable technical problems have been eliminated, a thorough systematic evaluation of the patient should be performed. Because many patients will have a "data bank" of current laboratory values available, coagulation profiles, liver and renal function studies, hemoglobin, hematocrit, and culture data should be reviewed. Any data not current at the time of the bleeding episode should be immediately obtained. Culture data become important in evaluating patients with septic foci as the bleeding source. Since many patients will be receiving or will have recently received broad-spectrum antibiotics, empiric administration of vitamin K should be considered. At least 6 units of cross-matched blood and any necessary blood components suggested by the coagulation profile should be readily available.

Patients who do not already have nasogastric tubes should have a large-bore sump tube placed. All coffee ground or bright red material should be as completely lavaged as possible. If bleeding ceases with lavage, urgent endoscopic examination is indicated. In the presence of a newly created gastric or gastroenteric anastomosis, this should be strictly coordinated with the operating surgeon. If lavage fails to clear, other diagnostic and therapeutic steps may be taken.

RADIOGRAPHIC CONTRAST STUDIES

Before flexible endoscopy was developed, barium examination of the upper gastrointestinal tract was the "gold standard" for establishing a diagnosis. Single-contrast gastrography has been reported to be accurate in only 42% of the cases. Although double-contrast gastrography in one series has nearly duplicated the diagnostic accuracy of endoscopy (80%), other studies have shown that active bleeding or signs of recent hemorrhage and the establishment of definitive diagnosis were possible in only 46% of cases. Single-contrast gastrointestinal examinations rarely demonstrate mucosal erosions or esophagitis and cannot accurately demonstrate signs of recent hemorrhage. Lesions located in the body of the stomach or at the cardia have a diagnostic error rate of approximately 22%. Double-contrast gastrointestinal examination is capable of showing signs of recent hemorrhage and definitions of lesions in the cardia with a diagnostic error rate of approximately 6%. The presence of blood adversely affects the ability of barium to coat the gastrointestinal mucosa and therefore negates the usefulness of double-contrast studies. To obtain accurate double-contrast studies, patients must be moved to the radiology suite, which may be ill-advised for those who are either too ill to cooperate with the examination or hemodynamically unstable. Should patients require angiography to establish a diagnosis or to effect therapeutic embolization, the presence of barium may significantly interfere with the performance of this study.

BARIUM ENEMA

Single- or double-contrast barium enemas have been relied on not only to establish the source of lower gastrointestinal bleeding but also to temporarily arrest hemorrhage. Although barium enemas may accurately reveal such lesions as diverticuli, polyps, carcinomas, or masses, the presence of large clots or retained feces may preclude the use of barium enemas in the acute situation. Mucosal and submucosal lesions such as angiodysplasias or arteriovenous malformations are not visualized with barium examinations.

ANGIOGRAPHY

Extended application of endoscopy in patients with gastrointestinal bleeding and the recent introduction of radionuclide localization of bleeding sites in patients with lower gastrointestinal bleeding have altered considerably the role of angiography.

Several prerequisites are necessary for the performance of angiography. A well-trained angiography team with appropriate radiologic apparatus is necessary. An appropriate patient transport team, including a physician plus nurse or respiratory therapist (depending on the patient's ventilatory status), is essential. It is generally agreed that barium studies probably have little place in the acute management of gastrointestinal bleeding and that endoscopy should be performed, if at all possible, before arteriography. For both upper and lower gastrointestinal bleeding, the study may be useful, not only in defining pathology but also in effecting definitive therapy, namely, angiographic embolization. In addition to embolization, placement of catheters for the purpose of direct interarterial vasopressin infusion may be accomplished at the time of the initial diagnostic study.

Angiographic embolization may be used to treat lesions of the upper and lower gastrointestinal tracts. Although less likely to be useful for purposes of angiographic embolization, angiography for cases of lower intestinal bleeding is valuable in identifying major bleeding of diverticular origin as well as bleeding from lesions such as vascular ectasias.

RADIONUCLIDE STUDIES

Radionuclide studies to determine the gastrointestinal bleeding site have been used primarily for lower gastrointestinal hemorrhage. Frequently lower gastrointestinal hemorrhage may be a frustrating problem because of difficulties in localization. Conventional radiographic studies have failed to document sources of lower gastrointestinal bleeding in 20% to 25% of patients. A recent study using ^{99m}Tc-labeled red blood cells revealed accurate localization in 94% of cases. The study using ^{99m}Tc-sulfur colloid provides an excellent methodology that is simple to perform, may be done portably, and is noninvasive. This particular modality is attractive for the critically ill patient because the patient does not have to leave the ICU.

ENDOSCOPY

Since the development and widespread application of fiberoptic endoscopy, accurate diagnosis of upper gastrointestinal bleeding sites approaches 90% to 95%. Even patients with known peptic ulcer disease or esophageal varices require a specific diagnosis because frequently the bleeding site will be from a lesion other than that from the known pathology. Such information becomes necessary in formulating a therapeutic plan. Two major questions emerge regarding the use of endoscopy: "What is the diagnostic accuracy rate?" and "Does the ability to establish a precise diagnosis and effect early therapeutic intervention appreciably alter morbidity and mortality?" In several large series, endoscopy was performed within 24 hours of admission. A documented site of bleeding was found in 70% of patients and a potential source of bleeding was found in over 90%. Many experienced endoscopists believe that patients with a history of hematemesis, except for a young individual's first occurrence suggestive of viral gastroenteritis or alcoholic gastritis, should undergo upper gastrointestinal endoscopy.

The value of upper gastrointestinal endoscopy in a patient with liver disease is obvious. The etiology of upper gastrointestinal bleeding with documented cirrhosis and esophageal varices in many studies actually varies in rates ranging from 28% to 72%. This confirms the need to identify precisely the bleeding site. Regardless of the bleeding site, the presence of gastrointestinal hemorrhage is an ominous sign in a cirrhotic patient. Clearly more important than the ability to diagnose the bleeding site is the presence of liver failure or the requirement for multiple blood transfusions. Considerable controversy exists as to whether the establishment of precise diagnosis alters morbidity and mortality. No study conclusively documents the efficacy or value of upper gastrointestinal endoscopy in altering morbidity and mortality.

It should be mentioned, however, that upper gastrointestinal endoscopy may identify subgroups of patients in whom conservative management of hemorrhage is unlikely to be successful. These subgroups of patients include those with a visible vessel in the base of an active ulcer, bleeding gastrointestinal neoplasms, and active arterial hemorrhage. Because many patients in these subgroups will have coexisting MOSF, it is important to identify these subgroups before prolonged resuscitative efforts render them poor operative candidates.

THERAPY OPTIONS

COAGULATION

With the advent of fiberoptic endoscopy and the ability to pass small electrodes or laser fiberoptic light bundles down a channel of the endoscope, coagulation of actively bleeding lesions has become commonplace. Considerable experience has been amassed over the past decades in the use of electrocoagulation in upper gastrointestinal hemorrhage. The technique is particularly attractive because electrocoagulation units are small and portable, which obviates the need to transport patients to a remote area.

Monopolar and dipolar electrodes have been used. Although highly successful, monopolar electrodes tend to cause more extensive tissue coagulation. In both experimental studies and clinical trials this has resulted in an appreciable incidence of transmural injury to the stomach. In carefully controlled studies, however, actively bleeding lesions were coagulated in over 90% of cases. Bipolar electrodes emit a more "focused" current, resulting in limited tissue necrosis and lessening the possibility of transmural necrosis. Success rates with bipolar coagulation approach those with monopolar electrodes.

In the hands of experienced endoscopists, the cost–benefit analysis of electrocoagulation is attractive. Of particular significance is the patient in whom a visible vessel can be identified in the base of the ulcer. In addition to being able to precisely identify the bleeding lesion, electrocoagulation in one study has resulted in the successful arrest of hemorrhage in 15 of 16 patients. One patient in the group did rebleed 3 days after electrocoagulation and required surgical intervention.

PHOTOCOAGULATION

Although an extensive discussion of the biomedical application of laser technology is beyond the scope of this chapter, a few basic principles deserve mention. Three types of lasers currently used most often are the carbon dioxide laser, argon laser, and the neodymium aluminum yttrium garnet (YAG) laser. Carbon dioxide lasers have had the widest application as cutting surgical instruments. Carbon dioxide lasers produce light in the infrared spectrum, invisible to the naked eye. This is a high-energy type of laser that rapidly vaporizes tissue. Therefore, its application in photocoagulation has been limited owing to the depth of tissue necrosis. The argon laser produces a continuous visible blue-green light. This particular type of laser light is not absorbed by nonpigmented tissue, is transmitted through clear tissue, and has a shallow depth of tissue penetration. It is ideally suited for coagulation of retinal lesions and for the obliteration of cutaneous lesions. It has also been used extensively to treat gastrointestinal lesions. The neodymium YAG laser is also a high-powered laser source whose energy is not selectively absorbed by red pigmentation or hemoglobin, and therefore is able to penetrate through a layer of blood. This makes it ideally suited for the coagulation of actively bleeding gastrointestinal lesions. Although this is a high-energy light source (energy five times that of the argon laser), extensive tissue necrosis has not been noticed in the energy levels required for hemostatic photocoagulation. In several studies, arrest of upper gastrointestinal hemorrhage has been achieved in 85% to 90% of patients. Lesions treated to date include bleeding esophageal varices, Mallory–Weiss tears, acute and chronic ulcers, angiodysplasias, and superficial gastric erosions. The one drawback of the technology is that it requires sophisticated equipment and technical support.

INJECTION SCLEROTHERAPY

Patients with bleeding esophageal varices, who are hemodynamically unstable or who are not candidates for immediate surgery, present a peculiar therapeutic dilemma. Although balloon tamponade has been successful in arresting early hemorrhage, a significant percentage of patients rebleed once the balloon tamponade has been terminated. Therefore, injection sclerotherapy has been used for both short-term and long-term therapy. This technique is probably not effective in patients with brisk hemorrhage. However, it may certainly be used as initial therapy.

In past trials, control of the upper airway with tracheal intubation and general anesthesia was necessary to use the rigid Jackson esophagoscope for sclerotherapy. With the advent of flexible fiberoptic endoscopy and the development of new sclerosing agents such as sodium morrhuate and sodium tetradecyl sulfate, patients may be treated (often at the bedside) without general anesthesia.

It is uncertain whether the severely ill cirrhotic patients with bleeding varices may be helped by any type of therapy because of the underlying liver disease. However, such therapy may indeed temporarily arrest hemorrhage to avoid depleting the blood bank supply of various blood products. This also avoids resorting to often futile surgery in which morbidity and mortality rates are exceedingly high.

VASOACTIVE INFUSION

Systemic infusion of vasopressin has become popular for managing acute gastrointestinal hemorrhage, particularly in patients who are poor operative candidates. Vasopressin constricts the arteries and contracts the bowel wall, thus reducing mucosal blood flow and allowing the natural sequence of thrombus formation to occur.

Vasopressin is given by regional perfusion through angiographically placed catheters or by systemic venous infusion. Commonly used doses vary from 0.2 to 0.3 U/min. However, doses as high as 0.9 U/min have been used systemically by central venous infusion. To control bleeding of arterial–capillary origin, vasopressin should be infused selectively into the vessel supplying the bleeding site. In many studies, the left gastric artery has been noted as the vessel from which most acute gastrointestinal hemorrhage occurs. The second most commonly bleeding vessel has been the gastroduodenal artery. Therefore, if these two vessels can be identified, selective vasopressin infusion may successfully decrease hemorrhage. With the exception of left-sided colonic lesions that have been controlled with intravenous infusion of vasopressin, little data support the hypothesis that intravenous infusion of vasopressin will alter the course of arterial–capillary hemorrhage.

In patients with portal hypertension or bleeding gastroesophageal varices, intravenous vasopressin infusion at low doses substantially reduces mesenteric arterial blood flow and, therefore, portal pressure. It is suggested that these infusions be delivered by a centrally placed line because extravasation of vasopressin into subcutaneous tissue may result in significant tissue slough.

The overall complication rate of vasopressin infusion among 599 patients studied at Massachusetts General Hospital was 9.5%. Major complications were cardiovascular. Readily reversible minor complications included dysrhythmias, oliguria, hyponatremia, pulmonary edema, and peripheral cyanosis. Vasopressin use may be precluded in patients with significant vascular disease.

TRANSCATHETER EMBOLIZATION

The other angiographic modality that has been successful is transcatheter embolization. This modality should be considered only when vasopressin infusion fails to control acutely bleeding lesions.

Various embolic substances have been used, including stainless steel coils, polyvinyl alcohol, and cyanoacrylate. Alternatively, pledgets of Gelfoam or Gelfoam plus thrombin have been used to accomplish transcatheter embolizations. In a recent review, 219 transcatheter embolizations were performed on patients with gastrointestinal bleeding, including tumors, arteriovenous malformations, and aneurysms. The reported incidence of major complications was only 5% and included gastric ischemia, peritonitis, aspiration, renal failure, and failure to control the bleeding source. Since many of these patients were considered poor surgical candidates, this may be considered an acceptable complication rate.

This therapy may be considered a primary mode of angiographic management in patients with a bleeding duodenal lesion and in those who are poor operative candidates. Bleeding from Mallory–Weiss lesions may be controlled either with vasopressin infusion in the left gastric artery or by embolization of surgical gelatin. Lesions in the small bowel, including arteriovenous malformations, leiomyomata, and mesenteric varices, have all been embolized successfully. The incidence of other lesions such as angiodysplasias has become more obvious with the refinement of angiographic techniques. The use of angiography in these patients, however, rests more with the establishment of diagnosis rather than effecting definitive therapy.

For more information, please see Chapter 107 in Civetta JM, Taylor RW, Kirby RR: Critical Care. *Philadelphia: J. B. Lippincott, 1988*

BIBLIOGRAPHY

Anthanasoulis CA: Angiography in the management of patients with gastrointestinal bleeding. *Adv. Surg* 1983; 16:1
Clouse RE, Costigan DJ, MIlls BA, et al: Angiodysplasia as a cause of upper gastrointestinal bleeding. *Arch Intern Med* 1985; 145:458
Cutler JA, Mendelhoff AI: Upper gastrointestinal bleeding: Nature and magnitude of the problem in the U.S. *Dig Dis Sci* July (suppl) 1981; 26(7):90s
Forde KA: Colonoscopy in the diagnosis and management of colonic bleeding. *Bull NY Acad Med* 1983; 59(3):301
Kauffman GL Jr: Mucosal damage to the stomach: How, when and why? *Scand J Gastroenterol* 1984; 19(suppl 105):19
Lieberman DA, Keller FS, Katon RM, et al: Arterial embolization for massive upper gastrointestinal tract bleeding in poor surgical candidates. *Gastroenterology* 1984; 86:876
Orecchia PM, Hensley EK, McDonald PT, et al: Localization of lower gastrointestinal hemorrhage: Experience with red blood cells labeled *in vitro* with technetium TC-99m. *Arch Surg* 1985; 120:621
Pingleton SK: Gastrointestinal hemorrhage. *Med Clin North Am* 1983; 67(6):1215
Silverstein FE, Gilbert DA, Auth DC: Endoscopic hemostasis using laser photocoagulation and electrocoagulation. *Dig Dis Sci* July (suppl) 1981; 26(7):31s
Wara P: Endoscopic control of major stress ulcer bleeding. *Scand J Gastroenterol* 1984; 19 (suppl 105):101
Wexler MJ: Emergency management of upper gastrointestinal bleeding. *Compr Ther* 1982; 8(8):7

60 Hepatobiliary Disease

Patients with acute, severe liver disease may be admitted to the ICU if reversibility of hepatic failure is considered possible. Since the advent of liver transplantation, this determination is more difficult because patients with irreversible liver disease who can be stabilized physiologically can be considered candidates for transplantation.

FULMINANT HEPATIC FAILURE

Approximately 1% of patients with icteric hepatitis develop massive necrosis of the liver. Most ICU patients will come from this subgroup. Hepatitis B patients present a high risk for transmission of the infection to ICU personnel. Vaccination is therefore recommended for personnel who have frequent contact with type B viral hepatitis or with patients' blood.

Hepatic failure can also result from drugs, Reye's syndrome, pregnancy, and Wilson's disease, among others. Prolongation of the prothrombin time by 10 seconds or more is the best laboratory parameter to predict massive necrosis of the liver. Supportive care should be directed to prevent hypoglycemia, correct precipitating factors or encephalopathy, and treat cerebral edema.

HEPATIC ABSCESS

Currently, management of liver abscesses has shifted to a predominantly medical approach. Patients are admitted when hypotensive and septic. The diagnosis can be established with ultrasonography, computed tomography (CT) scans, and needle aspiration in selected cases. Blood cultures and amebic titers should also be taken on admission. In addition to resuscitation and treatment of depressed cardiovascular function, broad-spectrum antibiotic coverage, including metronidazole effective against *Entamoeba histolytica* and anaerobes, should be used. Percutaneous catheter drainage may also be used in the initial stages of management. Surgical drainage is usually considered only if patients fail to respond to antibiotic therapy and catheter drainage. The clinical presentation of hepatic malignancy may mimic liver abscess.

CHOLESTASIS

Patients with clinical and laboratory signs suggestive of obstructive jaundice usually have features of bacteremia and septic shock when considered for admission to the ICU. Mechanical obstruction of the biliary tree must be differentiated from intrahepatic cholestasis. Surgery is necessary in the first instance and contraindicated in the second. Shaking chills and toxemia are more common with suppurative cholangitis. The differential diagnosis can be particularly difficult in the alcoholic patient because alcoholic hepatitis is also associated with nausea, vomiting, abdominal pain, fever, and jaundice. Liver biopsy may be diagnostic and may be performed if the prothrombin time is not greater than 4 seconds above control and if the platelet count is greater than $50,000/mm^3$. Direct cholangiography should be performed to prove the presence of mechanical obstruction before operation if alcoholic hepatitis is a serious consideration.

COMPLICATIONS OF CIRRHOSIS

If the patient is bleeding from gastroesophageal varices, intravenous pitressin should be used in a dose of 0.3 to 0.5 U/min. If the patient has coronary artery disease, nitroglycerin should be given to counteract the coronary vasoconstriction. Endoscopic sclerotherapy may be used whether or not the bleeding continues. If bleeding cannot be controlled, a Blakemore–Sengstaken tube should be inserted. An emergency surgical decompression may be necessary if these measures have not stopped the bleeding.

Paracentesis is mandatory to establish the diagnosis of spontaneous bacterial peritonitis. The white blood cell (WBC) count is usually greater than $500/mm^3$, predominantly polymorphonuclear leukocytes. Specimens should be cultured at the bedside. Broad-spectrum antibiotic coverage is necessary, but aminoglycosides should be avoided if at all possible.

Patients with hepatic encephalopathy may be admitted to the ICU. Except for fetor hepaticus, the clinical features mimic a spectrum of metabolic encephalopathies. In a cirrhotic patient, the precipitating factors should be investigated and eliminated if possible: central nervous system (CNS) depressants, electrolyte imbalance, azotemia, gastrointestinal bleeding, infection, and hypoxia. Lactulose may be given initially by enema and then by nasogastric tube.

Hepatorenal syndrome is characterized by a rising blood urea nitrogen (BUN) value and a low urine sodium level (less than 10 meq/liter). Patients usually have ascites refractory to oral diuretic therapy. Hepatorenal syndrome must be differentiated from volume depletion and acute tubular necrosis. Invasive cardiovascular monitoring may help identify the diagnosis and guide further fluid therapy. Intravenous albumin, 250 to 500 ml of 5% solution, furosemide, 20 to 60 mg, and mannitol, 200 ml of 20% solution, may promote diuresis. Paracentesis may be necessary if the ascites is tense and massive. Volume replacement may also be necessary. Peritoneal venous shunting may be considered in patients with reversible liver disease. Ultrafiltration of ascitic fluid, continuous arteriovenous hemofiltration, continuous ultrafiltration, and hemodialysis are other means of treating ascites in the hemodynamically unstable cirrhotic.

HEPATOBILIARY DYSFUNCTION IN THE CRITICALLY ILL PATIENT

The typical patient with multiple organ system failure (MOSF) has an increased pigment load, hypoxic injury to the liver, liver failure, and sepsis. Old bank blood represents an increased pigment load (250 mg bilirubin/U). Unconjugated hyperbilirubinemia occurs if the maximum capacity to transport unconjugated bilirubin is exceeded. Usually conjugated hyperbilirubinemia is present because the secretory step is rate limiting. Hypoxic injury may range from subtle liver chemical abnormalities to a clinical picture of fulminant hepatic failure with profound encephalopathy. Renal failure impairs the excretion of bilirubin, and hyperbilirubinemia will be disproportionately high for the magnitude of the liver dysfunction. Additionally, azotemia may precipitate or worsen encephalopathy due to the increased ammonia production created by urea diffusion into the gut. The jaundice of sepsis is not well characterized but is probably multifactorial. Endotoxin may compromise biliary secretion; associated renal failure and hypotension compound the impaired biliary secretion.

Postoperative jaundice is rarely due to common duct injury or halogenated anesthetic-induced hepatitis. It is usually the result of the four preceding mechanisms. If a cholestatic picture evolves, direct cholangiography should be used to prove mechanical obstruction. Non-A, non-B post-transfusion hepatitis may occur with a mean incubation period of approximately 50 days. The hepatitis induced by halogenated anesthetics is usually preceded by several days of fever and followed by a picture similar to viral hepatitis. Rash and eosinophilia may also be present. Jaundice due to common duct ligation or injury is usually not apparent for some days because the bilirubin rises only at a rate of 0.5 to 2 mg/dl/day.

CONCLUSION

A spectrum of hepatobiliary disorders should be cared for in an ICU. Paramount among these entities are fulminant hepatic failure, bleeding esophageal varices, severe hepatic encephalopathy, suppurative cholangitis with sepsis, and selected cases with spontaneous bacterial peritonitis. Significant hepatobiliary dysfunction may become apparent in patients with MOSF treated in an ICU. The characteristics and the severity of the hepatobiliary dysfunction in these patients are often a reflection of pigment load, hypoxia, renal failure, and sepsis.

For more information, please see Chapter 108 in Civetta JM, Taylor JW, Kirby RR: Critical Care. *Philadelphia: J. B. Lippincott, 1988*

BIBLIOGRAPHY

Bernuau J. Rueff B, Benhamou J–P: Fulminant and subfulminant liver failure: Definition and causes. *Semin Liver Dis* 1986; 6:97

Canalese J, Gimson AES, Davis C, et al: Controlled trial of dexamethasone and mannitol for the cerebral oedema of fulminant hepatic failure. *Gut* 1982; 23:625

Cello JP, Grendell JH, Grass RA, et al: Endoscopic sclerotherapy versus portacaval shunt in patients with severe cirrhosis and acute variceal hemorrhage. *N Engl J Med* 1987; 316:11

Epstein M: Renal complications in liver disease. In Schiff L, Schiff ER (eds): *Diseases of the Liver,* 6th ed, pp 903–923. Philadelphia, JB Lippincott, 1987

Kwatsuki et al: Liver transplantation for fulminant hepatic failure. *Am J Gastroenterol* 1986; 81:879

LaMont JT, Isselbacher KJ: Postoperative jaundice. *N Engl J Med* 1973; 288:305

McDonald MI, Corey GR, Callis HA, et al: Single and multiple pyogenic liver abscesses: Natural history, diagnosis and treatment, with emphasis on percutaneous drainage. *Medicine* 1984; 63:291

Mendenhall CL: Alcoholic hepatitis. In Schiff L, Schiff ER (eds): *Diseases of the Liver,* 6th ed, pp 669–686. Philadelphia, JB Lippincott, 1987

Schiff ER: Nonsurgical management of emergency hemorrhage for esophageal varices. In Zeppa R (ed): *Progress Symposium on Portal Hypertension. World J Surg* 1984; 8:50

61 Pancreatic Disease

DIAGNOSIS AND ADMISSION INDICATIONS

It is often difficult to make a conclusive diagnosis of pancreatitis or to separate it from other causes of acute abdominal pain. Specific diagnosis of the complications of pancreatitis is equally difficult. Historical features include similar attacks or previous hospitalizations along with associated etiologic factors such as alcohol and biliary tract disease. Once the patient develops peritoneal signs, there are no distinguishing features, although isolated head or tail disease may localize pain to the right or left upper quadrant and referred pain may be localized to subscapular areas if there is diaphragmatic irritation. An elevated serum amylase level is sensitive but not specific because hyperamylasemia is found in perforated or penetrating peptic ulcers, ruptured ectopic pregnancy, and intestinal obstruction or infarction. Radiographic diagnostic signs, again, are not specific but include duodenal ileus, jejunal ileus or "sentinel loop," or elevated hemidiaphragm and pleural effusion. Ultrasonography may be limited by this ileus, but it may be helpful in confirming the clinical diagnosis, detecting complications early, and identifying associated biliary tract disease. Computed tomography (CT) scans can be used to detect changes in gland size and abnormalities of pancreatic ducts and to identify peripancreatic fluid collections. It may also be used to differentiate pancreatic phlegmon from abscess.

Eleven clinical features identified by Ranson correlate with patient morbidity, length of stay in the intensive care unit (ICU), and eventual mortality. Five can be assessed on admission: age older than 55 years, blood glucose value greater than 200 mg/dl, white blood cell (WBC) count greater than 16,000/mm^3, serum lactic dehydrogenase (LDH) value greater than 350 IU/liter, and serum glutamic oxaloacetic transaminase (SGOT) greater than 250 Sigma Frankel units. The other six features are evaluated within 48 hours of admission: serum calcium level less than 8 mg/dl, arterial P_{O_2} less than 60 mm Hg, base deficit greater than 4 meq/liter, blood urea nitrogen (BUN) increase greater than 5 mg/dl, hematocrit fall greater than 10 percentage points, and fluid sequestration greater than 6 liters. Fewer than three of the criteria are usually correlated with the benign form and course of the disease. Therefore, admission to the ICU can be suggested for any patient with three or more of the criteria, those who need monitoring, large volume resuscitation, or ventilatory support, or those with metabolic imbalance, renal insufficiency, cardiovascular collapse, and sepsis with multiorgan system failure (MOSF).

CARE IMPLICATIONS OF PANCREATIC DISEASE

The overall therapeutic principles for acute pancreatitis include placing the pancreas "at rest," supporting the patient's metabolic and nutritional needs, and correcting the acute causes of mortality: cardiovascular collapse, respiratory insufficiency, and renal failure. Detecting the development of complications that require surgery and preventing and treating septic complications are also necessary.

Suppression of pancreatic function has been attempted by eliminating oral fluids and suppressing acid secretion, by gastric decompression, and by giving antacids, anticholinergics, and proteolytic enzyme inhibitors. None has been shown to alter the outcome of the disease significantly, but ileus and the risk of erosive gastritis justify stopping oral intake, using gastric suction and some form of acid suppression or neutralization.

Metabolic and nutritional support are necessary because of the duration of the illness and the increase in caloric requirements caused by septic complications. Because of the variations in glucose intolerance, insulin may be necessary using sliding scale coverage, drips, or direct administration with parenteral nutrition.

Given the volume of electrolyte-rich fluid loss, careful attention to both fluid and electrolyte balance is mandatory. Hypocalcemia is common although ionized calcium may not be decreased. Cardiovascular collapse and respiratory insufficiency, although similar in many respects to other acute illnesses, have some special features. Cardiac output may remain depressed despite adequate filling pressures; inotropic agents may be used in these situations independent of demonstrating myocardial depressant factor. Respiratory insufficiency may develop secondary to activation of C5a complement or degradation in pulmonary surfactant by activated pancreatic enzymes. Invasive cardiovascular monitoring is frequently used to differentiate myocardial depression from hypovolemia and to guide the effects of therapy. Ventilatory support with positive end-expiratory pressure (PEEP) may be necessary to correct acute hypoxemia; mechnical support may also be necessary to aid in the elimination of carbon dioxide.

Renal insufficiency may be related to massive fluid losses although, late in the disease, compromised renal function associated with septic complications is common.

Management of pancreatitis has two principal objectives: complete physiologic resuscitation and support and continued observation for complications that require special procedures or surgical intervention. Early in the course, surgery may be necessary when other "surgical" causes cannot be definitively excluded (bowel infarction) and for the treatment of biliary tract disease which initiated the episode of pancreatitis.

The treatment of developing complications requires continued vigilance to detect their onset, to diagnose them quickly, and to intervene effectively. Vascular complications include bleeding from pancreatic pseudocysts and ruptured pseudoaneurysms. These may present with melena or hypovolemia and abdominal pain subsequent to rupture into the peritoneal cavity. The diagnostic and therapeutic plan includes emergency upper gastrointestinal endoscopy, selective visceral angiography, ultrasound, and CT scanning. Temporary control can be effected by selective arterial catheterization and pitressin infusion, embolization, or electrocoagulation. These procedures may be considered temporizing measures until the patient can tolerate surgery. Portal venous thrombosis may be recognized by acute decompensation, hypotension with fluid sequestration, acidosis, hepatic enzyme elevation, alteration in clotting studies and, finally, venous infarction of the bowel.

Pseudocyst formation is not infrequent and may spontaneously resolve during the first 6 weeks. Pseudocysts that persist longer should have definitive treatment because of the increased frequency of complications and rare resolution. Complications include infection, visceral and biliary tract obstruction, free rupture into the peritoneal cavity, the bowel, or the pleural space, or hemorrhage. Diagnosis may be made with CT scans and can be followed using ultrasound. Infected pseudocysts can be confirmed by percutaneous needle aspiration. Pseudocysts may resolve after catheter drainage; otherwise, operative internal decompression may be required.

Biliary obstruction secondary to acute pancreatitis occurs frequently, and this resulting obstruction can be confused with the initiating etiology. If it does not resolve, ultrasonography, endoscopic retrograde choledochopancreatography, or percutaneous transhepatic cholangiography (PTC) may be necessary. To avoid an emergency operation, PTC and drainage may be used to decompress patients who develop acute cholangitis.

The most difficult and devastating complication is the development of pancreatic necrosis and abscess. It is rare to see septic complications in the first week, not unusual after the second week, and almost universal if the patient remains in the ICU for more than 3 weeks. Abdominal pain, fever, and leukocytosis associated with severe systemic deterioration strongly suggest the onset of this complication. Approximately one third of patients with three or more of Ranson's prognostic signs develop pancreatic sepsis. The problem is complicated by differentiating a pancreatic source of sepsis from the usual nosocomial infections that develop in long-term ICU patients, including pneumonia, urinary tract infection, and catheter-related infection. Sequential CT scanning is the best tool for diagnosing and following the disease process. Percutaneous techniques play little role in adequate drainage of a pancreatic abscess because the tissue is usually thick, stringy, necrotic, devitalized, and heavily contaminated, requiring widespread debridement and large sump drains. Recently, marsupialization of the lesser sac and open packing have permitted daily dressing changes, irrigation, and repacking in the ICU with the patient appropriately sedated. In this manner, development of recurrent abscesses with clinical deterioration and the necessity for multiple operations can be avoided.

Finally, prolonged tube drainage may result in intestinal fistulization into the colon and duodenum. The management of the controlled fistula probably carries less morbidity than the necessity for reoperation because of premature removal of lesser sac drains. Hemorrhage, a feared complication of this disease, may be difficult to control in the face of necrotic surrounding tissue. Open packing and radiographic embolization of the bleeding vessel may be necessary.

For more information, please see Chapter 109 in Civetta JM, Taylor RW, Kirby RR: Critical Care. *Philadelphia: J. B. Lippincott, 1988*

BIBLIOGRAPHY

Balslov JT, Jorgensen HE, Nielsen R: Acute renal failure complicating severe pancreatitis. *Acta Chir Scand* 1962; 124:348

Bradley EL III, Clements JL Jr, Gonzalez AC: The natural history of pancreatic pseudocysts: A unified concept of management. *Am J Surg* 1979; 137:135

Cameron JL, Kieffer RS, Anderson WJ, Zuidema GD: Internal pancreatic fistulas: Pancreatic ascites and pleural effusions. *Ann Surg* 1976; 183:587

Davidson ED, Bradley EL III: "Marsupialization" in the treatment of pancreatic abscess. *Surgery* 1981; 89:252

Harper PC, Gamelli RL, Kaye MD: Recurrent hemorrhage into the pancreatic duct from a splenic artery aneurysm. *Gastroenterology* 1984; 87:417

Imrie CW, Allam BF, Ferguson JC: Hypocalcaemia of acute pancreatitis: The effect of hypoalbuminaemia. *Curr Med Res Opinion* 1976; 4:101

Mayer AD, McMahon MJ, Benson EA, Axon ATR: Operations upon the biliary tract in patients with acute pancreatitis: Aims, indications and timing. *Ann R. Coll Surg* 1984; 66:179

Nunez D Jr, Yrizarry JM, Russel E, et al: Transgastric drainage of pancreatic fluid collections. AJR 1985; 145:815

Ranson JHC, Spencer FC: The role of peritoneal lavage in severe acute pancreatitis. *Ann Surg* 1978; 187:565

Salt WB II. Schenker S: Amylase—Its clinical significance: A review of the literature. *Medicine* 1976; 55:269

Satiani B, Stone HH: Predictability of present outcome and future recurrence in acute pancreatitis. *Arch Surg* 1979; 114:711

Trapnell JE, Duncan EHL: Patterns of incidence in acute pancreatitis. *Br Med J* 1975; 1:179

62
Inflammatory Bowel Disease

Inflammatory bowel disease produces a number of complications that may require admission to an intensive care unit (ICU). Fulminant colitis, toxic megacolon, perforation, and massive hemorrhage are the most serious of these complications from an acute life-threatening standpoint and may occur in ulcerative colitis, Crohn's disease, and various infections.

FULMINANT COLITIS AND TOXIC MEGACOLON

The terms severe or fulminant colitis and toxic megacolon are often used interchangeably, but the syndrome of toxic megacolon more appropriately refers specifically to colonic dilation superimposed on a toxic state of acute fulminant colitis. Although most commonly seen with ulcerative colitis, fulminant colitis and toxic megacolon may occur in Crohn's disease, amebic colitis, shigella and salmonella infection, pseudomembranous colitis, and ischemic bowel disease. Regardless of the cause, fulminant colitis can accelerate quickly toward perforation and death. This is a medical/surgical emergency that requires hospitalization and integrated multidisciplinary care. When strictly defined, toxic megacolon is a relatively rare complication, but perforation can occur without megacolon.

CLINICAL FEATURES

Patients with severe or fulminant colitis are usually quite ill with frequent, often bloody diarrheal stools, fevere, anemia, hypoalbuminemia, weakness, and severe general debility. Fulminant ulcerative colitis may occur as a complication in a patient with a short or long-standing history of inflammatory bowel disease and commonly occurs as the initial presentation of the illness. Toxic megacolon is defined as a severe attack of colitis with total or segmental dilatation of the colon and can be regarded as a phase of toxic colitis.

On physical examination, vital signs show fever and tachycardia. Toxicity may be further manifested by lethargy, pallor, hypotension, mental changes, and signs of dehydration. Abdominal distention may be present, and frequently the contour of the dilated transverse colon can be seen or felt during examination. Bowel sounds are usually diminished, and the abdomen is often tympanitic on percussion. Localized tenderness, especially in the left upper quadrant, implies local peritonitis and impending perforation. Generalized tenderness, rebound tenderness, guarding, and complaints of shoulder-tip pain indicate free perforation, but surprisingly few clinical signs of frank peritonitis may be present in some patients. Some of these findings may be modified or masked by concurrent steroid therapy or disturbances of the patient's sensorium. Toxic psychosis and delirium should be regarded as sinister signs and are a reflection of toxemia. Gram-negative septicemia may be present but unrecognized.

Anemia, leukocytosis, electrolyte disturbances, and hypoalbuminemia are frequently present. Hypokalemia secondary to gastrointestinal loss is common and may contribute to the development of colonic dilatation, whereas other investigators believe that a clear-cut relationship has not been shown. Hypoalbuminemia is usually evidence for chronicity or severity of illness, but a rapid drop implies increasing toxicity, and in one series a serum albumin value of less than 1.9 g/dl was associated with a high mortality.

In all patients suspected of having severe or fulminant colitis or toxic megacolon of any etiology, plain abdominal films are essential. Anteroposterior recumbent and upright or left lateral decubitus films should be obtained in all patients. Such films may not only provide some information on distribution and extent of involvement but also are particularly important for diagnosing perforation and toxic megacolon. The plain recumbent film is usually diagnostic in patients with toxic megacolon. Colonic dilatation may affect the entire colon but is usually segmental, with the transverse colon being the most prominently dilated segment. The descending and sigmoid colon are also often distended; the rectum is rarely distended. Although dilatation of the transverse colon on a plain supine abdominal radiograph is a most conspicuous finding, it does not have specific pathophysiologic significance. Distention of the transverse colon in toxic megacolon is the result of its anterior position, and repositioning the patient redistributes gas to other segments depending on the position used. Dilatation beyond 5.5 cm is generally considered abnormal, and attempts have been made to fix the definition of toxic megacolon on the basis of the diameter of the transverse colon. However, strict criteria cannot be applied because the caliber of the distended segments can vary greatly. It is best not to rely on a single measurement of this type but to consider the radiographic appearance as only one factor, with the clinical manifestations being of equal importance.

Haustra may be absent but may be thickened early and subsequently disappear. The mucosal surface may display multiple broad-based nodular intraluminal protrusions due to pseudopolyps. Occasionally, a radiolucent line paralleling the bowel lumen can be seen and is believed to represent intramuscular air dissection, suggesting that perforation may be imminent.

Although perforation is rare in the absence of toxic dilatation, for unclear reasons it is more likely to occur during the initial severe attack of ulcerative colitis. Perforation is most common in patients with pancolitis and is most frequent in the sigmoid colon. In most cases, free intraperitoneal air can be easily demonstrated on the upright or lateral decubitus films.

When the classical features of toxicity and colonic dilatation occur in a patient with known idiopathic inflammatory bowel disease, a confident diagnosis of fulminant colitis or toxic megacolon can be made. In other patients, the diagnosis may be less clear and sigmoidoscopy should be performed to exclude the other much less frequent etiologies that can present in the same fashion. Most patients with inflammatory bowel disease should undergo sigmoidoscopy to exclude a superimposed infectious colitis (e.g., amebiasis) since steroid therapy could have devastating results. Sigmoidoscopy should be done with gentle, minimal manipulation and without preparation or air insufflation.

There are few, if any, indications for performing a barium enema in patients with fulminant colitis, and it is not required for routine management. The role of a barium enema in precipitating toxic megacolon is unclear, but it is generally believed to be contraindicated in toxic megacolon. The interdiction of barium enema in patients with fulminant colitis and toxic megacolon still holds.

MANAGEMENT

Fulminant colitis and toxic megacolon are medical/surgical emergencies requiring hospitalization, usually in an ICU, and integrated multidisciplinary care. Regardless of the etiology, if the initial assessment reveals perforation, immediate surgical intervention is mandatory. If perforation is not present, a short trial of medical management is indicated. The goals of therapy are to

1 Replace fluid, blood, and electrolyte losses rapidly;

2 Institute aggressive medical therapy;

3 Avoid precipitating toxic megacolon;

4 Monitor very closely to avoid perforation; and

5 Use surgery early if prompt and sustained improvement is not achieved.

A number of factors have been implicated as contributing to toxic dilatation in patients with a severe attack of colitis. Various medications that interfere with gut motility such as opiates (codeine, diphenoxylate), anticholinergics, and synthetic antidiarrheal agents (loperamide) have been accused of predisposing to toxic megacolon, but this has never been proven. The possible relation of toxic megacolon to hypokalemia and barium enema has been mentioned, and colonoscopy can be considered to have the same status. Despite suggestive observations it is not uniformly agreed that a cause-and-effect relationship exists between these factors and development of toxic megacolon. However, these drugs and diagnostic procedures are rarely, if ever, required in the management of a patient with acute colitis and therefore should be avoided.

Treatment consists of general supportive measures and efforts to arrest the necrotic process in the colon. Oral intake is discontinued and a nasogastric tube (16 French) placed and connected to intermittent suction to aspirate swallowed air to minimize bowel distention. Rectal tubes should not be used because of the risk of perforation.

Because extensive ulceration may facilitate bacterial invasion with resultant bacteremia and because frank perforation is a constant danger, broad-spectrum antibiotics are recommended. Acceptable regimens are ampicillin-gentamicin-clindamycin or metronidazole and cefoxitin-gentamicin. When amebiasis is suspected, intravenous metronidazole should be used.

Most authors agree on the use of corticosteroids in the treatment of fulminant colitis or toxic megacolon from ulcerative colitis or Crohn's disease. For patients with fulminant colitis or toxic megacolon, parenteral steroids such as prednisolone, 60 mg/day in divided doses, should be used for 48 to 72 hours. Patients who do not respond promptly or those who develop colonic perforation or even suspected perforation require prompt surgical attention.

OBSERVATION

Thus far the patient has been diagnosed, resuscitated, and treated medically. At this point, immediate surgery is indicated for free perforation or signs of general peritonitis, impending perforation, or massive hemorrhage. In the absence of perforation a short period of medical treatment is justified and does not adversely affect surgical morbidity or mortality. If a patient is going to respond to medical management, response generally occurs within 24 to 72 hours. During this time the patient's condition can deteriorate rapidly and frequent reexamination (every 4–6 hours) is required.

The frequency, volume, and nature of diarrhea should be recorded. Improvement in the patient's diarrhea to the point of absolute constipation is a sinister feature and reflects diminished colonic evacuation. Misinterpretation of this change may be avoided by examining the abdomen, which reveals distention, diminished bowel sounds, and tenderness. A plain abdominal radiograph may confirm continued colonic dilatation, and perforation should be looked for by upright or left decubitus radiographs. The corollary is also true that recurrence of diarrhea during medical treatment of toxic megacolon implies improvement in the patient's condition. Serial abdominal girth measurements may be an additional useful objective parameter in assessing overall abdominal distention. Repeated abdominal examination a few times a day is essential. Serial flat and upright abdominal radiographs are needed (sometimes twice daily), particularly if megacolon was initially present. The various hematologic parameters, electrolytes, especially potassium, and blood chemistry values are regularly monitored. No single parameter, however, is ideal to follow. For example, dramatic response to medical treatment may occur in the absence of radiographic improvement. A synthesis of the *overall* clinical picture is essential for determining whether the patient is responding.

Signs of impending perforation include spiking fever, leukocytosis, tachycardia, hypotension, worsening abdominal pain or tenderness, abdominal distention, and, as mentioned, a decrease in diarrhea as an ileus occurs. Steroids may mask signs and symptoms, causing the so-called silent perforation. The physician or nurse examining the patient may notice increasing toxicity, restlessness, or lethargy.

SURGERY

The different views regarding the necessity of surgical treatment of toxic megacolon have already been mentioned. There is not uniformity of opinion as to the best type of operation, and each surgeon must assess the risks in his own setting and based on his own experience. The three commonly performed procedures for toxic megacolon are subtotal colectomy and ileostomy with rectal mucus fistula, total proctocolectomy and ileostomy, and diverting loop ileostomy with decompressive, skin level ("blow-hole") colostomy. Subtotal colectomy and ileostomy is the most widely used procedure because it is less technically demanding, easier, and quicker than proctocolectomy. Usually a second-stage procedure is required for subsequent removal of the rectum or ilealrectal anastomosis. If an experienced colonic surgeon is available, proctocolectomy may be the procedure of choice, particularly for the good operative risk patient without colonic perforation. The diverting ileostomy and decompressive colostomy is not widely used.

TOXIC MEGACOLON FROM INFECTIOUS CAUSES

Infectious agents (ameba, *Salmonella, Shigella, Clostridium*) may occasionally cause toxic megacolon. Management should follow exactly the same general principles as already outlined. This implies a trial of medical therapy with emergency colectomy if there is not a swift response. If an infective agent is known or suspected, even in an accessory role, appropriate antibiotic therapy should be used to cover surgery.

COLONIC PERFORATION/MASSIVE HEMORRHAGE

After adequate resuscitation, patients who present with perforation or develop this complication during medical treatment require surgery. Massive hemorrhage is rare in inflammatory bowel disease, usually subsides spontaneously, and only rarely requires colectomy for control of bleeding. The same general principles that pertain to the management of any gastrointestinal bleeding apply to these patients and have been discussed previously in Chapter 59.

For more information, please see Chapter 110 in Civetta JM, Taylor RW, Kirby RR: Critical Care. *Philadelphia: J. B. Lippincott, 1988*

BIBLIOGRAPHY

Bayless TM: Fulminant colitis and toxic megacolon. In Bayless TM (ed): *Current Therapy in Gastroenterology and Liver Disease 1984–1985,* p 311. Philadelphia, BC Decker, 1984

Cassidy D, Boyd WP Jr: Toxic megacolon. In Nord NJ, Brady PG (eds): *Critical Care Gastroenterology,* p 317. New York, Churchill Livingstone, 1982

Famer RG, Hamilton SR, Morson BC, et al: Ulcerative colitis. In Berk JE (ed): *Bockus Gastroenterology,* 4th ed, p 2137. Philadelphia, WB Saunders, 1985

Fazio VW: Toxic megacolon in ulcerative colitis and Crohn's colitis. *Clin Gastroenterol* 1980; 9:389

Kramer P, Wittenburg J: Colonic gas distribution in toxic megacolon. *Gastroenterology* 1981; 80:433

Meyers S, Janowitz HD: Systemic corticosteroid therapy of ulcerative colitis. *Gastroenterology* 1985; 89:1189

Perkel MS: Acute inflammatory bowel disease. CCQ 1982; 5:21

Smith JN, Winship DH: Complications and extraintestinal problems in inflammatory bowel disease. *Med Clin North Am* 1980; 64:1161

Truelove SC, Marks SG: Toxic megacolon. *Clin Gastroenterol* 1981; 10:107

63 The Esophagus

Esophageal bleeding, reviewed in Chapter 59 is usually dramatic, but other disorders may have subtle presentations.

General guidelines for evaluation and management emphasize

1 Protection of the airway from aspiration;

2 Consideration of aspiration and secondary pulmonary insult occurring *prior* to presentation;

3 Elimination of ongoing damage (as in the case of corrosives); and

4 Avoidance of long-term complications by careful initial management.

CORROSIVE INJURY

PRESENTATION

Clinical presentation is dependent on the type (alkali/acid) and nature (solid/liquid) of the caustic substance. Liquid alkali is swallowed rapidly, causing less oropharyngeal injury but extensive damage to the esophagus and stomach. Solid alkali causes severe burns to the oropharynx and induces severe pain and expectoration such that little corrosive is actually swallowed. Acid ingestion injury is more localized to the gastric antrum, but systemic acidosis and toxicity have been reported. Thus, mouth pain, hoarseness, dysphagia, odynophagia, or abdominal pain occurs as determined by the agent ingested and location of the injury. Stridor, aphonia, dyspnea, and hoarseness suggest laryngeal edema. Substernal, abdominal, or back pain raises concern for mediastinitis or peritonitis.

Physical examination of the lips, mouth, and pharynx can reveal a spectrum of injury from mild erythema to erosions, ulcers, and obvious severe burns. Some authors have graded the injury by the presence and severity of oropharyngeal findings at the time of admission. It is often possible to estimate the degree of esophageal injury from the state of the oropharynx and type of agent ingested, but esophageal damage has been seen in patients without oropharyngeal burns.

DIAGNOSIS

After the history and physical examination have been obtained, with particular attention devoted to the oropharyngeal and airway status, laboratory data are directed at determining complications of the ingestion such as renal or hepatic insufficiency or anemia. Chest and abdominal radiographs should be performed looking for evidence of aspiration, visceral perforation, or mediastinal air. After the patient has been stabilized, the extent and severity of disease can be evaluated by fiberoptic endoscopy. When endoscopy was initially introduced as a diagnostic procedure for evaluating caustic ingestions, concern was raised about the risk of perforation. Authors opposed using early endoscopy or recommended not passing the endoscope beyond the first burned area. Recent work suggests that endoscopy can be safely performed early and provides information about severity and extent of damage that may influence management. When possible, a complete endoscopic examination evaluating the esophagus, stomach, and duodenum should be accomplished.

Radiographic examination can be helpful particularly if endoscopy is not available or is dangerous because of suspected perforation. In these situations, water-soluble contrast agents should be used.

MANAGEMENT

Initial efforts are directed toward stabilizing the patient and replacing fluids and blood as appropriate. The need for careful assessment of the airway cannot be overemphasized. Translaryngeal intubation or tracheostomy may be necessary. Evidence of esophageal perforation requires early surgical intervention. The corrosive should be neutralized only if the patient is seen within an hour of ingestion. Milk or antacids are used for acid ingestions and water or vinegar for alkali ingestions. Nasogastric intubation should be avoided unless the tube is placed under direct vision.

Early endoscopy is used when feasible. Complete examination of the esophagus, stomach, and duodenum should be attempted. If no significant injury is found, the patient can be discharged. In patients with significant injury, hospitalization and careful management are necessary. The use of steroids or antibiotics is not routinely advocated. Broad-spectrum antibiotic coverage is used for signs of aspiration, infection, suspected perforation, or when deep ulcers are present and perforation seems imminent. Laryngeal edema is treated with short courses of high-dose steroids. Early bougienage using mercury-weighted rubber (Maloney) or polyvinyl dilators can be used in an attempt to prevent stricture and is usually started 2 to 3 weeks after the ingestion. Patients are kept NPO until they can swallow their saliva. Then, clear liquids are allowed, advancing the diet thereafter as tolerated. Parenteral nutrition should be started early after stabilization.

It must be remembered that corrosive injuries are often severe, causing full-thickness mucosal destruction and perforation. The patients must be carefully observed for the need of surgical intervention.

COMPLICATIONS

Chemical injury to the gastrointestinal tract and resultant complications depend on the nature of the agent, the quantity and concentration of the agent, and contact time duration. Liquid alkali such as "Liquid Plumber" was a 20% sodium hydroxide solution when introduced in the late 1960s and was subsequently reduced to a 5% solution after being implicated in 20% of reported caustic ingestions. Liquid alkalis have a high specific gravity and pass rapidly through the esophagus to the stomach. In dogs, violent regurgitation of gastric contents and pyloric and cricopharyngeal spasm cause a "seesaw" action that prolongs contact time. Solid alkali is usually in crystal form and causes severe pain that limits further ingestion. Crystals adhere to mucous membranes of mouth, pharynx, and upper esophagus, causing predominately proximal burns. Alkali produces injury by liquefaction necrosis. This type of injury enhances alkali penetration and prevents surface neutralization that results in full-thickness burns. Concentrated acids produce a coagulative necrosis that forms eschar, which, with the coagulum, limits penetration to deeper muscular coats. Surface sloughing and perforation are therefore common problems. Late complications relate to location and extent of injury. Gastric injury may result in pyloric obstruction, antral stenosis, or "hourglass" deformity. Esophageal stricture may be proximal or distal and despite careful management develops in 10% to 20% of patients with caustic ingestion. In these patients, esophageal cancer has an estimated incidence of 2% to 4%, with a 1000-fold increase over normal persons more than 20 years after the caustic burn.

In attempts to avoid cicatricial esophageal stenosis, several interventions have been tried with controversial results. Traditional approaches have used antibiotics, steroids, and early "prophylactic" dilations, but these cannot be supported by any well-controlled studies. Total parenteral nutrition, agents that impair collagen synthesis, penicillamine, and intraluminal splinting with large-bore Silastic tubes or nasogastric tubes have also been used, but the role of these techniques in stricture prevention remains unclear.

ESOPHAGEAL PERFORATION

PRESENTATION

Esophageal perforations may be iatrogenic or noniatrogenic. Iatrogenic causes occur as complications of instrumentation such as esophagoscopy, attempts at tracheal intubation or obturator airway placement, or esophageal tubes or stents. Dilatation procedures and surgical misadventures or leaks also lead to perforation of the esophagus. Noniatrogenic etiologies are usually barogenic ruptures. The most well-known "spontaneous" rupture occurred in the gluttonous Dutch admiral Baron Van Wassanaer. The admiral gorged himself and induced forceful vomiting for relief. His autopsy by Hermann Boerhaave was published in 1724 and described the pathologic findings of barogenic esophageal rupture. Resultant signs and symptoms are similar for Boerhaave's syndrome and iatrogenic perforations. Pain is a near universal experience and 30% of patients develop acute pain. Fever and leukocytosis are also common. Other presentations are influenced by the site of perforation. Patients with abdominal esophageal segment tears have had retroperitoneal air and vague epigastric pain. Patients with thoracic perforations often complain of abdominal and back pain. Cervical perforations are associated with subcutaneous emphysema and chest pain. Symptoms that occur during or shortly after an esophageal procedure should raise concern for iatrogenic perforations. Other clinical findings in patients with esophageal tears include pleural effusion, pneumothorax, dysphagia, cervical crepitus, hematemesis, and shock. However, asymptomatic perforations have been demonstrated radiographically, which emphasize the importance of an accurate history and a high index of suspicion.

DIAGNOSIS

The diagnosis of esophageal perforation may be fairly obvious particularly in the iatrogenic group. Plain chest radiographs may suggest perforation in over 90% of patients. Findings include mediastinal air, pneumothorax, pleural effusion, infiltrate, or subcutaneous emphysema. Hyperextended neck films can reveal widened spaces, air, or esophageal displacement. Fears of barium mediastinitis have traditionally led to the use of water-soluble contrast media. Recent work reports that iodinated water-soluble media radiographs may be normal in 20% to 25% of thoracic and 50% of cervical perforations. Therefore, negative or equivocal findings on water-soluble studies should be immediately reexamined with barium sulfate contrast radiographs. Other authors believe that barium does not potentiate mediastinal inflammation. Because it is more palatable than water-soluble agents and less dangerous if aspirated into the bronchial tree, many use dilute barium in the initial examination to take advantage of its better coating and definition. Regardless of the agent used, it is important to examine the entire esophagus in multiple positions.

MANAGEMENT

Early diagnosis is essential for successful management. Intravenous access should be obtained and intravenous hydration initiated. The patient is placed NPO, and high-dose, broad-spectrum antibiotic therapy is started. Nasogastric suction and parenteral nutrition are used. Some authors recommend treating small instrumental tears or pharyngeal perforations nonoperatively, but most large instrument tears, trauma, or spontaneous perforations require surgery. Prompt neck exploration is advised for large cervical perforations. Absolute indications for operative intervention include sepsis, shock, respiratory failure, pneumothorax, pneumoperitoneum, and mediastinal emphysema. Most thoracic surgeons advise exploration with primary repair and drainage as the procedure of choice.

For more information, please see Chapter 111 in Civetta JM, Taylor RW, Kirby RR: Critical Care. *Philadelphia: J. B. Lippincott, 1988*

BIBLIOGRAPHY

Ajalat GM, Mulder DG: Esophageal perforations—The need for an individualized approach. *Arch Surg* 1984; 119:1318

DiCostanzo J, Noirclerc M, Jouglard J, et al: New therapeutic approach to corrosive burns of the upper gastrointestinal tract. *Gut* 1980; 21:370

Foley MJ, Ghahremani GG, Rogers LF: Reappraisal of contrast media used to detect upper gastrointestinal perforations—Comparison of Jonic water-soluble media with barium sulfate. *Radiology* 1982; 144:231

Hine KR, Atkinson M: The diagnosis and management of perforations of esophagus and pharynx sustained during intubation of neoplastic esophageal strictures. *Dig Dis Sci* 1986; 31:571

Oakes DD, Sherck JP, Mark JBD: Lye ingestion—Clinical patterns and therapeutic implications. *J Thorac Cardiovasc Surg* 1982; 83:194

Phillips LG, Cunningham J: Esophageal perforation. *Radiol Clin North Am* 1984; 22:607

Richardson JD, Martin LF, Borzotta AP, Polk HC: Unifying concepts in treatment of esophageal leaks. *Am J Surg* 1985; 149:157

Tucker JA, Yarington CT: The treatment of caustic ingestion. *Oto Clin North Am* 1979; 12:343

VIII. Urologic Disease

64

Renal Function: Diagnosis

Preservation of renal function is more important than the treatment of lost function. When 50% or more of renal function is lost, fluid balance and composition are less well maintained, white blood cell (WBC) and platelet functions decline, and red blood cell (RBC) production decreases. Pneumonia and gastrointestinal bleeding increase. The overall mortality rate of acute renal failure is 50%, but in selected conditions, such as ruptured abdominal aortic aneurysm, it may be 90% or greater.

All critically ill patients must be watched carefully for the development of acute renal failure. Loss of renal function in a person who already has other organ systems compromised may lead to a 200% decrease in the chances of the patient's survival. The best overall screening procedures include the determination of the serum creatinine at least every other day and a careful measurement of all fluid intake and output. Two major events should make the physician more vigilant with regard to loss of renal function. The first is *any* cardiovascular problem that may lead to renal hypoperfusion, including decreased blood pressure, a major rhythm disturbance, or severe hypoxia. Such episodes may be brief, lasting only 10 minutes, yet have a severe impact on splanchnic blood flow. The second event is the use of potentially toxic medications, especially in patients with already decreased renal function. Such medications are frequently used for many days; during this time, the loss of kidney function may be subtle yet profound.

Renal function loss may occur without oliguria and present even as a polyuric state in its early stages, especially after aminoglycoside therapy. Other clues indicate possible loss of renal function. One is the development of refractoriness to previously effective diuretics. A second is the presence of a urinary sodium (Na^+) concentration between 40 and 80 meq/liter in a patient with renal hypoperfusion. Some patients with acute renal failure have renal potassium (K^+) wasting and develop hypokalemia. Others manifest renal tubular acidosis resulting from the toxic renal effects of certain drugs. Grossly abnormal-appearing urine from pigments such as bile, myoglobin, and hemoglobin frequently warns of a state that predisposes to the loss of renal function. Urine that is particularly frothy is often indicative of heavy proteinuria.

PRERENAL AZOTEMIA

The best test to confirm decreased blood flow to the kidneys is calculation of the fractional Na^+ excretion. A value less than 1% indicates that the renal tubules are not receiving adequate glomerular flow, the principal cause of which is decreased total blood flow. A value between 1% and 3% is equivocal and may indicate hypoperfusion as well as some damage to the renal parenchyma. A blood urea nitrogen (BUN) to creatinine ratio greater than 20:1, with creatinine usually less than 4 mg/dl, is strongly indicative of renal hypoperfusion. Urinary osmolality greater than 450 mOsm/liter and urine specific gravity greater than 1.015 also are consistent with this diagnosis.

Careful scrutiny of the patient's clinical status frequently suggests renal hypoperfusion, especially when the individual is known to have decreased left ventricular function or is hypovolemic. Severe hypoalbuminemia may also be a contributing feature. Note that hypovolemia results from several mechanisms of fluid loss (see Table 64-1). Factors such as acidosis may lead to cardiovascular failure because of profound venodilatation, decreased cardiac output, and hypotension refractory to both endogenous and exogenous catecholamines. In the traumatized patient, cardiac tamponade must be considered when cardiovascular failure is present.

PARENCHYMAL FAILURE

Numerous factors contribute to the more common causes of acute parenchymal renal failure (Table 64-2). At least 50% of patients with such loss of kidney function have ischemic damage. Forty-five percent have lost function from either endogenous or exogenous nephrotoxins, and only 5% have vasculitis or nontoxic interstitial nephritis. When a patient has a sudden loss of

TABLE 64-1 ETIOLOGIES OF ACUTE RENAL FAILURE

Hypovolemia
External fluid losses
Hemorrhage, profuse diaphoresis, diarrhea, diuretics
Internal fluid losses
"Third space" fluid, anaphylaxis, acute respiratory distress syndrome
Cardiovascular failure
Decreased cardiac output
Decreased left ventricular function, dysrhythmia, cardiac tamponade
Vascular pooling
Sepsis, severe acidosis, anaphylaxis
Emboli to kidneys
Macroscopic or microscopic
Parenchymal swelling
Interstitial nephritis, kidney transplant rejection
Hepatorenal syndrome

TABLE 64-2 CAUSES OF ACUTE PARENCHYMAL LOSS OF RENAL FUNCTION

- Ischemia
- Endogenous toxins
  - Hyperuricemia
  - Hypercalcemia
  - Hypokalemia
  - Hemoglobinuria
  - Myoglobinuria
- Exogenous toxins
  - Antibiotics
    - Aminoglycosides
    - Amphotericin
    - Penicillin
    - Sulfas
    - Cephalosporins
  - Radiocontrast dyes
  - Organic solvents
  - Heavy metals
    - Mercury, cadmium, lead
  - Anesthetics
    - Methoxyflurane
  - Nonsteroidal anti-inflammatory drugs
  - Angiotensin-converting enzyme inhibitors
- Vasculitis and glomerulonephritis
- Malignant hypertension
- Multiple myeloma
- Hepatorenal syndrome
- Severe acute pyelonephritis with papillary necrosis
- Cortical necrosis
- Vascular occlusion

kidney function, cardiovascular stability must be assessed immediately. If a Foley catheter is not already in place, it should be inserted to rule out urinary retention and to monitor the urine output carefully.

As the patient's circulation is stabilized, or determined to be adequate, 12.5 to 50 g mannitol should be infused in the first hour, depending on the determined safety of this measure. The principal concern is the mobilization of fluid from the intracellular to the extracellular compartment and subsequently to the vasculature. Shortly thereafter, 40 to 60 mg furosemide should be given intravenously over 20 minutes. An alternative medication is 1 to 3 mg bumetanide given intravenously. Both mannitol and loop diuretics are most effective when adequate renal blood flow is established before their use. The patient's drug list should be reviewed for all possible nephrotoxic medications, as well as those drugs likely to accumulate with azotemia. Restitution of urine output is important for at least two reasons: Good output allows greater flexibility with regard to administered fluids, and the prognosis of parenchymal acute renal failure is best for nonoliguric patients.

Patients with as little as 10 minutes of decreased blood pressure at a level

TABLE 64-3 RENAL FAILURE DUE TO HYPERURICEMIA

Associated with tissue catabolism or institution of drugs mobilizing uric acid
Serum uric acid 15 mg/dl and rapidly rising
Crystaluria—may be a normal finding
Aborted with alkaline diuresis
Intense delayed nephrogram on IVP
Uric acid to creatinine concentration ratio greater than on a spot urine
Responds well to hemodialysis

two thirds their normal value have been known to progress to severe oliguric acute renal failure lasting 7 to 10 days. During such moderate hypotensive episodes, renal blood flow and glomerular filtration rate (GFR) obviously are profoundly decreased. However, recent studies show that renal blood flow during septic shock may, in fact, be normal in individuals who subsequently develop severe renal failure. This observation suggests the presence of a circulating toxin that affects kidney function.

A fractional excretion of Na^+ greater than 3% associated with a rising BUN and creatinine is highly suggestive of acute parenchymal damage. The urine is usually isosmotic, with a specific gravity of 1.010 and osmolality of 300 mOsm/liter. Urinary sediment frequently shows pigmented casts. Rarely is more than 1+ to 2+ proteinuria indicated by dipstick testing.

The causes and characteristics of renal failure from other origins are listed in Tables 64-3 through 64-5.

POSTRENAL FAILURE

Possible obstruction to urine flow must be considered in the initial evaluation of a patient with acute renal function loss. A rectal and pelvic examination and placement of a Foley catheter in the urinary bladder quickly exclude obstruction of the lower urinary tract.

A variety of intrinsic and extrinsic causes of postobstructive renal failure are known (Table 64-6). Many patients with obstructive uropathy have a totally normal urine output with unremarkable urinary sediment. In the first 24

TABLE 64-4 MYOGLOBINURIC RENAL FAILURE

Reason for muscle damage
Dark orthotoluidine (dipstick occult blood) + urine pigmented casts
Markedly elevated creatine kinase, usually > 10,000 U
Hypocalcemia during renal failure
Hypercalcemia in recovery
Inordinately rapid rise in serum creatinine, phosphorus, and uric acid
May be aborted by high-volume diuresis
Usually a mild insult with good prognosis

TABLE 64-5 CAUSES OF NONTRAUMATIC RHABDOMYOLYSIS AND MYOGLOBINURIA

Acute exertion
Heat stress
Enzyme deficiencies
Carnitine palmityl transferase
Myophosphorylase (McArdle's disease)
Phosphofructokinase (Tarvi's disease)
Muscle disease
Muscular dystrophies
Polymyositis, dermatomyositis
Drugs
Alcohol
Heroin
Amphetamines
Phencyclidine
Toxins
Infectious agents
Hypokalemia

hours of obstructive uropathy leading to azotemia, the urinary Na^+ concentration may be low, with a fractional Na^+ excretion less than 1%. However, after this initial phase, the fractional excretion of Na^+ is usually greater than 3%. On occasion, the urine output increases with obstructive uropathy as the kidneys develop a form of nephrogenic diabetes insipidus. Patients with obstructive uropathy are rarely hypertensive from this problem.

TABLE 64-6 CAUSES OF OBSTRUCTIVE (POSTRENAL) RENAL FAILURE

Intrinsic to collecting system
Intraluminal
Within the kidney (uric acid crystals, sulfa crystals, myeloma proteins)
Outside the kidney (renal calculi, blood clots, fungus balls, sloughed papillae)
Intramural
(tumor, infection, strictures, urethral valves)
Extrinsic to the collecting system
Reproductive organ abnormalities
Prostatic cancer or benign prostatic hypertrophy
Uterine or ovarian masses
Gastrointestinal lesions
Diverticulitis with abscess formation or tumor
Vascular abnormalities
Abdominoaortic aneurysm
Aberrant renal vessels
Aberrant ovarian veins or vena cava
Retroperitoneal processes
Inflammation or fibrosis
Previous surgery
Tumor
Infection

TABLE 64-7 USUAL FEATURES OF PRERENAL, RENAL, AND POSTRENAL AZOTEMIA

	Prerenal	Renal	Postrenal
Urine output	0.6–1 liter	0.3 liter to normal	0 to normal
Sediment	1+ to 2+ protein	hyaline, granular casts many RBC, WBC, and epithelial cells	frequent–normal
UOSM	> 450 mOsm/liter	300 mOsm/liter	300 mOsm/liter
UNA$^+$	< 15 meq/liter	30–60 meq/liter	low, then 30–60 meq/liter*
FE NA$^+$	< 1%	> 3%	> 3%
U:P Creatinine	> 40:1	< 20:1	< 20:1
BUN:Creatinine	> 20:1	20:1	20:1

* For 24 hours after acute obstruction, the U Na$^+$ may be less than 10 meq/liter.

Careful monitoring of intravascular volume at the time of relief of obstructive uropathy is very important. If the obstruction was present for less than 2 weeks, a prompt return to normal renal function may be expected. In obstruction of several months' duration, weeks may be necessary for the maximum improvement in renal function. The final creatinine clearance may not return to a normal value.

The usual features of the prerenal, parenchymal, and postrenal azotemic states are summarized in Table 64-7. A mixture of two or three conditions may be present in any given patient, making discrimination difficult.

For more information, please see Chapter 112 in Civetta JM, Taylor RW, Kirby RR: Critical Care. *Philadelphia: J. B. Lippincott, 1988*

BIBLIOGRAPHY

Bennett WM: Drug therapy in renal disease. *Sci Am Med* 1986; App A:A1

Brown CB, Ogg CS, Cameron JJ: High dose furosemide in acute renal failure: A controlled study. *Clin Nephrol* 1981; 15:90

Hilberman M, Derby G, Spencer R, et al: Sequential pathophysiologic changes characterizing the progression from renal dysfunction to acute renal failure following cardiac surgery. *J Thorac Cardiovasc Surg* 1980; 79:838

Klahr S: Pathophysiology of obstructive uropathy. *Kidney Int* 1983; 23:414

Moore RD, Smith CR, Lipsky JJ, et al: Risk factors for nephrotoxicity in patients treated with aminoglycosides. *Ann Intern Med* 1984; 100:352

Oken DE: On the differential diagnosis of acute renal failure. *Am J Med* 1981; 71:916

Talner LB, Scheible W, Ellenbogen PH, et al: How accurate is ultrasound in detecting hydronephrosis in azotemic patients? *Urol Radiol* 1981; 3:1

65
Renal Function: Treatment

Awareness of the circumstances most likely to result in loss of renal function in the critically ill patient lessens the chances of this occurrence. A review of the preceding chapter suggests that at least half of the in-hospital cases of acute renal function loss can be prevented or decreased in severity with thorough, attentive renal care.

PREVENTION

The physician should carefully monitor the fluid status of any critically ill patient, both with regard to the total amount and distribution in the intravascular, interstitial, and intracellular compartments. This process cannot be adequately performed without a careful daily physical examination, precise recording of fluid balance, and measurement of body weight. A pulmonary artery (PA) catheter to assure adequate left ventricular filling pressure is essential in a patient with unstable circulation, falling urine output, and rising serum creatinine. In the more stable patient, a urine output of greater than 1 liter a day without diuretic therapy is reassuring but may be deceptive. Only by measuring the serum creatinine at least every other day can renal function stability be ascertained.

Review the status of renally excreted antibiotics both for possible nephrotoxic serum levels and for their accumulation in patients with already limited renal function. Clinical signs associated with kidney malfunction include unexplained fever, skin rash, sterile pyuria, flank pain, increased eosinophils in the blood or urine, polyuria, and unexplained hypokalemia.

Angiographic studies must be discussed with the radiologist, and only those that are absolutely necessary should be performed, using the least nephrotoxic radiographic dye in the smallest amounts possible. This precaution is particularly applicable to elderly patients with a decreased cardiac output, modest volume depletion, or diabetes mellitus.

If the patient remains oliguric despite adequate circulation and, by implication, normal renal blood flow, the administration of mannitol and a loop diuretic to establish a normal urine output is reasonable. The greater the urine output in a patient with acute renal function loss, the better the prognosis.

PRIORITIES OF CARE

Immediately obtain a fresh battery of all important kidney-related laboratory parameters in patients with newly diagnosed acute renal function loss. The pertinent blood tests include a complete blood count, creatinine, blood urea nitrogen (BUN), sodium (Na^+), potassium (K^+), chloride (Cl^-), bicarbonate (HCO_3^-), calcium, phosphorus, magnesium, and arterial gas partial pressures and *p*H. A urinalysis, urine culture, and urine Na^+, creatinine, and osmolality may be helpful.

If the patient is eating, the diet should be changed immediately to no added salt, low K^+, and low dairy product content. No more than 1 g/kg of high biologic value protein should be given. These dietary changes, when made as soon as renal function loss is noted, may prevent major problems with electroyte disturbances several days later. If the patient is euvolemic, protect this status by careful fluid restriction while assuring that intravascular volume is maintained. Use uncomplicated intravenous fluids so that inadvertent excesses of such substances as K^+, magnesium, or HCO_3^- are not administered. Because most body fluid losses are hypotonic and may be decidedly so should an individual be tachypneic or very febrile, the use of 5% dextrose in one half normal saline is recommended. This simple, basic intravenous fluid can be easily augmented in a patient-specific way when necessary.

By limiting the patient's K^+ intake immediately, future problems with this electroyte may be prevented. All sources of exogenous K^+ excess must be considered, including medications, intravenous fluids, and the patient's oral intake.

When a patient is known to have renal function loss, initially assume the worst-case scenario. Despite a normal urine output, the serum creatinine may rise from 1 to 2 mg/dl/day, indicating a creatinine clearance of less than 10 ml/min. Thus, at the time of the initial diagnosis, all medications should be adjusted to levels given to patients with *no* kidney function. Initial orders for a renal failure patient must include measurements of daily weight, intake, and output.

VOLUME MANAGEMENT

No good formula is available to calculate the amount of fluid needed when one patient is compared with another. In renal insufficiency patients, however, think of the urine output as being either absent or relatively unchanging in amount.

Two minor adjuncts to volume management include the double or quadruple strength mixing of all necessary intravenous medications. In addition, some additional urine output may be induced with the use of intravenous chlorothiazide, 500 mg every 12 hours, followed by a loop diuretic such as bumetanide, 1 to 3 mg, or furosemide, 40 to 80 mg intravenously, 2 hours later. In general, unless an increase in urine output of at least 500 ml occurs in the 4-hour period following the administration of these diuretics, do not continue the regimen.

HYPERKALEMIA

Potassium excess is the most life-threatening of all complications. Endogenous K^+ may contribute to an elevated serum K^+ as this electrolye is shifted from the intracellular to the extracellular compartment. This shift rarely causes a life-threatening elevation of serum K^+ except in the case of true tissue necrosis. Thus, a patient may die of hyperkalemia if the kidneys cannot excrete the K^+ released from a totally gangrenous lower extremity.

Treatment must be vigorous and immediate. Administer one ampule of $CaCl_2$ and one ampule of $NaHCO_3$, without specific regard for the patient's acid–base status. Subsequently, give one ampule of 50% dextrose in water and 10 units of regular insulin. Quickly review the patient's records, intravenous fluid summary, and diet for causes of hyperkalemia and reassess for possible tissue destruction (gastrointestinal bleeding, infarction of the small bowel, or vascular compromise of an extremity). Begin a regimen of sodium polystyrene sulfonate (Kayexalate) enemas with 50 g of Kayexalate in 100 ml of 10% sorbitol. This mixture is instilled in the rectum using a balloon catheter to ensure its retention for at least 1 hour.

HYPOKALEMIA

Patients with acute renal failure may be K^+ depleted because of clinical circumstances (*i.e.*, long-term diuretic therapy). Serum K^+ should be increased to greater than 4 meq/liter or a level at which no dysrhythmias related to hypokalemia are likely. However, be cautious about such replacement, using increments at one half the usual rate of replacement. No specific formula for K^+ replacement in this situation is available. If a patient has a normal serum pH and a serum K^+ less than 3 meq/liter, the total body K^+ deficit is greater than 200 meq.

HYPONATREMIA

Hyponatremia is common in acute renal failure. The most common cause is the administration of fluids that are too dilute, such as 5% dextrose in water when the body cannot rid itself of water excess. Fluid losses normally are hypotonic and equal to the loss of approximately one half normal saline. Thus, the administration of maintenance fluids to a patient with renal failure is best achieved by 5% dextrose in one half normal saline. This fluid can be adjusted to nearly normal saline with the addition of 1 ampule of $NaHCO_3$/liter, when indicated. Severe hyponatremia with serum Na^+ concentrations less than 115 meq/liter may be treatable only with dialysis if the patient is obtunded and having seizures.

HYPOCALCEMIA

Patients with acute renal failure can develop a decrease in total and ionized calcium. In addition, the formation of the active metabolite of vitamin D, 1,25-dihydrocholecalciferol may be reduced. Serum calcium is further depressed as the serum phosphorus rises. However, tetany is unusual in this circumstance. An unusual source of hypocalcemia may occur in the patient with rhabdomyolytic renal failure. In this circumstance calcium is deposited within the damaged muscle. In the diuretic phase calcium is released, and some patients may actually become hypercalcemic. Specific treatment usually is unnecessary.

HEMODIALYSIS

Hemodialysis is the preferred treatment of acute renal failure. Laboratory abnormalities and volume excess can be corrected in the early part of a 3- or 4-hour treatment. Because they are treated for only a portion of the day, patients are available for other therapy, diagnostic studies, or surgical procedures. Hemodialysis is most easily achieved with a subclavian double-lumen catheter placed percutaneously using the standard Seldinger technique. It may be kept open by filling the dual lumens with a heparin solution containing 5,000 U/ml. Between dialyses the catheter may be used for other purposes such as drug administration or central venous pressure measurement.

PERITONEAL DIALYSIS

Peritoneal dialysis is a less used technique in acute renal failure but can be instituted immediately with the percutaneous placement of a peritoneal catheter. A dialysis machine and technically trained personnel are not required. Because it is slower and takes place "around the clock," there is less likelihood of disequilibrium symptoms and hypotension. Patients with borderline low blood pressure or severely compromised left ventricular function may tolerate fluid removal with peritoneal dialysis better than with hemodialysis. The technique does not require systemic heparinization and, from a risk-of-bleeding standpoint, is safer.

CONTINUOUS ARTERIOVENOUS HEMOFILTRATION

A newer form of treatment uses the patient's arterial pressure to provide blood flow through a hemofilter. The hemofilter is much more porous than a hemodialysis cartridge. Loss of uremic toxins, fluid, and electrolytes results from bulk flow across the filter membrane, as opposed to diffusion with a dialysis cartridge. Replacement fluid must be administered in the venous line coming from the hemofilter to prevent marked hemoconcentration. Adequate blood flow can be assured by a simple calculation involving measurement of fluid ultrafiltration from the cartridge and the hematocrit of blood entering and leaving the cartridge. Measurement of activated clotting time allows safe heparin use with adequate anticoagulation of blood entering the filtration cartridge but little or no anticoagulation of the patient.

Continuous arteriovenous hemofiltration is particularly valuable for patients with volume overload, hemodynamic instability, or decreased serum proteins. It also can be used for those receiving large-volume parenteral nutrition. This technique is not effective in patients with a very high BUN level because it is much less efficient than hemodialysis. Because of the low blood flow, patients with high hematocrit, atherosclerotic peripheral arteries, or hypercoagulability are not well served by hemofiltration. The technique requires a reasonably sophisticated knowledge of heparin use, blood flow calculation, and fluid volume management.

For more information, please see Chapter 113 in Civetta JM, Taylor RW, Kirby RR: Critical Care. *Philadelphia: J. B. Lippincott, 1988*

BIBLIOGRAPHY

Abel RM, Beck CH, Abbot WM, et al: Improved survival from acute renal failure after treatment with intravenous essential amino acids and glucose. *N Engl J Med* 1973; 288:695

Anderson RJ, Linas SL, Berns AS, et al: Nonoliguric acute renal failure. *N Engl J Med* 1977; 296:1134

Bartlett RH, Mault JR, Deckert RE: Continuous arterial venous hemoperfusion: Improved survival in surgical acute renal failure? *Surgery* 1986; 100:400

Brown RS: Extrarenal potassium homeostasis. *Kidney Int* 1986; 30:116

Cohen RD, Woods HF: Lactic acidosis revisited. *Diabetes* 1983; 32:181

Conger JD: A controlled evaluation of prophylactic dialysis in posttraumatic acute renal failure. *J Trauma* 1975; 15:1056

Myers BD, Moran SM: Hemodynamically mediated acute renal failure. *N Engl J Med* 1986; 314:97

Solomon RJ: Ventricular arrhythmias in patients with myocardial infarct and ischaemia: Relationship to serum potassium and magnesium. *Drugs* 1985; (suppl 1)28:66

66
Urinary Tract Infections

Urinary tract infections (UTI) occur frequently in intensive care unit (ICU) patients. These infections can range from an incidental finding on admission to life-threatening pyelonephritis with gram-negative sepsis and shock.

CYSTITIS

Most of the patients admitted to the ICU with a UTI have asymptomatic bacteriuria as an incidental finding. This is particularly common in the elderly, in whom pyuria may be absent. Pyuria is defined as the presence of 10 or more leukocytes per high-power field in a urine sediment. Bacteriuria is found in about 10% of elderly men and 20% of women living at home and can increase to 25% in patients in nursing homes. Hospitalized elderly patients have an even higher probability of acquiring an infection. This increased risk occurs even if urinary catheterization is not done. Many patients in the ICU have urinary catheters for at least some period of time, further increasing the risk of infection.

Symptomatic UTIs require antimicrobial therapy, and commonly an empiric regimen is necessary pending the results of the urine culture. The urine Gram stain may be helpful and should be performed. Immunocompetent female patients with cystitis alone may be treated with single-dose oral therapy with 3.0 g amoxicillin or trimethoprim/sulfamethoxazole (two double-strength tablets), provided none of the following conditions exist: renal stones, prior infections with resistant organisms, or known urologic abnormalities (including urinary catheters). Treatment of immunocompromised patients or those with complicated UTI depends on the physician's clinical judgment. Choices range from oral ampicillin or trimethoprim/sulfamethoxazole to intravenous therapy with a third-generation beta-lactam antimicrobic, or the latter combined with an aminoglycoside. Patients requiring intravenous antimicrobics should have blood cultures done before therapy is started. If single-dose therapy is given, a urine culture should be repeated in 48 to 72 hours; if infection persists, more prolonged therapy is indicated.

PYELONEPHRITIS

Pyelonephritis is characterized by bacterial invasion of the renal interstitium resulting in an acute inflammatory response and suppurative necrosis. Pathologically, multiple areas of suppurative inflammation in the parenchyma, which are well demarcated from surrounding areas of uninvolved kidney, are seen. The areas of inflammation may be discrete focal abscesses or large, wedge-shaped areas of coalescent suppuration.

The diagnosis of pyelonephritis is usually not difficult, particularly in a young woman. Patients are almost always febrile, often with a temperature above 104°F, frequently appear "toxic," and complain of flank or low back pain. Nausea and vomiting, chills or rigors, and dysuria are frequently present. Some patients, especially the elderly, may be asymptomatic or have nonspecific complaints. Abdominal ileus may occur, but peritoneal signs are unusual. Other conditions such as renal infarction can mimic pyelonephritis.

A marked leukocytosis is usual, although with sepsis the leukocyte count may be low with a significant shift toward immature cells. The blood urea nitrogen (BUN) and creatinine values are normal unless shock or underlying renal disease is present. Urinalysis most commonly reveals pyuria and bacteriuria; white blood cell (WBC) casts indicate upper tract infection. Elderly patients may have an entirely normal urine sediment. Complete ureteral obstruction of the affected kidney may also result in a normal urinalysis. The urine culture almost always reveals the causative organism, but, in one study of bacteremia secondary to UTI, 19% of patients had fewer than 10^5 organisms on culture. The laboratory should be alerted to identify any isolated organisms when pyelonephritis is suspected.

In the ICU pyelonephritis can usually be diagnosed with little difficulty. Ureteral catheterization can definitively prove the diagnosis but may be difficult and time consuming, especially in a critically ill patient. Antibody-coated bacteria tests are relatively specific for upper tract disease but are available only at specialized laboratories and have not been standardized. Contrast studies (*e.g.*, excretory urograms) are not helpful in diagnosing acute pyelonephritis; ultrasound and computed tomography (CT) scans are also nonspecific. Gallium scans are abnormal but cannot be interpreted until 48 to 72 hours after injection. Indium-111-labeled autologous leukocyte scans are somewhat more helpful. Renal scanning with ^{99}Tc-DMSA is very sensitive for pyelonephritis and shows a specific pattern of striated or flare-diminished renal uptake. In addition, it is readily available and requires little time to perform. Thus, in a critically ill patient in whom the diagnosis of pyelonephritis is suspected but not proven, the ^{99}Tc-DMSA study is the preferred procedure.

Knowing antibiotic resistance patterns for bacterial microorganisms in each hospital is very important; these are usually summarized monthly or yearly by the microbiology laboratory or infection control service. Physicians should have this information available. There may be considerable variation in the susceptibility of an organism to a particular antimicrobic from one hospital to another (*e.g., P. aeruginosa* to the aminoglycosides). Up to 20% of community-acquired *E. coli* infections are resistant to ampicillin, and 30% of hospital-acquired strains are resistant to ampicillin and cefazolin; 20% to 30% of hospital-acquired *K. pneumoniae* organisms are resistant to cefazolin.

Knowledge of the antimicrobic spectrum of activity against the common urinary tract pathogens is crucial. Of the penicillins, ampicillin is the most commonly used and the least expensive. Because of increasing resistance, it cannot be relied on for treatment of most gram-negative bacteria, and its use empirically in the ICU should be limited to suspected enterococcal infections. Carbenicillin and ticarcillin have essentially been replaced with newer penicillins such as azlocillin, mezlocillin, and piperacillin, which have a much wider spectrum of activity and significantly lower sodium content. These antimicrobics are effective against most gram-negative bacteria, including *P. aeruginosa. In vitro,* piperacillin seems to be best for this organism, although the difference may not be clinically important. These drugs are also very good against enterococci, but not *S. aureus.*

The development of resistance has markedly diminished the role of first-generation cephalosporins also. Second-generation drugs such as cefamandole and cefuroxime have somewhat better gram-negative coverage against *E. coli* or *K. pneumoniae* and are probably adequate initial coverage for *S. aureus.* However, they have no activity against enterococci. The third-generation cephalosporins have broad-spectrum activity against gram-negative bacteria but are not reliable against *S. aureus.* For enterococci, only cefoperazone has *in vitro* activity, and its clinical efficacy is unproven. Ceftazidime and cefoperazone are active against *P. aeruginosa,* with the former having better *in vitro* data.

The aminoglycosides are excellent antimicrobics in ICU patients despite the risks of ototoxicity and nephrotoxicity. In most cases they should not be used alone, especially with enterococci or *P. aeruginosa.* Considerable variation in susceptibility within this group may exist among hospitals, but in general gentamicin remains commonly effective.

Trimethoprim/sulfamethoxazole also has an excellent spectrum of activity and is useful in patients with penicillin allergies. It is not effective against *P. aeruginosa* and enterococci. Imipenem has extremely broad coverage against gram-negative and positive organisms and should cover essentially all potential urinary tract pathogens. However, it is expensive, and there have been some concerns about induced bacterial resistance.

If the urine Gram stain suggests an enterococcal infection, appropriate therapy is ampicillin or piperacillin combined with an aminoglycoside. In the penicillin-allergic patient, vancomycin may be substituted. If *S. aureus* is strongly suspected, then oxacillin or nafcillin combined with an aminoglycoside is effective. If this organism is considered a somewhat less likely pathogen, then cefuroxime is reasonable therapy. Gram-negative bacilli seen on Gram stain are somewhat less helpful because a specific organism cannot be identified. The antibiotic regimen chosen depends on the clinical circumstances but in general includes either piperacillin/mezlocillin or a third-generation cephalosporin coupled with an aminoglycoside. Trimethoprim/sulfamethoxazole along with gentamicin is an excellent choice for a community-acquired infection. If *P. aeruginosa* is strongly suspected, then the cephalosporin used should be either ceftazidime or cefoperazone. If the urine Gram stain does not reveal an organism, the combination of piperacillin and an aminoglycoside is best because it is effective against enterococci as well.

NOSOCOMIAL INFECTIONS

Nosocomial UTIs are common and potentially serious problems in the ICU. Approximately 80% of nosocomial UTIs are due to urinary catheters. By definition, these infections are considered "complicated" (*i.e.,* the presence of an abnormality in the urinary outflow tract) and are often not properly managed. By the 10th day of catheterization, 50% of patients have a UTI. In general, ICU patients have the same risk of acquiring these infections as do other patients. It has been found that 40% of UTIs could have been prevented if the catheter had been removed at the appropriate time and that more than one third of the total catheterization days were unnecessary.

Using the usual cutoff point of more than 10^5 organisms to define a UTI is not appropriate in the catheterized patient. The presence of *any* amount of bacteria in a cultured urine specimen will progress to more than 10^5 organisms, usually within 3 days. It is very important that the microbiology laboratory be made aware of the importance of identifying any bacteria present in amounts equal to or greater than 10^2 in a patient with a urinary catheter.

Eighty-four percent of nosocomial UTIs are due to gram-negative rods, with *E. coli* causing less than half of these. *Proteus, Klebsiella, Pseudomonas, Enterobacter,* and *Serratia* are the other most common isolates. Most gram-positive infections are due to enterococci, followed by coagulase-negative staphylococci and *S. aureus;* the latter causes less than 2% of nosocomial UTIs.

Of importance to the ICU physician is that between 1% and 4% of patients with these infections will get a secondary bacteremia. *Serratia* and *Klebsiella* are the two organisms most often responsible and, along with *P. aeruginosa,* have the highest mortality rate. A study of 221 bacteremias secondary to nosocomial urinary tract infections revealed an overall direct mortality rate of 12.7%; all of the deaths occurred in patients with chronic or progressive underlying disease. If shock was present, the mortality rate was 35%. Thus, although many patients with asymptomatic nosocomial UTIs do not need antimicrobic therapy, those in an ICU usually will need aggressive treatment.

For more information, please see Chapter 114 in Civetta JM, Taylor RW, Kirby RR: Critical Care. *Philadelphia: J. B. Lippincott, 1988*

BIBLIOGRAPHY

Bryan CS, Reynolds KL: Hospital-acquired bacteremic urinary tract infection: Epidemiology and outcome. *J Urol* 1984; 132:494

Garibaldi RA, Burke JP, Dickman ML, et al: Factors predisposing to bacteriuria during indwelling urethral catheterization. *N Engl J Med* 1974; 291:215

Handmaker H: Nuclear renal imaging in acute pyelonephritis. *Semin Nucl Med* 1982; 12:246

Hartstein AI, Garber SB, Ward TT, et al: Nosocomial urinary tract infection: A prospective evaluation of 108 catheterized patients. *Infect Control* 1981; 2:380

Kaye D: Urinary tract infections in the elderly. *Bull NY Acad Med* 1980; 56:209

Krieger JN, Kaiser DL, Wenzel RP: Urinary tract etiology of bloodstream infections in hospitalized patients. *J Infect Dis* 1983; 148:57

Neu HC: The emergence of bacterial resistance and its influence on empiric therapy. *Rev Infect Dis* 1983; 5(suppl):S9

Stamm WE, Martin SM, Bennett JV: Epidemiology of nosocomial infections due to gram-negative bacilli: Aspects relevant to development and use of vaccines. *J Infect Dis* 1977; 136(suppl): S151

Stark RP, Maki DG: Bacteriuria in the catheterized patient: What quantitative level of bacteriuria is relevant? *N Engl J Med* 1984; 311:560

Strand CL, Bryant JK, Sutton KH: Septicemia secondary to urinary tract infections with colony counts less than 10^5 CFU/ml. *Am J Clin Pathol* 1985; 83:619

IX. Endocrine Disorders

67 Glucose Metabolism

DIABETIC KETOACIDOSIS

CLINICAL DESCRIPTION

The presentation of patients with diabetic ketoacidosis (DKA) is usually straightforward, and the diagnosis is not difficult. However, it is not well appreciated that approximately 80% of the episodes of DKA are recurrent and appear in patients previously known to have diabetes mellitus and that older diabetics constitute at least 75% of the patients with DKA. Fifty percent of the episodes of DKA are precipitated by coexistent medical illnesses, such as infection or myocardial infarction, and only 20% to 25% are due to the omission of insulin. Curiously, no precipitating factor can be identified in the remaining 25%, but emotional stress related to psychosocial issues is likely important.

LABORATORY FEATURES

The glucose concentration seldom exceeds 800 mg/dl and usually averages between 500 to 700 mg/dl. In 15% of episodes the glucose concentration is less than 350 mg/dl. Pregnancy and active alcoholism are associated with lower glucose concentrations than expected from the severity of insulin deficiency, the former because glucose consumption by the fetoplacental unit is not insulin dependent and the latter because alcohol inhibits gluconeogenesis.

The metabolic acidosis is typically associated with an increase in the anion gap (anion gap = $[Na - (Cl + HCO_3)] = 12 \pm 2$ meq/liter). The increase in the anion gap (*i.e.*, the calculated anion gap − 12) represents 80% or more (Δ anion gap/Δ bicarbonate ≥ 0.8) of the calculated reduction in the bicarbonate concentration (24 meq/liter − measured bicarbonate). However, patients may also present with varying degrees of hyperchloremia and may have a combined anion gap and hyperchloremic type of metabolic acidosis (Δ anion gap/Δ bicarbonate = 0.4–0.8) or a predominant hyperchloremic metabolic acidosis (Δ anion gap/Δ bicarbonate < 0.4). Patients with the anion gap metabolic acidosis pattern are more volume contracted (greater azotemia) and have retained the ketoacid anions, whereas those with hyperchloremic acidosis have maintained their volume status more effectively during the period of decompensation and have excreted the ketoacid anions in the urine with sodium and potassium. Occasionally, patients may have an increase in the anion gap that is greater than the calculated reduction in bicarbonate (Δ anion gap/reduction in $HCO_3 > 1.0$). These patients have a coexistent metabolic alkalosis, which should be suspected by the presence of hypochloremia and hypokalemia. Depending on the magnitude of the metabolic alkalosis and acidosis, such patients may have a normal *p*H if the disorders are of equal severity, be acidemic if the acidosis is predominant, or be alkalemic if the alkalosis is severe.

Water and electrolyte deficits can be extensive in patients with well-established DKA despite misleading plasma electrolyte concentrations:

1 Water: 100 ml/kg body wt

2 Sodium: 7–10 meq/kg body wt

3 Potassium: 3–5 meq/kg body wt

4 Magnesium: 0.5–1.0 meq/kg body wt

5 Phosphorus: 1 mM/kg body wt

Sodium deficiency and redistribution of water into the extracellular compartment lead to hyponatremia. Rarely hypertriglyceridemia may also contribute to hyponatremia. (This should be suspected when the plasma is lactescent.)

Although potassium deficits are substantial, the plasma potassium concentration is usually elevated. Hyperkalemia is usually attributed to the intracellular shift of hydrogen and a hydrogen–potassium exchange. More recently, the hyperkalemia has been attributed directly to insulin deficiency. Hypokalemia at presentation identifies patients with larger potassium deficits, who are at higher risk for morbidity and mortality. Such patients usually have a coexistent metabolic alkalosis due to diuretics or protracted vomiting.

The deficiency of magnesium that is present in DKA is seldom clinically important and usually requires no therapy, unless recovery from DKA is delayed and prolonged parenteral fluid administration is required. Rarely magnesium deficiency may be unmasked by administration of phosphate and precipitation of hypocalcemia. It manifests itself as tetany and paresthesias.

Despite phosphorus deficiency, most patients are hyperphosphatemic at presentation, often strikingly so. Nonetheless, the deficiency of phosphorus is mild (only $\pm$ 60–70 mM from a total body pool of 6000–8000 mM) unless the patient has had coexistent diarrhea or protracted diuresis.

Patients with DKA often have hyperamylasemia associated with abdominal pain and other features suggesting an acute surgical abdomen. Careful correlation reveals that patients with DKA and abdominal pain may have normal amylase values, patients with hyperamylasemia may be asymptomatic, and some patients may have both hyperamylasemia and abdominal pain. Recently, hyperamylasemia has been demonstrated to be a feature of nondiabetic metabolic acidosis and is due to an increase in a nonpancreatic amylase isozyme. Lipase measurements should be obtained if pancreatitis is suspected clinically. The diagnosis of pancreatitis should not be made simply because of abdominal pain and hyperamylasemia, unless there is other supportive clinical evidence.

TREATMENT

The treatment of DKA requires the administration of adequate amounts of insulin, correction of fluid and electrolyte deficits, and identification and treatment of coexistent medical illnesses. The details are summarized in Table 67-1. Most experts recommend use of low doses of insulin, but it should be understood that these are still not physiologic doses, and substantial insulin resistance exists in these patients.

COMPLICATIONS

There are relatively few complications of DKA therapy. A hyperchloremic nonanion gap metabolic acidosis usually replaces the anion gap metabolic acidosis present at the initiation of therapy. When this occurs a therapeutic plan must be ready for returning the patient to his or her regular insulin dose and diet. The kidney will adjust and restore the chloride and bicarbonate concentrations to normal over several days. The reasons for the development of the hyperchloremic state are complex and include loss and continued excretion of ketones in the urine during therapy, which serve as substrate for regeneration of bicarbonate, and bicarbonate and buffer losses in excess of the ketone bodies retained in the extracellular space.

The development of cerebral edema, once considered idiosyncratic, seems to occur in all treated patients, suggesting that this dreaded complication is quantitative and not qualitative. Avoidance of rapid and excessive reduction of the blood glucose concentration is usually recommended. The appearance of drowsiness, lethargy, and particularly headache during successful therapy is ominous and suggests that aggressive management of incipient cerebral edema with mannitol and large doses of glucocorticoids be undertaken, although there are no data to support the effectiveness of this regimen.

Acute noncardiac or low-pressure pulmonary edema has occurred in the treatment of DKA causing severe gas exchange abnormalities.

TABLE 67-1 TREATMENT OF DIABETIC KETOACIDOSIS

Insulin

1. 10 U regular insulin IV as loading dose followed by 5–10 U/hr (0.1 U/kg body wt) thereafter until glucose concentration is 250–300 mg/dl and the pH $\geq$ 7.3 or $HCO_3 \geq$ 18 meq/liter.

or

2. 10 U regular insulin IV as loading dose followed by 5–10 U/hr IM.
3. When control achieved:
   a. Return to previous insulin regimen, if known and if satisfactory.
   b. Use regimens recommended by White (modified closed-loop system) or by Alberti, for perioperative treatment of diabetes, if an interim strategy is necessary.

Fluids

1. Isotonic saline.
2. Infuse at rate of 1–2 liters for the first hour; 1 liter/hr for hr 2–4, based on intake and output measurements, clinical assessment of hydration state. Where indicated use hemodynamic monitoring, make decisions based on pressure measurements.
3. When the plasma glucose reaches 250–300 mg/dl, administer glucose at a rate of 5–20 g/hr, either as separate infusion or combined with isotonic saline. If volume requirements remain high, "piggyback" dextrose and water through IV line; if volume replacement for correction of hypovolemia and dehydration no longer necessary, use 5–10% dextrose and saline at 100 mg/hr.

Potassium

1. Measure potassium and obtain EKG before adding potassium to parenteral fluids.
2. If the potassium is 4–5 meq/liter incorporate 20 meq K^+ into each liter of isotonic saline and infuse at 1 liter/hr.
3. Maintain K^+ between 4–5 meq/liter.
   a. If 4–5 meq/liter continue K^+ at rate of 20 meq/hr.
   b. If 5–6 meq/liter decrease to 10 meq/hr.
   c. If > 6 meq/liter stop K^+.
   d. If 3–4 meq/liter increase K^+ to 30 meq/hr.
   e. If $\leq$ 3 meq/liter increase K^+ to 40–60 meq/hr.

Bicarbonate

1. Not recommended for routine treatment of DKA.
2. Consider if other indications present.

Phosphate

1. Not routinely recommended.
2. Deficit is approximately 1.0 mM/kg body wt.
3. Replace 25–50% in first 24 hr if serum $PO_4 \leq$ 1.0 mg/dl.
4. 1.5–2.5 mM phosphate/hr as the potassium salt (some circumstances might justify use of the sodium salt).

HYPEROSMOLAR HYPERGLYCEMIC NONKETOTIC DIABETES

CLINICAL DESCRIPTION

Hyperosmolar hyperglycemic nonketotic diabetes, also known as the hyperosmolar hyperglycemic syndrome (HHS), tends to occur in older patients who have no history of diabetes mellitus or in whom the diabetes has been mild. It is usually precipitated by coexistent illness (infections, pancreatitis, burns, hemodialysis), by medications (glucocorticoids, diuretics, beta-blockers, phenytoin), or by other conditions associated with hypokalemia. Following recovery, many patients can be controlled by diet alone or diet plus an oral hypoglycemic agent. Because of the absence of severe metabolic acidosis, the prodrome of this syndrome is prolonged and greater deficits of body water develop, leading to more severe hyperglycemia. The older age of these patients may also predispose them to greater water deficits than in DKA, because of altered thirst and impaired renal conservation of water. Hyperglycemia is often accentuated because of the ingestion of glucose-containing liquids. Metabolic acidosis is usually mild and is attributed to poor tissue perfusion and lactic acidosis. However, the lactate concentration never entirely accounts for the increased anion gap, and coexistent beta-hydroxybutyric acid acidosis is likely in view of the negative nitroprusside reaction (acetest). Altered mental consciousness and focal neurologic symptoms suggesting cerebral thrombosis are frequently part of the presenting signs and symptoms of the disorder. The neurologic symptoms and signs may be variable.

LABORATORY FEATURES

Moderate to very marked hyperglycemia (range: 600–2700 mg/dl; average 1200 mg/dl) and hyperosmolality (range: 327–416 mOsm/kg; average, 373 mOsm/kg) in the absence of ketoacidosis are distinguishing features of this disorder. Hyperosmolality and hyperglycemia, though of lesser magnitude, are also features of DKA; thus it is the absence of ketoacidosis and not the hyperosmolality that distinguishes this disorder. Acidemia, if present, is usually mild (pH range; 6.81–7.49; average 7.26) and attributed to lactic acidosis, even though the increase in the anion gap is greater than the lactate concentration. Mixed acid–base disturbances may be present in these patients with a metabolic alkalosis due to diuretic use, coexisting with a metabolic acidosis due to decompensated diabetes or lactic acidosis. The plasma sodium concentration varies over a wide range (120–180 meq/liter; average, 140 meq/liter). The plasma potassium concentration is usually low (range: 2–4 meq/liter), and body deficits of potassium are comparable or greater than those seen in DKA. Because of the extreme degree of hypovolemia, prerenal azotemia is frequently present.

TREATMENT

Most of the principles described for treatment of DKA apply to the treatment of this syndrome. However, the deficit of water and potassium is often greater than that in DKA. Because of severe water depletion and hypovolemia, these patients may be hypotensive and require more aggressive fluid resuscitation. Under these circumstances 0.9% saline is the preferred replacement fluid and is an excellent fluid to use in the early phases of treatment even in the absence of hypotension, because it is hypotonic to the osmolality of plasma. When adequate volume is reestablished, 0.45% saline can be used for hypernatremia. The rates of fluid administration should be determined by assessing the hydration state of the patient.

In treating fluid deficits, it is important to protect volume even at the expense of composition. If severe volume depletion is initially present, the blood glucose concentration may fall precipitously just from rehydration and dilution and from reestablishment of glomerular filtration with excretion of glucose in the urine. If the patient is not hypotensive and the plasma sodium level is elevated, then 0.45% saline can be used. If hypotension occurs during therapy, then 0.9% saline should be substituted for 0.45% saline. Isotonic saline should be used in patients with normal or reduced serum sodium concentrations, and 0.45% saline should be used in hypernatremic patients unless they are hypotensive.

When the initial plasma sodium value is normal or elevated, correction of the hyperglycemia and simultaneous infusion of 0.9% saline may be associated with the development of significant hypernatremia (*i.e.*, plasma Na of 160–170 meq/liter). This may be viewed as beneficial because it buffers rapid changes in extracellular osmolality, but there are no data on this point. Frequent measurements of the sodium concentration and hemodynamic evaluation should allow the proper use of 0.9% and 0.45% saline.

Insulin is probably best utilized as in DKA, but because rehydration can contribute significantly to the reduction in the hyperglycemia, the blood glucose level should be carefully monitored, and the rate of insulin infusion should be adjusted appropriately. Excessive rates of fall of the glucose concentration and the plasma osmolality should be avoided, and the guidelines suggested for DKA should be followed.

The serum potassium concentration must be followed closely because potassium deficits may be large in these patients. The guidelines for DKA can be used in the treatment of this disorder.

COMPLICATIONS

The mortality rate in patients with this disorder is high (40–50%) owing to coexistent serious medical problems and complications such as cerebral edema, cerebral bleeding, thromboembolism, acute tubular necrosis, and myocardial infarction.

For more information, please see Chapter 120 in Civetta JM, Taylor RW, Kirby RR: Critical Care. *Philadelphia: J. B. Lippincott, 1988*

BIBLIOGRAPHY

Adrogue HJ, et al: Diabetic ketoacidosis: Role of kidney in the acid–base homeostasis re-evaluated. *Kidney Int* 1984; 25:591

Adrogue HJ, Wilson H, Boyd AE, et al: Plasma acid–base patterns in diabetic ketoacidosis. *N Engl J Med* 1982; 307:1603

Adrogue HJ, Lederer ED, Suki WN, et al: Determinants of plasma potassium levels in diabetic ketoacidosis. *Medicine* 1986; 65:163

Alberti KGMM: Insulin therapy in diabetic ketoacidosis and surgery. Insulin Update, p 260. Amsterdam, Excerpta Medica, 1982

Arieff AI, Carroll JH: Nonketotic hyperosmolar coma with hyperglycemia: Clinical features, pathophysiology, renal function, acid–base balance, plasma–cerebrospinal equilibrium and the effects of therapy in 37 cases. *Medicine* 1972; 51:73

Barrett EJ, DeFronzo RA, Bevilacqua S, et al: Insulin resistance in diabetic ketoacidosis. *Diabetes* 1982; 31:923

Beigelman PM: Potassium in severe diabetic ketoacidosis. *Am J Med* 1973; 54:419

Fisher JN, Kitabchi AE: A randomized study of phosphate therapy in the treatment of diabetic ketoacidosis. *J Clin Endocrinol Metab* 1983; 57:177

Foster DW, McGarry JD: The metabolic derangements and treatment of diabetic ketoacidosis. *N Engl J Med* 1983; 309:159

Krane EJ, Rockoff MA, Wallman JK, et al: Subclinical brain swelling in children during treatment of diabetic ketoacidosis. *N Engl J Med* 1985; 312:1147

Stacpoole PW: Lactic acidosis: The case against bicarbonate therapy. *Ann Int Med* 1986; 105:276

White NH, Skur D, Santiago JV: Practical closed-loop insulin delivery. Ann Intern Med 1982; 97:210

68
Diabetes Insipidus

Central diabetes insipidus (DI) is caused by inadequate secretion of antidiuretic hormone (ADH) by the neurohypophysis. Lack of ADH leads to the dramatic onset of polyuria because the patient is unable to produce a concentrated urine. If the intake of water is insufficient, this condition will lead to hypertonic encephalopathy due to hypernatremia, circulatory collapse due to volume depletion, or both.

The neurohypophysis extends from the hypothalamus to the posterior pituitary. Antidiuretic hormone is produced by the neurosecretory cells concentrated in the supraoptic and paraventricular nuclei of the hypothalamus, transported in neurosecretory granules down the cell's axon, and stored in terminal dilatations of the axon. On its release into the bloodstream, ADH functions as a true hormone. Although most axons terminate in the posterior pituitary, a large minority terminate high in the pituitary stalk and release their hormone into the portal venous system that drains into the anterior pituitary. Destruction of the hypothalamic neurosecretory cells or high transection of the stalk is associated with permanent DI. Distal stalk transection or removal of the posterior pituitary produces only transient polyuria because sufficient hormone can be released from axons terminating higher in the pituitary stalk to prevent permanent DI.

DIAGNOSIS

CENTRAL DI

Patients with central DI generally describe the abrupt onset of polyuria and polydipsia. Urine volumes of 10 to 12 liters/day are common. Nocturia is present; the patient may complain of fatigue due to disturbed sleep. If the underlying disease that destroyed the neurohypophysis causes no symptoms, the patient may appear surprisingly well. With an intact thirst mechanism and free access to water, the patient will match his intake to his output and maintain a normal serum sodium and osmolality. The inability to obtain free water, which frequently occurs following head trauma or anesthesia, may lead to life-threatening hypernatremia. A careful record of urine volumes and serum osmolalities in patients with CNS trauma will prevent this complication. Rarely, the patient with central DI may also have destruction of the thirst receptors in the hypothalamus. These patients must be taught to take fluids at regular intervals to prevent the development of hypernatremia.

Patients who develop permanent DI after surgical destruction of the neurohypophysis may undergo a characteristic response consisting of an initial 4- to 5-day period of polyuria immediately after the surgery followed by a 5- to 6-day period of oliguria before the polyuria and polydipsia of permanent central DI supervene. This triphasic response parallels the neurosecretory cell's response to injury. The initial trauma causes a shock paralysis of neurosecretory function, and ADH is not released. During the oliguric phase, cellular degeneration causes release of preformed hormone into the circulation. Finally, neurosecretory cell death causes permanent DI to appear. Failure to appreciate this sequence of events may lead to the following two common management errors. First, water intoxication may develop during the oliguric phase if hypotonic fluids routinely given postoperatively are not appropriately restricted. Second, the patient's ability to concentrate his urine 6 to 10 days postoperatively may be mistakenly interpreted as a sign of permanent recovery of neurohypophyseal function. Fortunately, most patients have lesser damage to the neurohypophysis and recover fully. The physician managing an early case of postsurgical DI should avoid premature judgments regarding the permanence of the condition.

Since only 15% of the neurohypophyseal secretory capacity is required to maximally concentrate the urine, DI following trauma is most often transient. Idiopathic DI may occur at any age and affect either sex. It is second only to trauma as a cause of central DI. Intracranial neoplasms are the third most common cause of central DI. In children, craniopharyngiomas predominate; metastatic lung or breast carcinomas are the common offenders in adults. Interestingly, pituitary tumors rarely cause central DI because they seldom reach sufficient size to disrupt the neurosecretory function of axons terminating high in the stalk. Therefore, if a patient with DI also has an abnormal sella, the tumor is more likely to be of suprasellar origin with extension downward into the sella rather than a primary pituitary neoplasm. Granulomatous diseases infiltrating the hypothalamus, CNS infections, vascular lesions, and an inherited form of central DI should also be considered in the differential diagnosis of DI.

NEPHROGENIC DI

The kidney may be unable to respond to ADH because of metabolic or structural derangements. Both hypercalcemia and hypokalemia interfere with the action of ADH on the renal tubule. The concentrating ability returns when these metabolic abnormalities are corrected. Since the production of a concentrated urine requires normal renal tubular function, chronic pyelonephritis, cystic kidney disease, or renal failure from any cause may produce hyposthenuria. Measurement of the blood urea nitrogen (BUN), creatinine, and glomerular filtration rate (GFR) will identify these patients. In the rare patient with familial nephrogenic DI, the disturbance is manifest shortly after birth and is usually transmitted in an X-linked recessive pattern.

PSYCHOGENIC WATER DRINKING

Any condition which stimulates the thirst center when the serum osmolality is below the threshold for ADH release results in a state of primary polydipsia. These patients "washout" their medullary interstitial gradient with large volumes of water and are subsequently unable to concentrate the urine effectively. Patients in this category can usually be identified by an absence of nocturia, a 24-hour urine volume in excess of 20 liters, and a plasma osmolality less than 285 mOsm/kg.

WATER DEPRIVATION TEST

Occasionally, the diagnosis of DI can be made with certainty only by performing a formal water deprivation test. Patients are deprived of water until the urine osmolality is maximized, that is, increases less than 30 mOsm/kg in an hour. Plasma osmolality is then determined and 5 U aqueous vasopressin is injected subcutaneously. The urine osmolality is determined 60 minutes after the vasopressin injection. Patients with DI may require as little as 3 hours to maximally concentrate the urine, whereas most other patients must be water deprived 16 to 18 hours to achieve maximal urine concentration.

In patients with central DI, urine osmolality will be less than plasma osmolality with water deprivation, but the urine osmolality will increase by at least 50% after the vasopressin injection. Patients who have nephrogenic DI also have a urine osmolality that is less than plasma osmolality, but vasopressin injection fails to cause a significant increase in urine osmolality. In patients with partial defects in ADH secretion, initial urine osmolality is greater than plasma osmolality, and following vasopressin injection, the urine osmolality increases by 10% to 50%. Normal subjects will maximally concentrate the urine in response to dehydration and show no further increase following vasopressin injection. Patients with primary polydipsia are able to concentrate the urine only slightly during water deprivation due to a "washed-out" renal medullary interstitium. However, since they have maximally stimulated the endogenous ADH secretion, urine osmolality will not increase after vasopressin injection. Once the diagnosis of DI has been established, consultation with an endocrinologist is appropriate to delineate the etiology and extent of the disease.

MANAGEMENT

The preferred medication for the treatment of central DI is 1-desamino-8-arginine vasopressin (DDAVP). The drug is administered by nasal insufflation.

The desired dose is drawn into a J-shaped catheter. The end containing the medication is placed into the nose and a quick puff of air blown into the other end of the catheter deposits the medication onto the nasal mucosa where it is readily absorbed into the circulation. Patients who have "colds" need only blow their noses before DDAVP administration because absorption will usually be satisfactory. The initial dose of DDAVP should be small, about 50 μg. The urine output and osmolality should be monitored. When polyuria returns, the dose may be increased to 100 μg and the duration of action determined. Most patients require a dose before bedtime to prevent nocturia and a dose in the morning to allow normal daily activity without frequent interruptions. Excessive amounts of DDAVP may produce water retention, hyponatremia, and natriuresis. If nasal packing prevents intranasal administration, DDAVP may be given subcutaneously or intravenously. When administered subcutaneously or intravenously, similar antidiuretic effects are seen at less than 10% of the intranasal dose. Therefore, 0.5 to 1.0 μg should be tried initially. This will produce antidiuresis for 8 to 12 hours.

Vasopressin tannate in oil is a long-acting preparation that should not ordinarily be used in critically ill patients. Water intoxication is common due to its long duration of action (up to 72 hours). Its relatively potent vasoconstrictive properties are of concern in the patient with cardiovascular disease. When this drug is used, it is important to realize that the "brown stuff" at the bottom of the vial is the active hormone, which must be dissolved in the oil vehicle. Hand-warming the vial facilitates the process.

Patients with partial defects in ADH secretion may only require free access to water. Occasionally, drugs that stimulate endogenous ADH release (clofibrate) or enhance ADH action on the renal tubule (chlorpropamide) are useful in these patients. No specific drug therapy exists for nephrogenic DI, but thiazide diuretics may decrease urine volume by creating a total body sodium deficit. This causes enhanced resorption in the proximal tubule and secondarily decreases fluid delivery to the collecting duct.

Patients with unrecognized DI may develop hypertonic encephalopathy that requires emergency treatment. Rapid infusion of hypotonic solutions may produce cerebral edema and generalized seizure activity in up to 40% of these patients. Normal saline should be administered if there are signs of circulatory collapse until the patient is no longer orthostatic. Hypotonic saline solutions may then be used cautiously. Generally speaking, the serum sodium level should be normalized over 36 to 48 hours.

For more information, please see Chapter 121 in Civetta JM, Taylor RW, Kirby RR: Critical Care. *Philadelphia: J. B. Lippincott, 1988*

BIBLIOGRAPHY

Barlow ED, DeWardener HE: Compulsive water drinking. *Q J Med* 1959; 28:235

Blotner H: Primary or idiopathic diabetes insipidus: A system disease. *Metabolism* 1958; 7:191

Coggins CH, Leaf AL: Diabetes insipidus. *Am J Med* 1967; 42:807

Rado JP, Marosi J, Fischer J: Comparison of the antidiuretic effects of single intravenous and intranasal doses of DDAVP in diabetes insipidus. *Pharmacology* 1977; 15:40

Randall RV, Clark EC, Dodge HW, et al: Polyuria after operation for tumors in the region of the hypophysis and hypothalamus. *J Clin Endocrinol* 1960; 20:1614

Sawyer WH, Acosta M, Balaspiri L, et al: Structural changes in the arginine vasopressin molecule that enhance antidiuretic activity and specificity. *Endocrinology* 1974; 95:140

Williams RH, Henry C: Nephrogenic diabetes insipidus: Transmitted by female and appearing during infancy in males. *Ann Intern Med* 1947; 27:84

Zimmerman EA, Robinson G: Hypothalamic neurons secreting vasopressin and neurophysin. *Kidney Int* 1976; 10:12

69 Adrenal Insufficiency and Glucocorticoid Medications

ADRENAL HORMONE INSUFFICIENCY

Hypoadrenalism can occur on the basis of diseases which involve the adrenal gland directly (primary adrenal insufficiency), or because of the lack of stimulation by ACTH of an otherwise normal adrenal gland (secondary adrenal insufficiency). Although the treatment of these two problems is similar, they have widely divergent causes and some differences in clinical presentation.

DIFFERENTIAL DIAGNOSIS

The most common cause of primary hypoadrenalism in the United States is autoimmune adrenalitis, which is responsible for almost 70% of the cases described. This disorder is associated with numerous other autoimmune-mediated endocrinopathies. In adults, these include thyroiditis and diabetes mellitus (Schmidt's syndrome). Occasionally, other autoimmune disorders such as hypogonadism, vitiligo, and pernicious anemia may be present.

The second most common cause of primary adrenal insufficiency is destruction of the gland secondary to *Mycobacterium tuberculosis*. This rarely occurs except in the presence of other extrapulmonary tuberculosis, especially with involvement of the genitourinary system. In contrast with autoimmune adrenalitis, tuberculosis adrenal disease is not associated with other endocrine diseases. In addition, the adrenal glands are frequently enlarged and may be calcified in this disorder in contrast to the atrophied, noncalcified glands seen with autoimmune involvement.

Other much less common etiologies of primary hypoadrenalism include acquired immunodeficiency syndrome, bilateral hemorrhage of the glands secondary to bacterial infection with sepsis and shock, other granulomatous diseases such as sarcoidosis and systemic fungal infections, metastatic malignancies, and amyloidosis.

The differential diagnosis of secondary hypoadrenalism involves disorders of the hypothalamus or the pituitary. The most common disorders involving these organs are pituitary adenomas and hypothalamic neoplasms such as craniopharyngiomas. Metastatic carcinomas, most commonly from the lung or breast, or lymphoproliferative malignancies with involvement of the pituitary or hypothalamus can also produce adrenal insufficiency. Pituitary infarction in the immediate postpartum state (Sheehan's syndrome), traumatic lesions such as basilar skull fractures, infections such as tuberculosis, nocardiosis, and actinomycosis, and other infiltrative diseases such as sarcoidosis, hemochromatosis, and amyloidosis have also been known to produce a similar condition. Overall, however, the most common cause of secondary adrenal insufficiency in this country is iatrogenic. The common use of high-dose glucocorticoid medications sufficient to suppress the HPA axis and increasing use of pituitary surgery and irradiation frequently result in adrenal insufficiency.

Although the symptoms, signs, and general laboratory results seen in adrenal insufficiency are nonspecific, taken together they form a pattern of findings which should suggest the possibility of hypoadrenalism (Table 69-1).

Hormonal testing is necessary to confirm the diagnosis of adrenal insufficiency. Serum cortisol levels increase significantly in normal patients who are in shock, and the finding of a cortisol level less than 20 μg/dl in the setting of shock is highly suggestive of compromised adrenal function. As a rule, however, baseline serum and urine hormonal measurements are inadequate to confirm the diagnosis. Adrenal insufficiency can be determined effectively by ACTH stimulation tests. The short ACTH stimulation test is an excellent screening examination for adrenal insufficiency and may be performed without difficulty in an ICU patient. Serum cortisol samples are obtained just prior to and 30 to 60 minutes after an intravenous injection of 250 μg of synthetic ACTN (cosyntropin). A normal response is defined as an increase

TABLE 69-1 CLINICAL FINDINGS IN ADRENAL INSUFFICIENCY

Symptoms
Weakness/fatigue
Anorexia
Gastrointestinal symptoms
Orthostatic symptoms
Myalgias/arthralgias
Signs
Weight loss
Orthostatic hypotension
Hyperpigmentation
Vitiligo
General laboratory findings
Hyponatremia
Hyperkalemia
Acidosis
Prerenal azotemia
Lymphocytosis/eosinophilia
Hypoglycemia

in the cortisol level of at least 7 μg/dl over the basal level and a rise in serum cortisol to an absolute level of at least 20 μg/dl. Note that both conditions must be met for a normal response. The short ACTH stimulation test is a simple, effective test for evaluating adrenal insufficiency. It does not, however, distinguish between primary and secondary hypoadrenalism. If results are abnormal, this test should therefore be followed by the long ACTH stimulation test.

MANAGEMENT

The management of adrenal insufficiency is dependent on whether the patient complains of mild symptoms suggestive of chronic hypoadrenalism and is felt to have normal cardiovascular hemodynamics, or presents in shock with symptoms of acute adrenal insufficiency (adrenal crisis). Management of acute adrenal insufficiency is outlined in Table 69-2.

TABLE 69-2 MANAGEMENT OF ACUTE ADRENAL CRISIS

I. Initial management—*all patients*
    1. Obtain baseline blood samples for cortisol, electrolytes, glucose, BUN, and creatinine while establishing IV lines for therapy.

II. Glucocorticoid therapy
    A. For patients with *diagnosis well established*
        1. Administer hydrocortisone hemisuccinate 100-mg IV bolus.
        2. Establish hydrocortisone hemisuccinate IV infusion at 75–100 mg every 6 hr.
        3. After resuscitation, taper to standard replacement doses (hydrocortisone 30 mg/24 hr) as rapidly as patient's condition allows.
    B. For patients with *diagnosis not established*
        1. Administer dexamethasone phosphate 4-mg IV bolus.
        2. Establish dexamethasone phosphate IV infusion at 4 mg every 8 hr.
        3. Switch to hydrocortisone hemisuccinate after diagnostic procedures are completed.

III. Fluid management—*all patients*
    1. Administer isotonic saline IV in volumes sufficient to support blood pressure.
    2. If patient is hypoglycemic, use 5% dextrose in isotonic saline.
    3. Assume patient will have at least 20% of extracellular fluid depleted.
    4. Hemodynamic monitoring is advised.

IV. Diagnostic procedures
    A. For patients with *diagnosis well established*
        1. No special diagnostic procedures are necessary.
    B. For patients with *diagnosis not established*
        1. Perform short ACTH stimulation test after therapy is initiated.
        2. If the short ACTH test is abnormal, perform long ACTH stimulation test after stabilization.

V. Other supportive measures—*all patients*
    1. Mineralocorticoid replacement is not usually necessary as long as isotonic saline is administered as required.
    2. Treat underlying problem that precipitated the episode of adrenal crisis.
    3. Prophylactic antibiotic use is not indicated.

The proper dose for a particular glucocorticoid medication (Table 69-3) is determined largely by the indications for its use. The choice of a particular steroid and its dose becomes a matter of reported clinical experience, pharmacologic (versus physiologic) effects, and prescribing habits. For example, glucocorticoids are commonly used for acute trauma to the central nervous system (CNS) in doses which are orders of magnitude beyond those which produce maximum glucocorticoid effects. Despite this, a dose–response relationship exists between the dose of a glucocorticoid and the clinical outcome. The pharmacology of glucocorticoids in these massive doses is not well understood, and their use is guided by clinical experience and experimental data from animal models where they have been beneficial.

A principal guideline in using steroid hormone medications is to accomplish the therapeutic end point while using the least amount of glucocorticoid for the shortest length of time. This is done to minimize the side-effects and complications of glucocorticoid therapy, as well as to prevent suppression of the hypophyseal-adrenal axis (HPA). In addition to their well-known metabolic and immunologic effects, glucocorticoids have been associated with various complications, such as glaucoma, posterior subcapsular cataracts, benign intracranial hypertension, psychiatric symptoms, pancreatitis, edema, aseptic necrosis of bone, and poor wound healing, among others.

A major concern in the use of large doses of glucocorticoids is suppression of the HPA axis, placing the patient at risk for adrenal insufficiency in times of stress. In general, doses of glucocorticoids equivalent to 20 to 30 mg of prednisone daily for a week probably do not cause clinically important adrenal suppression. For larger doses or more prolonged usage, the physician can assume some degree of adrenal suppression has occurred. This is supported by abnormal findings on ACTH stimulation or insulin tolerance tests. Realizing that these laboratory findings may not correlate with clinically significant adrenal suppression, common practice is to treat patients as if they have adrenal insufficiency in times of stress for at least a year after cessation of prolonged or high-dose glucocorticoid therapy, unless the HPA axis has been shown to be functioning properly.

TABLE 69-3 DAILY REPLACEMENT DOSES FOR SEVERAL COMMON GLUCOCORTICOID MEDICATIONS

Medication	Daily Dose (mg)
Hydrocortisone	30
Cortisone acetate	38
Prednisone	5
Prednisolone	5
Methylprednisolone	4
Dexamethasone	1

The decision to stop glucocorticoid therapy can be a major clinical problem. If there is any doubt as to the functional capability of the HPA axis, the medications should be tapered rather than abruptly discontinued. The rate at which the taper occurs will vary in different clinical situations. The choice of a particular tapering schedule must take into account the duration and magnitude of therapy to estimate to what degree the HPA axis has been suppressed: the more the suppression, the slower the taper. In addition, the underlying disease process must be considered; a self-limited acute allergic reaction might require only 3 days of large doses with no taper, whereas an aggressive inflammatory arthritis might require a taper lasting months to prevent a disease flare-up.

Typically, a steroid taper follows these general guidelines. First, drug administration should be switched from an intravenous to an oral route. Next, a change should be made from divided doses of glucocorticoids to a single morning dose using a short-acting medication. Of the commonly used glucocorticoids, dexamethasone has the longest duration of action while hydrocortisone and cortisone acetate have the shortest durations of action. Use of short-acting agents allows some ecape from the ACTH-suppressive effects of the drug in the early morning hours, allowing the HPA axis to be stimulated. The absolute amount of glucocorticoid that can be withdrawn depends in some measure on the total amount of steroid the patient is taking. In general, for glucocorticoid doses greater than 40 mg of prednisone or its equivalent, individual decrements of 10 mg can be used; when the prednisone dose is 20 to 40 mg, decrements should be limited to 5 mg; when the prednisone dose falls below 20 mg, individual decrements of no more than 2.5 mg should be attempted. Finally, the timing of each decrement may vary from a day to several weeks, depending on the clinical situation. The glucocorticoid dose is tapered only as rapidly as the patient's clinical condition permits to prevent relapse of the underlying disease state.

For more information, please see Chapter 122 in Civetta JM, Taylor RW, Kirby RR: Critical Care. *Philadelphia: J. B. Lippincott, 1988*

BIBLIOGRAPHY

Axelrod L: Glucocorticoid therapy. *Medicine* 1976; 55:39

Baxter JD, Forsham PH: Tissue effects of glucocorticoids. *Am J Med* 1972; 53:573

Byyny RL: Withdrawal from glucocorticoid therapy. *N Engl J Med* 1976; 295:30

Graber AL, Ney RL, Nicholson WE, et al: Natural history of pituitary–adrenal recovery following long-term suppression with corticosteroids. *J Clin Endocrinol* 1965; 25:11

Meuleman J, Katz P: The immunologic effects, kinetics, and use of glucocorticosteroids. *Med Clin North Am* 1985; 69:805

Nerup J: Addison's disease—clinical studies: A report of 108 cases. *Acta Endocrinol* 1974; 76:127

Nugent CA, Nichols T, Tyler FH: Diagnosis of Cushing's syndrome. *Arch Intern Med* 1965; 116:172
Plumpton FS, Besser GM: The adrenocortical response to surgery and insulin-induced hypoglycemia in corticosteroid-treated and normal subjects. *Br J Surg* 1969; 56:216
Rose LI, Williams GH, Jagger PI, et al: The 48-hour adrenocorticotropin infusion test for adrenocortical insufficiency. *Ann Intern Med* 1970; 73:49
Spiegel RJ, Vigersky RA, Oliff AL, et al: Adrenal suppression after short term corticosteroid therapy. *Lancet* 1979; 1:630

70
Thyroid Disease

HYPERTHYROIDISM

PRESENTATION

The presentation of an anxious, perspiring, thin young woman with proptosis and goiter is a rather easy diagnostic challenge for most clinicians. Table 70-1 lists the common symptoms and signs of thyrotoxicosis. However, intensive care unit (ICU) physicians are more likely to be confronted with patients with nonclassic presentations of Graves' disease, hyperthyroidism manifested primarily by severe dysfunction of one organ system, or thyrotoxicosis of non-Graves' etiology.

Multiple etiologies other than Graves' disease exist for thyrotoxicosis. Toxic multinodular goiter is seen more often in the elderly than in the young. The goiter should be appreciated by the careful examiner unless it is substernal. In this case, the displaced thyroid tissue will be apparent on chest radiograph. Patients who have recently received contrast material for radiographic procedures may present with iodine-induced thyrotoxicosis. The antidysrrhythmic agent, amiodarone, may also cause hyperthyroidism, presumably due to its high iodine content. Rarely patients will present with exogenous thyroid hormone ingestion as the etiology of their hyperthyroidism. If the patient has preexisting thyroid disease, a goiter may be present.

Hyperthyroidism may present in the elderly with only alterations in mental status, cardiac tachydysrhythmias, CHF, or weight loss (so called "apathetic thyrotoxicosis"). The physician must have a low threshold for suspicion of thyroid disease in elderly patients and embark on appropriate testing. Failure to make a timely correct diagnosis in these patients may make treatment of nonthyroidal manifestations of the disease ineffective. Furthermore, diagnostic and therapeutic maneuvers may place the patient with unrecognized thyrotoxicosis at risk for thyroid storm, a situation with catastrophic potential.

Patients treated with beta-blockers may have masking of some of the

TABLE 70-1 COMMON SYMPTOMS AND SIGNS OF HYPERTHYROIDISM

Symptoms	Signs
Weight loss	Hyperkinesis
Increased appetite	Ophthalmopathy (if Graves' disease)
Nervousness	Lid retraction
Heat intolerance	Lid lag
Sweating	Goiter
Palpitations	Thyroid bruit (if Graves' disease)
Dyspnea	Warm, moist palms
	Smooth skin
	Fine hair
	Tachycardia
	Tremor

classic signs and symptoms of hyperthyroidism. In particular, hyperadrenergic manifestations (lid retraction, lid lag, tachycardia, tremor, and sweats) may be virtually absent in some hyperthyroid patients who receive beta-blockers. The patient treated with these agents should not be considered to lack thyroid disease simply because of absence of a classic presentation.

DIAGNOSIS

The diagnosis of hyperthyroidism can usually be made by either a direct measurement of serum free thyroxine (FT_4) or an approximation of this measurement by calculating the serum free thyroxine index (FT_4I) from a measurement of total thyroxine (T_4) and some measurement of binding capacity such as the resin triiodothyronine (T_3) uptake (RT_3U) test. The FT_4I is calculated $FT_4I = T_4 \times RT_3U$. Occasionally values for these tests will be normal, but the diagnostic suspicion will be so high that the measurement of serum T_3 will be indicated to consider the possibility of "T_3 toxicosis." An elevation of the serum free T_3 index ($FT_3I = T_3 \times RT_3U$) will then be indicative of hyperthyroidism in these cases. However, "T_4 toxicosis" (FT_4I elevated, FT_3I normal) is probably much more common than "T_3 toxicosis" in severely ill patients. Most authorities recommend using a thyrotropin-releasing hormone (TRH) stimulation test in borderline cases, particularly in patients with atrial fibrillation. Whether "occult" thyrotoxicosis should be searched for by TRH testing in all patients with atrial fibrillation is unclear. It should be remembered that a "flat" TRH test may not always indicate frank hyperthyroidism, particularly in older men, patients with multinodular goiter, patients with severe nonthyroidal illness, and patients treated with dopamine. However, a normal TRH test rules out hyperthyroidism in such cases.

Nonendocrine laboratory test findings are nonspecific in thyrotoxicosis. Abnormalities of liver function tests and occasionally marked hyperbilirubinemia may be seen. Serum cholesterol levels are frequently low. Mild anemia and agranulocytosis can occur. Impaired glucose tolerance is occasionally seen. Hypercalcemia may occur in as many as 25% of patients.

In patients who do not have nodular goiters, Graves' disease can usually be differentiated from other forms of thyroid disease by measuring the radioactive iodine uptake. The patient with a diffuse goiter or no goiter and an elevated radioactive iodine uptake most likely has Graves' disease as the etiology of hyperthyroidism (though patients with preexisting thyroid disease and amiodarone-induced thyrotoxicosis may have elevated values as well). Patients with very low radioactive iodine uptake values usually have subacute or silent thyroiditis, postpartum thyroiditis, iodine-induced thyrotoxicosis, or exogenous thyroid hormone ingestion. Patients should be taken off antithyroid drugs 48 to 72 hours before this test. Thyroid scintiscanning is only necessary if a solitary toxic nodule is suspected.

TREATMENT

Graves' disease, toxic nodular goiter, and iodine-induced thyrotoxicosis can be treated acutely with antithyroid drugs. More definitive treatment, such as with radioactive iodine, should be deferred if immediate therapy is necessary. In most cases 300 to 600 mg propylthiouracil daily in three divided doses or 30 to 60 mg methimazole daily in divided doses is begun with gradual return of the patient to a euthyroid state. Although propylthiouracil is probably the preferred agent in patients with thyroid storm due to its inhibition of T_4-to-T_3 conversion and in pregnancy due to the association of methimazole with fetal skin defects, the drugs are probably otherwise equally useful in the hospitalized patient. Since the incidence of adverse side-effects with these agents (fever, rash, or a granulocytosis) may be dose dependent, the smallest dose possible to control the disease should be used in patients who do not have life-threatening illness. Beta-blockers relieve some of the discomfort associated with hyperthyroidism. However, in patients who are critically ill, particularly those with severe cardiac manifestations of thyrotoxicosis, the restoration of the euthyroid state should be as immediate as possible. In this setting, other drugs may be considered. Antithyroid drugs, iodides, and glucocorticoids are useful (see section on thyroid storm for dosage). The use of beta-blockers in patients with overt heart failure is controversial, but usually helpful. Although cardiac function may decline with use of these agents, the negative chronotropic effects of these drugs may more than make up for the adverse inotropic effects. Therapy with digoxin is often indicated for supraventricular tachydysrhythmias and CHF.

Although beta-blockers have been used as sole preparation for surgery in thyrotoxic patients, it is probably best to defer surgery until a euthyroid state is achieved. In emergency situations requiring immediate surgical intervention, hyperthyroid patients should be aggressively treated with all available forms of treatment to minimize the risk of thyroid storm.

THYROID STORM

When extreme manifestations of hyperthyroidism coexist with fever, tachycardia out of proportion to the fever, and central nervous system (CNS) dysfunction, diagnosis of thyroid storm is made. Since thyroid storm is life-threatening, therapy should begin immediately without awaiting the results of thyroid hormone tests.

The "classic" patient may have all of the symptoms outlined in Table 70-1. Physical examination reveals lid retraction and lid lag, hand and tongue tremor, warm moist skin, a hyperdynamic precordium, tachycardia, and hyperreflexia. The signs and symptoms are more severe than in most patients with hyperthyroidism. A goiter is frequently present as is a thyroid bruit if Graves' disease is the etiology for thyroid storm. Fever greater than 100°F is necessary to make the diagnosis of thyroid storm. Tachycardia is usually out of proportion to the fever. The patient may be comatose, highly agitated, or present with seizures or other manifestation of CNS disturbance. Gastrointestinal findings (hyperdefecation or liver function test abnormalities) may also be present in these patients.

An underlying precipitating factor for thyroid storm should be vigorously sought (Table 70-2). Infection is probably the most common event now that surgery on thyrotoxic patients is less common, and those patients who do have surgery have better preoperative preparation than a few decades ago.

TABLE 70-2 PRECIPITATING FACTORS FOR THYROID STORM

Precipitating factors
Infection
Thyroid Manipulations
Surgery
Radioactive therapy
Vigorous palpitation
Withdrawal of iodine therapy
Institution of iodine therapy
Metabolic
Diabetic ketoacidosis
Hypoglycemia
Medical Emergencies
Myocardial infarction
Pulmonary embolus
Surgical Emergencies
Trauma
Abdominal catastrophe
Medication Overdosage
T_4
Haloperidol
Digitalis
Other
Labor and delivery
Diagnostic procedures
? stress

The diagnosis of thyroid storm is clinical; therefore, laboratory tests cannot be relied on to make a diagnosis acutely since treatment must be initiated immediately. The patient should have blood specimens obtained for measurement of serum T_4 and RT_3U values (or direct measurement of serum FT_4). Serum T_3 values may also be of interest. Although FT_4 values have been reported to be higher in patients in thyroid storm than in those with uncomplicated hyperthyroidism, no laboratory values are definitively diagnostic of this disorder. Treatment for this disorder is outlined in Table 70-3.

HYPOTHYROIDISM

PRESENTATION

Hypothyroidism is less likely than hyperthyroidism to be encountered as a significant problem by the ICU physician. This disparity exists for two reasons. First, hypothyroidism is less common than hyperthyroidism. Second, many cases of hypothyroidism are mild. Hypothyroid patients rarely present with potential catastrophic manifestions. Nonetheless, this disease process should be familiar to the critical care physician since patients with coexistent coronary artery disease or coexistent adrenal insufficiency require particular care and management.

Common symptoms and signs of hypothyroidism are listed in Table 70-4. The symptoms are nonspecific, and the degree of severity of these symptoms and signs is quite varied from patient to patient. Goiter may or may not be

TABLE 70-3 TREATMENT OF THYROID STORM

Treat Underlying Cause
Supportive Care
- Hydration with glucose-containing solutions
- Multivitamins
- Reduce temperature
- Digoxin for CHF or supraventricular tachycardia

Inhibit Hormonal Biosynthesis
- Propylthiouracil 800–1200 mg orally, then 200–300 mg every 6 hr
- If oral route not possible use rectal methimazole 80–100 mg initially then 30 mg every 8 hr

Inhibit Hormone Release
- Iodides (SSKI 5 drops orally every 8 hr or sodium iodide 1 g IV over 30 min every 12 hr)
- Dexamethasone 2 mg every 6 hr

Antagonize Peripheral Effects of Thyroid Hormone
- Propranolol 40 mg orally every 6 hr or 1 mg IV every 5 min up to 10 mg maximum dose. Titrate dose to achieve appropriate effect.
- If propranolol contraindicated, use cardioselective beta-blockers or reserpine (1–5 mg IM after test dose, then 1–2.5 mg IM every 4–6 hr), or guanethidine (1–2 mg/kg orally daily)

TABLE 70-4 COMMON SYMPTOMS AND SIGNS OF HYPOTHYROIDISM

Symptoms	Signs
Weakness	Dry and coarse skin
Lethargy	Coarse hair
Weight gain	Periorbital edema
Dry skin	Bradykinesia
Cold intolerance	Peripheral edema
Hoarseness	Delayed relaxation phase of deep tendon reflexes
Constipation	Bradycardia
Paresthesias	

present depending on the cause of the hypothyroidism. Of particular note to ICU physicians is the fact that hypothyroid patients, like patients with other endocrine deficiency states, may not display a fever when an infectious process is present.

DIAGNOSIS

Though screening for primary hypothyroidism in outpatients can be accomplished by measuring the TSH level, it is probably wise to measure the FT_4I or FT_4 directly in addition to the TSH level in severely ill patients since interpretation of the clinical picture and thyroid tests in these patients may be difficult. Measuring serum T_3 has no place in the evaluation of hypothyroidism. Most hypothyroid patients have a low FT_4I (or FT_4) and a significant elevation of TSH. The metabolic status of patients with normal FT_4I but mild elevation in TSH is debatable (though I frequently err on the side of calling such patients hypothyroid). In severely ill patients the TSH may be found to be transiently elevated during recovery from nonthyroidal illness as the patient's serum T_4 level returns to normal. Serum TSH may also be elevated in adrenal insufficiency.

Most ICU physicians are aware of the diagnostic dilemma presented by the finding of a low serum T_4, low FT_4I, and normal TSH level. Statisitically, the overwhelming majority of these patients will have the "euthyroid sick syndrome." However, secondary hypothyroidism is a possibility. If other signs and symptoms point to possible pituitary disease in such patients, do a TRH stimulation test (500 μgTRH given intravenously, with TSH and prolactin values obtained at times 0, 15, 30, 60 and 120 min). Prolactin measurements also should be obtained to ensure that the pituitary responds to a potent secretagogue. If there is no TSH response or a delayed response, then the possibility of secondary hypothyroidism should be considered. Keep in mind that this test result is also consistent with severe nonthyroidal illness. Limit TRH stimulation testing to patients with clear evidence of pituitary or hypothalamic disease. A more useful test may be an assessment of adrenal function. If ACTH stimulation shows inadequate adrenal reserve, the patient should be assumed to have hypothalamic–pituitary disease. Complete testing of the pituitary should be carried out when the patient is not gravely ill.

TREATMENT

L-Thyroxine is the appropriate treatment for hypothyroidism. There is no indication for the use of combination T_4/T_3 preparations or for using T_3 alone since T_3 is formed in peripheral tissues from T_4. Presumably the body can more appropriately regulate T_3 levels than the physician. The usual oral replacement dose of L-T_4 is approximately 100 μg daily. (Note that this dose is lower than that given in many references before 1985 due to recent reformulation of T_4 tablets.) Patients with normal or near-normal FT_4I (or FT_4) and elevated TSH levels can be treated with full replacement doses with impunity. However, special care is necessary in hypothyroid patients where gradual replacement is deemed appropriate. Specifically, patients with possible coexistent coronary artery disease, long-standing hypothyroidism, or possible coexistent primary or secondary adrenal insufficiency deserve cautious treatment. Consider all hypothyroid patients over the age of 40 at risk for coronary disease. These patients should receive initially a low dose of T_4 which gradually is increased until full replacement is achieved. An initial dosage of 25 μg daily L-T_4 is used. The daily dosage is increased each month by 25 μg. For patients with known heart disease, a more cautious replacement schedule may be in order. Dosage is increased until the TSH level is in the normal range. A small number of patients will never be able to have full replacement due to incapacitating angina. Concomitant antianginal therapy or coronary artery bypass surgery may be necessary to allow full replacement in these patients.

Surgery can be carried out in hypothyroid patients, though minor complications may be increased. The anesthesiologist must pay careful attention to altered drug metabolism in these patients.

MYXEDEMA COMA

Myxedema coma is fortunately a rare manifestation of hypothyroidism. It is usually seen in elderly patients during the winter months. Metabolic decompensation is apparently due to nonthyroidal factors. The clinician should be alert to the recognized precipitants of myxedema coma listed in Table 70-5. Pulmonary infection is the most common such factor. Since most series of this disorder are from decades prior to accurate measurement of thyroid and other parameters, the reader can rightly question whether some of these factors were causal of the metabolic disaster or merely results of the underlying disease process.

The hallmarks of myxedema coma are severe depression of the sensorium and hypothermia, though one fifth of reported patients have normal temper-

TABLE 70-5 PRECIPITATING FACTORS OF MYXEDEMA COMA

Infection
Drugs (phenothiazines, barbiturates, narcotics, anesthetics)
Respiratory failure
CHF
Cerebrovascular accident
Trauma
Exposure to cold
Gastrointestinal hemorrhage
Metabolic disturbances (hypoglycemia, hyponatremia, hypoadrenalism)
Surgery
Seizures

atures. A normal temperature in such a patient may indicate bacterial infection. Most comatose, hypothermic patients will not have myxedema coma. However, the risk of missing myxedema coma far outweighs the risks of unnecessary T_4 treatment. Thus, the ICU physician should have a lower threshold to consider this diagnosis. It should be remembered that as many as half the cases of myxedema coma in some series have occurred after hospitalization, emphasizing the risks of therapeutic maneuvers in the undiagnosed severely hypothyroid patient.

If information from the patient's family is available, the physician should inquire carefully about a previous history of radioiodine treatment or T_4 therapy. Questioning family members about past signs and symptoms of hyperthyroidism is quite useful. Naturally, inquiry regarding previous thyroidectomy should be made. Family members should be questioned about symptoms of hypothyroidism. A recent change in mental or emotional state or presence of seizures is especially noteworthy.

The typical patient has dry, scaly skin, periorbital puffiness, thinning hair and eyebrows (lateral third), yellowish skin, and bradycardia. Most patients are comatose though occasionally some arousal may be seen. Temperatures below 80°F have been reported, so measurements should be made with a thermometer which registers below 94°F. Myxedema coma patients do not shiver. Survival is inversely proportional to body temperature.

Patients may present in cardiovascular collapse or be hypertensive. If respiratory failure has not yet occurred it may be impending due to airway obstruction, decreased sensitivity of central nervous respiratory centers to hypoxic and hypercapnic drives, or respiratory muscle weakness. The examiner should look closely for the possibility of a thyroidectomy scar. Goiters are rarely seen in patients with myxedema coma.

Pleural and pericardial effusion and ascites may be present. The patient may appear to have bowel obstruction due to decreased gastrointestinal motility. Localizing neurologic signs may be seen.

None of the usual laboratory tests are pathognomonic for myedema coma. Leukocytosis may not occur despite overwhelming infection. Hyponatremia (due to decreased free water excretion) and hypoglycemia may be

TABLE 70-6 TREATMENT OF MYXEDEMA COMA

Treat underlying cause
Passively warm patient
Treat hypotension with fluids
Use pressors, if needed, cautiously
Secure the airway and mechanically ventilate if necessary
Hydrocortisone 100 mg IV every 8 hr
T_4 500 μg IV followed by:
100 μg T_4 IV daily, or
25 μg T_3 IV every 6 hr

present. Hypercalcemia rarely is seen. The patient may have respiratory acidosis due to respiratory failure or metabolic acidosis if hypoperfusion is present. The cerebrospinal fluid (CSF) protein content may be quite elevated. Changes in cardiac enzymes and the EKG induced by hypothyroidism may complicate the diagnosis of myocardial infarction in these patients.

Treatment of this disorder is outlined in Table 70-6.

For more information, please see Chapter 123 in Civetta JM, Taylor RW, Kirby RR: Critical Care. *Philadelphia: J. B. Lippincott, 1988*

BIBLIOGRAPHY

Brent GA, Hershman JM: Thyroxine therapy in patients with severe nonthyroidal illnesses and low serum thyroxine concentration. *J Clin Endocrinol Metab* 1986; 63:1

Chopra IJ, Hershman JM, Pardridge WM, et al: Thyroid function in nonthyroidal illness. *Ann Intern Med* 1983; 98:946

Cooper DS: Antithyroid drugs. *N Engl J Med* 1984; 311:1353

Forester CF: Coma in myxedema. *Arch Intern Med* 1963; 111:734

Forfar JC, Muir AL, Sawers SA, et al: Abnormal left ventricular function in hyperthyroidism: Evidence for a possible reversible cardiomyopathy. *N Engl J Med* 1982; 307:1165

Klein I, Levey GS: Unusual manifestations of hypothyroidism. *Arch Intern Med* 1984; 144:123

Macklin JF, Canary JJ, Pittman CS: Thyroid storm and its management. *N Engl J Med* 1974; 291:1396

Shenfield GM: Influence of thyroid dysfunction on drug pharmacokinetics. *Clin Pharmacol* 1981; 6:275

Slag MR, Morley JE, Elson MK, et al: Hypothyroxinemia in critically ill patients as a predictor of high mortality. *JAMA* 1981; 245:43

Tibaldi JM, Barzel US, Albin J, et al: Thyrotoxicosis in the very old. *Am J Med* 1986; 81:619

X. Allergic/Immunologic Disorders

71 Anaphylaxis

Serious anaphylactic and anaphylactoid reactions are usually manifested as critical destabilization of the cardiovascular and respiratory systems, in addition to suggestive dermatologic signs and symptoms. The two syndromes, which are clinically indistinguishable, are often fatal without immediate treatment. Fulminant hypotension, bronchospasm, or laryngospasm occurs within seconds to minutes after exposure to a provocative agent. Frequently associated symptoms include pruritus, flushing, urticaria, rhinorrhea, metallic taste, nausea, headache, a feeling of impending doom, and tachycardia (Table 71-1).

The physician's response to suspected anaphylaxis must be immediate and correct. Evaluation and management must be initiated rapidly and simultaneously (Table 71-2). The first priorities are to correctly identify and treat the most life-threatening possibilities. With anaphylaxis, these are shock and laryngeal obstruction. Epinephrine is the mainstay of initial treatment and should be given in a dose of 0.3 ml to 0.5 ml SC or IM of a 1:1000 solution. In cases of severe hypotension or laryngospasm, 3 ml to 5 ml of a 1:10,000 solution may be given intravenously (less if cardiac risks carry considerable weight); the dose for children is 0.1 ml/kg of 1:10,000 epinephrine. If an intravenous catheter is not in place, 0.5 ml of 1:1000 epinephrine is given intramuscularly or 10 ml of 1:10,000 epinephrine can be administered through the endotracheal tube. Inhaled epinephrine from an aerosol (three inhalations of 0.16–0.20 mg epinephrine per inhalation, repeated every 5 minutes as needed) or nebulizer (8–15 drops of 2.25% epinephrine in 2 ml normal saline, administered every 5 minutes as needed), may help bronchospasm and laryngospasm. For laryngospasm, aerosolized epinephrine should be administered against a closed glottis (three activations), as well as inhaled (three more activations). If laryngospasm is refractory to these measures, a needle catherter cricothyroidotomy or emergency surgical cricothyroidotomy may be necessary. The necessary apparatus for a needle catheter cricothyroidotomy is available on most hospital wards (Figures 71-1 and 71-2). Following epinephrine, H_1 and H_2 blockers should be administered: diphenhydramine, 1 mg/kg IV, plus ranitidine, 1 mg/kg IV, is recommended (intravenous cimetidine causes substantial short-term hypotension).

TABLE 71-1 CLINICAL MANIFESTATIONS OF ANAPHYLAXIS AND ANAPHYLACTOID REACTIONS

System	Manifestation
Major Contributors to Lethality	
Respiratory	Bronchospasm, laryngospasm, bronchorrhea
Cardiovascular	Shock, tachycardia, dysrhythmias, capillary leak
Frequent Nonlethal Manifestations	
Skin	Pruritus, urticaria, angioedema, erythema
Neurologic	Dizziness, fear of death, syncope, perineal burning, lethargy, weakness, seizure, metallic taste
Eye	Conjunctival suffusion, lacrimation, pruritus
Nose	Rhinorrhea, pruritus, congestion, sneezing
Gastrointestinal	Nausea, vomiting, abdominal pain, diarrhea (may be bloody)

(Modified from Kaliner M: Anaphylaxis. *New England and Regional Allergy Proceedings* 1984; 5[4]:324)

The unconscious patient with signs suggestive of anaphylaxis should be intubated (or cricothyroidotomy performed if rapid intubation is impossible). Conscious patients may be stabilized with injected or inhaled epinephrine. Hypotensive patients should be placed in the Trendelenburg position, receive fluid challenges (5 ml/kg over 1–2 minutes) of crystalloid (which infuses more quickly than colloid), and be transferred to an intensive care unit. If stabilization and improvement do not occur within minutes of initial resuscitative measures, intra-arterial and pulmonary arterial catheters should be inserted and dopamine administered (5–20 μg/kg/min). If dopamine fails to support blood pressure, L-norepineprine, 3 μg/min, should be initiated and titrated to support a mean arterial pressure $\geq$ 60 mm Hg.

Emergency evaluation must accompany initial treatment measures. Infusions of possible etiologic agents must be stopped and the contents saved for analysis. Local epinephrine should be injected next to a subcutaneous or intramuscular injection site that is suspected of dispersing anaphylatoxin. In such cases, a tourniquet should be placed proximal to the injection site, and pressure applied to occlude venous return. Following administration of epinephrine, H_1 and H_2 blockers, and steroids, the tourniquet can be released cautiously for 1 minute every 15 minutes. The tourniquet should be removed as soon as release does not further aggravate life-threatening symptoms.

Leading differential diagnostic possibilities include vasovagal collapse, pulmonary embolism, acute bronchospasm, acute pulmonary edema, and an acute panic attack. Rarer diagnostic considerations include angioedema, carcinoid syndrome, pheochromocytoma, systemic mastocytosis, and the capillary leak syndrome. Rapid auscultation of the chest, combined with interpretation of the clinical setting and a triage history, including overview of the patient's problem list (if available), will allow the physician to direct treatment to the most likely etiologic factors.

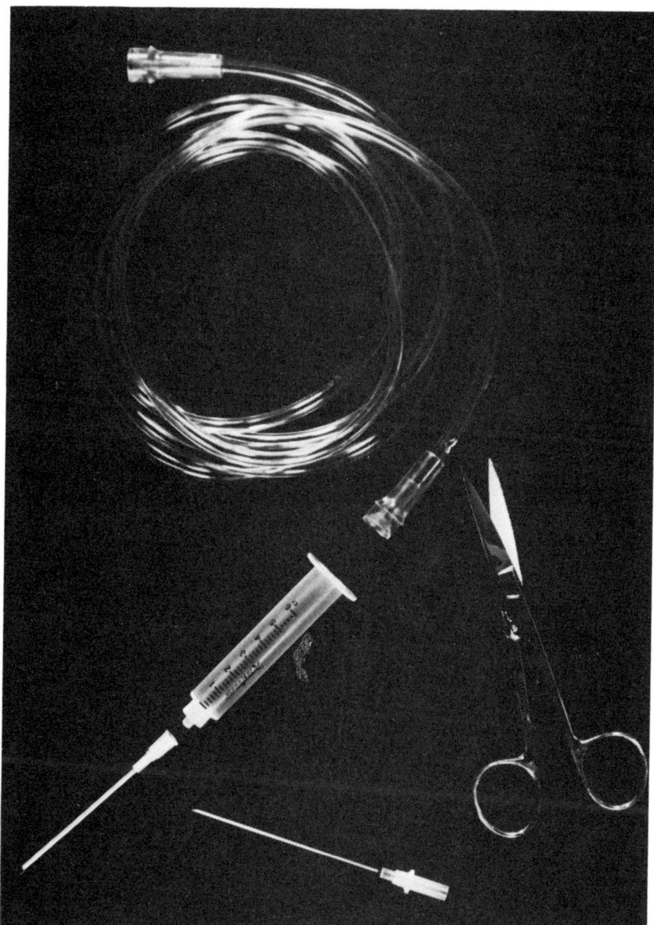

Figure 71-1 Equipment for a needle-catheter/cricothyroidotomy is readily available on most medical wards and all ICUs. The end of standard oxygen tubing should be forced snugly into an empty 6-ml disposable plastic syringe barrel (it can be taped in place). A 2 × 2-mm hole should be cut in the tubing as shown, to form an orifice that the thumb can be placed over to force wall oxygen (flowing at 15 liters/min) into the tracheal catheter, or which can allow most of the oxygen to be vented when the thumb is released for expiration.

TABLE 71-2 ACUTE MANAGEMENT OF ANAPHYLACTIC AND ANAPHYLACTOID REACTIONS*

Time	Evaluation	Management
Immediate	Conscious: determine severity of shortness of breath, lightheadedness; observe respirations, skin color; palpate pulse; check BP Unconscious: BLS algorithm with early anaphylaxis regimen	1. Establish likelihood of anaphylactoid syndrome 2. Establish one or more reliable IVs 3. Place tourniquet proximal to antigen exposure site 4. Stop possible provocative agent infusions 5. Use Trendelenburg position if hypotensive 6. If assistance is insufficient, call a code
0–2 Minutes	Determine degree of dyspnea or hypotension frequently (every minute); collaborate likelihood of precipitating agents; clinically exclude similar diagnostic possibilities (see text)	1. Give epinephrine IV, IM, SC or IT (see text for dosages) 2. Administer 100% inhaled oxygen 3. Use early inhaled aerosolized epinephrine or intubation for severe dyspnea (RR > 40); consider cricothyreotomy 4. Arterial BP monitoring if hemodynamic instability or shock not reversed within minutes or pressors required to keep MAP > 60 mm Hg 5. Infiltrate 0.1–0.3 ml of 1:1000 epinephrine at antigen injection site if identifiable

2–5 Minutes	Correlate important historical items; begin simultaneous diagnostic measures to evaluate management (AGBs; consider pulmonary artery catheter and intra-arterial pressure monitoring) and coexisting diagnostic possibilities	1. Diphenhydramine (dose as in text) IV; IM is route of second choice 2. For bronchospasm: 4 mg/kg aminophylline over 20 minutes, followed by 0.9 mg/kg/hr infusion† 3. For shock: dopamine 5–20 μg/min followed by L-norepinephrine drip: begin at 3 μg/min and titrate up or down to keep MAP > 60; consider volume challenges (5 ml/kg crystalloid × 1 or 2) over 5 minutes as well as early pulmonary artery catheter insertion unless prompt improvement occurs 4. Give hydrocortisone, 1.5 mg/kg IV push, then every 6 hours
5 Minutes	If still unstable, transfer to ICU	1. Keep MAP > 60 by optimizing preload (PAOP goal = 15–18 mm Hg) and afterload (SVRI > 400 by norepinephrine) 2. Endotracheal tube, arterial catheter, and pulmonary artery catheter indicated unless prompt resolution occurs 3. Consider inhaled β-agonists 4. Consider glucagon if patient is on β-antagonists

* Abbreviations: BLS = basic life support; RR = respiratory rate; ABG = arterial blood gases; IT = intratracheally; PAOP = pulmonary artery occlusion pressure; MAP = mean arterial pressure.
† Adjust infusion for individuals' theophylline clearance.

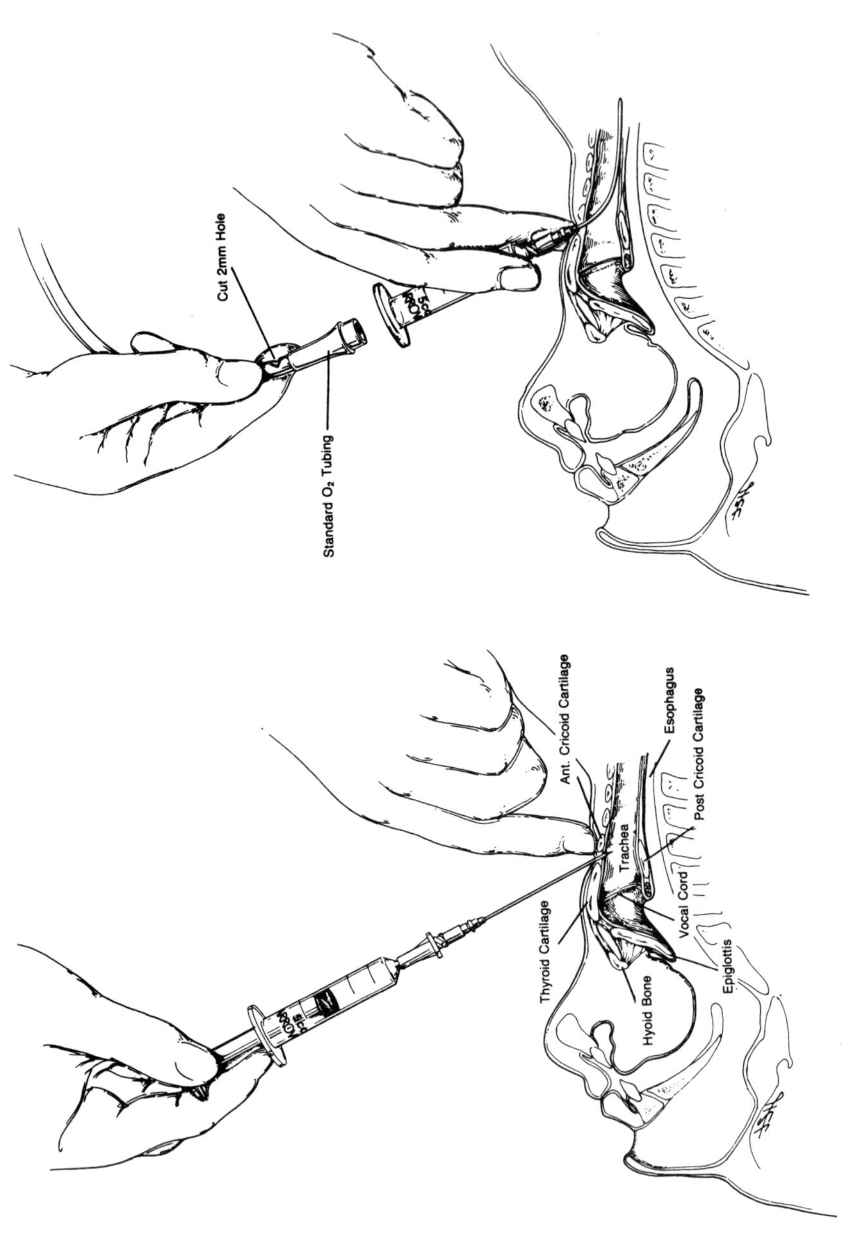
Cut 2mm Hole
Standard O_2 Tubing
Thyroid Cartilage
Ant. Cricoid Cartilage
Trachea
Esophagus
Post Cricoid Cartilage
Vocal Cord
Hyoid Bone
Epiglottis

Figure 71-2 Procedure for needle catheter cricothyroidotomy. The operator should cannulate the trachea between the thyroid cartilage and the cricoid ring, withdraw the needle, confirm placement by withdrawing air through the catheter, and then place the syringe barrel–oxygen tubing assembly into the catheter hub. When wall oxygen is turned on to 15 liters/min or more, the lungs are insufflated by occluding the hole in the oxygen tubing briefly. Exhalation will usually occur successfully past the larynx that is obstructed to inspiration. This is a temporizing measure that must be emergently followed by incisional cricothyreotomy or tracheostomy.

More thorough management and evaluation, including steroids (1.5 mg/kg hydrocortisone every 6 hours), can be undertaken after initial resuscitation measures. Milder cases of anaphylaxis, manifested primarily by flushing and urticaria alone, may require only antihistamines plus subcutaneous epinephrine. Mild bronchospasm can be treated with theophylline plus epinephrine. The physician should be prepared to institute the entire treatment regimen, however, in the event that progressive symptoms are seen.

A thorough follow-up evaluation, with institution or reinforcement of preventive measures, is always appropriate. For patients who must be reexposed to antigens or agents that have caused reactions previously, desensitization can be instituted using standard regimens. Although reexposure to iodinated intravenous contrast media usually fails to reinduce an anaphylactoid reaction in people who have had a previous life-threatening reaction, (*i.e.*, sensitization does not occur) prophylactic corticosteroid administration is recommended.

For more information, please see Chapter 126 in Civetta JM, Taylor RW, Kirby RR: Critical Care. *Philadelphia: J. B. Lippincott, 1988*

BIBLIOGRAPHY

Kaliner M: Anaphylaxis. *New England and Regional Allergy Proceedings* 1984; 5(4):324

Parrillo JE: Intravenous cimetidine administration commonly produces a decrease in arterial pressure in critically ill patients. *Update in Critical Care Medicine* 1986; 1(7):5

Whitten DM: Reaction to urographic contrast media. *JAMA* 1975; 231:974

72 Vasculitis and Collagen Vascular Disorders

Vasculitis is an inflammatory process that damages blood vessels and leads to organ damage. The presentation of vasculitis is invariably complex: laboratory data can be conflicting and diagnostic tests are often inconclusive. The differential diagnosis remains lengthy until histopathologic examination reveals the ravages of an untreated vasculitis. The first step in making the diagnosis of a vasculitis is to consider it in the differential. Vasculitis must always be considered in the critically ill patient presenting with multisystem disease (Table 72-1). Specific clues to a possible vasculitis in ICU patients include fever, fleeting pulmonary infiltrates, altered mental status, abdominal pain, seizures, congestive heart failure, arthralgias, hypertension, skin lesions, limb ischemia, weakness, renal failure, or deterioration of visual acuity. Vasculitis should be considered if these clinical features are unexplained, uncontrolled, or progressive. One should "think vasculitis" in a young person with unexplained multiple organ compromise or in an elderly patient with constitutional symptoms that are out of proportion to findings on physical examination.

DIAGNOSIS

It is an advantage in the ICU to have access to rapid and frequent radiographs that can detect fleeting pulmonary infiltrates and cavitations (Fig. 72-1). Interval monitoring detects changes in specific organ functions that are typical of a vasculitis. Pulmonary artery catheter placement may indicate a pericardial effusion or evidence of the diffuse cardiac compromise seen in systemic lupus erythematosus (SLE). Focal cardiac dysfunction is seen in polyarteritis nodosa (PAN) or giant cell arteritis. An echocardiogram is useful in separating diffuse from focal cardiac muscle dysfunction and clarifying a pericardial effusion. Other parameters that warrant repeat monitoring are the CBC, creatinine, BUN, and a urinalysis to discover red blood cell casts. The goal of all such monitoring is to rapidly identify significant organ damage and to establish the pattern of unexplained multisystem disease that is common in a necrotizing vasculitis.

TABLE 72-1 MULTISYSTEM MANIFESTATIONS OF VASCULITIS

General	Profound malaise, fever, hypertension, pain
Cardiovascular	Jaw or limb claudication, aneurysms, diminished pulses, myocardial infarction, cardiomyopathy, congestive heart failure, pericarditis
Respiratory	Sinusitis, pulmonary hemorrhage and infiltrates, asthma, pleural effusion
Gastrointestinal	Hematochezia, abdominal pain, pseudo-obstruction, ruptured viscus
Central nervous system	Headache, amaurosis fugax, seizures, mononeuritis multiplex, cerebrovascular accident, organic brain syndrome, coma, myelopathy
Musculoskeletal	Arthralgia/arthritis, myalgia/myositis, weakness
Genitourinary	Proteinuria, hematuria, cellular casts
Mucocutaneous	Purpura, rash, nodules, ulcers, embolic lesions

Once the diagnosis of vasculitis is considered in a specific organ, a biopsy can be obtained. Biopsy evidence of a vasculitis should be sought vigorously before initiating potentially life-threatening therapy. In general, needle biopsies yield inadequate tissue, but an open muscle biopsy of a symptomatic muscle will be diagnostic in 40% of patients with PAN (Fig. 72-2). An electro-

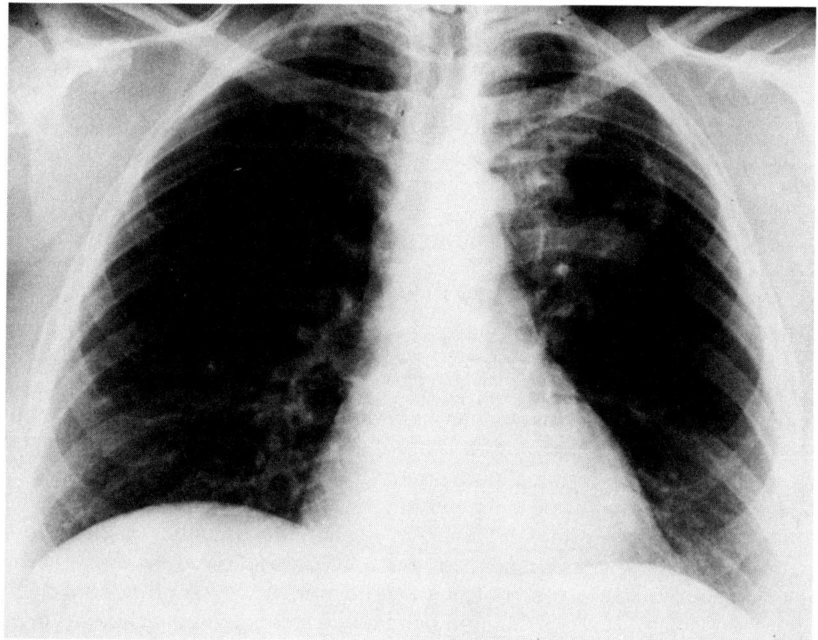

Figure 72-1 A cavitary lesion of the left upper lobe typical of Wegener's granulomatosis.

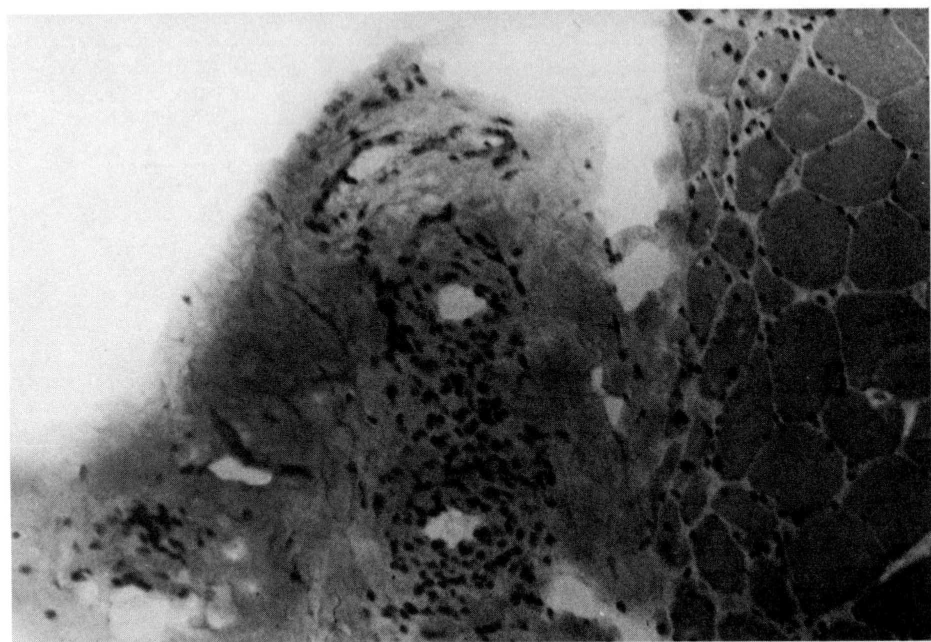

Figure 72-2 Note the vessel inflammation revealed in this muscle biopsy, diagnostic of a vasculitis.

myogram (EMG) can assist in localizing an abnormal muscle group; however, it can also induce artifactual tissue changes. Therefore, the biopsy must be taken distant from the EMG needle insertions or taken from the contralateral muscle group. Biopsy of the sural nerve may be diagnostic if conduction velocity studies of this nerve are abnormal. A biopsy of the vessels of the epineurium can reveal a vasculitis. Other cutaneous nerves that are accessible for biopsy include the superficial peroneal and superficial radial nerve.

Biopsy of the kidney yields a high frequency of positive results when urine sediment abnormalities are present. A biopsy may identify a glomerulonephritis or a small vessel vasculitis seen in SLE, Wegener's granulomatosis, and PAN. A needle biopsy of the kidney may be diagnostic, but an open biopsy is safer in the critical care unit patient. This is particularly true in PAN, where an aneurysm may be inadvertently biopsied.

A needle biopsy of the lung may diagnose infection or malignancy but often does not yield sufficient tissue to identify a vasculitis. An open lung biopsy of an abnormal area on a chest radiograph gives the best results. The lingula should not be routinely used simply because of its convenient anatomic location. Occasionally, it does not reflect pathologic changes present in the rest of the lung.

Testicular biopsies will demonstrate vascular inflammation in 86% of patients with a necrotizing vasculitis when the entire testis is sectioned. Needle biopsy of the testis is positive in 20% of patients. Any tissue removed during abdominal surgical procedures should be examined carefully for evidence of vasculitis (Fig. 72-3). Remember that necrotizing vasculitis can cause infarctions of the intestine, appendix, gall bladder, liver, and spleen and can produce massive bloody stools, pancreatitis, and hepatitis.

Leukocytoclastic vasculitis of the skin can be clarified by a biopsy performed at the bedside. The specimen should be sent for culture and immunofluorescence for immunoglobulin and complement. In addition to regular histopathology, special stains are required to identify an infection. Vasculitis in a medium-sized vessel can occasionally be identified by a deep dermal skin biopsy.

In the absence of a positive tissue biopsy, other diagnostic tests should be undertaken, even though these tests lack sensitivity or specificity. A computerized tomography (CT) scan of the brain can reveal evidence of major vessel infarction. A single infarct or a pattern of multiple smaller infarcts can be seen in vasculitis. A nuclear brain scan can identify a diffuse smaller vessel cerebritis or a focal abnormality. Magnetic resonance imaging (MRI) of the brain can identify a pattern of multiple small vessel lesions consistent with a vasculitis

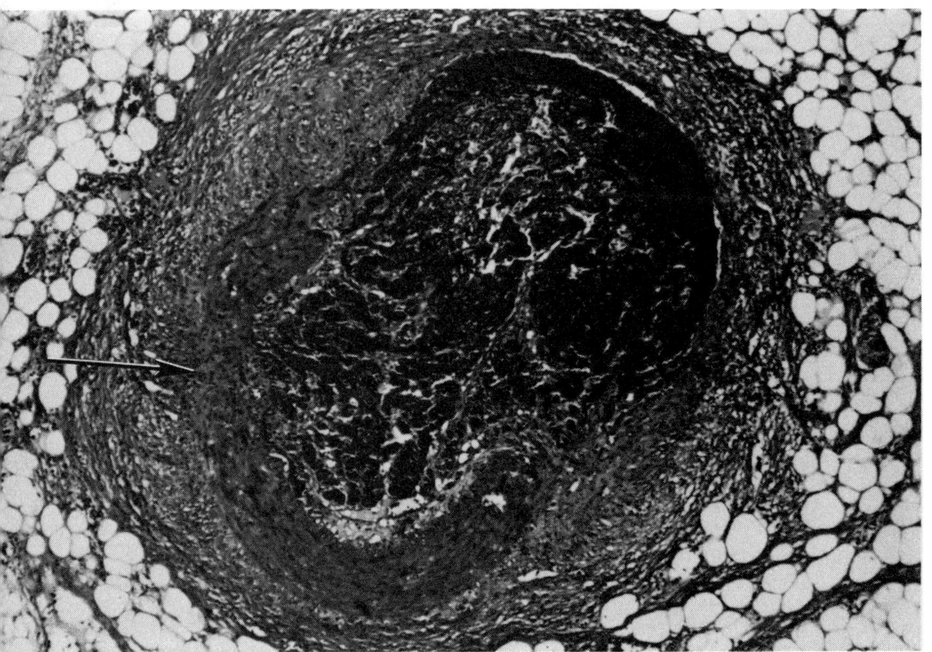

Figure 72-3 Mesenteric artery biopsy in a patient with PAN reveals a transmural cellular infiltrate and fibrinoid necrosis.

(Fig. 72-4) that may not be apparent on CT scan or angiogram. These lesions can mimic those seen in patients with multiple sclerosis.

Angiography is an important diagnostic tool in assessing medium and larger vessel vasculitis and may be abnormal in 70% of cases. In the PAN group, cut-off lesions, vessel narrowing, and saccular or fusiform aneurysms are seen (Fig. 72-5). In the giant cell arteritis group, diffuse vessel narrowing can be identified (Fig. 72-6); this can present clinically with extremity claudication. In the granulomatous vasculitis group, a cerebral angiogram may be the preferred way to diagnose angiitis of the CNS (Fig. 72-7). A normal angiogram does not completely rule out a vasculitis because small arterioles and postcapillary venules are not normally visible. A small vessel CNS vasculitis is occasionally diagnosed only by a leptomeningeal and brain biopsy.

TREATMENT

For the patient in the ICU, time is the critical consideration. How long can the patient wait for a diagnosis to be made before suffering irreparable organ damage? The answer to this question at the time of initial assessment will separate vasculitis that is a medical emergency from less fulminant disease.

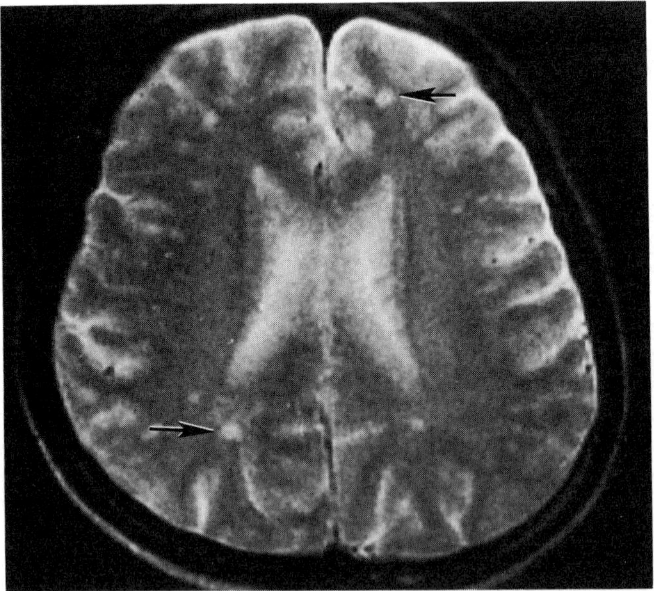

Figure 72-4 A magnetic resonance image of the brain demonstrates multiple hypodense periventricular lesions in a patient with SLE vasculitis. A CT scan and angiogram of this same area were normal.

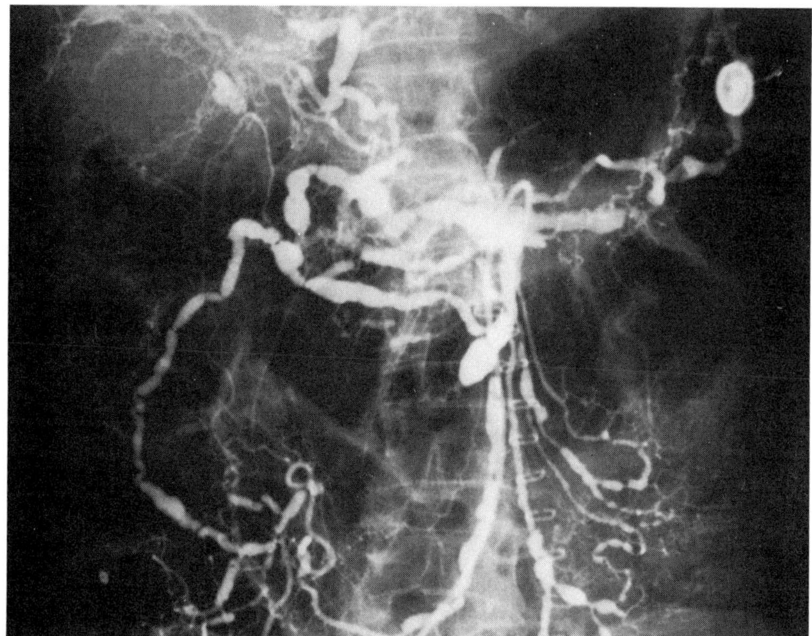

Figure 72-5 A visceral angiogram in PAN demonstrates aneurysms in the hepatic, splenic, celiac, and mesenteric circulations.

Fulminant disease can present with blindness, pulmonary hypoxemia, altered mental status, bowel ischemia, progressive neuropathy, or renal failure. Diagnostic procedures are not a substitute for experience; however, decisions about therapeutic intervention in these patients may have to be made with very few data available. The diagnosis of a systemic vasculitis can still be justified when all available investigative procedures are nondiagnostic. For example, severe visceral vasculitis can exist when biopsy and angiographic studies are negative. The benefits and risks of empirical therapy must be carefully weighed, and consultation with a physician experienced in these disorders is strongly advised before initiating therapy.

Corticosteroids are the mainstay of vasculitis therapy because their function is to decrease inflammation and the immunologic events associated with it. Prednisone (or equivalent) is given in a dose of 1 mg/kg/day in four divided doses. This dose should be maintained until there is evidence of a clinical response, which may take 7 to 30 days. When a response is observed, a split dose can be consolidated to a daily dose. Split-dose therapy for longer than 14 days requires a gradual consolidation to a single dose and then a slow tapering over months. Later in the patient's course, alternate-day corticosteroid therapy can be used. Patients or consenting family members

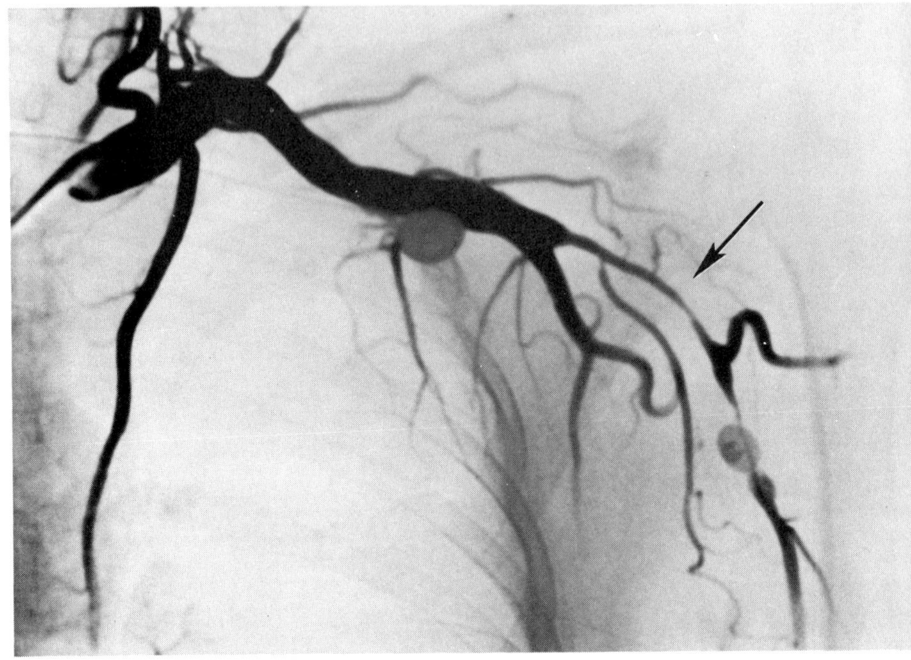

Figure 72-6 A left subclavian artery angiogram demonstrates vessel narrowing in a patient with giant cell arteritis.

should be counseled about the myriad of corticosteroid toxicities. In patients who develop a bacteremia, the corticosteroid dose should be rapidly consolidated to a daily dose to minimize granulocyte inhibition. Pulse dose methylprednisolone can be used as an initial adjuvant to therapy: 1 g of methylprednisolone in 100 ml D_5W is given intravenously over 30 minutes, and this dose is repeated every 24 hours for a total of three doses. Particular attention is given to monitoring the blood pressure and electrolytes. Hypokalemia is a contraindication to the use of pulse methylprednisolone. A patient is considered a steroid failure if the disease does not become inactive, if it progresses, or if steroid side-effects become intolerable.

Cytotoxic drugs should be considered next. There are numerous cytotoxic drugs, but cyclophosphamide, an alkylating agent, has been reported more often in the treatment of vasculitis. To obtain control of a vasculitis, doses of 1 to 4 mg/kg/day of cyclophosphamide are given intravenously or orally. The effect of cyclophosphamide therapy may not be observed for up to 14 days. The white blood cell count should be maintained above 3000 cells/mm^3 and the neutrophil count above 1500 cells/mm^3. Potential toxicities include marrow suppression, hemorrhagic cystitis, hair loss, sterility, delayed onset malignan-

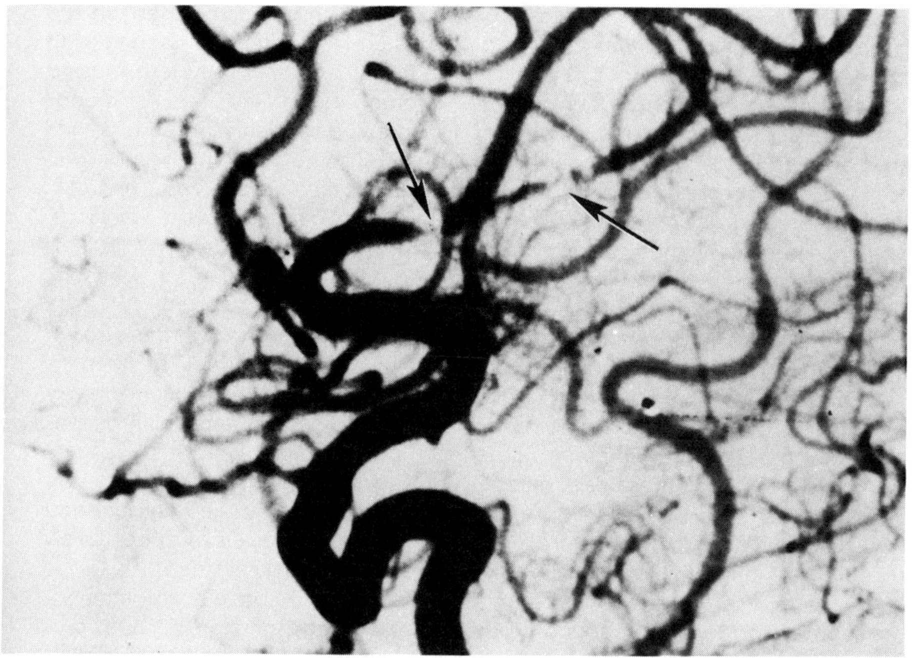

Figure 72-7 Granulomatous angiitis of the central nervous system is evident on a carotid angiogram. Note the segmental nature of the lesions.

cies, and an increased risk of herpes infection. Also, cyclophosphamide can be sequestered in effusions or ascitic fluid and then be released slowly, causing prolonged marrow suppression. Patients must maintain an adequate urine output to avoid hemorrhagic cystitis. Chlorambucil, another alkylating agent, is not associated with hemorrhagic cystitis and can be used in doses of 1 to 4 mg/day. A monthly pulse dose of cyclophosphamide, 0.5 to 1 g/m^2, has been used successfully in SLE, but the role of this therapy in vasculitis is unclear. It may be of more use as a maintenance therapy once control is established.

Fulminant vasculitis warrants high-dose corticosteroids and cyclophosphamide. Pulse methylprednisolone, split-dose prednisone, and 2 to 3 days of cyclophosphamide at 4 mg/kg/day can be combined. Cyclophosphamide is then changed to 2 mg/kg/day and the dose is adjusted over the next 14 days to maintain a white blood cell count greater than 3000 cells/mm^3. In life-threatening multisystem vasculitis or with evidence of persistent immune complex damage despite steroid and cyclophosphamide therapy, consider adding plasma exchange therapy. Plasma exchange is controversial and has been debated in the literature. Only experienced clinicians should attempt its use. The possible role of plasma exchange in vasculitis is based on the rationale that it removes immune complexes and low-affinity antibodies, and helps restore the clearing function of the reticuloendothelial system. Plasma exchange is acceptable therapy under appropriate circumstances for Goodpasture's syndrome and for thrombotic thrombocytopenic purpura. It has been reported in uncontrolled studies to show some favorable response in Henoch–Schönlein purpura, cryoglobulinemia, rheumatoid vasculitis, SLE, Wegener's granulomatosis, PAN, and fulminant LCV. In each of these settings, it has been combined with corticosteroid and cytotoxic drug therapy. Patients may undergo 1.5- to 2-liter exchanges on a daily or alternate-day schedule, depending on response.

Colloidal replacement can be given with 5% albumin or with fresh frozen plasma. The use of albumin is preferred to minimize the risk of hepatitis exposure. However, when albumin replacement is used, the patient's levels of other proteins, including immunoglobulins, fibrinogen, and antithrombin-III, will fall. The most common side-effect is citrate toxicity, which may present with circumoral paresthesis, muscle twitching, chills, nausea, vomiting, and syncope. These side-effects are related to low plasma ionized calcium and can occur in up to 15% of procedures. Serum calcium levels must be closely followed, and platelet counts maintained above 50,000 cells/mm^3.

Theoretically, if plasma exchange is used without concomitant immunosuppressive drugs, a rebound production of antibody–antigen immune complexes may develop and contribute to a worsening of the patient's clinical state. It is also important to note that plasma protein fraction contains no cholinesterase and that resynthesis after plasma exchange is delayed. This may lead to prolonged periods of apnea as a complication of anesthesia induced within 72 hours of plasma exchange. Plasma exchange should not be considered in the setting of active bleeding. Transfusions of fresh red blood cells may improve a patient's clearance of immune complexes. The surfaces of red blood cells have C3b receptors that may assist in carrying immune complexes to be cleared.

For more information, please see Chapter 127 in Civetta JM, Taylor RW, Kirby RR: Critical Care. *Philadelphia: J. B. Lippincott, 1988*

BIBLIOGRAPHY

Austin HA III, Klippel JH, Balow JE, et al: Therapy of lupus nephritis: Controlled trial of prednisone and cytotoxic drugs. *N Engl J Med* 1986; 314:614

Conn DL, Hunder GG: Necrotizing vasculitis. In Kelley WN, Harris ED Jr, Ruddy S, et al (eds): *Textbook of Rheumatology*, p 1137. Philadelphia, WB Saunders, 1985

Dyck PJ, Thomas PK, Lambert EH, et al: *Peripheral Neuropathy*, p 765. Philadelphia, WB Saunders, 1984

Fan PT, Davis JA, Somer T, et al: A clinical approach to systemic vasculitis. *Semin Arthritis Rheum* 1980; 9:248

Fauci AS: Vasculitis. *J Allergy Clin Immunol* 1983; 72:211

Hazards of apheresis. *Lancet* 1982; 2:1025

Klein HG, Balow JE, Dau PC, et al: Clinical applications of therapeutic apheresis. *J Clin Apheresis* 1986; 3:33

Lightfoot RW Jr: The vasculitis syndromes. In McCarty DJ (ed): *Arthritis and Allied Conditions: A Textbook of Rheumatology*, p 723. Philadelphia, Lea & Febiger, 1985

Lockwood CM, Worlledge S, Nicholas A, et al: Reversal of impaired splenic function in patients with nephritis or vasculitis (or both) by plasma exchange. *N Engl J Med* 1979; 300:524

Parris T: Vasculitis. In Beary JF III, Christian CL, Sculco TP, et al (eds): *Manual of Rheumatology and Outpatient Orthopedic Disorders: Diagnosis and Therapy*, p 273. Boston, Little, Brown & Co, 1981

XI. Hematologic/ Oncologic Disorders

73 Hematologic Diseases

REDUCED BLOOD COUNTS

ANEMIA

In the patient with hypovolemia due to blood loss, the clinical indications for transfusion are tachycardia and hypotension or instability of the heart rate and blood pressure with exertion or changes in position. The indications for transfusion to alleviate inadequate oxygen delivery include tachypnea and evidence of specific organ anoxia, such as mental confusion, angina pectoris, and indications of anaerobic (hypoxic) metabolism, such as lactic acidosis. The hematocrit or hemoglobin level associated with these changes varies widely among individuals depending on the oxygen demand, cardiac output, distribution of blood flow, and the affinity of hemoglobin for oxygen.

Patients with severe aplastic anemia may be candidates for bone marrow transplantation. Because prior transfusion of blood products diminishes the success rate of this therapy, transfusion should be avoided or minimized in such patients. What diagnostic studies should be obtained before transfusion? The reticulocyte count, corrected for the degree of anemia and early release of erythroid cells from the marrow, is the "reticulocyte index" which provides an estimate of red blood cell production. In the absence of acute blood loss, a reticulocyte index greater than 2 indicates hemolysis. Other laboratory tests, such as serum bilirubin, haptoglobin, or lactic acid dehydrogenase, are not necessary to demonstrate hemolysis as the mechanism of the anemia. If a hemoglobinopathy is suspected, a blood sample for hemoglobin electrophoresis should be obtained before transfusion.

Autoimmune Hemolytic Anemia

Autoimmune hemolytic anemia (AIHA) presents signs and symptoms of decreased oxygen delivery. Mild jaundice may also be present. Initial laboratory data show an elevated reticulocyte index, and the blood smear shows increased numbers of diffusely basophilic (polychromatophilic) red cells (reflecting the increased reticulocytes) and variable numbers of microspherocytes and fragmented cells. Once hemolysis is suspected or demonstrated, a direct Coombs' (antiglobulin) test should be ordered.

It is of immediate importance to determine whether the hemolysis is drug-related and whether it is due to warm-reacting or cold-reacting antibodies. The mainstay of treatment of AIHA due to warm-reacting antibodies is corticosteroids, given in dosages equivalent to 60 to 80 mg/day of prednisone. In patients who do not respond to steroids, splenectomy or treatment with immunosuppressive drugs may be useful. Steroids are less effective in AIHA that is due to cold-reactive antibodies (cold agglutinin disease), but responses have been observed using larger doses. Warming usually prevents or alleviates symptoms, but in a small percentage of cases plasmapheresis to reduce the concentration of the offending IgM antibodies may be required. In drug-induced immune hemolysis, discontinuing the drug is usually the only treatment needed.

In the patient with AIHA who has a critical degree of anemia, it may be impossible to find "compatible" red blood cells by the usual crossmatching procedures, and transfused cells may be subject to rapid antibody-mediated destruction. A test dose of ^{51}Cr-labeled donor red cells to determine survivability may be helpful. Transfusion of plasma, which contains complement, should be avoided because hemolysis is complement-mediated and may be limited by depletion of complement *in vivo*.

Hemolytic Anemia Due to G-6-PD Deficiency

Red blood cell glucose-6-phosphate dehydrogenase (G-6-PD) deficiency is inherited as an X-linked recessive disorder. Hemolysis may occur with exposure to certain drugs or with certain illnesses. Among the former are some sulfonamides, nitrofurantoins, and antimalarials, such as primaquine. Illnesses that may trigger hemolysis include acute infections and diabetic acidosis. Infectious hepatitis, in particular, has been associated with severe hemolytic episodes in G-6-PD-deficient individuals. Heinz bodies may be identified in red cells by special staining methods. These precipitates of oxidatively denatured hemoglobin provide a useful diagnostic clue, and should be looked for if G-6-PD deficiency is suspected as a cause of acute hemolysis. The red cell enzyme deficiency may be readily detected by laboratory assay when the patient is in a stable state but may be more difficult to demonstrate during a hemolytic episode. If the diagnosis is suspected, any potentially offending drugs should, of course, be stopped. Otherwise, supportive care is usually all that is necessary.

Mechanical Hemolytic Anemia

The two major categories are malfunctioning intravascular prosthetic devices (e.g., heart valves, vascular grafts and shunts) and disorders affecting blood vessels to produce so-called microangiopathic hemolytic disease (e.g., disseminated intravascular coagulation, thrombotic thrombocytopenic purpura, hemolytic uremic syndrome, and various vasculitides). On accasion a badly malfunctioning prosthesis, such as an artificial heart valve, may require replacement, but this is more often necessary to correct a life-threatening hemodynamic abnormality than to alleviate severe hemolysis.

Sickle Cell Anemia

Many of the complicating syndromes occurring in the sickle cell disorders are labeled "crises" and present as problems requiring critical care (Table 73-1). "Hemolytic crisis" is not mentioned; worsening of anemia due to accelerated hemolysis is not characteristic of sickle cell diseases. If hemolysis does increase significantly, a second disorder, such as G-6-PD deficiency or AIHD, should be sought.

The discussion here is directed primarily toward homozygous sickle cell disease. Patients with related, commonly occurring, doubly heterozygous conditions, such as sickle cell–hemoglobin C disease and sickle cell–β-thalassemia, may have similar complications. It is important to recognize that sickle cell trait, the heterozygous sickle cell state, is very infrequently associated with symptoms, signs, or laboratory abnormalities.

Painful Crisis. The painful or vaso-occlusive crisis is the most common symptomatic event in sickle cell disease. There are no pathognomonic signs or diagnostic laboratory tests or radiographs. Treatment of the painful crisis is supportive. Dehydration, acidosis, and hypoxemia all promote red cell sickling and should be prevented or corrected.

Lungs. The term "chest syndrome" is used to describe the clinical situation in which painful crisis is accompanied by pleuritic chest pain, fever, and a pulmonary infiltrate on chest radiograph. Arterial blood gases must be followed closely in this situation, and if the Pa_{O_2} cannot be maintained above 75 mm Hg, transfusion or exchange transfusion must be considered. There are no proven guidelines for the extent of transfusion therapy required, but a hematocrit of 25% to 30% with 50% non-hemoglobin-S-containing red cells is an acceptable goal.

TABLE 73-1 COMPLICATIONS OF SICKLE CELL DISORDERS

Painful (vaso-occlusive) crisis
Chest syndrome
Hepatic crisis
Cholelithiasis
Aseptic necrosis of bone
Bone marrow necrosis and fat embolism
Cerebral vascular occlusion
Hematuria
Priapism
Splenic infarction and sequestration
Postsplenectomy sepsis

Liver. A modest increase in conjugated serum bilirubin is commonly seen in sickle cell crises, presumably as a result of intrahepatic sickling and cholestasis. Rare patients may go on to hepatic failure and death. Anecdotal experience suggests that these patients may benefit from timely exchange transfusion. If abdominal symptoms are present, the possibilities of cholecystitis and complications of cholelithiasis must be considered.

Bone and Bone Marrow. Bone marrow infarction may produce a syndrome manifested by severe bone pain, fever, neurologic abnormalities, and respiratory distress, and is frequently fatal. Treatment by exchange transfusion may be lifesaving.

Central Nervous System. Strokes occur in a significant percentage of sickle cell patients. Treatment should be by exchange transfusion.

Genitourinary System. Hematuria occurs as a complication of the sickle cell diseases, including sickle cell trait, and may be severe. Supportive treatment with hydration, and perhaps urinary alkalinization, is often sufficient for this self-limited complication. Transfusion or exchange transfusion is rarely required. Priapism, a frequent and very painful complication of sickle cell disease, arises from vaso-occlusion that produces congestion and sickling in the corpora cavernosa. It may resolve spontaneously, and initial conservative treatment with analgesics, hydration, and alkalinization is appropriate. Exchange transfusion and various surgical procedures hae been successful in terminating priapism.

Spleen. The spleen, for unknown reasons, suddenly traps a large proportion of the red cell mass, causing left upper quadrant pain, a rapid fall in hematocrit, shock, and occasionally death. Transfusion reverses the process rapidly and should be administered immediately. By adulthood, almost all patients with sickle cell disease have undergone "autosplenectomy" due to repeated infarctions and therefore are not susceptible to this syndrome. The functional asplenia of most sickle cell patients renders them susceptible to fulminant septicemia caused by encapsulated organisms, such as *Streptococcus pneumoniae* and *Haemophilus influenzae*. Preventive strategies include prophylactic penicillin in children and administration of polyvalent pneumococcal vaccine to children and adults.

Aplastic Crisis in Hemolytic Anemia

Sudden intensification of anemia in hemolytic disease as a result of precipitous reduction in the rate of red cell production is known as aplastic crisis. Patients characteristically have fever, anorexia, nausea, and vomiting; abdominal pain and headache are common. The "aplastic" nature of the anemia is demonstrated by very low reticulocyte counts and marked reduction in erythroid precursors in the bone marrow.

Treatment is transfusion with red blood cells. The volume given should be sufficient to alleviate signs or symptoms of inadequate tissue oxygenation; that amount need not be exceeded because episodes are self-limited, and the patient's hematocrit will return rapidly to its baseline level.

LEUKOPENIA

Leukopenia refers to a circulating granulocyte count below $1500/mm^3$. Agranulocytosis implies very severe neutropenia or complete absence of granulocytes. The clinical importance of granulocytopenia lies in the associated increased risk of bacterial infection. This risk is slightly increased if the absolute neutrophil count is 500 to $1000/mm^3$. If neutrophil counts below $500/mm^3$ persist, bacterial infection becomes the rule.

Malignant Disease

Malignant diseases involving the bone marrow, particularly those of hematopoietic origin, commonly produce neutropenia, and the cytotoxic therapy currently used to treat these diseases almost invariably does so.

When the patient with severe neutropenia (absolute granulocyte count $< 500/mm^3$) develops fever above 101°F in the absence of other possible pyrogenic influences (*e.g.*, transfusion of blood products), infection must be assumed to be the cause. The common effects of bacterial infections—purulent sputum in pneumonia, pyuria in urinary tract infection, or abscess formation—may be absent. Cultures of blood, sputum, and urine should be obtained in all patients and other sites cultured as indicated in individual patients. Because infections that may be rapidly fatal, such as *Pseudomonas* septicemia, occur in these patients, antibiotics must be given promptly on an empirical basis before the results of the cultures are available. The choice of antibiotic regimen is predicated on the knowledge that most bacterial infections in these neutropenic subjects are due to aerobic, gram-negative bacilli and that combination regimens containing bactericidal agents provide the best outcome.

If cultures are negative, empirical therapy should be continued if the patient remains febrile and neutropenic. Even if the patient becomes afebrile, it is advisable to continue antibiotics for a minimum course of 7 to 10 days. When fever continues and the patient's general condition deteriorates, prescribe empirical treatment with amphotericin B because of the frequency of fungal infections. Granulocyte transfusion remains a final therapeutic option.

Bone Marrow Aplasia

Some cases of aplastic anemia appear to have an autoimmune basis; in others, a drug or chemical exposure may be suspected as etiologic. Benzene and its derivatives are potentially toxic to the bone marrow, and many other chemicals, such as DDT and other insecticides, are suspect. Toluene exposure in glue-sniffers may be associated with aplastic anemia. Drugs for which an etiologic role seems likely include chloramphenicol, phenylbutazone, indomethacin, diphenylhydantoin, sulfonamides, and gold preparations.

Immune Granulocytopenia

Phenylbutazone, sulfonamides, and antithyroid drugs may produce granulocytopenia. The characteristic clinical syndrome, includes high fever, chills, and severe sore throat ("agranulocytic angina") due to bacterial infection. Oral and pharyngeal ulcers, necrotizing tonsilitis, pharyngeal abscesses, and bacteremia may occur. The blood shows virtual absence of granulocytes. The bone marrow appears devoid of intermediate and mature granulocytes. After discontinuation of the drug, recovery occurs over a period of about 1 week. Because this disease can be fatal, early recognition and appropriate antibiotic and supportive therapy are important.

THROMBOCYTOPENIA

The earliest hemorrhagic lesions due to thrombocytopenia are typically petechiae in dependent body parts. With severe thrombocytopenia, epistaxis, menometrorrhagia, hematuria, and gastrointestinal and intracranial bleeding may be seen. Bleeding with ordinary trauma ("easy bruising") rarely occurs unless the count is less than 50,000/mm^3, and severe spontaneous bleeding is seen only at counts less than 10,000/mm^3 unless other defects are present.

Examination of the bone marrow for the presence of megakaryocytes is frequently necessary to distinguish between increased destruction (megakaryocytes present) and decreased production (megakaryocytes absent). The presence of splenomegaly raises the possibility of sequestration. When thrombocytopenia is due to destruction or sequestration of the patient's own platelets, transfused platelets will be subject to the same fate. Chronically transfused patients may become refractory to platelet transfusions from random donors because of alloimmunization. In such cases, platelets obtained from family members by plateletpheresis may still be effective.

Idiopathic (Autoimmune) Thrombocytopenic Purpura, (ITP)

The mechanism of the thrombocytopenia is established by the presence of ample megakaryocytes on bone marrow examination, and the presumptive diagnosis of ITP is made by excluding other possible causes of accelerated platelet destruction.

Platelet transfusions are used only in the case of serious (life-threatening) hemorrhage. The initial therapy is with corticosteroids in a dosage equivalent to 1 mg/kg/day of prednisone. If the platelet count does not rise substantially within 2 to 4 weeks, splenectomy is usually the next step.

The 10% to 20% of patients who fail to respond to splenectomy may benefit from treatment with vincristine or immunosuppressive agents like cyclophosphamide. The anabolic steroid danazol, when given for periods of several months, has also been effective in some cases of ITP. Newly available preparations of gamma globulin, which can be given intravenously, have also increased platelet counts in ITP perhaps through blockade of reticuloendothelial sites of platelet destruction.

Thrombotic Thrombocytopenic Purpura

Like the hemolytic-uremic syndrome and postpartum renal failure, which are closely related disorders, thrombotic thrombocytopenic purpura (TTP) may be catastrophic and rapidly fatal. Thus, prompt recognition and therapy are often crucial. The causes of TTP remain unknown, but some pathogenetic features have been elucidated. Factors in the plasma of some patients with TTP enhance platelet aggregation, and this effect may be inhibited by factors in normal plasma. In patients with chronic relapsing TTP, there is evidence that unusually large multimers of von Willebrand's factor, perhaps arising from endothelial cells and persisting abnormally in the plasma, contribute to platelet aggregation. Other factors and mechanisms have been postulated. Whatever the underlying and initiating factor(s), platelet aggregation and occlusion of arterioles and capillaries by hyaline thrombi are important features of the disease. The thrombi contain platelets and fibrin-like material, but disseminated intravascular coagulation is not characteristically present. The mortality rate is high in TTP, and early death is the rule in untreated patients.

When the diagnosis is made, corticosteroid therapy is begun with prednisone at a dosage of 1 mg/kg/day (or the equivalent dosage of another steroid). Arrangements are made for plasmapheresis to be started as soon as possible. If it will be more than 2 to 4 hours before the procedure transfusion with several units of fresh frozen plasma should be started. During plasmapheresis, the removed plasma should be replaced with fresh frozen plasma.

INCREASED BLOOD COUNTS

ERYTHROCYTOSIS

Polycythemia Vera (PV)

Criteria for the diagnosis of PV are an increased red cell mass and oxygen saturation of arterial blood over 92%, plus splenomegaly or two of the following: platelet count > 400,000/mm^3; white blood cell count > 12,000/mm^3 (without infection); and leukocyte alkaline phosphatase score > 100, serum vitamin B_{12} level > 900 pg/ml, or serum unbound vitamin B_{12} binding capacity > 2200 pg/ml.

Symptoms due to decreased cerebral blood flow, such as headache, dizziness, and changes in vision, are the most common manifestations of hyperviscosity. Hemorrhage or thrombosis can affect almost any body part. Peptic ulcer disease with bleeding is common. Thromboses may be arterial or venous. Surgery poses an enormous risk in the patient with uncontrolled PV. The mainstay of such therapy is phlebotomy to reduce the red cell mass. This may be done as rapidly as 1 unit of blood every other day. Electrolyte solutions or plasma expanders should be administered to avoid sudden changes in blood volume. Cytotoxic chemotherapy may be needed. Hydroxyurea may begin in an initial dose of 15 to 30 mg/kg/day.

ALTERED BLOOD RHEOLOGY

SERUM PROTEIN ABNORMALITIES

The disease most commonly associated with increased serum viscosity is Waldenström's macroglobulinemia, in which a malignant proliferation of plasmacytoid lymphocytes results in overproduction of monoclonal macroglobulin. These IgM molecules, because of their molecular size and shape, frequently produce increased serum viscosity and the clinical picture of the "hyperviscosity syndrome." A lower incidence of the hyperviscosity syndrome is seen in multiple myeloma, the malignant plasma cell dyscrasia in which monoclonal IgA or IgG is overproduced. Because of its greater tendency to aggregate, IgA is more often associated with hyperviscosity than is IgG. Hyperviscosity may occur in cryoglobulinemia, in which cold-precipitable immunoglobulins or immune complexes are responsible for the abnormalities.

The most common manifestations of the hyperviscosity syndrome are headache, visual disturbances, hearing loss, vertigo, altered consciousness (ranging from stupor to coma), paresis, seizures, and peripheral neuropathy bleeding tendency may exist due to associated thrombocytopenia or interference by the abnormal protein with the function of platelets or plasma coagulation factors. Careful examination of the optic fundi is important because the presence of alternating bulges and constrictions in the column of blood in retinal veins (so-called "boxcar" or "sausage-link" abnormalities) is highly suggestive of hyperviscosity. Direct measurement of serum viscosity can be carried out in the laboratory. The most rapidly effective form of therapy for hyperviscosity due to serum protein abnormalities is plasmapheresis.

OTHER HEMATOLOGIC DISEASES REQUIRING CRITICAL CARE

TUMOR LYSIS SYNDROME IN HEMATOLOGIC MALIGNANCIES

Hyperuricemia, hyperphosphatemia, and hyperkalemia are the major abnormalities. The malignancies most often associated are undifferentiated lymphoproliferative diseases. The tumor lysis syndrome commonly appears 1 to 2 days after chemotherapy is initiated and persists for 4 to 7 days. Acute increase of uric acid may produce acute oliguric or anuric renal failure. Allopurinol may be given orally in a dosage of 300 to 800 mg/day. It acts within 1 to 3 days. Vigorous hydration should be undertaken, with the goal of achieving a urine flow of 100 ml/hr. Alkalinization of the urine to a *p*H of 7 may be pursued by addition of 50 to 100 meq sodium bicarbonate to each liter of intravenous fluids. Acetazolamide, in doses of 250 to 500 mg/day, has been used to aid in alkalinization of the urine. Dialysis may be necessary in a patient with established renal failure. Hyperphosphatemia may occur because of the release of phosphates from destroyed cells. Hyperkalemia is rare, but deaths due to cardiac dysrhythmias have been reported to result from this complication.

BONE MARROW TRANSPLANTATION AND GRAFT-VERSUS-HOST DISEASE (GVHD)

Acute GVHD occurs usually within the first 2 months; chronic GVHD occurs later. Immunosuppressive therapy recently shown to be beneficial includes methotrexate given for a period of days after transplantation and cyclosporine administered for 6 months. Skin rash is often the first sign. Gastrointestinal manifestations include esophageal symptoms of dysphagia and heartburn, as well as chronic diarrhea, steatorrhea, and malabsorption. Hepatocellular and cholestatic abnormalities of liver function may be present. Ocular manifestations include photophobia, blurred vision, dryness (keratoconjunctivitis sicca), and uveitis.

The most common treatment that has been applied is prednisone in dosages of 1 to 2 mg/kg/day. Other therapies that have been used include large "pulse" doses of steroids, antithymocyte globulin, cyclosporine, and other immunosuppressive agents. The multiplicity of clinical manifestations of chronic GVHD is illustrated by the list of diseases it may mimic, such as scleroderma, systemic lupus erythematosus, Sjögren's syndrome, primary biliary cirrhosis, and lichen planus. The skin involvement, as in acute GVHD, takes many forms. Biopsy of affected tissues helps to verify the diagnosis of chronic GVHD and estimate its severity. Chronic GVHD has been treated with corticosteroids and various other immunosuppressive agents.

For more information, please see Chapter 132 in Civetta JM, Taylor RW, Kirby RR: Critical Care. *Philadelphia: J. B. Lippincott, 1988*

BIBLIOGRAPHY

Berk PD, Goldberg JD, Donovan PB, et al: Therapeutic recommendations in polycythemia vera based on polycythemia vera study group protocols. Semin Hematol 23:132, 1986.

Bloch KJ, Maki DG: Hyperviscosity syndromes associated with immunoglobin abnormalities. Semin Hematol 10:113, 1973.

Bukowski RM: Thrombotic thrombocytopenic purpura: A review. Prog Hemost Thromb 6:287, 1982.

Camitta BM, Storb R, Thomas ED: Aplastic anemia. Pathogenesis, diagnosis, treatment, and prognosis. N Engl J Med 306:645, 1982.

Charache S: Treatment of sickle cell anemia. Annu Rev Med 32:195, 1981.

Cohen LF, Balow JE, Magrath IT, et al: Acute tumor lysis syndrome. A review of 37 patients with Burkitt's lymphoma. Am J Med 68:486, 1980.

Estey E, Maksymiuk A, Smith T, et al: Infection prophylaxis in acute leukemia. Comparative effectiveness of sulfamethoxazole and trimethoprim, and ketoconazole, and a combination of the two. Arch Intern Med 144:1562, 1984.

Mills ML: Life-threatening complications of sickle cell disease in children. JAMA 254:1487, 1985.

Schreiber AD, Herskovitz BS, Goldwein M: Low-titer cold-hemagglutinin disease. Mechanism of hemolysis and response to corticosteroids. N Engl J Med 296:1490, 1977.

Sheehan RG: Thrombopoiesis and thrombokinetics—An approach to the evaluation of thrombocytopenia. Am J Med Sci 289:168, 1985.

Slater SD, Rahman M, Lindsay RM: Renal function in chronic intravascular haemolysis associated with prosthetic cardiac valves. Clin Sci 44:511, 1973.

Sullivan KM, Shulman HM, Strob R, et al: Chronic graft-versus-host disease in 52 patients: Adverse natural course and successful treatment with combination immunosuppression. Blood 57:267, 1981.

Sullivan KM, Deeg HJ, Sanders J, et al: Hyperacute graft-vs-host disease in patients not given immunosuppression after allogeneic marrow transplantation. Blood 67:1172, 1986.

Worlledge SM: Immune drug-induced hemolytic anemias. Semin Hematol 10:327, 1973.

74 Coagulation Disorders

AN APPROACH TO THE PATIENT WITH AN ACTUAL OR SUSPECTED COAGULATION DISORDER

Specific questions regarding bleeding should investigate the occurrence of any of the following: spontaneous, easy, or disproportionately severe bruising; intramuscular hematoma formation (either spontaneous or related to trauma); spontaneous or trauma-induced hemarthrosis; spontaneous mucous membrane bleeding; prior problems with bleeding related to surgery (including dental extractions, tonsillectomy, and circumcision); the need for transfusions in the past; menstrual history; and, finally, current medications.

Patients with primary hemostatic defects tend to manifest "capillary type bleeding"—oozing from cuts or incisions, mucous membrane bleeding, or excessive bruising. In contrast, individuals with dysfunction of secondary hemostasis have "large vessel bleeding," characterized by hemarthroses, intramuscular hematomas, and the like.

The physical examination should answer several basic questions: Is the process localized or diffuse? Is it related to an anatomic or surgical lesion? Is there mucosal bleeding? Are there signs of thrombosis (either arterial or venous)? An enlarged spleen coupled with thrombocytopenia suggests splenic sequestration. Liver disease (e.g., portal hypertension, ascites), points to decreased factor synthesis.

Findings of disseminated malignancy suggest disseminated intravascular coagulation (DIC). Venous and arterial telangiectasias may be seen in von Willebrand's disease and liver disease, respectively. Table 74-1 summarizes several major categories of hemorrhagic disorders and the tests that are characteristically abnormal in each. The suspicion that DIC is present in certain situations (Table 74-2) usually stems from one of two situations: unexplained, generalized oozing or bleeding, or unexplained abnormal laboratory parameters of hemostasis. The differential diagnosis includes conditions listed in Table 74-3.

Liver disease and several other conditions can have presentations similar to DIC. Measurement of fibrin degradation products (FDP) in the serum is

TABLE 74-1 HEMORRHAGIC SYNDROMES AND ASSOCIATED LABORATORY FINDINGS

Clinical Syndrome	Screening Tests	Supportive Tests
DIC	Prolonged PT, aPTT, TT; decreased fibrinogen, platelets	(+) FDPs, D-dimer; decreased factors V, VIII, and II (late)
Massive transfusion	Prolonged PT, aPTT; decreased fibrinogen, platelets +/− Prolonged TT	All factors decreased; (−) FDPs, D-dimer (unless DIC develops); (+) transfusion history
Anticoagulant overdose		
Heparin	Prolonged aPTT, TT; +/− prolonged PT	Toluidine blue/protamine corrects TT; reptilase time normal
Warfarin (same as vitamin K deficiency)	Prolonged PT; +/− prolonged aPTT (severe); normal TT, fibrinogen, platelets	Vitamin-K-dependent factors decreased; factors V, VIII normal
Liver disease		
Early	Prolonged PT	Decreased factor VII
Late	Prolonged PT, aPTT; decreased fibrinogen (terminal liver failure); normal platelet count (if splenomegaly absent)	Decreased factors II, V, VII, IX, and X; decreased plasminogen; +/− FDPs unless DIC develops
Primary fibrinolysis	Prolonged PT, aPTT, TT; decreased fibrinogen +/− platelets decreased	(+) FDPs, (−) D-dimer; short euglobulin clot lysis time

helpful in confirming the presence of DIC, particularly when they are present in concentrations greater than 40 μg/ml. The primary treatment for DIC is correction of the underlying problem that led to its development. Supportive therapy includes the use of several component blood products. Cryoprecipitate contains a much higher concentration of fibrinogen than whole blood

TABLE 74-2 UNDERLYING DISEASES ASSOCIATED WITH DISSEMINATED INTRAVASCULAR COAGULATION

Sepsis	Retained placenta
Liver disease	Hypertonic saline abortion
Shock	Amniotic fluid embolus
Penetrating brain injury	Retention of a dead fetus
Necrotizing pneumonitis	Eclampsia
Tissue necrosis/crush injury	Localized endothelial injury
Intravascular hemolysis	(aortic aneurysm, giant hemangiomata, angiography)
Acute promyelocytic leukemia	
Thermal injury	Disseminated malignancy
Freshwater drowning	(prostate, pancreatic)
Fat embolism syndrome	

TABLE 74-3 DIFFERENTIAL DIAGNOSIS OF DISSEMINATED INTRAVASCULAR COAGULATION

Liver disease	Thrombotic thrombocytopenic purpura (TTP)
Massive transfusion	Heparin therapy
Fibrinolysis	Dysfibrinogenemia/afibrinogenemia

or fresh frozen plasma (FFP). Fresh frozen plasma effectively repletes other coagulation factors except fibrinogen.

Pharmacologic therapy for DIC has two primary aims: to "turn off" ongoing coagulation and to impede thrombus formation. The most widely used drug is heparin. A bolus dose of 25 units/kg is given, followed by a continuous infusion of 10 units/kg/hr. Clinical signs of improvement include decreased bleeding and improved organ function. Platelet counts, plasma fibrinogen levels, and specific coagulation factor levels (*e.g.*, factor V) should improve when heparin therapy is successful.

LIVER DISEASE AND HEPATIC INSUFFICIENCY

The most common problem in patients with liver disease and a prolonged PT is due to decreased factor VII. Plasma concentrations of the vitamin-K-dependent coagulation proteins also decrease, as do those of factor V (which is not vitamin-K-dependent). Factor II (fibrinogen) is maintained until the disease approaches the terminal phase. Fresh frozen plasma provides the most immediate source of specific coagulation factors (*i.e.*, factor VII). Vitamin K replacement may be needed (typically requires longer than 12 to 24 hours.) Platelet transfusions may also be required, depending on the clinical situation.

VITAMIN K DEFICIENCY

The most common cause of a prolonged PT in the intensive care unit is vitamin K deficiency. The differential diagnosis of an isolated prolongation of the PT is primarily liver disease. The management of vitamin K deficiency consists primarily of its repletion. Therapy should not await the development of bleeding or oozing. The usual dose of vitamin K is 5 mg–10 mg IV. If the PT does not correct within 72 hours following three daily doses of vitamin K, intrinsic liver disease should be suspected. When the patient is actively bleeding, it is not sufficient to give vitamin K alone. Fresh frozen plasma usually contains sufficient amounts of vitamin-K-dependent coagulation proteins to stem further bleeding.

MASSIVE TRANSFUSION SYNDROME

The patient who is bleeding as a consequence of massive transfusion or washout presents with diffuse oozing and bleeding from all surgical wounds and puncture sites. Laboratory abnormalities include prolonged PT, aPTT, and TT. Fibrinogen levels and platelet counts are typically decreased; FDP are not usually increased unless concurrent DIC is present. Platelet administration may help stem bleeding from anatomic wounds. When the patient continues to bleed despite what should be adequate therapy for massive transfusion syndrome, the possibility of DIC should be investigated.

ANTICOAGULANT OVERDOSE

Heparin

Heparin affects coagulation through its influence on antithrombin III. Heparin–antithrombin III complex then inactivates thrombin, as well as factors VII, IX, X, and XI. When one "reboluses" or increases a heparin infusion rate in response to insufficient anticoagulation (*i.e.*, inadequate prolongation of the aPTT), a point will be reached when further small increments in the heparin infusion rate result in a substantially greater prolongation of the aPTT.

Serious bleeding associated with heparin overdose can be rapidly reversed by protamine sulfate. As a general rule, 1 mg of protamine will neutralize approximately 100 units of heparin (specifically, 90 USP units of bovine heparin, or 115 USP units of porcine heparin). The dose of protamine needed is estimated from the original heparin dose and the typical half-life for that infusion rate. The drug should be given by slow intravenous push over 8 to 10 minutes. A single dose should not exceed 50 mg. No more than 100 mg should be given as a cumulative dose without rechecking coagulation parameters.

Warfarin

Several drugs and pathophysiologic conditions are associated with potentiation of warfarin's effects on coagulation (Table 74-4). When over-anticoagulation with warfarin presents as a bleeding problem, the treatment of choice is FFP. Four to six units of FFP are usually sufficient. Vitamin K may also be administered in situations that are less acute.

Warfarin necrosis is characterized pathologically by the thrombosis of small blood vessels in the fat and subcutaneous tissues. Protein C is also a vitamin-K-dependent protein, and is subject to the effects of warfarin as well. In some situations (particularly when an initial dose of warfarin greater than 10–15 mg is given), levels of protein C may actually fall before those of the vitamin-K-dependent coagulation proteins. Under these conditions, thrombosis may be precipitated. This can generally be avoided if heparin and warfarin therapy are overlapped until "coumadinization" is complete, and if large loading doses of warfarin are avoided.

PLATELET DISORDERS

Platelet disorders are a common cause of clinical bleeding in the ICU (Table 74-5.)

TABLE 74-4 DRUGS THAT POTENTIATE THE ANTICOAGULANT EFFECTS OF WARFARIN

Antibiotics	Phenylbutazone (oxyphenbutazone)
Broad-spectrum antibiotics (especially cephalosporins)	Sulfinpyrazone
Griseofulvin (oral)	Other Drugs
Metronidazole	Cimetidine
Sulfonamides	Clofibrate
Trimethoprim sulfamethoxazole	Disulfiram
Anti-inflammatory Drugs	Phenytoin
Steroids (anabolic, in particular)	Thyroxine (both D- and L-isomers)
Acetylated salicylates	Tolbutamide

TABLE 74-5 PLATELET DISORDERS SEEN IN THE ICU

Quantitative	Qualitative
Increased Destruction	*Drugs*
Immune	Antiinflammatory agents
Thrombotic thrombocytopenic purpura/hemolytic uremic syndrome	Aspirin (irreversible)
Idiopathic thrombocytopenic purpura	Nonsteroidal anti-inflammatory agents
Systemic lupus erythematosus	Corticosteroids
Acquired immunodeficiency syndrome	Antibiotics
Durgs (gold salts, heparin, sulfonamides, quinidine, quinine)	Penicillins (*e.g.*, ampicillin, carbenicillin, ticarcillin, penicillin-G)
Sepsis	Cephalosporins (*e.g.*, cephalothin)
Nonimmune	Nitrofurantoin
Mechanical destruction (*e.g.*, cardiopulmonary bypass, hyperthermia)	Chloroquine, hydroxycholoroquine
Consumption (*i.e.*, DIC)	Phosphodiesterase inhibitors
Decreased production	Dipyridamole
Marrow suppression	Methylxanthines (*e.g.*, theophylline)
Chemotherapy	Other drugs
Viral illness (*e.g.*, cytomegalovirus, Epstein–Barr virus, herpes simplex, parvovirus)	Antihistamines
Drugs (thiazides, ethanol, cimetidine)	α-Blockers (*e.g.*, phentolamine)
Marrow replacement	β-Blockers (*e.g.*, propranolol)
Tumor	Dextran
Myelofibrosis	Ethanol
Other conditions	Furosemide
Splenic sequestration	Heparin
Dilution (see massive transfusion syndrome)	Local anesthetics (*e.g.*, lidocaine)
	Phenothiazines
	Tricyclic antidepressants
	Nitrates (*e.g.*, sodium nitroprusside, nitroglycerin)
	Metabolic Causes
	Uremia
	Stored whole blood
	Disseminated intravascular coagulation (*i.e.*, FDPs)
	Hypothyroidism

Quantitative disorders

A decrease in the number of circulating platelets reflects either increased peripheral destruction/sequestration, decreased marrow production, or a combination of these factors. Chronic idiopathic thrombocytopenic purpura (ITP) often requires therapy. Steroids may be given (1–2 mg/kg/day of prednisone or its equivalent). Splenectomy may also be required to avert serious bleeding complications in those patients who do not respond to steroids. Agents such as vincristine/vinblastine and cyclophosphamide have also been used as immunosuppressants, with variable success. Recently, high doses of intravenous gamma globulin (1–2 g/kg given over 2–5 days) have been useful in producing at least transient elevations in platelet counts.

Drug-induced immune-mediated platelet destruction is a common cause of thrombocytopenia seen in the ICU. Fortunately, it is usually reversible; withdrawal of the offending drug prevents further immune-medicated platelet destruction. Acute nonidiosyncratic heparin-induced thrombocytopenia is seen in approximately 10% to 15% of patients receiving heparin. It usually remits despite continued use of the drug. Heparin need not be stopped in these patients. Idiosyncratic heparin-induced thrombocytopenia is of much greater clinical consequence. It is less frequent, (fewer than 5%). Arterial thrombosis is the usual problem, and may be life threatening (*i.e.*, by causing myocardial infarction, cerebrovascular accident, or pulmonary embolism). The mechanism of thrombosis is thought to be a consequence of the deposition of platelet aggregates in the microcirculation. The diagnosis of heparin-induced thrombocytopenia is usually one of exclusion. It is almost exclusively associated with the use of bovine lung heparin. Cancer chemotherapeutic agents currently used may adversely influence thrombopoiesis.The thiazide diuretics, cimetidine, ethanol, and several of the cephalosporin and penicillin antibiotics have similar effects.

Qualitative Disorders

These disorders are particularly important in the ICU, where virtually all drugs used can be potential causes of qualitative platelet dysfunction. All unnecessary drugs should be viewed as suspect and discontinued in patients with evidence of qualitative platelet dysfunction. Terminating these drugs usually results in a restoration of normal platelet functional activity.

TABLE 74-6 THE THROMBOTIC DISORDERS

Thrombotic thrombocytopenic purpura/hemolytic uremic syndrome
Deep venous thrombosis
Pulmonary embolism syndrome
Heparin-induced thrombocytopenia
Thrombotic disseminated intravascular coagulation
Coronary thrombosis/acute myocardial infarction
Stroke
Peripheral vascular disease/arterial thrombosis

The relationship of thrombocytopenia to clinical bleeding is relative, that is, it is difficult to identify a specific, arbitrary platelet count (threshold) beyond which bleeding is likely to occur. Several conditions, such as massive transfusion syndrome and DIC, may respond to empirical platelet transfusion at counts as high as 80,000 or even 100,000 platelets/μl. With other causes, such as thrombocytopenia seen with cancer chemotherapy and bone marrow aplasia, therapy may not be required until counts fall below 20,000/μl.

THROMBOTIC SYNDROMES

Thrombotic disorders are listed in Table 74-6.

For more information, please see Chapter 129 in Civetta JM, Taylor RW, Kirby RR: Critical Care. *Philadelphia: J. B. Lippincott, 1988*

BIBLIOGRAPHY

Barton JC, Poon MC: Coagulation testing of the Hickmann catheter blood in patients with acute leukemia. *Arch Intern Med* 1986; 146:2165

Bloom AL: Intravascular coagulation and the liver. *Br J Haematol* 1975; 30:1

Clouse LH, Comp PC: The regulation of hemostasis: The protein C system. *N Engl J Med* 1986; 314:1298

Colman RW, Robboy SJ, Minna JD: Disseminated intravascular coagulation: A reappraisal. *Annu Rev Med* 1979; 30:359

Gastineau DA, Kazmier FJ, Nichols WL, et al: Lupus anticoagulant: An analysis of the clinical and laboratory features of 219 cases. *Am J Hematol* 1985; 19:265

Gralnick HR: Massive transfusion. In Colman RW, Hirsh J, Marder VJ, et al (eds): *Hemostasis and Thrombosis: Basic Principles and Clinical Practice*. Philadelphia, JB Lippincott, 1982

Gralnick HR, Bagley J, Abrell E: Heparin treatment for the hemorrhagic diathesis of acute promyelocytic leukemia. *Am J Med* 1972; 52:167

Janson PA, Jubelirer SJ, Weinstein MJ, et al: Treatment of the bleeding tendency in uremia with cryoprecipitate. *N Engl J Med* 1980; 303:1318

Kazmier FJ, Bowie EJW, Hagedorn AB, et al: Treatment of intravascular coagulation and fibrinolysis (ICF) syndromes. *Mayo Clin Proc* 1974; 49:665

Kelton JG: Heparin-induced thrombocytopenia. *Haemostasis* 1986; 16:173

Livio M, Mannucci PM, Vigano G, et al: Conjugated estrogens for the management of bleeding associated with renal failure. *N Engl J Med* 1986; 315:731

Mannucci PM, Remuzzi G, Pusineri F, et al: Deamino-8-D-arginine vasopressin shortens the bleeding time in uremia. *N Engl J Med* 1983; 308:8

Mant MJ, King EG: Severe, acute disseminated intravascular coagulation: A reappraisal of its pathophysiology, clinical significance, and therapy based on 47 patients. *Am J Med* 1979; 67:557

O'Reilly RA: Anticoagulant, antithrombotic, and thrombolytic drugs. In Gilman AG, Goodman LS, et al (eds): *The Pharacological Basis of Therapeutics,* 7th ed. New York, MacMillan, 1985

Phillips LL: Transfusion support in acquired coagulation disorders. *Clin Hematol* 1984; 13:137

Salzman EW, Deykin D, Shapiro RM, et al: Management of heparin therapy. A controlled prospective trial. *N Engl J Med* 1975; 292:1046

Schwartz BS, Williams EC, Conlan MG, et al: Epsilon-aminocaproic acid in the treatment of patients with acute promyelocytic leukemia and acquired alpha-2-plasmin inhibitor deficiency. *Ann Intern Med* 1986; 105:873

Thompson AR, Harker LA: *Manual of Hemostasis and Thrombosis*. Philadelphia, FA Davis, 1983

Walls WD, Losowsky MS: The hemostatic defect of liver disease. *Gastroenterology* 1971; 60:108

75
Transfusion Therapy

ACUTE MASSIVE HEMORRHAGE

CASE HISTORY

You have just been told that your patient, a 60-year-old man, has been transferred directly from the emergency room to the ICU with an upper gastrointestinal (GI) bleed. On initial examination, you note the patient to be somewhat stuporous; he is cold and clammy, has a heart rate of 130 beats/min, and his systolic blood pressure is 80 mm Hg by palpation. Fresh blood and blood clots are in the emesis basin that accompanied him to the ICU. He tells you that he suffers from arthritis, for which he takes aspirin three times daily, and that he had a heart attack last year. He began vomiting blood an hour earlier. Clearly this is not the time to obtain an extensive history and physical examination. You have already determined that the patient has an upper GI bleed, which may be complicated by a platelet defect as a result of aspirin ingestion, and that he is markedly hypovolemic (> 40% blood loss). The rest of the history and physical examination should be performed while treatment is being administered.

MECHANICS OF TREATMENT

As always, first ascertain that the airway is adequate, then insert a large 14- to 16-gauge catheter (preferably 14 gauge) in the upper extremity (Table 75-1). Using a 20-ml syringe to start the intravenous (IV) infusion allows you to draw blood samples immediately. Fill the syringe and then attach the IV tubing with a macrodrip chamber to the cannula. Initially, give normal saline or lactated Ringer's solution "wide open." Use a pressure bag or a stopcock and 50-ml syringe to achieve high flow rates (> 100 ml/min). The initial blood specimen must be sent for type and crossmatch (red-top tube); complete blood count (CBC) (purple top); prothrombin time (PT) and partial thromboplastin time (PTT) (blue top); and blood urea nitrogen (BUN), creatinine, sodium, potassium, chloride, and bicarbonate (usually red top). Other studies

TABLE 75-1. ALGORITHM FOR MASSIVE HEMORRHAGE

1. Establish an adequate airway.
2. Obtain initial vital signs.
3. Insert a large (14 to 16 gauge) intravenous catheter, preferably in an arm vein. Simultaneously obtain a blood sample and request type and crossmatch, CBC, PT, PTT, BUN, creatinine, sodium, potassium, chloride, and bicarbonate.
4. Give 1 to 2 liters of crystalloid rapidly (> 100 ml/min) until blood pressure rises and is stable.
5. Put direct pressure on the site of hemorrhage when possible. If intra-abdominal hemorrhage is suspected, apply military antishock trousers (MAST). Evaluate the need for surgery now!
6. Estimate the present volume deficit and the deficit in 40 to 60 minutes at present rate of hemorrhage. Order the appropriate number of RBC units.
7. Insert a second large intravenous cannula.
8. If hemorrhage continues, give crossmatched packed RBCs as soon as they are available.
9. If hemorrhage is massive, order universal donor packed cells (O-positive for males, O-negative for females) (ready in 10 minutes). Type-specific red cells (20 minutes) also can be ordered.
10. Heat the room, warm all solutions (crystalloid and blood products), and use a warming blanket. Maintain body temperature at 37°C!
11. After 6 to 8 units of packed RBCs are transfused, give FFP at a ratio of 1 to 2 units for each additional 2 units of packed cells. Fresh frozen plasma must be ordered 35 to 45 minutes before it is needed. Anticipate!
12. After replacing 8 to 10 units of packed red cells, give platelets at a ratio of 1:1 (*i.e.*, 6 units of platelets with the 14th, 20th, and 26th units of RBCs). Fresh platelets or liquid stored platelets < 48 hours old are recommended.
13. If the patient had a deficiency in plasma volume, red cell mass, platelets, or clotting factors prior to the hemorrhagic event, replace them at the initiation of resuscitation.
14. Measure hematocrit, PT, PTT, Ca^{2+}, and platelet count periodically and modify therapy as necessary.
15. Give one ampule of calcium *slowly* after every 4 to 6 units of packed RBC's *only* if the rate of infusion approaches 1 unit every 5 minutes. Follow Ca^{2+} levels when possible; otherwise, monitor QT intervals.
16. Consider surgical or interventional radiologic methods to stop the hemorrhage.
17. Consider using a blood salvage system.
18. Maintain patient temperature.

may also be useful, so save any extra blood in a red-top tube. It is your responsibility to be certain that the tube for type and crossmatch is properly labeled. The second most common cause of major transfusion reactions is failure to label this tube properly. Also, the blood bank will not release blood for your patient unless the labeling is complete.

Considerations of speed and safety strongly favor the use of arm veins. If no suitable arm vein can be found, the femoral vein is a second choice. Internal jugular or subclavian vein approaches have greater risks, take longer, require the Trendelenburg position, and in general use smaller catheters incapable of the rapid flow rates that can be obtained through 4-cm-long 14-gauge or 16-gauge catheters. A single 16-gauge catheter has a larger cross-sectional area and allows higher flow rates than two 18-gauge catheters. During the 15 minutes it takes to infuse the first 2 liters of fluid, insert a second large-bore IV catheter and ascertain pertinent information regarding allergies, medication, and past medical history. Aspirin, warfarin, nonsteroidal anti-inflammatory agents such as ibuprofen, and other drugs may profoundly affect bleeding and therapy. The pulse rate is misleading in patients taking β-adrenergic blocking drugs, and cardiac output may not increase in response to anemia. The patient's premorbid state of health and nutrition should be assessed to determine any preexisting volume or red cell deficits. Patients with signs and symptoms of malnutrition may be hypovolemic and anemic on the basis of a catabolic state. Those losses must be replaced in addition to the measured and estimated losses caused by the acute hemorrhagic event.

ESTIMATING THE ACUTE DEFICIT

If the deficit is estimated to be 1 unit of blood (10% of normal blood volume), blood replacement probably is unecessary (Table 75-2). On the other hand, if the initial deficit is estimated to be 3 to 4 units and brisk bleeding continues, at least 8 units of blood should be requested for the first crossmatch, and additional components—fresh frozen plasma (FFP) and possibly platelets—also should be ordered. An acute blood loss of 15% of the normal blood volume is manifested clinically by minimal tachycardia and essentially no change in blood pressure, pulse pressure, respiratory rate, or capillary blanch. In a 70-kg man, a 15% blood loss is approximately 1.5 units of blood and can be replaced with crystalloids.

A 15% to 30% blood loss (1.5 to 3 units of blood) results in tachycardia, tachypnea, and a decrease in pulse pressure. The majority of such patients require transfusion. However, they can be easily stabilized with crystalloid during the initial resuscitation. An acute blood loss of 30% to 40% of blood volume (3 to 4 units) results in a reduction in systolic blood pressure, significant tachycardia, and tachypnea. Transfusion is always required. A loss of more than 40% (over 4 units of blood) is potentially life threatening, with symptoms including marked tachycardia, significant depression of systolic blood pressure, very narrow pulse pressure, and frequently unobtainable auscultatory diastolic pressure. The skin is cold and pale.

Our hypothetical patient has a blood loss greater than 40% with no evidence that the bleeding has stopped. Eight units of packed cells should be ordered immediately and the transfusion begun as soon as the blood is available. Crystalloids should be infused rapidly in the interim period. Colloid therapy is controversial and has not proven to be more efficacious than crystalloid infusion. It is also significantly more expensive. Give 1 to 2 liters of crystalloid and, if the blood pressure rises, continue this infusion until red cells are available. If the blood pressure falls again, or fails to rise with rapid infusion of 2 liters of crystalloid, order type-specific or universal donor blood. The use of such blood is associated with a less than 1% incidence of com-

TABLE 75-2 ESTIMATED FLUID AND BLOOD REQUIREMENTS IN A 70-KG MALE*

	Initial Presentations			
	Class I	**Class II**	**Class III**	**Class IV**
Blood loss (ml)	< 750	750–1500	1500–2000	≥ 2000
Blood loss (% BV)	< 15%	15%–30%	30%–40%	≥ 40%
Pulse rate	< 100	> 100	> 120	≥ 140
Blood pressure	Normal	Normal	Decreased	Decreased
Pulse pressure (mm Hg)	Normal or increased	Decreased	Decreased	Decreased
Capillary blanch test	Normal	Positive	Positive	Positive
Respiratory rate	14–20	20–30	30–40	> 35
Urine output (ml/hr)	30 or more	20–30	5–15	Negligible
CNS—mental status	Slightly anxious	Mildy anxious	Anxious and confused	Confused and lethargic
Fluid replacement (3:1 rule)	Crystalloid	Crystalloid	Crystalloid + blood	Crystalloid + blood

(*Advanced Trauma Life Support Course, Instructor Manual.* American College of Surgeons (ACS) Committee on Trauma, 1983/1984)

* Applied blindly, these guidelines can result in excessive or inadequate fluid administration. For example, a patient with a crush injury to the extremity will have hypotension out of proportion to his or her blood loss and will require fluids in excess of the 3:1 guidelines. In contrast, a patient whose ongoing blood loss is being replaced will require less than 3:1. The use of bolus therapy with careful monitoring of the patient's response can moderate these extremes.

plications. Nevertheless, most patients in the ICU can be stabilized long enough to wait for fully crossmatched blood.

If stabilization is not easily achieved and more than 10 to 12 units of blood probably will be required because of continued bleeding, order FFP and platelets. It takes 30 to 45 minutes to thaw, prepare, and deliver FFP, and 1 to 3 hours may be needed to obtain platelets. Accordingly, early anticipation of the patient's needs prevents significant delays in treating a coagulopathy that results from platelet and other clotting factor deficits. Platelets should be ordered earlier if any antiplatelet drugs have been ingested (*e.g.*, aspirin, ibuprofen). At least 2 units of FFP and 10 mg of subcutaneous vitamin K should be administered if warfarin has been taken recently.

Hypothermia may have a significant negative effect on the success of resuscitation. With a volume deficit of 40%, the skin is cool (near room temperature) because of vasoconstriction. With rehydration, warmer core blood flows through the periphery and is rapidly cooled, effectively reducing the core temperature. Platelets have a marked, but reversible, functional impairment as a result of hypothermia. In addition, the complex chemical reactions of the clotting mechanism are temperature dependent. Thus, hypothermia may inhibit hemostasis. All fluids should be warmed to 37° C and efforts made to maintain body temperature from the outset. The most practical means of raising body temperature include increasing the room temperature, using blood warmers for all intravenous solutions, and applying a hyperthermia blanket. However, these measures are very inefficient in warming a cold patient, serving only to help maintain the current temperature.

SUBACUTE BLOOD VOLUME DEFICIENCY

CASE HISTORY

You have been asked to evaluate a 45-year-old man scheduled for drainage of a pelvic abscess. Two weeks earlier he underwent emergency sigmoid colon resection and colostomy for perforated diverticulitis and initially did well. On day 5 he began eating, but he developed nausea and vomiting 2 days later. On day 9, parenteral nutrition was initiated. A computed tomography (CT) scan reveals a small pelvic abscess. The patient has no history of cardiac, renal, or pulmonary disease. He feels well, has had several loose bowel movements, has taken some oral fluids, and has a temperature of 37.5° C. Examination suggests that he is well-hydrated, has clear lungs, a nontender abdomen, and slight peripheral edema. His hematocrit is 34%, white blood count is 10,000, and serum albumin is 3.6 g/dl; the rest of his laboratory studies are normal. You determine that this man is a good operative risk, needs no preoperative ICU evaluation, and wonder why you were asked to see him, given that antibiotics have already been started.

At 3 a.m., the patient is transferred on an emergency basis to the ICU with a temperature of 39.5° C and a blood pressure of 70 mm Hg by palpation.

You rule out bleeding and cardiogenic shock, and do all the appropriate things to treat sepsis. The patient responds, and by 7 a.m. he is alert and hemodynamically stable, with a normal urine output, cardiac output, and pulmonary artery occlusion pressure. To your astonishment his hematocrit is now 23%, and his albumin is 2.8 g/dl. Where did all that blood go?

DISCUSSION

Blood volume deficiency (see algorithm in Table 75-3) in the hospitalized and chronically ill patient results from poor nutrition, GI losses, fever or inadequate volume replacement, and chronic vasoconstriction. Routine, frequent phlebotomy to obtain blood for diagnostic tests reduces blood volume significantly. The deficit can be as much as 20% to 40% of normal blood volume. Routine clinical assessment, including heart rate, systolic and diastolic pressure, respiratory rate, hematocrit, and urine output are generally near normal. The diagnosis of blood volume deficit can be assessed more accurately using ^{51}Cr-labeled red cells, but this test is not readily available.

The deficit should be suspected in any chronically ill hospitalized patient. Accordingly, you must have a high index of suspicion and assume a preexisting deficit, especially when relatively small hemorrhagic events or stress cause greater than expected changes in physiological parameters. Crystalloid infusions increase urine output but do not expand blood volume. Indirect confirmation of this syndrome occurs when infusion of 1 to 2 units of packed red blood cells fails to increase the hematocrit. Presumably, the red cells

TABLE 75-3 ALGORITHM FOR SUBACUTE BLOOD VOLUME DEFICIENCY

1. Chronic blood volume deficiency is common in hospitalized, chronically ill patients.
2. The deficit is difficult to diagnose; it can be 20% to 30% or more of the normal blood volume.
3. Heart rate, systolic and diastolic blood pressure, respiratory rate, hematocrit, albumin, urine output, central venous pressure, occlusive pressure, and cardiac output can be near normal.
4. The diagnosis can be made by measuring blood volume using ^{51}Cr-labeled red cells, a test often not readily available. High index of suspicion must prevail.
5. Subacute deficiencies are almost routine in patients with mild chronic sepsis, prolonged bowel preparations, intestinal fistulae, long-term total parenteral nutrition, advanced cancer, prolonged ICU stays, and poor nutrition.
6. Patients with marked subacute deficiencies tolerate anesthesia, hemorrhage, and stress poorly.
7. The most effective treatment is replacement with packed red cells; such therapy is controversial.
8. Treatment with crystalloid or colloid increases urine output without increasing blood volume.
9. Assume a subacute deficiency is present if a relatively small stress or hemorrhage causes a greater than expected physiological derangement.
10. Be prepared to transfuse packed cells early in patients undergoing second operations or those who are in the ICU for prolonged periods.

expand the peripheral circulation and recruit plasma proportionately, resulting in an unchanged hematocrit. Clinicians often are reluctant to transfuse patients with hematocrits over 30%. This is a rational decision, provided that the plasma volume is normal. However, if a *total* volume deficit of 30% is present, restoration of the *plasma* volume yields a hematocrit of only 21%. (Total blood volume equals 75 ml/kg × 70 kg or 5250 ml. A 30% deficit, or 5250 ml × 70% of normal, yields a 3675-ml blood volume. If the measured hematocrit is 30%, the red cell mass is 1100 ml. When blood volume is expanded to normal, the new hematocrit is 1100/5250 × 100 = 21%.) Few would argue against transfusion when the "true" hematocrit is 21%.

Be sure to anticipate the need to transfuse packed cells early in patients undergoing secondary operations or those requiring prolonged stays in the ICU. For the syndrome described, therapy continues to be controversial. No prospective studies demonstrate the efficacy of restoring red cell mass and plasma volume to normal in critically ill patients. Disease transmission through blood products has reduced the enthusiasm for transfusion. Prospective studies are now in progress to determine if these large, subacute deficiencies require treatment. Until the risk of transfusion is proven to be justified in these relatively asymptomatic patients, you should realize that 20% to 40% blood volume deficits may exist and be prepared to transfuse immediately if patients become symptomatic.

CHRONIC ANEMIA

This problem is not of major concern in the ICU. An algorithm for its evaluation and treatment is summarized in Table 75-4.

TABLE 75-4 ALGORITHM FOR CHRONIC ANEMIA

1. In an asymptomatic patient with no major stress, no treatment is indicated until the cause is determined. Determine iron, iron binding capacity, B_{12}, folate, red cell indices, Coombs' test, and reticulocyte count. A thorough history and physical examination, including stool guaiac, often reveal the cause.
2. Young, previously healthy patients can tolerate a stable hematocrit of 20% following an acute hemorrhagic event.
3. If further stress is anticipated in an asymptomatic anemic patient (e.g., rebleed, second operation, sepsis), give oral iron.
4. If further stress is anticipated, transfuse to a hematocrit of 30% prior to surgery.
5. Patients with chronic renal failure tolerate hematocrits of 18% to 22% well and do not require transfusion prior to surgery. Patients who have received 2 to 3 units of packed red cells depleted of 2,3-DPG for an acute hemorrhagic event may no longer have an elevated P_{50}. They may require higher hematocrit during and immediately following the acute hemorrhagic event for adequate oxygen transport.
6. Patients with severe coronary artery disease may need a hematocrit of 35% to control angina.
7. Patients with severe chronic lung disease often have hematocrits above 50% and often need hematocrits above 40% to wean from ventilator support.

For more information, please see Chapter 130 in Civetta JM, Taylor RW, Kirby RR: Critical Care. *Philadelphia: J. B. Lippincott, 1988*

BIBLIOGRAPHY

Counts RB, Haisch C, Simon TL, et al: Hemostasis in massively transfused trauma patients. *Ann Surg* 1979; 190:190

Gould SA, Rice CL, Moss GS: The physiologic basis of the use of the blood and blood products. *Surg Annu* 1984; 16:13

Isbister JP: Haemotherapy for acute haemorrhage. *Anaesth Intens Care* 1984; 12:217

Schwab CW, Shayne JP, Turner J: Immediate trauma resuscitation with Type O uncrossmatched blood: A two year prospective experience. *J Trauma* 1986; 26:897

Valeri CR, Altshule MD: *Hypovolemic Anemia of Trauma: The Missing Blood Syndrome.* Boca Raton, CRC Press, 1981

76
Oncologic Emergencies

CANCER HYPERCALCEMIA

Serum calcium levels above 13 mg/dl or a clinical picture consistent with hypercalcemia, regardless of the serum calcium concentration, warrant urgent intervention.

CLINICAL PRESENTATION

Hypercalcemic crisis presents with nausea, vomiting, abdominal pain, lethargy, dehydration, and renal failure. Contraction alkalosis with progressive dehydration may lead to further renal impairment, and frank renal failure is seen, especially in the patient with underlying multiple myeloma. Three quarters of patients complain of weakness and have demonstrable sensory deficits. Most patients have bladder or bowel dysfunction.

THERAPY

The only effective long-term means of reversing malignancy-associated hypercalcemia is tumor ablation or a reduction in the tumor burden. Restoration of intravascular volume in patients who are dehydrated usually increases urinary calcium excretion by 100 to 300 mg/day. A urine output of 1.5 to 2 ml/kg/min is sought. Calciuresis is enhanced by a provoked natriuresis with furosemide, a loop diuretic.

Calcitonin decreases plasma calcium levels by inhibiting bone resorption. Eight MRC units/kg IV or IM every 6 hours usually produces a partial and mild response in lowering calcium level. Single administration usually does not result in normal levels. Plicamycin, an osteoclast cytotoxic agent in dosages of 25 μg/kg IV over 4 to 6 hours, can be expected to lower serum calcium levels in 6 to 12 hours after injection, and certainly by 48 hours. The effect usually lasts 4 to 6 days. Plicamycin may be associated with thrombocytopenia; mild, usually reversible, hepatic dysfunction, hemorrhagic diathesis; and nephrotoxicity. Plicamycin should be used with calcitonin for life-threatening hypercalcemia because calcitonin, although less effective, has a much more rapid onset of action.

Intravenous phosphates uniformly and promptly lower calcium levels in a dose-dependent manner. This route of administration is extremely toxic and is associated with extra-skeletal calcification of the lung, kidney, or both. Administered at a daily dose of 200 mg/m^2 for 5 days, gallium nitrate lowers serum calcium levels to normal limits in approximately 85% of all cancer patients. It appears to be well tolerated. Ethanehydroxydiphosphonate and dichloromethylene diphosphonate administered parenterally may prove efficacious in acute cancer hypercalcemia. Despite their frequent clinical use, there are no data supporting the use of corticosteroids or prostaglandin inhibitors such as indomethacin for acute hypercalcemia.

Dexamethasone, 100 mg IV followed by 24 mg IV every 6 hours for 72 hours and then tapered over 2 weeks, offers substantial amelioration of pain, often within hours in the majority of patients. Consultation for external beam radiation therapy to the involved area should be obtained immediately. Surgery should not be considered in the patient who presents with paraplegia because the outlook for neurologic recovery is dismal. When diagnosis is in doubt, the nature of the tumor is unknown, or a bone protrusion causes the block, surgery is indicated. Relapse when no further radiation can be administered, and progression of symptoms despite radiation, are indications for surgery.

ACUTE TUMOR LYSIS SYNDROME

CLINICAL MANAGEMENT

Patients with bulky abdominal tumors, markedly elevated plasma lactic dehydrogenase levels, evidence of renal dysfunction, or metabolic alterations require careful monitoring and renal prophylaxis during the induction of antineoplastic therapy to prevent ARF.

The mainstay in prophylaxis is vigorous hydration. If diuresis cannot be achieved by saline alone, an infusion of dopamine, 1.5 μg/kg/min, is useful in initiating and maintaining urine flow. If this is unsuccessful, patients may be given either an intravenous bolus of furosemide, 80–120 mg, or mannitol, 12.5 g of a 25% solution. Diuresis can be maintained by continuous infusion of furosemide, 3 to 5 mg/kg/day, or mannitol, 5 g/hr. Allopurinol, 10 mg/kg PO or IV, is given to control hyperuricemia. While the patient remains hyperuricemic, the urine *p*H can be maintained at or above 7 with IV sodium bicarbonate. Acetazolamide, 250 mg to 500 mg IV, alkalinizes the urine without bicarbonate administration. The potassium, phosphorus, calcium, uric acid, magnesium, arterial *p*H, creatinine, and blood urea nitrogen (BUN) levels should be measured at least once daily. Serum electrolytes should be measured twice daily.

Calcium is not administered unless there is a positive Chvostek's or Trousseau's sign, other sign of impending tetany, or significant electrocardiographic (EKG) abnormalities. Hyperphosphatemia should be anticipated and phosphate-binding antacids started prior to therapy. Hypertonic glucose and insulin administered intravenously or the initiation of total parenteral nutrition may help control hyperphosphatemia and hyperkalemia. Dialysis should be initiated if oliguria develops or there is significant hyperkalemia or other electrolyte imbalance.

OBSTRUCTIVE SYNDROMES

ACUTE AIRWAY OBSTRUCTION

Extrathoracic Upper Airway and Intrathoracic Tracheal Obstruction

Obstruction due to a bulky oropharyngeal tumor is best managed with elective tracheotomy because trauma or hemorrhage associated with oral or nasotracheal intubation may create complete obstruction in an already compromised patient. If the obstruction is due to an external compression of the trachea by lymphoma or other tissue highly sensitive to radiation or chemotherapy, then nasal or orotracheal intubation may be performed to maintain airway patency until the tumor mass shrinks.

Intrathoracic Obstruction

Lymphomas may cause compression of the airway. These tumors are extremely sensitive to radiation and chemotherapy and may regress rapidly, regardless of initial size. All attempts to adequately oxygenate and ventilate these patients are thus warranted. Intrathoracic obstruction is suspected when a patient complains of dyspnea, wheezing, and chest discomfort. Examination may reveal tachycardia, tachypnea, and occasionally a significant pulsus paradox.

TOXICITY OF ANTINEOPLASTIC THERAPY

Respiratory failure may present as an acute hypersensitivity reaction, chronic insidious pulmonary fibrosis, and occasionally, although rarely, as noncardiogenic pulmonary edema. Patients with a history of bleomycin therapy and respiratory failure should be managed with as low an F_{IO_2} as clinically possible.

Cardiac toxicity is seen with anthracycline antibiotics such as adriamycin. Chronic administration may be associated with subclinical ventricular dysfunction or overt congestive heart failure. Acute toxicities of anthracyclines can present with EKG abnormalities, myocarditis-pericarditis, or transient deterioration of left ventricular function. Cyclophosphamide is ordinarily lethal at doses above 50 to 100 mg/kg, although this amount is routinely administered as preparation for bone marrow transplantation. Invasive monitoring to optimize hemodynamic function is usually required, and continuous arteriovenous hemofiltration is necessary to manage congestive heart failure should it occur.

For more information, please see Chapter 133 in Civetta JM, Taylor RW, Kirby RR: Critical Care. *Philadelphia: J. B. Lippincott, 1988*

BIBLIOGRAPHY

Ahman F: A reassessment of the clinical implications of the superior vena caval syndrome. *J Clin Oncol* 1984; 2:8

Bajorunas D: Disorders of endocrine function in the critically ill cancer patient. In Howland WS, Carlon GC (eds): *Critical Care of the Cancer Patient,* pp 143–149. Chicago, Year Book Medical Publishers, 1985

Gilbert RW, Kim JH, Posner JB: Epidural spinal cord compression from metastatic tumor: Diagnosis and treatment. *Ann Neurol* 1978; 3:40

Goldiner PL, Carlon GC, Cvitkovic E, et al: Factors influencing post-operative morbidity and mortality in patients treated with bleomycin. *Br Med J* 1978; 1:1664

Goldiner PL: Airway problems in head and neck cancer. In Howland WS, Carlon GC (eds): *Critical Care of the Cancer Patient,* pp 35–38. Chicago, Year Book Medical Publishers, 1985

Gottdiener JS, Applebaum FR, Ferrans VJ, et al: Cardiotoxicity associated with high dose cyclophosphamide therapy. *Arch Intern Med* 1981; 141:758

Greenberg HS, Kim JH, Posner JB: Epidural spinal cord compression from metastatic tumor: Results with a new treatment protocol. *Ann Neurol* 1980; 8:361

Nealon N: Neurologic complications in the cancer patient. In Howland WS, Carlon GC (eds): *Critical Care of the Cancer Patient,* pp 31–32. Chicago, Year Book Medical Publishers, 1985

Rodichok L, Harper GR, Ruckdeschel JC, et al: Early diagnosis of spinal epidural metastasis. *Am J Med* 1981; 70:1181

Siegel T, Siegal T, Robin G, et al: Anterior decompression of the spine for metastatic epidural compression: A promising avenue of therapy? *Ann Neurol* 1982; 11:28

Turnbull A (ed): *Surgical Emergencies in Oncology.* Chicago, Year Book Medical Publishers, 1987

Turnbull AD, Carlon G: Airway management in the thrombocytopenic cancer patient with acute respiratory failure. *Crit Care Med* 1979; 7:76

XII. Skin and Muscle Disorders

77
Common ICU Skin Disorders

DRUG ERUPTIONS

MORBILLIFORM

Typical morbilliform eruptions occur within the first 7 days of initiation of therapy, although they may occur up to 28 days (ampicillin). The eruptions are maculopapular, and initially they occur on the trunk or in dependent areas, especially in ICU patients. The erythematous macules and papules are usually symmetrical and tend to become confluent.

Make a list of the patient's medications and temporally relate them to the onset of the rash. If necessary, continue a drug in the face of a morbilliform eruption without fear of precipitating an anaphylactic episode. In some instances, the eruption will fade with continued therapy. Pruritus, usually the only complication, can be treated with topical antipruritics: For cutaneous therapy, use open wet dressings, total body if applicable, followed by a mild steroid ointment, either hydrocortisone or a nonfluorinated steroid.

URTICARIAL

Urticarial eruptions may occur within minutes of administration of the drug as part of an anaphylactic reaction. Treatment consists of identifying and discontinuing the offending medication. Oral antihistamines of the H_1 type are the mainstay of therapy. Combinations consisting of two or three H_1 antihistamines can be used in the more difficult cases. Doxepin hydrochloride (Sinequan) is used in difficult cases. Severe urticarial reactions associated with wheezing, laryngeal edema, and circulatory collapse may require subcutaneous epinephrine, tracheal intubation, and systemic corticosteroids.

BULLOUS

Bromides, iodides, mercury, arsenic, salicylates, phenolphthalein, minoxidil, and penicillamine are associated with generalized bullous reactions. Therapy consists of discontinuing the causative agent and using supportive skin care.

ERYTHEMA MULTIFORME

Clinically, erythema multiforme (EM) erupts with a sudden onset of erythematous macules and papules. The center may progress to a vesiculobullous lesion with a dusky hue. When surrounded by a paler edematous ring with peripheral erythema, it completes the so-called target. The eruption is symmetrical with a predilection for the dorsal aspect of the hands and feet, palms and soles, and extensor extremities. Sulfonamides, hydantoins, barbiturates, penicillins, and phenolphthalein are the most common drug offenders. Herpes simplex virus and *Mycoplasma pneumoniae* are the most common infections.

Laboratory tests are not diagnostic; a confirmatory diagnosis can be made with a skin biopsy. Removal of the offending drug usually brings about recovery. Oral mucous membrane involvement may be treated with mild mouthwashes. Milder topical steroids are beneficial for pruritus. Oral corticosteroids are unwarranted in uncomplicated EM.

PURPURA

SENILE

Perhaps the most common type of purpura seen in an ICU is senile purpura, occurring in 14% of elderly patients. There is no specific therapy. However, if the skin becomes too fragile and tears, an antibiotic ointment should be applied to prevent secondary infection. Corticosteroids, either topical or oral, appear to compound the situation.

DRUG-INDUCED

Some medications (*e.g.*, aspirin) impair platelet function, whereas others cause vasculitis. Any new medication should be discontinued and a comparable medication of different chemical structure administered.

VASCULITIC

Leukocytoclastic vasculitis (LCV), generally presents as palpable purpura of the lower extremities, occasionally with edema. The morphologically round purpuric papules form the so-called vasculitic pattern of purpura. This is an extremely important clinical finding. Opposed to this is the infarctive pattern.

The finding of palpable purpura implies a vasculitis until proven otherwise. A skin biopsy confirms the diagnosis, and the laboratory tests listed in Table 77-1 should be obtained. There are four main etiologies of LCV—infections, especially streptococcal and viral influenza, medications, foreign proteins, and systemic disease, (*e.g.*, collagen vascular diseases and malignancies).

TABLE 77-1 LABORATORY WORK-UP FOR LEUKOCYTOCLASTIC VASCULITIS

Skin biopsy
Urinalysis
Antistreptolysin O titer
Antinuclear antibody, rheumatoid factor
Sedimentation rate
Complete blood count
Chest radiograph
Hematest stool
Hepatitis-associated antigen
Cryoglobulins
Total complement
Throat culture, if indicated

If the patient is asymptomatic and the blood test results are normal, no therapy is indicated. Antihistamines to decrease vascular permeability and aspirin for its anti-inflammatory and antichemotactic activity may be used. If the kidneys are involved, oral corticosteroids are indicated. If the patient's condition deteriorates, cyclophosphamide (2 mg/kg/day) should be used.

INFARCTIVE

Four basic pathophysiologic mechanisms are involved in infarctive lesions (Table 77-2). Blood work, cultures, and skin biopsy are usually required immediately. Treatment varies with the underlying disease.

COUMARIN NECROSIS

Coumarin necrosis is a well-defined entity. Classically, between day 3 and day 10 of coumarin loading the symptoms begin. A sudden onset of pain is followed by purpura, bulla formation, and necrosis. The usual sites are those with significant areas of subcutaneous adipose tissue, such as the breasts, buttocks, abdomen, or thighs. The lesions do not progress with continued use of the medication.

TABLE 77-2 PATHOGENESIS OF INFARCTIVE PATTERN OF HEMORRHAGE

Hypoperfusion—cardiac failure
Vasospasm—medications, Raynaud's disease, cold injury, livedo vasculitis
Embolic—septic, cholesterol, cryoglobulins, disseminated intravascular coagulation, hemoglobinopathies
Inflammation surrounding the vessel—polyarteritis nodosa, Wegener's granulomatosis, allergic granulomatosis

HEPARIN NECROSIS

Skin necrosis secondary to heparin usually occurs at the injection site, but has been documented at distant locations. Obese, middle-aged, diabetic women are particularly vulnerable.

The diagnosis is suggested by skin biopsy. It is extremely important to obtain a platelet count in these patients. Heparin can induce the development of a platelet aggregating factor. Skin necrosis can then be a harbinger of a dangerous triad consisting of skin necrosis, thrombocytopenia, and myocardial infarciton.

SPECIFIC DISEASE ENTITIES

ACQUIRED IMMUNE DEFICIENCY SYNDROME (AIDS)

Various skin findings have been reported in AIDS (Table 77-3). The "bottom line" in these immunocompromised patients is that any skin eruption may appear atypical. It is essential then that any suspicious lesion be biopsied. Moreover, any infectious agent should also be cultured and aggressively treated because of its ability to rapidly disseminate.

CONTACT DERMATITIS

A very common consultation to the ICU is a request to rule out contact dermatitis. First, obtain a history for any substance applied to the skin. This includes topical medications, cleansing agents, and even tape. Then examine the patient.

Clinically, vesicles on an erythematous base, in a linear arrangement, are the hallmark of contact dermatitis. The physician should also look for sharply

TABLE 77-3 CUTANEOUS SKIN FINDINGS ASSOCIATED WITH AIDS

Kaposi's sarcoma
Thrombocytopenic purpura
Seborrheic dermatitis
Viral disease—molluscum contagiosum, herpes simplex, herpes zoster, verruca vulgaris, condyloma acuminatum
Oral candidiasis
White, hairy oral leukoplakia
Evanescent maculopapular eruption
Eosinophilic pustular folliculitis
Chronic acne-like follicular inflammation (often in the axilla)
Impetigo in neck and beard area
Dermatophyte infections
Acquired keratoderma of soles
Acquired icthyosis

angulated arrangements and right angles in an eruption. These signal an "outside contact" as opposed to a systemic finding. The eruption is localized to the area of the contact. Treatment consists of discontinuing the topical medication or irritant and finding an alternative. Open wet dressings followed by a topical steroid ointment are indicated. Antihistamines titrated to eliminate pruritus may also be necessary, especially at night. Oral corticosteroids are indicated in acute contact dermatitis if the reaction is widespread. Use a 3-week tapering course of prednisone and prescribe 60 mg orally for 1 week, then 40 mg orally the second week, followed by 20 mg daily the final week, in an average-sized individual.

For more information, please see Chapter 136 in Civetta JM, Taylor RW, Kirby RR: Critical Care. *Philadelphia: J. B. Lippincott, 1988*

BIBLIOGRAPHY

Adam RM. Fischer AA: Contact allergen alternatives: 1986. *J Am Acad Dermatol* 1986; 14:951

Braverman IM: *Skin Signs of Systemic Disease,* 2nd ed, p 378. Philadelphia, WB Saunders, 1981

Grossman ME, Silvers DN, Walther RR, et al: Cutaneous manifestations of disseminated candidiasis. *J Am Acad Dermatol* 1980; 2:111

Levine LE, Bernstein JE, Soltani K, et al: Heparin-induced cutaneous necrosis unrelated to injection sites. *Arch Dermatol* 1983; 119:400

Murray JC: Miscellaneous blistering diseases. *Dermatol Clin* April 1983; 1(2):318

Sams WM: Necrotizing vasculitis. *J Am Acad Dermatol* 1980; 3:1

Tan PL, Barnett BS, Flowers FP, et al: Current topical corticosteroid preparations. *J Am Acad Dermatol* 1986; 14:79

Tonnesen MG, Soter NA: Erythema multiforme. *J Am Acad Dermatol* 1979; 1:357

Wintroub BU, Stern R: Cutaneous drug reactions: Pathogenesis and clinical classification. *J Am Acad Dermatol* 1985; 13:167

78 Life-Threatening Dermatologic Conditions

ERYTHEMA MULTIFORME

Erythema multiforme (EM) is a cutaneous or multisystem hypersensitivity reaction pattern to an etiologic factor. The reaction is self-limited and benign in most patients; it usually resolves spontaneously within a 2-week period. Patients with severe forms may require intensive inpatient care, and death from septicemia or pneumonia is possible. Stevens–Johnson syndrome is a severe form of EM with marked oral mucosal and ocular involvement. These patients may develop extensive epidermal necrosis with large denuded areas simulating toxic epidermal necrolysis. Drugs and infections are the most common etiologies of EM (Table 78-1).

Therapy is mainly supportive because the condition generally is self-limited and mild. Some dermatologists use systemic corticosteroid therapy in severely ill patients because it may cause a dramatic resolution of the patient's symptoms. However, the frequency of complications and patient morbidity may be increased. Oral prednisone or its intravenous equivalent is given in an initial adult dose of 60 to 100 mg/day and a pediatric dose of 30 to 60 mg/day. Once the skin lesions begin to involute, this dosage should be tapered gradually. Cessation of therapy after a total course of approximately 2 to 3 weeks is recommended.

TOXIC EPIDERMAL NECROLYSIS

Toxic epidermal necrolysis is manifested by a severe vesiculobullous cutaneous reaction to an etiologic agent (Table 78-2), most commonly a drug, followed by infection and preexisting multisystem illness. The prodrome is sudden with fever, malaise, skin tenderness, and prostration, followed by focal or confluent erythema, urticarial plaques, papules, or vesiculobullous lesions. The skin findings rapidly evolve toward extensive epidermal necrosis with a positive Nikolsky's sign (lateral shearing pressure on normal-appearing skin adjacent to a vesiculobullous lesion rubs off the epidermis leaving a moist erosion).

TABLE 78-1 CAUSATIVE AGENTS OF ERYTHEMA MULTIFORME

Medications
Sulfa preparations
Phenytoin
Penicillin
Barbiturates
Tetracycline
Infections
Herpes simplex labialis
Hepatitis B
Mycoplasma pneumonia
Influenza
Streptococcal pharyngitis
Histoplasmosis
Vaccinations/immunizations
Multisystem diseases
Collagen–vascular
Physical agents
Sunlight
Radiotherapy of tumors

A rotating bed frame is helpful in providing access to all affected skin areas. Topical wet dressings with Burow's solution or weak silver nitrate preparations (0.25–0.5%) reduce the accumulation of crusts and also act as a local antiseptic.

Silver sulfadiazine (Silvadene) cream provides a soothing cover that counteracts the colonization of bacteria on the open skin. If a sulfa drug is sus-

TABLE 78-2 TOXIC EPIDERMAL NECROLYSIS—ETIOLOGY

Drugs
Sulfonamides
Phenylbutazone barbiturates
Phenytoin
Penicillin derviatives
Infections
Viral
Immunizations
Polio
Diphtheria
Tetanus
Preexisting diseases
Collagen–vascular
Graft-versus-host disease
Stevens–Johnson syndrome
Neoplasia (lymphoma)
Physical agents
Radiotherapy of tumors

pected as the etiologic factor do not use silver sulfadiazine or silver nitrate because either one may cross-react. Periodic examination of the denuded areas with a Wood's lamp may provide early evidence of pseudomonas infections.

Corticosteroid therapy can be given at an early stage before extensive epidermal necrosis occurs. At an advanced stage, such therapy appears to be associated with increased morbidity and mortality. The drugs are usually administered intravenously. Use a prednisone equivalency level of 80 to 160 mg/day depending on severity. Plasmapheresis has been used successfully in a limited number of patients.

STAPHYLOCOCCAL SCALDED SKIN SYNDROME

The staphylococcal scalded skin syndrome is a self-limited disease whose clinical manifestations are caused by an epidermolytic exotoxin most commonly produced by a nasopharyngeal source of *Staphylococcus aureus* group 2, phage types 3A, 3B, 3C, 55, and 71. The disease runs a self-limited course of 10 to 14 days. The epidermal necrosis is superficial and, therefore, usually no serious problems occur with fluid–electrolyte losses or superimposed bacterial infections. Most patients are treated with topical astringent soaks (Burow's solution). They should be treated with penicillin derivatives or erythromycin. Corticosteroids are not indicated.

GENERALIZED PUSTULAR PSORIASIS (VON ZUMBUSCH)

The abrupt onset of fever and prostration precedes or accompanies a peculiar generalized eruption. The primary skin lesions are pustules, which arise on erythematous skin or psoriaform plaques. Chills and leukocytosis are common. The majority of cases are classified as idiopathic (Table 78-3).

The therapy for generalized pustular psoriasis includes supportive measures as well as specific measures to correct fluid and electrolyte disturbances and treat superimposed bacterial infections. Long-term psoralen and long-wave ultraviolet light photochemotherapy have been effective in some patients. The oral administration of synthetic retinoids, etretinate (0.5 mg/kg/day–1.0 mg/kg/day) and isotretinoin (1.5 mg/kg/day–2.0 mg/kg/day), has provided an alternative to methotrexate or systemic corticosteroids in the management of severe cases.

ERYTHRODERMA

The most common cause of erythroderma is the exacerbation of a preexisting dermatologic disease. Other causes are listed in Table 78-4. The patient may suffer from fever, skin tenderness, and paroxysmal shivering. Patches of ery-

TABLE 78-3 CAUSES OF GENERALIZED PUSTULAR PSORIASIS

Systemic corticosteroid therapy and its subsequent withdrawal
Other medications
  Sulfa drugs
  Penicillin
  Cough medicine
  Salicylates
  Potassium iodide
Infections
  Bacterial—skin infections, dental abcesses
  Viral—upper respiratory infections
Pregnancy
  Impetigo herpetiformis?
Postsurgical hypoparathyroidism
Idiopathic
  No preexisting psoriasis or identifiable extraneous precipitating factor

thema become confluent and cutaneous edema becomes a prominent clinical feature. Pruritus may be intense, especially if the underlying process is an eczematous or lymphoproliferative disorder. Excoriations may lead to erosions with secondary impetiginization, lichenification, and hyperpigmentation. A "leathery" skin appearance, generalized hair loss, and loss of nails are commonly seen in the patient with chronic erythroderma.

There is no universally effective therapy for erythroderma. Psoralen and long-wave ultraviolet photochemotherapy and tar–ultraviolet light therapy have been helpful in patients with underlying psoriasis or eczema.

TABLE 78-4 CAUSES OF ERYTHRODERMA AND EXFOLIATIVE DERMATITIS

Exacerbation of preexisting dermatologic disease
  Dermatophyte infections
  Eczema
  Lichen planus
  Pemphigus foliaceous
  Pityriasis rubra pilaris
  Psoriasis
  Scabies
Malignancies
  Leukemia
  Lymphoma
Contact dermatitis
Drugs
  Barbiturates
  Gold
  Penicillin
  Sulfonamides
Idiopathic
  No preexisting disease or identifiable precipitating factor

Systemic corticosteroids are reserved for patients with a rapidly deteriorating physiologic status. Once corticosteroids are discontinued, the erythroderma usually recurs. Wet compresses with saline or tap water are of value in the acute phase of erythroderma. In patients with severe exfoliation, emollient creams and ointments (Eucerin, Aquaphor, petrolatum) are beneficial.

PEMPHIGUS VULGARIS

Pemphigus is an autoimmune blistering disorder affecting the skin and mucous membranes. It is more prevalent in Jewish people and most commonly affects persons in their fourth or fifth decade of life.

The primary lesions in pemphigus are vesicles and bullae which break, leaving painful denuded areas. The diagnosis is based on the clinical picture and histologic changes showing loss of cohesiveness between keratinocytes in the stratum malpighii (acantholysis) and a "tombstone" appearance of the cells of the basal layer. Direct immunofluorescence of normal patient skin will demonstrate deposition of IgG antibodies in the intercellular space between keratinocytes.

Without corticosteroid therapy, pemphigus vulgaris is invariably fatal. The painful oral lesions result in inadequate fluid intake and nutrition. Debility combined with superimposed infections and epidermal fluid and electrolyte losses contribute to the patient's death.

A high corticosteroid dose (200–400 mg/day of prednisone orally) is used for several weeks until the disease activity decreases significantly (no new blisters or very few blisters). Prednisone dosage may then be reduced to about 40 mg/day, and an immunosuppressant is usually added (azathioprine 100 mg/day) in hopes of reducing total steroid dosage. After three weeks the corticosteroid dose is changed to an alternate day schedule of 40 mg for 1 year.

DISSEMINATED VIRAL INFECTIONS

ECZEMA HERPETICUM (KAPOSI'S VARICELLIFORM ERUPTION)

A condition first described by Kaposi in 1894, eczema herpeticum results from the inoculation of inflamed skin by herpes simplex virus. A similar pathophysiologic process was responsible for the dissemination of vaccinia virus in atopic patients (eczema vaccinatum) when smallpox vaccination was a common practice in this country. The infection is usually seen in patients with severe, eczematous atopic dermatitis and is characterized by the presence of multiple superficial crusted lesions which evolve from small umbilicated vesicles or pustules. Superimposed bacterial infection may lead to septicemia with subsequent mortality.

The Tzanck test is helpful in diagnosis and can be peformed rapidly. The base of a vesicular lesion is scraped using a #15 surgical blade, the blade is rubbed against a glass slide, the slide is air dried, and undiluted Giemsa stain (or Wright stain) is applied. After 30 seconds, the excess stain is removed with gently flowing tap water. The slide is blotted dry with filter or towel paper, and a cover slip is applied. It is examined under low and high power to locate multinuclear epidermal squamous cells (epithelial giant cells), which demonstrate abundant basophilic nuclear material. This test is also positive in varicella–zoster infections.

Acyclovir provides effective therapy. The drug should be given orally or intravenously in a weight-adjusted dosage (Table 78-5). Antibiotic therapy should be instituted for those patients with superimposed bacterial infections. Astringent soaks (Burow's) are helpful in decreasing exudation and crust formation from ruptured vesicles or pustules.

VARICELLA–ZOSTER INFECTIONS

Cough, respiratory difficulty, chest pain, or neurologic abnormalities may be clinical signs of varicella–zoster virus dissemination in a patient with antecedent dermatomal herpes zoster or chickenpox. Multiple vesicular lesions occurring away from the original dermatome of involvement are the dermatologic sign of dissemination in patients with herpes zoster. In most instances, they represent increased viral activity due to the host's immunocompromised status.

The correlation between the clinical picture and a positive Tzanck smear from an active lesion is usually diagnostic. Viral cultures provide confirmation of the initial clinical impression. Intravenous administration of acyclovir or vidarabine has been helpful in these patients (see Table 78-5).

For more information, please see Chapter 137 in Civetta JM, Taylor RW, Kirby RR: Critical Care. *Philadelphia: J. B. Lippincott, 1988*

TABLE 78-5 THERAPY FOR LIFE-THREATENING VIRAL INFECTIONS

Eczema herpeticum
- Acyclovir
  - 25 mg/kg/day orally for 5 days; give individual doses every 4 hr, 5 times/day
  - 5 mg/kg/8 hr IV for 5 days*
- Antibiotics
  - IV or orally for treatment of superimposed bacterial infections

Disseminated varicella–zoster infections with organ involvement (encephalitis or pneumonitis)
- Acyclovir
  - 10 mg/kg/day IV for 10 days*
- Vidarabine
  - 10 mg/kg/day IV for 5 days

*Infuse over at least 1 hour to prevent crystallization in renal tubules. Monitor creatinine clearance during therapeutic course.

BIBLIOGRAPHY

Baker H, Ryan TJ: Generalized pustular psoriasis: A clinical and epidemiological study of 104 cases. *Br J Dermatol* 1968; 80:771

Elias PM, Fritsch P, Epstein EH: Staphyloccocal scalded skin syndrome: Clinical features, pathogenesis and recent microbiological and biochemical developments. *Arch Dermatol* 1977; 113:207

Huff JC, Weston WL, Tonnesen MG: Erythema multiforme: A critical review of characteristics, diagnostic criteria and causes. *J Am Acad Dermatol* 1983; 8:763

Kamanabros D, Schmitz–Laudgraf W, Czarnelzki BM: Plasmapheresis in severe drug induced toxic epidermal necrolysis. *Arch Dermatol* 1985; 121:1548

Lever WF, Schaumburg–Lever G: Treatment of pemphigus vulgaris. Results obtained in 84 patients between 1961 and 1982. *Arch Dermatol* 1984; 120:44

Lyell A: A review of toxic epidermal necrolysis in Britain. *Br J Dermatol* 1967; 79:662

Shepp DH, Dandliker PS, Meyers JD: Treatment of varicella–zoster virus infection in severely immunocompromised patients. A randomized comparison of acyclovir and vidarabine. *N Engl J Med* 1986; 314:208

Shuster S: The metabolic and haemodynamic effects of skin disease. *Ann Clin Res* 3:135; 1971

Whitley R, Soong SJ, Alford CA, et al: Treatment of biopsy proven herpes simplex encephalitis: Vidarabine versus acyclovir. *Clin Res* 1985; 33:422a

79 Rhabdomyolysis

Rhabdomyolysis is a clinical and laboratory syndrome resulting from skeletal muscle injury with release of cell contents into the plasma. The causes of rhabdomyolysis are legion (Table 79-1).

DIAGNOSIS

Following massive muscle injury, the release of potassium into the free circulation can cause overwhelming hyperkalemia, and lethal dysrhythmias may ensue, especially during the first 1 to 3 days. Additionally, metabolic acidemia and decreased renal clearance of potassium are often present, both of which may exacerbate serum hyperkalemia. Hypocalcemia occurs frequently in rhabdomyolysis. Typically this is seen early in the clinical course, and at a time when measured serum proteins such as albumin are often elevated. Hypercalcemia may be seen in patients with myoglobinuria who develop acute renal failure and who are in the diuretic phase of their illness.

Hyperuricemia is usually present and is marked in those patients with postexertional rhabdomyolysis. Patients with rhabdomyolysis and acute renal failure have an anion gap metabolic acidosis. Like potassium, phosphorus leaks from injured muscle cells. Skeletal muscle breakdown also results in the release of creatine. Creatinine, in turn, is the metabolic waste product of creatine degeneration. In rhabdomyolysis, creatinine formation exceeds its filtration rate, such that measured serum creatinine levels increase out of proportion to the BUN levels. As a result, the calculated BUN/creatinine ratio is typically quite low. The measured serum CK is invariably elevated in rhabdomyolysis. Although the degree of CK elevation roughly correlates with the degree of muscle necrosis, it does not predict those patients at risk to develop pigment-induced renal failure. Generally, CK levels achieve their peak within the first 24 hours following injury. Thereafter, levels should decrease at a rate of 50% each 48 hours. If a second rise is seen in serial CK determinations, recurrent or on-going muscle injury and necrosis should be considered, and the possibility of a compartment syndrome should be investigated.

TABLE 79-1 ETIOLOGIC FACTORS IN RHABDOMYOLYSIS

Traumatic
Crush syndrome
Prolonged compression
Ischemia (embolization)
Postexertional
Seizures
Heat stroke
Malignant hyperthermia
Electric shock/burns

Nontraumatic
Metabolic disorders
- Myophosphorylase deficiency
- Phosphofructokinase deficiency
- Carnitine palmityltransferase deficiency
- Diabetic ketoacidosis
- Hyperosmolar coma
- Hypo/hyperthyroidism

Electrolyte deficiencies
- Hypokalemia
- Hypophosphatemia
- Hypomagnesemia

Inflammatory muscle disease
- Polymyositis
- Dermatomyositis
- Arteritis/vasculitis

Infection
- Hepatitis
- Influenza/coxsackie viruses
- Shigellosis
- Salmonellosis
- Gram-negative septic shock
- Legionella
- Leptospirosis
- Rocky Mountain spotted fever
- Trichinosis
- Tetanus
- Gas gangrene

Toxins
- Alcohol
- Snake/spider venom
- ϵ-aminocaproic acid
- Glutethimide
- Clofibrate
- Sedatives (i.e., prolonged compression)
- Amphotericin-B
- Amphetamines
- Carbenoxolone
- Steroids
- Glycyrrhizate (licorice)
- Carbon monoxide

In rhabdomyolysis, myoglobin is released from injured skeletal muscle and may appear in the urine when serum levels exeed 1500 to 3000 ng/ml. Myoglobin may be measured quantitatively in both the urine and serum, or it may be detected with the use of an orthotolidine dipstick method or a stool guaiac card.

THERAPY

Adequate maintenance of the circulating plasma volume is the most important aspect of treating a patient with rhabdomyolysis. Additional therapy is aimed at any contributing or underlying cause of this disorder (e.g., carbon monoxide poisoning, infection) to control such problems as hyperkalemia. Research in vitro suggests that alkalinization of a patient's urine may inhibit the process of myoglobin dissociation and liberation of toxic ferrihemate and aid in the prevention of renal failure.

The use of either loop diuretics, such as furosemide, or osmotic agents, such as mannitol, is also thought to be beneficial in preventing the renal failure of rhabdomyolysis by maintaining urine flow, and thereby decreasing tubular concentrations of hematin. A renewed elevation of CK activity should also alert the clinician to the possibility of a developing compartment syndrome. Measurement of the intracompartmental pressure can be performed using a probe and transducer. Intracompartmental pressures greater than 30 mm Hg generally require a fasciotomy to prevent neurovascular damage. The tibialis anterior, in particular, is susceptible to this complication because it is normally a tight compartment with little room for expansion.

COMPLICATIONS

Muscular swelling, and the resultant compression of intracompartmental muscles within the fascial sheath, poses a substantial risk in severe rhabdomyolysis. Fasciotomy may be required to relieve intracompartmental tension.

Life-threatening ventricular dysrhythmias can result with the severe hyperkalemia seen in rhabdomyolysis. In this setting, calcium administration may be of some benefit in limiting the dysrhythmogenic effects of hyperkalemia. The otherwise indiscriminate use of calcium may further complicate the clinical picture by potentiating muscle cell injury and worsening rhabdomyolysis.

For more information, please see Chapter 138 in Civetta JM, Taylor RW, Kirby RR: Critical Care. *Philadelphia: J. B. Lippincott, 1988*

BIBLIOGRAPHY

Cadnapaphornchai P, Taher S, McDonald FD: Acute drug-associated rhabdomyolysis: An examination of its diverse renal manifestations and complications. *Am J Med Sci* 1980; 280:66

Eneas JF, Schoenfeld PY, Humphreys MH: The effect of infusion of mannitol–sodium bicarbonate on the clinical course of myoglobinuria. *Arch Intern Med* 1979; 139:801
Gabow PA, Kaehny WD, Kelleher SP: The spectrum of rhabdomyolysis. *Medicine* 1982; 61:141
Haller RG, Knochel JP: Skeletal muscle disease in alcoholism. *Med Clin North Am* 1984; 68:91
Whiteside TE, Haney TC, Morimoto K, et al: Tissue pressure measurements as a determinant for the need of fasciotomy. *Clin Orthop* 1975; 113:43

XIII. ICU Infections

80
The Febrile Patient

IMMEDIATE CONCERNS

Fever in critically ill patients often creates a sense of urgency to find the etiology. This is understandable because most critically ill surgical patients and many medical intensive care unit (ICU) patients die of complications of sepsis. The approach to evaluating febrile episodes, however, is often difficult to justify based on existing data from the literature. Infection must always be considered as a cause for fever in critically ill patients, but a rational approach to evaluation should be used rather than rote ordering of expensive and nonspecific laboratory tests and radiographs. An exhaustive treatise on every potential cause for fever is beyond any single textbook chapter. Rather, a rational clinical approach to evaluating fever in critically ill patients is presented.

The evaluation process should be "therapy-directed" so that tests which have no major impact on clinical management are avoided early in the clinical course. An initial febrile episode should be evaluated with a careful review of the patient's history and a thorough physical examination. If this fails to identify a source, then no further procedures are necessary unless the patient is severely immunocompromised or there is a high probability of bacteremia. If a second febrile episode occurs, further testing for various infections must be considered. Figure 80-1 provides guidelines for evaluating infectious sources for fever.

If pneumonia is suspected, then sputum Gram stain should precede any cultures. Urinalysis should always precede urine culture, which should be ordered only if bacteria and more than ten white blood cells per high powered field are present on urinalysis. Venous or arterial catheter-related infection is virtually nonexistent during the first 48 hours of catheter use if the catheter is placed under the usual sterile conditions. Central venous catheters are an infrequent source for fever unless usage exceeds 72 hours. An approach to managing potential catheter-related febrile episodes is outlined in Figure 80-2. Fever in the immediate postoperative period requires careful inspection of all surgical or traumatic wounds. Gas gangrene and necrotizing fasciitis

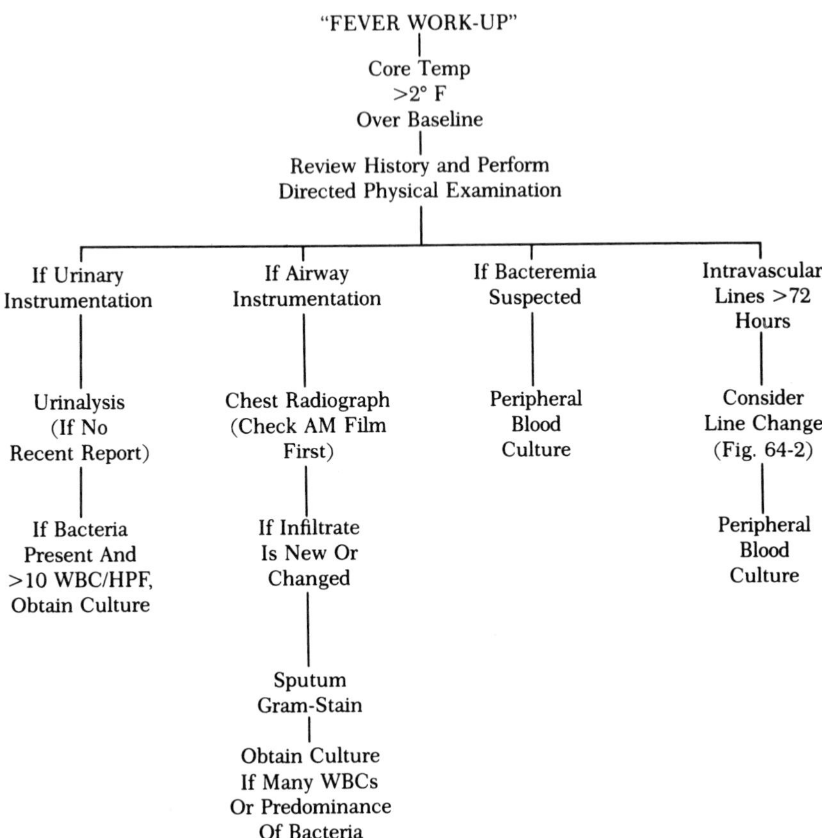

Figure 80-1 Guidelines for evaluating infectious sources of fever.

from clostridial or streptococcal organisms can occur within the first 48 hours postoperatively. Other types of infections occur later, but most can usually be diagnosed with careful inspection and palpation of the wound. Crush injury syndrome and tetanus, although infrequent, can be causes for fever in the postoperative trauma patient.

Meningitis is an infrequent cause of fever in surgical ICU patients, but must be considered in any critically ill patient who develops an altered mental status associated with high fever.

Because of limitations with conventional radiographs, ultrasound, and nuclear scans, computed tomography (CT) has become the preferred method of diagnosing intra-abdominal abscess as a possible cause for fever. However, CT scanning in critically ill patients is not as sensitive, specific, or beneficial as has been reported in general hospital populations. Scanning can

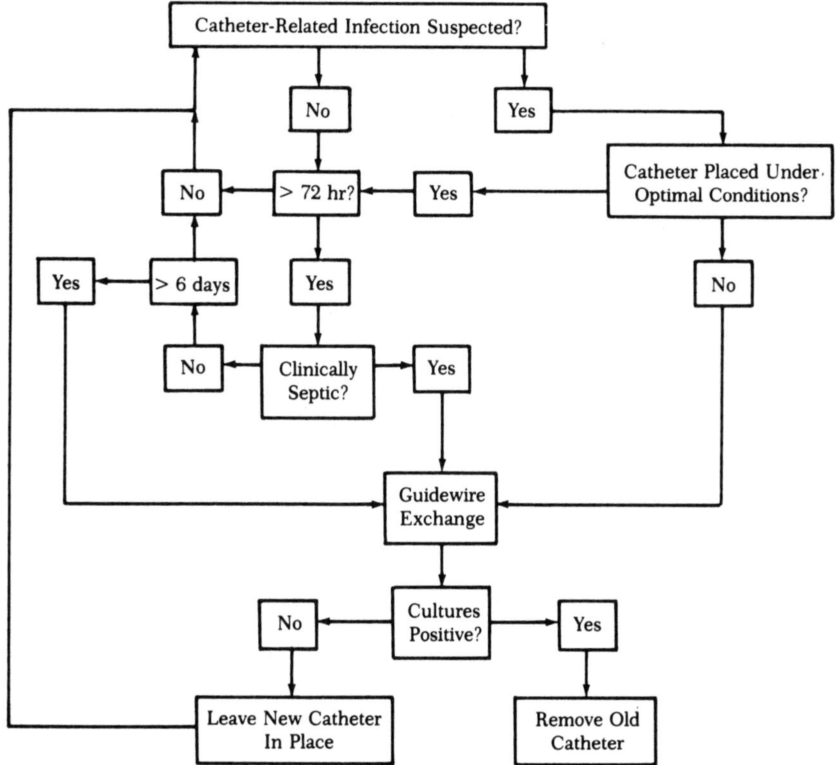

Figure 80-2 An approach to the management of potential catheter-related febrile episodes.

be helpful but should not be used as a tool to search blindly for a source of sepsis as part of a fever work-up. Abdominal reexploration may be necessary in some patients, especially those who develop unexplained single organ system failure.

Other critical etiologies for fever must be considered under certain clinical conditions. Approximately 15% of hospitalized patients experience some type of adverse drug reaction. Fever may be an isolated symptom (drug fever) or the first sign of anaphylaxis or serum sickness. Drugs which are associated with a high probability of allergic reactions should be replaced with other suitable drugs if possible.

About 90% of blood transfusion reactions are allergic or febrile. However, fever may also accompany acute hemolytic reactions, with the first manifestation being sudden diffuse oozing of blood from multiple sites. If fever develops within 20 to 30 minutes after beginning a blood product transfusion, then this potential life-threatening complication must be ruled out.

Malignant hyperthermia, which is classically observed during administration of general anesthesia, may not develop until the patient reaches the ICU. Early symptoms can be confused with thyrotoxicosis, undiagnosed pheochromocytoma, or the neuroleptic malignant syndrome.

Acute adrenocortical insufficiency is a rare cause of fever in critically ill patients. This should be considered in patients who are being weaned from high steroid dosages who suddenly develop fever and hypotension.

Adverse physiologic side-effects of fever cause major alterations in oxygen consumption which may be detrimental to critically ill patients if they are elderly or otherwise have limited ability to increase oxygen delivery. Fever should therefore be treated aggressively in these patients.

For more information, please see Chapter 64 in Civetta JM, Taylor RW, Kirby RR: Critical Care. *Philadelphia: J. B. Lippincott, 1988*

BIBLIOGRAPHY

Bernheim HA, Block LH, Atkins E: Fever: Pathogenesis, pathophysiology, and purpose. *Ann Intern Med* 1979; 91:261

Deutschman CS, Wilton P, Sinow J, et al: Paranasal sinusitis associated with nasotracheal intubation: A frequently unrecognized and treatable source of sepsis. *Crit Care Med* 1986; 14:111

Machiedo GW, Tikellia J, Suval W, et al: Reoperation for sepsis. *Am Surg* 1985; 51:149

Mandel SR, Boyd D, Jaques PF, et al: Drainage of hepatic, intra-abdominal, and mediastinal abscesses guided by computerized axial tomography. *Am J Surg* 1983; 145:120

Martin EC, Karlson KB, Fankuchen EI, et al: Percutaneous drainage of postoperative intra-abdominal abscesses. *Am J Radiol* 1982; 138:13

Martinez OV, Civetta JM, Anderson K, et al: Bacteriuria in the catheterized surgical intensive care patient—a prospective study of 100 patients. *Crit Care Med* 1986; 75:1298

Majeski JA, Alexander JW: Complications of wound infections. In Greenfield LJ (ed): *Complications in Surgery and Trauma,* p 27. Philadelphia, JB Lippincott, 1984

Rutledge R, Sheldon GF, Collins ML: Massive transfusion. *Crit Care Clin* 1986; 2:791

Shires GT, Dineen P: Sepsis following burns, trauma, and intra-abdominal infections. *Arch Intern Med* 1981; 142:2012

Stevens JJ: A case of thyrotoxic crisis that mimicked malignant hyperthermia. *Anesthesiology* 1983; 59:263

Weinberg S, Twersky RS: Neuroleptic malignant syndrome. *Anesth Analg* 1983; 62:848

81
Nosocomial Infections

Hospital-acquired infections are a major problem for physicians who treat critically ill patients and remain a major cause of death among hospitalized patients. Epidemiologic data may be misleading when applied to critically ill ICU patients. Since sources of sepsis are difficult to find and etiologies are often obscure, even the definition of nosocomial infection (*i.e.*, one that is neither present nor incubating at the time of admission to the hospital) may be difficult to apply.

Nosocomial infections in ICU patients are primarily respiratory tract or catheter-related infections; urinary tract sources are less frequent. In 20% of cases, multiple pathogens are causal. Although it is not difficult to obtain positive cultures from various sites in septic ICU patients, it is unclear whether these cultures constitute a true nosocomial infection, a fact which may be obscured in large epidemiologic studies.

Pneumonia is considered the most common fatal hospital-acquired infection. Diagnosis can be very difficult because virtually 100% of patients intubated for 48 hours or longer become colonized with gram-negative bacteria. High mortality rates may reflect inaccurate diagnoses and altered patient immune defenses rather than problems with therapy. Clinical findings of fever, leukocytosis, purulent secretions, and radiographic pulmonary infiltrates are often nonspecific in the ICU population, and diagnostic interventions that are most likely to provide a true diagnosis should be applied. For example, cultures obtained bronchoscopically using the plugged telescopic catheter (PTC) brush are considered more accurate for diagnosing nosocomial pneumonia. In most cases, antibiotic therapy is started empirically, based on a clinical suggestion of pneumonia, but broad-spectrum therapy may be reduced to more specific regimens if certain pathogens are cultured from PTC brush specimens, peripheral blood, or pleural fluid.

Although urosepsis is a common problem epidemiologically, the urinary tract is not a frequent source for systemic sepsis in critically ill ICU patients. Bacteriuria and pyuria on urinalysis should alert the physician to the possibility of urosepsis, and only then should urine cultures be obtained. Urosepsis is much more common in patients with urinary tract obstruction or instrumentation. Frequent catheter changes and routine microbiologic monitoring of the urine are not helpful.

Physical examination must also rule out nosocomial wound infections that may develop following both clean and clean-contaminated operations. Infections from gram-positive and gram-negative organisms usually present within different time frames with distinctly different clinical pictures.

Evaluating catheter-related nosocomial infections is often difficult because of the many different and important clinical questions with few specific data for answers (see Chapter 80). Catheter-related infections must be considered in terms of the interacting factors of the host, the organisms causing the infection, and the surrounding environment. "Catheter infection" is an imprecise term—clearly, inanimate objects cannot become infected. Confusion surrounding such terms has arisen from early erroneous interpretations of clinical studies. Blood cultures obtained through catheters are too sensitive and may result in the unnecessary removal of the catheter that is not really contributing to a nosocomial infection. Semiquantitative cultures of catheter segments, preferably the intracutaneous portion, should be obtained to diagnose catheter-related nosocomial infection. If more than 15 colonies of organisms are identified, the catheter should be removed. This recommendation is based on the original studies by Maki and associates, which showed a 16% incidence of peripheral bacteremia or local infection associated with such colony counts. There were no associated cases of bacteremia or local infection in that study if 15 or fewer colonies were identified by semiquantitative culture.

Current definitions and considerations indicate that replacement of an indwelling central catheter using a guidewire exchange method and semiquantitative culture of the intracutaneous segment removed is an appropriate diagnostic measure. The diagnosis of "line" sepsis therefore can be made by either obvious clinical signs of local infection (which should be an infrequent means, since such signs occur relatively late in the course of catheterization) or by positive semiquantitative culture of a removed catheter segment. It is recommended that in septic patients catheters for venous access and hemodynamic monitoring be exchanged over a guidewire after 3 days, with culture of the intracutaneous segments. In "clean" patients, the duration of catheterization may be extended to 4 days, at which time the catheter is changed over a guidewire and the intracutaneous segment and catheter tip semiquantitatively cultured. The use of a second guidewire exchange has not proven beneficial. This approach is a method of diagnosing catheter-related nosocomial infections and is not considered a form of therapy. If the catheter segment cultures are positive, then the exchanged catheter should be removed and a new catheter inserted at a different anatomic site.

Hyperalimentation catheters may be left in place indefinitely as long as the site of entry shows no obvious clinical signs of infection. If a hyperalimentation catheter is a suspected source of nosocomial infection, it should be removed over a guidewire and replaced with a new catheter through the same site. If subsequent semiquantitative cultures of the removed catheter segment are positive, then this new catheter should be removed and replaced with a new catheter at a different site.

At present there are few data concerning the use of multiple-lumen catheters and the incidence of nosocomial infection with prolonged usage. Until more data are collected, it seems prudent to treat multiple-lumen catheters in the same fashion as pulmonary artery catheters, with guidewire exchange (on the third day in septic patients and the fourth day in nonseptic patients), followed by semi-quantitative cultures of the intracutaneous segment to determine the possibility of catheter-related nosocomial infection.

Arterial catheters are an infrequent source of nosocomial infection, and can be left in place for extended periods if the entry site remains clean and free of induration or erythema.

Disposable pressure transducer systems and closed injectate systems for measuring cardiac output by thermodilution have also significantly reduced the incidence of nosocomial infections from external component system sources.

For more information, please see Chapter 65 in Civetta JM, Taylor RW, Kirby RR: Critical Care. *Philadelphia: J. B. Lippincott, 1988*

BIBLIOGRAPHY

Band JD, Maki DG: Infections caused by arterial catheters used for hemodynamic monitoring. *Am J Med* 1979; 67:735

Civetta JM, Hudson-Civetta JA: Cost effective use of the ICU. In Eisman B (ed): *Cost Effectiveness in Surgery.* Philadelphia, WB Saunders 1987; 3:13

Crouch TW, Higuchi JH, Coalson JJ, et al: Pathogenesis and prevention of nosocomial pneumonia in a non-human primate model of acute respiratory failure. *Am Rev Respir Dis* 1984; 130:502

Johanson WG, Pierce AK, Sanford JP, et al: Nosocomial respiratory infections with gram-negative bacilli. *Ann Intern Med* 1972; 77:701

Lushkin RL, Weinstein RA, Nathan C, et al: Extended use of disposable pressure transducers: A bacteriologic evaluation. *JAMA* 1986; 255:916

McGowan JE: Changing etiology of nosocomial bacteremia and fungemia and other hospital-acquired infections. *Rev Infect Dis* 1985; 7(suppl 3):357

Maki DG, Weis CE, Sarafin HW: A semiquantitative culture method for identifying intravenous cather-related infections. *N Engl J Med* 1977; 296:1305

Martinez OV, Civetta JM, Anderson K, et al: Bacteriuria in the catheterized surgical intensive care patient—A prospective survey of 100 patients. *Crit Care Med* 1986; 14:188

Platt R, Polk BF, Murdouk B, et al: Mortality associated with nosocomial urinary tract infection. *N Engl J Med* 1982; 307:637

Podnos SD, Toews GB, Pierce AK: Nosocomial pneumonia in patients in intensive care units. *West J Med* 1985; 143:622

Sitzman JV, Townsend TR, Siler MC, et al: Septic and technical complications of central venous catheterization. *Am Surg* 1985; 202:766

Tunn UW, Thieme H: Sepsis associated with urinary tract infection. *Arch Intern Med* 1982; 142:2035

Wimberley NW, Bass JB, Boyd BW, et al: Use of a bronchoscopic protected catheter brush for the diagnosis of pulmonary infections. *Chest* 1982; 81:556

82
Infections in the Immunocompromised Host

One of the most difficult clinical challenges for critical care physicians is the immunocompromised patient. Multisystem disease is common, as are complications involving multiple organ systems. Owing to advances in the treatment of previously fatal or untreatable chronic illnesses, the numbers of immunocompromised patients have increased dramatically in the past 30 years. Supportive measures, many of which are provided by critical care physicians, are partly responsible for the prolonged survival of these patients. Thus, familiarity with the presentation of immunocompromised patients and the complications they may experience is a necessity for the critical care physician. Infection is a common complication of immunosuppression. The immunosuppressed state may be a manifestation of the underlying disease or a result of therapy. Infections are often more severe and fulminant in immunocompromised patients than in normal hosts. An aggressive evaluation is mandatory to determine the infectious etiology so that specific therapy can be instituted as rapidly as possible.

The spectrum of infectious diseases manifested in immunocompromised patients is extensive. For example, the differential diagnosis of a pulmonary infiltrate includes not only the usual bacterial pathogens but also fungi, viruses, mycobacteria, *Nocardia, Legionella,* and protozoa. Certain infections are more commonly associated with particular subsets of immunocompromised hosts. For example, cryptococcal meningitis is almost exclusively seen in patients with defects in cellular immunity either as a manifestation of their underlying disease (Hodgkin's disease, lymphoma, or acquired immunodeficiency syndrome) or as a result of corticosteroid therapy for collagen vascular diseases or renal transplantation. Thus an understanding of the immune defects involved will enable the clinician to narrow the differential diagnosis to a smaller group of more likely etiologies. Based on these multiple factors, diagnostic efforts can then be directed toward specific suspected pathogens.

This chapter begins with an approach to the immunocompromised host with infectious complications. Particular emphasis is placed on those elements of the history, physical examination, and diagnostic procedures that are of special importance in these patients. Subsequent sections outline the infectious complications of the immunocompromised hosts most often seen in intensive care units: granulocytopenic patients, corticosteroid-treated patients, renal transplant receipients and, bone marrow transplant recipients. Patients with acquired immunodeficiency syndrome (AIDS) are discussed in Chapter 83. Many of the specific infectious diseases discussed here are also addressed elsewhere in the volume. This chapter emphasizes infectious diseases that are either common among or unique to each of the subsets of immunocompromised hosts. An outline of the diagnostic evaluation, including specialized procedures, tests, and options for therapy, is provided. The format is designed to assist the critical care clinician in the acute management of infections in the immunocompromised host.

APPROACH TO THE IMMUNOCOMPROMISED HOST

The evaluation of an immunocompromised patient with a suspected infectious complication is similar to the approach to any febrile patient (see Chap. 80). Certain aspects of the evaluation deserve special emphasis for immunocompromised hosts. Historical data should include underlying diseases and medications—particularly recent corticosteroid or cytotoxic chemotherapy, which may impact on the degree or type(s) of immune defects. A thorough epidemiologic history, including travel, exposure to ill persons, pet or animal contact, occupation, avocations, and environment at onset of the infectious process (community or hospital), may provide useful clues to possible etiologies. Often, infectious diseases present with a paucity of symptoms and signs in immunocompromised patients. Thus particular importance must be placed on any symptoms reported or elicited, particularly headache, localized pain or irritation, and dyspnea. These subtle complaints may be the only evidence localizing an occult infectious process.

The physical examination should emphasize the organ systems most frequently involved with infectious complications, such as the central nervous system (CNS), the urinary tract, the integument, and the lungs. Fundoscopy should be performed to look for retinal changes that may suggest candidal endophthalmitis or cytomegalovirus and toxoplasma chorioretinitis. The sinuses should be assessed, particularly in nasally intubated patients, for occult infection. The perirectal area should be examined carefully for local erythema or tenderness, as this is often an occult source of fever and bacteremia in granulocytopenic patients. Special attention should be given to the skin examination, as dermatologic lesions are frequently the first manifestation of a systemic infection. In a recent review, more than 50% of skin lesions were caused by fungi. Demonstration of the pathogen through skin biopsy may lead to improved survival with the prompt initiation of antifungal therapy.

Certain laboratory tests can be useful in evaluating the extent of immunosuppression and providing evidence of multisystem involvement. The absolute granulocyte count (polymorphonuclear cells and bands) is easily obtained from the complete blood count and is important in defining the extent of immunodeficiency. Liver function tests, such as aspartate transaminase and bilirubin, may reflect a systemic rather than localized process. The serum creatinine, as a marker of renal function, is important because many antimicrobial agents are metabolized or excreted by the kidneys and require dosage adjustments based on the creatinine clearance. A chest radiograph is an indispensible diagnostic tool for the immunocompromised host owing to the frequent lack of symptoms in patients with active pulmonary processes.

Once the patient has been assessed for the immune defects, organ system involvement, and epidemiologic background, a differential diagnosis of the likely etiologies can be constructed. A diagnostic plan can then be initiated to confirm or rule out these possibilities. This database will help the clinician decide whether to begin empirical therapy for the most likely pathogens while awaiting diagnostic procedures, or to defer therapy until more information is available.

The diagnostic pathway leading to the choice of therapy should be pursued aggressively for several reasons. First, immunocompromised patients as a group are less tolerant of delays in diagnosis owing to their tenuous clinical status. Second, the differential diagnosis often includes several pathogens with totally different therapeutic options (*e.g., Cytomegalovirus, Aspergillus, Pneumocystis*) and a diagnostic procedure may be able to direct specific therapy, avoiding toxicity from nonessential therapy. Finally, in some cases there are multiple pathogens involved in the infectious process, and optimal outcome depends on the proper treatment regimen. Thus it is important to make a microbiologic or tissue diagnosis.

Biopsy of involved tissue for culture, special staining, and histopathology should be considered for each patient individually. The importance of a thorough evaluation of any body fluid or tissue specimen obtained from an immunocompromised host must not be overlooked. The microbiology laboratory should be alerted to the specimen's arrival so that it can be Gram-stained and processed for bacterial, mycobacterial, viral, and fungal cultures. At this time, if a fastidious organism such as *Legionella* is suspected, special media can be requested and the cultures can be held for 14 days. Also, rapid diagnostic tests such as direct immunofluoresence for *Legionella* can be performed. It is important that part of the specimen be sent for cytology or histopathology. Coordination with the pathologist allows the preparation of special stains that may detect pathogens not recovered in culture. Discussions with a consultant in infectious diseases are useful to determine what rapid diagnostic tests are readily available and also to provide guidance for specimen collection and transportation.

THE GRANULOCYTOPENIC PATIENT

The granulocytopenic patient is probably the most commonly seen immunocompromised host. This is because of the increased use of myelotoxic chemotherapy for hematologic and solid tumors. The primary immune defect is a decreased number of the phagocytic cells responsible for defense against bacterial and some fungal pathogens. Absolute granulocytopenia is defined as ≤ 500/mm polymorphonuclear cells and bands. If the leukocyte count is falling because of recent chemotherapy, many would consider 1000 cells/ mm^3 as indicative of granulocytopenia.

PRESENTATION

The onset of infection in these patients may be fulminant but more frequently it is insidious. Usual signs and symptoms of infection may be lacking. Fever is an almost universal sign. Erythema and pain may be the only evidence of a localized process such as pharyngitis or cellulitis. Clinical symptoms of a urinary tract infection (dysuria, frequency) or pneumonia (cough, purulent sputum production) are not reliable. Clinical suspicion of infection in the febrile granulocytopenic patient must be very high, and a thorough examination is essential. A good skin examination is very important, and prompt biopsy of any new lesions, particularly those which are discolored or necrotic, is essential. It is the granulocytopenic patient who is most likely to have occult anorectal infection without fluctuance or ulceration because of the inability to form an acute inflammatory response. The most common sites of infection are the sinopulmonary and urinary systems as well as any mucosal barrier whose integrity has been violated. Cytotoxic drugs often cause mucosal sloughing throughout the gastrointestinal tract. This predisposes to local invasion by the colonizing microflora, resulting in pharyngitis, esophagitis, bacteremia, and anorectal cellulitis/abscess. These patients often have intravenous catheters for chemotherapy, hyperalimentation, and medication administration. These catheters may be peripheral but are more often central venous lines (Hickman or Broviac). Triple-lumen central venous catheters are also becoming more popular for simultaneous hyperalimentation and infusion of blood products and medication. All catheters breach the natural barrier to microbial invasion provided by the skin.

The most common organisms causing bacteremia in these patients are gram-negative rods, notably *Escherichia coli, Klebsiella pneumoniae,* and *Pseudomonas aeruginosa.* However, in the past decade there has been a significant rise in the isolation of gram-positive pathogens in cases of bacteremia and serious infections, particularly *Corynebacterium, Staphylococcus aureus,* and *Staphylococcus epidermidis.* Granulocytopenic patients are also at risk for opportunistic fungal infections. Other predisposing factors include hematologic malignancy, corticosteroid therapy, mucosal barrier breakdown, and, possibly, increased colonization resulting from antibacterial therapy. The most frequent isolates include *Candida, Aspergillus, Zygomycetes* (e.g., *Mucor, Rhizopus*) and *Cryptococcus.* However, any fungus isolated from a sterile site or biopsy culture in these patients should be considered a pathogen.

DIAGNOSIS

The diagnosis of infection in granulocytopenic patients requires a high index of suspicion combined with a willingness to perform procedures that may provide useful information. At the onset of fever, the basic laboratory evaluation should include a complete blood count with differential, a urinalysis and urine Gram stain and culture, blood cultures, and cultures with Gram stains of any site of suspected infection based on the presentation. A chest radiograph may identify an infiltrate when the patient has minimal or no pulmonary symptoms. Pulmonary infiltrates should be evaluated systematically yet aggressively, including consideration of transbronchoscopic lavage and biopsy or open lung biopsy if indicated. Any suspicious skin lesions should be biopsied as noted above.

THERAPY

Once the patient is evaluated and cultures have been obtained, antibacterial therapy should be initiated. If a source of the fever is discovered and a Gram stain or other procedure has indicated a likely pathogen, specific therapy directed against the organism can be started. However, more often the source of fever is occult or there is no specimen to guide therapy, and empirical therapy must be initiated. Experience with febrile granulocytopenic patients has demonstrated that the 48-hour mortality of untreated cases is unacceptable and can be markedly reduced through the use of empirical therapy. Currently accepted therapy includes the combination of a semisynthetic antipseudomonal penicillin such as carbenicillin or ticarcillin and an aminoglycoside. Other alternative penicillins are mezlocillin or piperacillin, which have increased *in vitro* activity against *Klebsiella* species. The choice of which penicillin and aminoglycoside to use should be based on a combination of the *in vitro* susceptibility patterns for the gram-negative bacillary strains endemic at a given institution and cost analysis of each drug. To date, there are no clinical data demonstrating a survival advantage for any particular regimen compared to the others.

The drug of choice for fungal infections is intravenous amphotericin B (AMB). The question of when to initiate empirical AMB for suspected fungal superinfection is troublesome, particularly in a critical care setting where any increased toxicity impacts adversely on other organ systems. The diagnosis of systemic fungal infection is difficult to make, and blood cultures are infrequently positive in disseminated mycoses other than *Candida*. Most fungal infections are not diagnosed until autopsy, yet it is the persistently febrile granulocytopenic patient on broad-spectrum antibacterial therapy who is at highest risk for fungal infection. Thus most centers advocate the use of empirical AMB if there is continued granulocytopenia and fever unresponsive to 7 days of antibacterial therapy.

Recently there has been interest in alternative empirical therapy for granulocytopenic patients. This is largely due to the development of a number of broad-spectrum β-lactams and to concern regarding the nephrotoxicity and ototoxicity of the aminoglycosides. One approach is to combine a penicillin and a cephalosporin or two cephalosporins that have broad gram-negative coverage—the double β-lactam combination. In reports to date, double β-lactam combinations have shown equal efficacy to the β-lactam and aminoglycoside combination, with less toxicity. However, the number of patients treated to date remains small. A second alternative is monotherapy with one of the broad-spectrum cephalosporins (ceftazidime, cefoperazone) or carbapenems (imipenem-cilastatin). A recent randomized comparative trial in cancer patients with granulocytopenia and fever demonstrated that ceftazidime monotherapy was a safe alternative to standard combination empirical therapy in achieving patient survival through the period of granulocytopenia. An open trial of imipenem-cilastatin as empirical therapy for febrile cancer patients achieved an overall response rate of 67%, which is similar to standard combination therapy. The results of monotherapy have been encouraging but inconclusive, and there have been disturbing reports of the emergence of resistance to the single agent while on therapy. Currently, combination empirical therapy with a β-lactam and an aminoglycoside is recommended. Aztreonam is the first agent of a new class of antimicrobial agents, the monobactams. The *in vitro* spectrum is similar to the aminoglycosides (aerobic gram-negative rods, including *P. aeruginosa*). Aztreonam may be an effective alternative agent for combination therapy, avoiding the potential nephrotoxicity of the aminoglycosides.

THE CORTICOSTEROID-TREATED PATIENT

The number of patients treated with corticosteroids is constantly rising and includes those with malignancies, collagen vascular diseases, autoimmune disorders and various forms of pulmonary disease. The number of immunosuppressed hosts at risk for infection has similarly expanded. Corticosteroids predominantly affect the mononuclear cell population causing a monocytopenia and relative lymphopenia by redistributing the T cells from the circulation, thus impairing their access to inflammatory sites. Various effects on the polymorphonuclear cell have been attributed to corticosteroids *in vitro*; however, *in vivo* prednisone has no discernible effect on polymorphonuclear function except at pharmacologic doses. The overall immune defect induced by corticosteroids is an impairment of cellular immunity, thus placing the host at risk for fungal, viral, and protozoal infection as well as several otherwise uncommon bacterial infections. Corticosteroids can also reactivate dormant mycobacterial and fungal infections by impairing the cellular immunity responsible for their control. Pathogens to consider when dealing with the steroid-treated patient include; *Pneumocystis carinii, Nocardia, Listeria,* and *Legionella.*

THE RENAL TRANSPLANT RECIPIENT

Renal allograft recipients are dependent on the chronic administration of drugs such as prednisone, azathioprine, cyclophosphamide, and cyclosporine for the maintenance of graft function. Currently, the most common regimen is a combination of cyclosporine and prednisone. During periods of acute rejection, these agents are given in higher doses in attempts to reverse the process. The combined effect of these drugs is one of constant immunosuppression, particularly of cellular-mediated immunity. Infection is a frequent complication for these individuals. Certain infectious syndromes can be expected to occur at different time periods after transplantation. The early transplant period is complicated predominantly by bacterial pathogens as well as herpes simplex virus and hepatitis B virus. Central nervous system infection is rare in the first month after transplant but is significant in the following months. Generally, the period after the first posttransplant month is associated with opportunistic fungal, protozoal, and bacterial infections. There are certain factors that can, to some degree, determine which infectious complications are likely to be encountered, including the types of immunosuppression employed, the underlying disease of the transplant population and, most importantly, the epidemiology of various microbial agents (*e.g., Legionella* or *Aspergillis* species) unique to a given region or institution.

BONE MARROW TRANSPLANT RECIPIENT

Recipients of allogeneic bone marrow transplantation (BMT) are the epitome of the immunosuppressed host. As a result of the preconditioning therapy, which involves high-dose cytotoxic chemotherapy and frequently total body irradiation, bone marrow elements are ablated and both humoral and cellular immunity are eradicated. Thus in the period immediately after the bone marrow transplant, the patient is devoid of most host defenses. The natural mucosal barriers also are interrupted by the effects of the preparative therapy. Thus it is not surprising that these patients are at high risk for infectious complications. Like renal transplant recipients, patients undergoing bone marrow transplants have characteristic infectious complications that reflect the immune defects present at each stage of the process. Bacterial, fungal, and viral infections are of concern.

For more information, please see Chapter 67 in Civetta JM, Taylor RW, Kirby RR: Critical Care. *Philadelphia: J. B. Lippincott, 1988*

BIBLIOGRAPHY

Barnes SG, Sattler FR, Ballard JO: Perirectal infections in acute leukemia. Improved survival after incision and debridement. *Ann Intern Med* 1984; 100:515

Bodey GP: Fungal infection and fever of unknown origin in neutropenic patients. *Am J Med* 1986; 80(suppl 5C):112

Meyers JD, Flournoy F, Thomas ED: Nonbacterial pneumonia after allogeneic marrow transplantation: A review of ten years' experience. *Rev Infect Dis* 1982; 4:1119

Rubin RH, Cosini AB, Tolkoff-Rubin NE, et al: Infectious disease syndromes attributable to cytomegalovirus and their significance among renal transplant recipients. *Transplantation* 1977; 24:458

Shepp DH, Dandliker PS, Meyers JD: Treatment of varicella-zoster virus infection in severely immunocompromised patients. A randomized comparison of acyclovir and vidarabine. *N Engl J Med* 1986; 314:208

Sickles EA, Greene WH, Wiernik PH: Clinical presentation of infection in granulocytopenic patients. *Arch Intern Med* 1975; 35:715

Wingard JR, Santos GW, Saral R: Late onset interstitial pneumonia following allogeneic bone marrow transplantation. *Transplantation* 1985; 39:21

Wolfson JS, Sober AJ, Rubin RH: Dermatological manifestations of infections in immunocompromised patients. *Medicine* 1985; 64:115

83
The Acquired Immune Deficiency Syndrome

Acquired immunodeficiency syndrome (AIDS) is a condition of cellular immune deficiency that results in life-threatening opportunistic infections and malignancies of which the etiologic agent is human immunodeficiency virus (HIV), also known as human T-cell leukemia virus-3 (HTLV-3), lymphadenopathy virus (LAV), and AIDS-related virus (ARV). Recent data suggest an HIV variant (HIV-2) may cause AIDS in African and European patients and that a number of related retroviruses such as HTLV-1, HTLV-2, and HTLV-4 may act as co-factors or rarely cause AIDS themselves.

Individuals with HIV infection and a chronic syndrome of fevers, night sweats, weight loss, adenopathy, or diarrhea and evidence of abnormal cell-mediated immunity are referred to as having AIDS-related complex (ARC). It is generally thought that ARC is an earlier or milder clinical manifestation of HIV infection than is AIDS, and, although the individual prognosis of a patient with ARC is unknown, it is believed that at least 30%, and possibly all, of these patients will progress to AIDS. The Centers for Disease Control (CDC) has classified HIV-associated disease into four groups (Table 83-1). In this classification, group I includes individuals with an acute mononucleosis-like syndrome from HIV, group II includes asymptomatic but infected individuals, group III includes those with persistent adenopathy, and group IV includes those with HIV-associated symptomatic clinical disease. Subgroup IV.A includes ARC patients, subgroup IV.B those patients with CNS complications, and subgroup IV.C those persons with secondary infection. Category C-1 includes infections diagnostic of AIDS, category C-2 includes oral hairy leukoplakia (associated with papilloma and Epstein–Barr viruses), multidermatomal herpes zoster, recurrent salmonella bacteremia, nocardiosis, tuberculosis (TB), and oral candidiasis. Subgroup IV.D includes secondary cancers—Kaposi's sarcoma, non-Hodgkin's lymphoma (small, noncleaved or immunoblastic sarcoma)—and primary lymphoma of the brain. Subgroup E includes miscellaneous conditions associated with HIV disease or cellular immunodeficiency such as chronic lymphoid interstitial pneumonia, conditions that do not fit into other groups.

DIAGNOSIS

Individuals infected with HIV are generally antibody positive for HIV (HIV Ab+), as detected by ELISA and Western blot testing. They exhibit viremia in the presence of antibody and should be considered as both infected and infectious. Unfortunately, HIV antibody testing is imperfect, and individuals who are antibody (+) but noninfected (false-positives), or antibody (−) but infected (false-negatives), exist. Diagnostic tests for HIV antibody using cloned HIV antigens, and tests for HIV antigen itself, are recent developments in this field.

Although the immunologic consequences of HIV infection are varied, the basic pathophysiologic derangement is a gradual and progressive depletion of T-helper lymphocytes or T4 cells, which leads to progressive cellular immunodeficiency. These changes are reflected in lymphopenia, by an abnormally low helper-supressor ratio, and by cutaneous anergy. Nonspecific activation of B cells occurs (possibly due to HIV or Epstein–Barr virus), leading to polyclonal gammopathy, and a variety of autoimmune epiphenomena, such as rashes and immune cytopenias. Human immunodeficiency virus also infects the nervous system directly, leading to a variety of complications, including a severe subacute encephalopathy (see CNS Complications of HIV).

EPIDEMIOLOGY

At a recent U.S. Public Health Service Conference on AIDS planning, it was estimated that between 1.5 and 3 million people in the United States are currently infected with HIV. To date, more than 75,000 cases of AIDS have been reported in the United States, and it is estimated that 270,000 individuals will have AIDS or will have died from it by 1991. In addition, it appears that infected individuals who do not develop AIDS may remain at risk indefinitely for HIV myeloencephalopathy, resulting in paralysis and dementia. In the United States the direct cost of medical care in 1991 for these people is conservatively estimated between 8 and 16 billion dollars, with an indirect economic cost of lost manpower and productivity several times that high.

When AIDS was first defined in 1981, it was widely recognized that homosexuals, IV drug abusers, transfusion recipients, and hemophiliacs were at high risk. It is now clear that HIV is spread in largely the same manner as hepatitis B virus—through parenteral and sexual exposure. Whether differences in efficiency of transmission exist between different sexes, partners, and practices remains problematic.

In Central Africa, the male-to-female ratio of AIDS is 1.1:1 and heterosexual transmission is common. There is, in addition, a high prevalence of HIV antibody positivity in prostitutes, female sexual partners and spouses of IV drug abusers, hemophiliacs, and transfusion-associated AIDS cases. These data suggest that the virus can be spread into the heterosexual U.S. population. A recent nationwide Department of Defense study of recruit applicants showed a prevalence of 1.5 HIV + individuals per 1,000 tested, with a male-to-female ratio of 3:1. As with AIDS cases, minority groups were especially at risk, with blacks 4 times and Hispanics 2.6 times as likely as whites to be HIV Ab+. As expected, prevalence was highest in large coastal urban areas. Because urban minorities are disproportionately in lower socioeconomic classes, which are also at the highest risk for infectious diseases of poverty, sexually transmitted diseases, and violent or traumatic injury, it can be seen that a large number of occultly HIV positive individuals will be emergently admitted to the ICU setting. Because the ICU is geared toward invasive measures of monitoring and resuscitation, it is imperative that ICU personnel protect themselves from accidental exposure to infectious blood and body fluids.

THERAPY

To date, no curative therapy for HIV infection or AIDS is available. Early attempts at therapy with thymosin, interferons, interleukins, and bone marrow transplants and other immunoadjuvants were unsuccessful. Suramin proved too toxic. Trials with ribavirin have yielded conflicting and controversial results. Current interest centers on azidothymidine (AZT or Zidovudine) and related antivirals. A multicenter, double-blinded placebo controlled trial with this agent revealed a significant survival advantage and fewer opportunistic infections in the AZT treated group versus placebo. As a result the controlled study was terminated and the drug approved by the FDA. Current concerns are that the drug [1] is virostatic, not curative; [2] has significant hematologic, and unknown long-term, toxicities; [3] is very expensive (currently a year's supply costs about $10,000); and [4] is only approved for patients with far advanced disease (T_4 counts less than 200 cells/mm^3 with symptomatic ARC, or patients with AIDS).

Areas of current interest in anti-HIV and retroviral therapeutics include the use of mismatched double-stranded RNA fragments (Ampligen), which act as an RNA chain terminator with anti-retroviral activity; other AZT-like nucleoside derivatives such as dideoxycytidine (DDC), which appears to have less marrow toxicity; and monoclonal antibodies directed against subunits of the viral genome and its gene products. In addition, recently cloned biologically active peptide cytokines such as tumor necrosis factor (TNF), erythropoietin (EP), and granulocyte-macrophage colony stimulating factors (GM-CSF) are being investigated as immunoadjuvants and marrow stimulators.

Development of a vaccine for HIV is of the highest priority, and research centers are identifying and cloning highly conserved and immunogenic subunits of the virion. Unfortunately, the end-product—a safe and effective vaccine—may be several years away.

TABLE 83-1 SUMMARY OF CLASSIFICATION SYSTEM FOR HUMAN IMMUNODEFICIENCY VIRUS

Group I.	Acute infection
Group II.	Asymptomatic infection*
Group III.	Persistent generalized lymphadenopathy*
Group IV.	Other disease
Subgroup A.	Constitutional disease
Subgroup B.	Neurologic disease
Subgroup C.	Secondary infectious diseases
Category C-1.	Specified secondary infectious diseases listed in the CDC surveillance definition for AIDS†
Category C-2.	Other specified secondary infectious diseases
Subgroup D.	Secondary cancers†
Subgroup E.	Other conditions

(Classification system of human T-lymphotropic virus type III/lymphadenopathy-associated virus infections. *MMWR* 1986; 35:334)
*Patients in Groups II and III may be subclassified on the basis of a laboratory evaluation.
†Includes those patients whose clinical presentation fulfills the definition of AIDS used by CDC for national reporting.

At present, the only effective means of preventing further spread of HIV is through widespread education to minimize sexual contact with infected individuals and to prevent contact, especially parenteral, with infected body fluids. The virus survives poorly outside the body, it is killed by traditional disinfection procedures, and there is no evidence that it is spread by casual contact.

For more information, please see Chapter 68 in Civetta JM, Taylor RW, Kirby RR: Critical Care. *Philadelphia: J. B. Lippincott, 1988*

BIBLIOGRAPHY

Additional recommendations to reduce sexual and drug abuse-related transmission of human T-lymphotropic virus type III/lymphadenopathy-associated virus. *MMWR* 1986; 35:152–155

Barnes D: News and comment: Grim projections for AIDS epidemic. *Science* 1986; 232:1589

Classification system of human T-lymphotropic virus type III/lymphadenopathy-associated virus infections. *MMWR* 1986; 35:334–339

Health and Public Policy Committee, American College of Physicians, and the Infectious Disease Society of America: Position paper: Acquired immunodeficiency syndrome. *Ann Intern Med* 1986; 104:575–581

Human Retrovirus Subcommittee: Human immunodeficiency viruses (letter). *Science* 1986; 232:697

Human T-lymphotropic virus type III/lymphadenopathy-associated virus antibody prevalence in U.S. military recruit applicants. *MMWR* 1986; 35:421–425

Marx J: Research news: Probing the AIDS virus and its relatives. *Science* 1987; 236:1523–1525

Steinbrook R, Lo B, Moulton J, et al: Preferences of homosexual men with AIDS for life-sustaining treatment. *N Engl J Med* 1986; 314:457–460

Update: Immunodeficiency virus infections in health care workers exposed to blood of infected patients. *MMWR* 1987; 36:286–295

Wachter RM, Luce JM, Turner J, et al: Intensive care of patients with the acquired immunodeficiency syndrome: Outcome and changing patterns of utilization (abstr). *Am Rev Respir Dis* 1986; 134:891

Yarchoan, R, Broder S: Special report: Development of antiretroviral therapy for the acquired immunodeficiency syndrome and related disorders. *N Engl J Med* 1987; 316:557–564

84
Antimicrobial Agents

ANTIBIOTIC SELECTION

The ideal antibiotic is one that is effective against the etiologic agent, is nontoxic, does not disturb the normal flora of the patient, and is inexpensive. Antibiotic therapy usually involves compromise of one or more of these factors. The selection of antibiotics has become more complex because of the introduction of a bewildering variety of antimicrobial agents, with subtle distinctions conferring therapeutic advantages in specific situations, as well as the increasing emphasis on the importance of antimicrobial costs and toxicities and the emergence of multi-drug-resistant nosocomial pathogens. Initial therapy is based on the goal of the antibiotic therapy and the special characteristics of the host in terms of drug toxicity or metabolism. The goal of therapy should be defined in terms of prevention (prophylaxis) versus treatment of infection, the target infectious organisms, and the site of proven or suspected infection. Special host characteristics include age, underlying disease, drug allergies, or organ dysfunction that may influence drug pharmacokinetics or predispose to drug toxicity. Antibiotic therapy should also be considered a dynamic process, with continual review of new information from the laboratory and, most importantly, assessment of the patient's response, which may dictate changes in therapy.

The tempo and vigor of the diagnostic work-up and therapy are determined by the site and virulence of the infection and by the underlying host defects. In patients with mild to moderate infections and normal host defenses, therapy can often be safely delayed until a specific diagnosis is made by use of noninvasive techniques. This allows the selection of an effective, nontoxic therapy aimed at the specific etiologic agent. In patients with life-threatening infections or those who are profoundly immunosuppressed, empirical therapy often must be initiated immediately, based on a presumptive diagnosis. Empirical antibiotic therapy does not obviate aggressive attempts to establish a precise anatomic and etiologic diagnosis, which may require the use of invasive techniques. Knowledge of the etiologic agent may allow institution of more specific therapy and discontinuation of unnecessary and toxic antimicrobial agents. A precise diagnosis may also dictate critical ancillary treatment measures, such as drainage of localized infection, relief of obstruction, and removal of infected foreign bodies. Prolonged therapy with broad-spectrum antibiotics increases the risk of superinfection, especially with fungi. Widespread use of antibiotics in an ICU also contributes to the emergence of multi-drug-resistant organisms.

THE INFECTING ORGANISM

Identification of the infecting organism allows prediction of an effective antimicrobial agent (Table 84-1). Laboratory sensitivity testing confirms the predicted sensitivity pattern, identifies isolates with unusual resistance, and often permits selection of less toxic antibiotics that would not otherwise be predictably effective. Information about local sensitivity patterns is a valuable adjunct to published drug sensitivity data. This is particularly true in ICUs, which have an increased frequency of pathogens with unusual resistance patterns, often due to transmissible drug resistance plasmids.

THE SITE OF INFECTION

The site of infection influences its seriousness, the likelihood of specific etiologic agents, and drug delivery. Almost all antibiotics are delivered effectively to infections of the soft tissues and tissue spaces such as joints and pleural and peritoneal cavities. Some antimicrobials have a limited ability to penetrate certain sites, especially the central nervous system (CNS). In the presence of obstruction, delivery of antibiotic to an infected urinary, biliary, or respiratory tract is poor, and clinical response depends on appropriate drainage. Some urinary tract antimicrobials, such as nitrofurantoin, depend on high urinary concentrations and are ineffective in systemic infections or in patients with renal failure. Infected sites where there is necrosis or an impaired blood supply respond to antibiotics poorly, if at all, without adjunctive therapy. This is due in part to impaired delivery of antibiotic, as well as to altered *p*H and defective host response. Therapy of these sites must include debridement, drainage, and possibly revascularization.

MANIFESTATIONS OF INFECTION

A carefully performed history and physical examination, supplemented with appropriate laboratory and radiologic studies, still remains the basis for diagnosis and treatment of infectious diseases. The history should focus on predisposing host factors, exposure to potential sources of infection, localizing symptoms of infection, and host factors relating to potential antibiotic toxicities. The physical examination of the intensive care patient should emphasize not only those sites of potential infection suggested by history but also the areas at special risk in this setting, such as intravenous catheter sites, wounds (surgical and traumatic), and the respiratory tract. Initial laboratory examination should include a complete blood count to assess lymphocyte count and polymorphonuclear response. Basic tests also include an assessment of liver and renal function to allow predictions of probable drug pharmokinetics and toxicity.

The problem of diagnosis is complicated by the difficulty of obtaining diagnostic specimens that represent the etiologic organism. At least two sets of blood cultures should be done with an additional set if the likelihood of bacteremia is high. A fresh Gram-stained specimen from potential infected sites permits a judgment as to whether the specimen is free of contamination with normal flora and thus is likely to give meaningful culture results, and may provide an early clue to the etiology of the infection. An adequate specimen of urine, sputum, or wound exudate is characterized by a paucity of squamous epithelial cells and the presence of polymorphonuclear cells with a predominance of a single organism.

Radiographs of potentially infected sites, especially the chest, are helpful in defining the extent and nature of the infection, and some patterns are suggestive of certain types of infection.

HOST FACTORS

Sources of Infection

Exposure to infectious disease hazards may occur before or after hospitalization. Common sources of outpatient exposure include infectious diseases circulating in the community, travel to an area of endemic disease, exposure to illnesses in the family unit, and common source outbreaks. Recognition of these exposures may suggest specialized diagnostic techniques or allow early suspicion of infections that are not adequately treated by usual broad-spectrum therapy, such as mycoplasma, legionellosis, or influenza. Commonly, intensive care patients are placed at risk for infection by inpatient therapy, such as intubation and ventilatory support, intravenous catheters, and invasive monitoring.

Host Immune Defense

Mechanisms of protection against infection include mechanical barriers to invading organisms (skin and respiratory cilia), humoral factors (antibodies), cellular (T-cell dependent) immune functions, and phagocytic factors (granulocytopenia). Defects in these host defense mechanisms lead to increased rates of infection, with specific defects predisposing to specific types of infection. Classic immunodeficiencies include congenital defects, which may involve cellular, humoral, or combined defects; malignancies such as multiple myeloma (humoral) and Hodgkin's disease (cellular); and chemotherapy with steroids and cytotoxic drugs (combined defects). Patients with AIDS are emerging as an important new group with severe cellular immunodeficiency. Most of these patients are members of a high-risk group (male homosexuals or bisexuals, intravenous drug abusers, or patients with hemophilia). The number of AIDS patients is increasing rapidly, and it is clear that in the future

TABLE 84-1 DRUGS OF CHOICE IN SERIOUS INFECTIONS*

Organism	Drug of Choice	Alternate Drugs
Gram-Positive Cocci		
Staphylococcus aureus or S. epidermidis		
Penicillin sensitive	Penicillin G	Cephalosporin, vancomycin, or clindamycin†
Penicillinase producing	Oxacillin or nafcillin	Cephalosporin, vancomycin, or clindamycin†
Methicillin resistant	Vancomycin	TMP/SMZ‡
Nonenterococcal streptococci	Penicillin G	Cephalosporin, vancomycin, or clindamycin†
Enterococci	Penicillin or ampicillin + aminoglycoside	Vancomycin + aminoglycoside
Pneumoccoccus	Penicillin G	Cephalosporin, vancomycin, chloramphenicol§, erythromycin
Gram-Positive Bacilli		
Listeria monocytogenes	Ampicillin	Chloramphenicol§, tetracycline
Bacillus anthracis	Penicillin	Tetracycline, erythromycin
Clostridium difficile	Vancomycin"	Metronidazole
Clostridium tetani	Penicillin#	Tetracycline
Clostridium perfringens	Penicillin[xx]	Chloramphenicol, clindamycin, metronidazole, tetracycline
Corynebacterium diphtheriae	Erythromycin#	Penicillin
Corynebacterium, JK	Vancomycin	
Proprionobacterium species	Penicillin	Clindamycin, erythromycin
Actinomyces israeli	Penicillin G	Tetracycline
Nocardia asteroides	Sulfonamide	TMP/SMZ, minocycline, ampicillin + erythromycin
Gram-Negative Cocci		
Branhamella catarrhalis	Amoxicillin–clavulanic acid	TMP/SMZ, ceftriaxone, erythromycin, tetracycline
Neisseria gonorrhea	Penicillin G	Spectinomycin
Neisseria meningiditis	Penicillin G	Chloramphenicol§, cefuroxime, TMP/SMZ
Enteric Gram-Negative Bacilli		
Bacteroides		
Oral flora	Penicillin	Clindamycin, cefoxitin, metronidazole

TABLE 84-1 *(continued)*

Organism	Drug of Choice	Alternate Drugs
Bowel strains	Clindamycin or metronidazole	Cefoxitin, mezlocillin, piperacillin, chloramphenicol, imipenem
Citrobacter	Gentamicin, cephalosporin	Gentamicin, amikacin, chloramphenicol, piperacillin, aztreonam, imipenem
Enterobacteriaceae	Gentamicin, cephalosporin	Gentamicin, amikacin, chloramphenicol, piperacillin, aztreonam, imipenem
Escherichia coli	Gentamicin, cephalosporin	Gentamicin, ampicillin, amikacin, imipenem, aztreonam, piperacillin
Klebsiella	Gentamicin, cephalosporin	Gentamicin, amikacin, chloramphenicol, piperacillin, aztreonam, imipenem
Proteus		
P. mirabilis	Ampicillin	Gentamicin, cephalosporin, tobramycin, amikacin, chloramphenicol, piperacillin
Other Proteus species	Cephalosporin, gentamicin	Tobramycin, amikacin, chloramphenicol, piperacillin, aztreonam, imipenem
Providenia	Second- or third-generation cephalosporin	Getamicin, amikacin, piperacillin, aztreonam, imipenem, TMP/SMZ
Salmonella typhosa	Chloramphenicol	Ampicillin, TMP/SMZ
Other Salmonella	Ampicillin††	Chloramphenicol, TMP/SMZ
Serratia	Gentamicin	Cephalosporin, imipenem, aztreonam, piperacillin, TMP/SMZ
Shigella	TMP/SMZ	Ampicillin, chloramphenicol
Yersinia enterocolitica	TMP/SMZ	Gentamicin, tetracycline, third-generation cephalosporin
Other Gram-Negative Bacilli		
Acinetobacter	Gentamicin	Imipenem, amikacin, piperacillin, TMP/SMZ, tetracycline
Eikenella corrodens	Ampicillin	Erythromycin, tetracycline

(Continued on page 642)

TABLE 84-1 *(continued from page 641)*

Organism	Drug of Choice	Alternate Drugs
Francisella tularensis	Streptomycin	Tetracycline, chloramphenicol
Fusobacterium	Penicillin	Clindamycin, metronidazole, chloramphenicol
Haemophilus influenzae	Chloramphenicol	Ampicillin, cephalosporin, TMP/SMZ
Legionella	Erythromycin	Rifampin, tetracycline
Pasturella multocida	Penicillin	Tetracycline, cephalosporin
Pseudomonas aeruginosa	Antipseudomonal penicillin + gentamicin	Aztreonam or cephalosporin + amikacin
Pseudomonas cepacia	TMP/SMZ	Chloramphenicol
Spirillum minus	Penicillin G	Tetracycline, streptomycin
Streptobacillus moniliformis	Penicillin G	Tetracycline, streptomycin
Vibrio cholerae	Tetracycline‡‡	TMP/SMZ
Yersinia pestis	Streptomycin	Tetracycline, chloramphenicol
Chlamydia		
C. trachomatis	Tetracycline	Erythromycin, sulfonamide
C. psittaci	Tetracycline	Chloramphenicol
Mycoplasma	Erythromycin	Tetracycline
Rickettsia	Tetracycline	Chloramphenicol
Spirochetales		
Treponema pallidum	Penicillin	Tetracycline, erythromycin
Borrelia	Penicillin	Tetracycline

* This table does not consider minor infections that may be treated with oral agents, single-agent therapy or less toxic drugs. Sensitivity testing should be done to confirm the usual sensitivity pattern of most organisms.
† First-generation cephalosporins are most active. If endocarditis is suspected, do not use clindamycin; some authorities recommend the addition of an aminoglycoside for endocarditis caused by nonenterococcal streptococci or tolerant staphylococci.
‡ Methicillin-resistant staphylococci should be assumed resistant to cephalosporins even if disk testing suggests sensitivity.
§ Drug of choice in meningitis for penicillin-allergic patients.
" In antibiotic-associated colitis, discontinue the offending drug. Oral vancomycin is the drug of choice; oral or parenteral metronidazole is also effective.
As an adjunct to passive and active immunization.
xx As an adjunct to debridement of infected tissue.
†† Uncomplicated salmonella enteritis should not be treated with antibiotics.
‡‡ Primary treatment is fluid and electrolyte replacement.

heterosexual transmission will become an increasingly important factor in the spread of human immunodeficiency virus (HIV). A history of blood transfusion, particularly between the years of 1979 and 1985, or of multiple heterosexual relationships provides important clues to this diagnosis. Serologic confirmation of HIV should be sought in patients presenting with puzzling or unusual infections, even if they do not seem to fit the classic risk groups. These patients may present with a variety of opportunistic pulmonary infections, particularly *Pneumocystis carinii* but also including *Cytomegalovirus, Cryptococcus neoformans,* and atypical mycobacteria.

Initial therapy in these patients should include those organisms that are classically associated with specific defects in host defense (Table 84-2). In the granuocytopenic host, infections progress rapidly and local signs of infection are often minimal or absent, requiring initiation of therapy before a definitive diagnosis is reached. The most common forms of infections in these patients are primary bacteremia, pneumonia, urinary tract infection, and cellulitis (often perirectal). The most common etiologic organisms are gram-negative rods, and initial therapy usually consists of an antipseudomonal penicillin and an aminoglycoside. Patients who respond to empirical therapy should have therapy continued until the granulocytopenia resolves or for at least 2 weeks, regardless of whether an etiologic agent is isolated. When patients fail to respond and an isolate resistant to initial therapy has been identified, therapy should be modified according to laboratory information. Consideration should be given to administering two synergistic drugs against gram-negative isolates that are causing bacteremia or pneumonia. If a patient fails to respond within 3 to 5 days and no isolate has been obtained, the risk of fungal infection is high and the addition of amphotericin B therapy should be considered.

Other patients have more subtle defects. Alcoholic patients often have deficiencies in polymorphonuclear function and delayed hypersensitivity. Uremic patients have defects in humoral and cell-mediated immunity and are also at risk for dialysis-related infections. Diabetic patients frequently have vascular compromise, defects in skin integrity, and polymorphonuclear dysfunction, with increased frequencies of both common infections, such as

TABLE 84-2 PATHOGENS ASSOCIATED WITH IMMUNE DEFICITS

Immune Deficit	Usual Pathogens	Typical Settings
Granulocytopenia	Aerobic gram-negative bacilli, *Candida, Aspergillus*	Hematologic malignancy
Cell-mediated immunosuppression	*Cytomegalovirus, Pneumocystis,* herpes zoster, *Nocardia, Listeria, Cryptococcus, Legionella, Strongyloides*	Acquired immunodeficiency syndrome, renal transplantation, Hodgkin's disease
Hypogammaglobulinemia or dysgammaglobulinemia	*S. pneumoniae, H. influenzae*	Chronic lymphocytic leukemia, multiple myeloma, congenital hypogammaglobulinemia

cellulitis and osteomyelitis, and uncommon infections, such as zygomycosis and malignant otitis externa. Malnutrition is associated with defects in cellular immunity and predisposes patients to a variety of infections. Aging also increases the risk of infection, particularly urinary tract and respiratory infections. Residence in a special care unit influences the type of organisms causing infection and the severity of the infection. Initial therapy should consider prevailing strains and resistance patterns in the special care unit.

ANTIBIOTICS IN PREGNANCY

Pregnancy is a special case for the use of any drug, in that consideration must be given to both the altered metabolism in the mother and possible risks to the fetus. Of special concern is that the teratogenic effects of most drugs have not been studied systematically. Maternal volume of distribution, glomerular filtration rate, and hepatic metabolism are increased, leading to lower drug levels. A balance must be struck between the maxim that no drug should be given to pregnant women in the absence of a firm indication and the recognition that untreated infection can be disastrous to the maternal-fetal unit. Preference is often given to the use of older classes of drugs (such as β-lactams), for which the risks are well established, in preference to newer, less well studied agents (Table 84-3).

DOSE, ROUTE, AND FREQUENCY OF ADMINISTRATION

The preferred dose of antimicrobial is designed to reliably deliver an inhibitory concentration of the drug to the site of infection, while avoiding toxicity. Fortunately, for most antibiotics, there is a sufficiently wide gap between therapeutic and toxic concentrations that differences in the MICs of different organisms can be ignored and a standard dose given. In general, higher doses are given for severe infections and for infections at sites where drug penetration is limited (e.g., meningitis), while lower doses suffice for urinary tract infection. Special attention is required in patients with renal insufficiency because many drugs are excreted by the kidneys, and some drugs may cause further deterioration of renal function. Drugs that have common or severe dose-related side-effects may require monitoring of serum levels, especially in patients at higher risk for toxicity or with impaired excretion. Routine monitoring of serum levels is recommended only for the aminoglycosides, with optional monitoring of at-risk patients receiving vancomycin, chloramphenicol, and sulfonamides.

Antibiotics may be given orally, intramuscularly, or intravenously. The intramuscular route is limited by patient discomfort, local complications, and unreliable absorption of some drugs. It is usually chosen for drugs that are designed to be absorbed slowly from an intramuscular depot (benzathine penicillin) or when intravenous administration is impractical.

For more information, please see Chapter 66 in Civetta JM, Taylor RW, Kirby RR: Critical Care. *Philadelphia: J. B. Lippincott, 1988*

TABLE 84-3 ANTIBIOTIC USE IN PREGNANCY

Antimicrobial	Maternal Toxicity	Fetal Toxicity	Breast Milk
	Contraindicated, or safer alternatives available		
Erythromycin estolate	Cholestasis	None known	Yes
Nitrofurantoin	Neuropathy, hemolysis	Hemolysis	Trace
Tetracycline	Liver necrosis	Tooth staining and dysplasia	Chelated
Trimethoprim-sulfamethoxazole	Allergic reactions	Kernicterus, teratogenicity	Yes
Trimethoprim	Allergic reactions	Teratogenicity in rats	Yes
	Caution: Use only for strong indication and lack of suitable alternatives		
Acyclovir	Nephrotoxicity	None known	?
Aminoglycosides	Ototoxicity and nephrotoxicity	8th nerve toxicity	Trace
Amphotericin B	Anemia, hepatotoxicity	Azotemia, hypokalemia	?
Chloramphenicol	Aplastic anemia	Gray-baby syndrome	Yes
Clindamycin	Allergy, colitis	None known	Yes
Flucytosine	Marrow depression	Potentially teratogenic	?
Isoniazid	Hepatotoxicity	Possible neuropathy and seizures	Yes
Metronidazole	Blood dyscrasia	None known	Yes
Sulfonamides	Allergic reactions	Kernicterus, hemolysis	Yes
Vancomycin	Ototoxicity and nephrotoxicity	None known	?
	Probably safe		
Erythromycin base	Gastrointestinal intolerance	None known	Yes
Penicillins	Allergic reactons	None known	Trace
Cephalosporins	Allergic reactions	None known	Trace

(Adapted from Chow AW, Jewesson PJ: Pharmokinetics and safety of antimicrobial drugs during pregnancy. *Rev Infect Dis* 1985; 7:287)

BIBLIOGRAPHY

Adams HG, Jordan C: Infections in the alcoholic. *Med Clin North Am* 1984; 68:179

Bennett WM, Aronoff GR, Morrison G, et al: Drug prescribing in renal failure: Dosing guidelines for adults. *Am J Kidney Dis* 1983; 3:155

Gaya H: In vitro considerations in monotherapy and combination therapy for severe infections. *Am J Med* 1986; 80(Suppl 5C):75

Gordon JE, Scrimshaw NS: Infectious disease in the malnourished. *Med Clin North Am* 1970; 54:1495

Levy SB: Microbial resistance to antibiotics: An evolving and persistent problem. *Lancet* 1982; 2:83

McCracken GH: Management of bacterial meningitis: Current status and future prospects. *Am J Med* 1984; 76(5A):215

Pizzo PA, Hathorn JW, Hiemenz J, et al: A randomized trial comparing ceftazidime alone with combination antibiotic therapy in cancer patients with fever and neutropenia. *N Engl J Med* 1986; 315:552

Rubin RH, Wolfson JS, Cosimi AB, et al: Infection in the renal transplant patient. *Am J Med* 1981; 70:405

Schimpff S, Satterlee W, Young VM, et al: Empiric therapy with carbenicillin and gentamicin for febrile patients with cancer and granulocytopenia. *N Engl J Med* 1971; 284:1061

XIV. Environmental Hazards

85
Substance Abuse and Withdrawal

ETHANOL

Ethanol (ethyl alcohol) is the most abused drug in this country and is therefore a major medical and social problem. Ethanol is the active ingredient in beer, wine, whiskey, gin, vodka, and a wide array of other beverages.

ACUTE TOXICITY

Common features of ethanol intoxication are shown in Table 85-1. Ethanol is a sedative-hypnotic drug and exerts its primary effects on the central nervous system. Intoxication depends on the rate of rise of the blood alcohol level and the length of time over which it is maintained. Blood alcohol levels of 20 mg/dl to 30 mg/dl are often associated with a mild euphoria, delayed reaction time, decreased inhibition, and alteration in judgment. Most individuals exhibit gross intoxication at levels above 150 mg/dl. Obtundation develops at levels above 300 mg/dl, and death may result from respiratory depression or cardiovascular collapse when levels exceed 400 mg/dl to 500 mg/gl.

TREATMENT OF ACUTE INTOXICATION

Treatment of acute ethanol intoxication is largely supportive. If the patient presents with an altered mental status, 50 mg to 100 mg of thiamine, 25 g of glucose, and 2 mg of naloxone should be administered intravenously. If the patient responds to the administration of glucose or if blood glucose levels are depressed, a continuous infusion of 10% glucose should be given. The airway should be intubated in the obtunded or comatose patient. Positive pressure ventilation should be instituted if alveolar hypoventilation is present. Ipecac or gastric lavage is useful only if performed within 2 hours of ingestion or if multidrug ingestion is suspected. As previously mentioned, alcoholic ketoacidosis is treated with intravenous administration of glucose and saline. Insulin is *not* indicated. Hypothermia should be corrected (see Chapter 86).

TABLE 85-1 CLINICAL MANIFESTATIONS OF ALCOHOL INTOXICATION

Central nervous system
Decreased inhibition
Slowed reaction time
Visual disturbance
Incoordination
Slurred speech
Diplopia
Nystagmus
Lethargy, stupor, coma
Cardiovascular
Vasodilation
Cardiac dysrhythmias
Myocardial depression
Respiratory
Hypoventilation
Aspiration
Metabolic
Electrolyte abnormalities
Hypoglycemia
Hypophosphatemia
Hypomagnesemia
Acid–base disturbance
Respiratory acidosis
Metabolic alkalosis (vomiting)
Metabolic acidosis (alcoholic ketoacidosis)
Gastrointestinal
Gastritis
Increased incidence of peptic ulcer
Pancreatitis
Alcoholic hepatitis
Hematologic
Suppression of all bone marrow cell lines
Other
Suppression of ADH (diuresis)
Increased sweating
Altered temperature regulation

Fluid, electrolyte, and acid–base disturbances are corrected depending on the clinical presentation. Hemodialysis has been used in cases of massive ethanol ingestion.

TREATMENT OF WITHDRAWAL

Clinical manifestations of alcohol withdrawal are shown in Table 85-2. Treatment strategies for alcohol withdrawal depend on the severity of signs and symptoms and therefore must be individualized. In all cases, close observation and reevaluation of response to therapy are necessary. The patient with mild withdrawal should receive thiamine, 50 mg to 100 mg, and an initial

TABLE 85-2 CLINICAL MANIFESTATIONS OF ALCOHOL WITHDRAWAL

Fever
Tremulousness
Diaphoresis
Seizures
Hallucinations
Tachycardia
Tachypnea
Cardiovascular instability
Agitation and confusion

oral dose of chlordiazepoxide, 50 mg to 100 mg, followed by a dose of 25 mg PO q.i.d. for approximately 4 days.

Work done by Thompson and others indicates the value of intravenous diazepam in severe withdrawal. The dosage is 10 mg IV, followed by 5 mg IV every 5 minutes until the patient is calm: 50 mg to 100 mg or more may be required to initially calm the patient. When the patient is calm, diazepam is given at a dose of approximately 5 mg IV every 4 hours and may be required for 2 to 4 days. The patient must be closely observed for evidence of respiratory or cardiovascular depression during this time. Special caution should be exercised in the patient with pulmonary disease who is withdrawing from alcohol.

COCAINE

Manifestations of cocaine intoxication are summarized in Table 85-3. The powder form of cocaine is commonly used intranasally ("snorting"). Because the drug causes intense vasoconstriction, its absorption by this route becomes limited over time. It is common practice to snort 30 mg to 60 mg of cocaine or more into each nostril and to repeat the process several times an hour over several hours. The euphoric effects of cocaine used in this fashion usually last 1 to 5 hours beyond the last administration.

Smoking cocaine freebase has become a widespread practice. This is usually done with a water pipe or by mixing cocaine freebase with tobacco and rolling the mixture into a cigarette. Vaporized cocaine is then presented to the rich pulmonary vascular bed, and cocaine plasma levels rise rapidly. The euphoric effect with this method only lasts 20 to 30 minutes. Because cocaine hydrochloride decomposes when heated, it cannot be used by this route.

Cocaine is often injected intravenously (usually 16–32 mg) as a single agent or mixed with other drugs such as heroin ("speedball"). Subcutaneous and intramuscular injections are also occasionally seen. Cocaine is readily absorbed from most mucosal surfaces; hence, it is also, although less often, administered orally, sublingually, vaginally, or rectally.

TABLE 85-3 CLINICAL MANIFESTATIONS OF COCAINE USE

Anesthetic effect
Localized numbness
Central neuronal depression
Coma
Central nervous system
Euphoria
Alertness
Tremor
Sleeplessness
Agitated behavior
Paranoia
Psychosis
Seizures
Intracerebral hemorrhage
Stroke
Inhibition of neuronal uptake of catecholamines
Sympathetic stimulation
Vasoconstriction (end-organ ischemia)
Muscular hyperactivity
Cardiovascular
Tachycardia
Supraventricular and ventricular tachydysrhythmias
Asystole
Hypertension
Myocardial infarction
Myocarditis
Aortic rupture
Respiratory
Pulmonary edema
Pulmonary hypertension
Respiratory arrest
Septic pulmonary emboli
Pulmonary vascular occlusion
Pneumothorax
Pneumomediastinum
Metabolic/other
Weight loss
Hyperthermia
Rhabdomyolysis
Local and systemic infections
Endocarditis
Nasal mucosal injury
Nasal septum perforation
Chronic rhinitis
Local infections
Obstetric complications

TREATMENT OF ACUTE INTOXICATION

The agitation and psychosis of cocaine overdose can usually be managed with titrated doses of intravenous diazepam (5–20 mg) or haloperidol (5–20 mg). Paralysis with pancuronium bromide (0.1 mg/kg) may be required in patients with persistent muscular activity or hyperthermia. Tracheal intubation and mechanical ventilation are, of course, required in this setting. Seizures are controlled in the usual manner with intravenous diazepam or other standard antiepileptics.

Hyperthermia should be aggressively treated with cool water, fanning, and other measures (see Chapter 66). Hypertension can be effectively treated with nitroprusside (0.5–10 μg/kg/min) or labetalol, 20 mg to 40 mg IV in a titrated fashion. Myocardial infarction and cardiac dysrhythmias are managed in the usual manner. Since the dysrhythmias are frequently secondary to enhanced sympathetic stimulation, β-blockers such as propranolol are usually effective. Calcium channel blockers may be effective in reversing some of the cardiotoxic effects of cocaine.

CLINICAL MANIFESTATIONS OF WITHDRAWAL

Psychological and biochemical dependency on the drug may be intense. Cocaine causes unusual activation of the dopamine system and blocks reuptake especially in the pleasure centers of the brain. Dopamine is trapped in the synapse, where it is metabolized rather than reused, and dopamine reserves become depleted. The result is that normal, basic instinctual needs, such as hunger, thirst, and the sex drive, cannot be met without cocaine. The brain becomes dopamine-deficient, and even a short period of cocaine abstinence results in a very real withdrawal state.

The clinical effects of cocaine withdrawal include depression, irritability, sleep and appetite dysfunction and, worst of all, an intense desire for more cocaine. To the addict, cocaine often is no longer used to feel good but to avoid feeling bad. A supportive environment and professional drug counseling are clearly warranted for the cocaine addict.

OPIOIDS

Illicit administration of opioids occurs in a variety of colorful ways. They may be swallowed, snorted, smoked, or injected subcutaneously ("skin-popping"), intramuscularly, or intravenously. The primary toxic manifestations of opioids are mediated via the mu and kappa receptors in the CNS. The typical patient with opioid intoxication presents in coma, with miotic pupils and shallow respirations. Common clinical effects of these drugs are shown in Table 85-4.

TREATMENT OF ACUTE INTOXICATION

Since the usual cause of death from opioid overdose is ventilatory failure, the most urgent intervention is airway management and ventilation. Intravenous access should be obtained as soon as possible. This may be a difficult task because intravenous drug addicts go to extreme lengths to obtain access. Peripheral veins may not be available, requiring central ve-

TABLE 85-4 CLINICAL MANIFESTATIONS OF OPIOID INTOXICATION

Central nervous system
Analgesia
Apathy
Lethargy
Seizures
Coma
Ventilatory depression
Nausea
Emesis
Miosis
Respiratory
Histamine release—bronchospasm
Pulmonary edema
Cardiovascular
Venous dilation
Preload reduction
Hypotension
Gastrointestinal
Decreased peristalsis
Decreased hydrochloric acid secretion
Constipation
Genitourinary
Urinary retention
Integument
Histamine release—urticaria, pruritus

nous cannulation. Titrated volume expansion should be administered to the hypotensive patient.

Naloxone, a pure opioid antagonist, reverses all of the opioid-induced CNS and ventilatory depressant effects. The dose required to reverse opioid effects depends on the amount of opioid administered. Intravenous naloxone in a dose of 0.4 mg to 0.8 mg is recommended for the obtunded patient without signs of ventilatory depression. An initial dose of 2 mg is recommended in patients with ventilatory depression. Larger doses may be required in patients who have administered large quantities of opioids. Some opioids (codeine, propoxyphene, diphenoxylate, pentazocine, butorphanol and nalbuphine) require more naloxone than others for reversal of depressant effects. If the altered mental status is not reversed in several minutes, larger doses of naloxone are indicated. Naloxone can be given in doses of 2 mg IV every 4 minutes as necessary, to a total dose of 20 mg. If CNS depression is not reversed by 20 mg of naloxone, alternate etiologies should be aggressively addressed (*e.g.*, hypoglycemia, hypothermia, head trauma). Close observation of the patient following naloxone administration is warranted because of its short half-life. After 20 to 30 minutes, toxic opioid side effects often reappear. The patient may require repeated bolus injections of naloxone, or a continuous infusion may be started. The initial amount of naloxone required to reverse the CNS effects is given each hour as a continuous infusion. Additional boluses may be required as the infusion is started.

CLINICAL MANIFESTATIONS OF WITHDRAWAL

Early signs and symptoms of opioid withdrawal usually occur 4 to 10 hours after the last dose of drug and progress through fairly predictable stages (Table 85-5). The timing of withdrawal symptoms varies with different drugs and from person to person. Heroin withdrawal symptoms begin as early as 4 hours after the last dose, while symptoms of methadone withdrawal may not begin for 2 days. If untreated, symptoms of opioid withdrawal may last from 1 to 3 weeks. Naloxone may abruptly precipitate life-threatening withdrawal symptoms in opioid addicts. Therefore, the minimal dose required to reestablish consciousness should be used in these patients. Oral clonidine is often effective in eliminating the subjective symptoms of opioid withdrawal. It has been successfully coupled with naltrexone as a means of withdrawal from methadone therapy (clonidine 5 μg/kg PO t.i.d.; naltrexone 1 mg PO on day 1, titrated to a 50-mg maintenance dose on day 5).

TABLE 85-5 CLINICAL MANIFESTATIONS OF OPIOID WITHDRAWAL

Early (4–10 hours)
Yawning
Lacrimation
Rhinorrhea
Sneezing
Sweating
Intermediate (12–18 hours)
Restless sleep
Piloerection
Restlessness
Irritability
Anorexia
Flushing
Tachycardia
Tremor
Hyperthermia
Late (> 24 hours)
Fever
Nausea
Vomiting
Abdominal pain
Diarrhea
Difficulty sleeping
Muscle spasm
Joint pain
Involuntary ejaculation
Suicidal ideation

For more information, please see Chapter 61 in Civetta JM, Taylor RW, Kirby RR: Critical Care. *Philadelphia: J. B. Lippincott, 1988*

BIBLIOGRAPHY

Cregler LL, Mark H: Medical complications of cocaine abuse. *N Engl J Med* 1986; 315:1495

Duberstein JL, Kaufman DM: A clinical study of an epidemic of heroin intoxication and heroin-induced pulmonary edema. *Am J Med* 1971; 51:704

Friedman HS, Lieber CS: Cardiotoxicity of alcohol. *Cardiovasc Med* 1977; 2:111

Isner JM, Estes NAM II, Thompson PD, et al: Acute cardiac events temporally related to cocaine abuse. *N Engl J Med* 1986; 315:1438

Johnston RE, Reier CE: Acute respiratory effects of ethanol in man. *Clin Pharmacol Ther* 1973; 14:503

Lowenfels AB, Miller TT: Alcohol and trauma. *Ann Emerg Med* 1984; 13:1056

Olson KR, Benowitz NL: Life-threatening cocaine intoxication. In Dellinger RP (ed): *The Substance Abuser: Problems in Critical Care*, p 95. Philadelphia, JB Lippincott, 1987

Sellers EM, Kalant H: Drug therapy: Alcohol intoxication and withdrawal. *N Engl J Med* 1976; 294:757

Thompson WL, Johnson AD, Maddrey WL, et al: Diazepam and paraldehyde for treatment of severe delirium tremens: A controlled trial. *Ann Intern Med* 1975; 82:175

Uhde TW, Redmond DE Jr, Kleber HD: Clonidine suppresses the opioid abstinence syndrome without clonidine-withdrawal symptoms: A blind inpatient study. *Psychiatry Res* 1980; 2:37

86
Temperature-Related Injuries

HYPOTHERMIA

Hypothermia is defined as a core body temperature less than 35°C (95°F). A listing of causes of hypothermia is included in Table 86-1.

The exact incidence of hypothermia is not known. However it is generally thought to be an underrecognized condition, particularly in the elderly. In the United States, clinically significant hypothermia is most commonly seen in alcoholic patients. Any clinical history suggestive of disorders listed in Table 86-1 mandates an accurate assessment of body temperature. Many thermometers in widespread hospital use are not calibrated below 35°C, and may contribute to underdiagnosis.

CLINICAL PRESENTATION

Mild hypothermia is characterized by a core body temperature between 35°C and 32°C. Blood pressure, heart rate, and respiratory rate are initially increased, but may later decline as the syndrome progresses. Muscle tone is increased and is frequently accompanied by active shivering. The level of consciousness may also be depressed and is typically manifest as stupor or confusion. Peripheral vasoconstriction is evidenced by diminished pulses, pallor or acrocyanosis, and coolness of the extremities to touch. Cardiac output falls as the heart cools and myocardial contractility decreases.

As the hypothermic condition worsens, it reaches a moderate state at a body temperature between 32°C and 28°C. These patients are more obtunded and are often incoherent, when they are capable of verbal expression. Coma usually supervenes at body temperatures less than 30°C. At this point, all vital signs are invariably subnormal. Compensatory mechanisms such as shivering are now absent, and muscle tone is quite rigid. Bowel sounds are absent. If coupled with stiff or "boardlike" abdominal musculature and a dropping blood pressure, hypothermia may mimic intra-abdominal sepsis, particularly if the body temperature is not accurately measured.

Hypothermia is considered severe at body temperatures less than 28°C.

TABLE 86-1 ACCIDENTAL HYPOTHERMIA—CLINICAL CAUSES

Anatomic	*Pathophysiologic Events*
Central nervous system	Metabolic
Head trauma	Hypoglycemia
Tumor	Hypothyroidism
Stroke	Hypoadrenalism
Wernicke's encephalopathy	Panhypopituitarism
Shapiro's syndrome	Diabetic ketoacidosis
Sarcoidosis	Anorexia nervosa (protein calorie malnutrition)
Spinal cord transection	Loss of dermal integrity
Environmental	Burns
Exposure	Erythroderma
Outdoor activities/exhaustion	Ichthyosis
Cold water immersion	Psoriasis
Inadequate indoor heating (particularly in the elderly)	Infection
	Generalized sepsis
Drug Related	Chronic health status
Ethanol	Advanced age (impaired thermoregulatory mechanisms)
Anesthetic agents (paralytic)	Chronic heart failure
Phenothiazines	Chronic renal failure
Barbiturates	Chronic hepatic insufficiency

In addition to the apparent absence of higher neurologic function, brain stem and deep tendon reflexes also cannot be demonstrated. The patient is either apneic or has an agonal respiratory pattern. Lack of a pulse is most frequently due to spontaneous ventricular fibrillation and less frequently to an agonal rhythm or asystole.

As the core body temperature falls, the basal metabolic rate decreases from a respiratory quotient of 0.82 at 37°C to 0.65 at 30°C. This results in decreased renal tubular cell reabsorptive function and the so-called "cold diuresis," which usually persists until intravascular volume depletion occurs.

Laboratory findings include evidence of hemoconcentration (elevated hemoglobin and hematocrit levels), an elevated serum glucose concentration, a decreased serum potassium concentration, and elevated serum aminotransferase and serum amylase levels. Metabolic acidosis also develops as a result of extremity hypoperfusion and increased energy consumption with shivering, both of which contribute to lactate generation. The oxyhemoglobin dissociation curve shifts to the left as a direct effect of the lowered temperature. In addition, blood gas measurement of the *p*H is depressed and the Pa_{O_2} increased if the gas solubility coefficients are not corrected for temperature. The EKG demonstrates progressive prolongation of the PR, QRS, and QT intervals as hypothermia worsens. The Osborn J wave following the QRS complex is pathognomonic of hypothermia, but is frequently absent. Ventricular and supraventricular ectopy are commonly seen, and further, the threshold for ventricular fibrillation is decreased and may be precipitated by excessive handling of the patient.

THERAPY

The mainstay of clinical therapy for these patients is the return of core body temperature to normal. However, a controversy exists as to how this should be achieved. Other means of supportive therapy should aggressively continue.

Passive external rewarming consists of adding an insulating layer to the patient (*i.e.,* a blanket) and allowing his own heat-generating mechanisms to restore body temperature. This method is adequate only in selected situations of mild hypothermia in which complications of the disorder are not yet evident and rapid rewarming is not required.

Active external warming uses devices which are placed in contact with the hypothermic patient (*i.e.,* hot water bottles, submersion in a tank of warm water, or heating blankets). Active external and core rewarming techniques are necessary for resuscitation from severe forms of hypothermia. The definitive method in humans is not clear, however. Early reports with active external rewarming describe hypotension or "rewarming shock" associated with peripheral vasodilatation and intravascular volume depletion as rewarming proceeded. These problems are for the most part obviated if volume repletion is promptly established and maintained during rewarming.

Invasive core rewarming methods include peritoneal dialysis, hemodialysis, partial cardiopulmonary bypass, thoracotomy with mediastinal irrigation, rectal and gastric lavage, and mechanical ventilation with warm, humidified air. In theory, these techniques afford core rewarming which occurs in parallel with cardiac rewarming. As a result, the cardiac output, and therefore tissue perfusion, should be reestablished in proportion to increasing cellular metabolic demands as the respiratory quotient returns toward normal. Notably, core rewarming shortens the interval during which cardiopulmonary resuscitation is required in those patients who suffer cardiopulmonary arrest, and it decreases the volume of fluids required for repletion of the intravascular volume, but does not appear to affect outcome.

HEAT STROKE SYNDROME

Heat stroke syndrome has been characterized diagnostically in various ways, but may generally be considered as a heat-related illness with a documented body temperature equal to or greater than 41.1°C (106°F), or as a syndrome with a body temperature of 40.6°C (105°F) or greater, anhidrosis, altered mental status, or both. The syndrome may be further considered as either exertional or nonexertional (classic heat stroke). *Exertional heat stroke* is typically seen in healthy young adults who overexert themselves during times of unusually high ambient temperatures or in an environment to which they are not acclimatized. Their thermoregulatory mechanisms are intact, at least initially; however, endogenous heat production outstrips heat-dissipating mechanisms. *Classic heat stroke,* in contrast, is nonexertional and is seen in elderly or debilitated individuals with chronic underlying diseases. These patients also present during times of increased ambient temperatures; however, their thermoregulatory mechanisms are impaired from the start. A number of other conditions and drugs are associated with the development of heat stroke syndrome and are included in Table 86-2.

CLINICAL PRESENTATION

Although the typical history for the patient with exertional heat stroke syndrome may seem self-evident, little or no clinical warning may precede the onset of classic heat stroke. As thermoregulatory mechanisms fail, the body temperature rapidly climbs, and the patient can quickly lapse from the apparent baseline health status to coma or obtundation with a high core body temperature.

In addition to an elevated body temperature, anhidrosis/hypohidrosis, and mental status changes, a number of characteristic laboratory features have also been described, depending on the severity of the pathophysiologic derangements. Significant dehydration is particularly seen in those patients suffering from exertional heat stroke syndrome and may be reflected as elevated blood urea nitrogen and creatinine levels, as well as hemoconcentration. Sodium, potassium, phosphate, calcium, and magnesium serum con-

TABLE 86-2 HEAT STROKE SYNDROME–ASSOCIATED FACTORS AND CAUSES

Exertional
- Environmental
  - Supranormal ambient temperatures
  - Increased humidity levels
- Physiologic
  - Lack of physical conditioning (overexertion; *i.e.,* military recruits)
  - Lack of acclimatization

Nonexertional
- Environmental
  - Supranormal ambient temperatures
  - Increased humidity levels
  - Lack of air-conditioning
  - Lack of shrubbery/trees around dwelling
  - Height of home floor above ground level
- Physiologic (impaired thermoregulation)
  - Advanced age
  - Chronic disease
    - Alcoholism
    - Congestive heart failure
    - Renal insufficiency
    - Diabetes mellitus
    - COPD
    - Dementia/schizophrenia
    - Cystic fibrosis
  - Thryotoxicosis
  - Hypokalemia
  - Dehydration

Drugs
- Alcohol
- Diuretics
- Phenothiazines
- Anti-Parkinsonians
- Anticholinergics
- Beta-blockers
- Tricyclic antidepressants
- Amphetamines
- Hallucinogens
- Butyrophenones

centrations are frequently low early in the clinical course of the syndrome. Sodium, potassium, and magnesium losses occur primarily through increased sweating and can be massive. Hypokalemia may also decrease the ability of the patient to secrete sweat, along with decreasing skeletal muscle blood flow, both of which may impair the dissipation of heat. Hyperkalemia may ensue, however, if significant skeletal muscle damage and cellular lysis develop. Hypocalcemia is usually seen in those patients with significant rhabdomyolysis, and is primarily a result of calcium salt precipitation and deposition in injured skeletal muscle (see Chap. 79). Some degree of creatine kinase (CK) elevation is invariably present and is considered by some to be a necessary diagnostic feature of the syndrome. These elevations may be extreme in cases of severe rhabdomyolysis.

Hematologic findings regarding the white and red blood cell counts are inconstant. Disseminated intravascular coagulation (DIC) is uncommonly seen but is a poor prognostic marker when present. A mixed acid–base disorder of metabolic acidosis and respiratory alkalosis is most common. Hyperthermia alone can cause hyperventilation and a primary respiratory alkalosis. However, the presence of hypoperfusion, tissue hypoxia, and anaerobic metabolism all lead to lactic acidosis with respiratory compensation.

A number of specific complications may arise in association with heat stroke and must be considered because they have particular therapeutic needs. These include myocardial failure and dysrhythmias, acute renal insufficiency, rhabdomyolysis, seizures, hepatic failure, and DIC. Their presence may be suggested by the laboratory findings discussed above.

THERAPY

Survival of heat stroke depends on promptly recognizing the syndrome and immediately lowering the core body temperature. Indeed, survival appears to be inversely related to the intensity and the duration of hyperpyrexia, with duration being of greater significance.

Effective lowering of the core body temperature usually requires only external cooling techniques. These include immersion in an ice water bath or simply wetting the skin with either cold water or alcohol, followed by the use of fans to facilitate evaporation and heat dissipation. Gastric or peritoneal lavage with iced saline are only rarely required in case of refractory temperature elevation or when thermogenesis is ongoing (as in malignant hyperthermia, discussed below). Vigorous skin massage should accompany immersion cooling techniques to prevent dermal stasis of cooled blood as local cutaneous vasoconstriction occurs. As the temperature approaches 39°C, efforts to cool the patient should be terminated, as the body temperature will continue to fall 1°C to 2°C. From a practical perspective, cooling by immersion may prove unsatisfactory when cardiac monitoring, therapy for events such as seizures, or airway protection are needed. Evaporative methods are equally effective and allow the patient to be placed on a bed and treated as the usual intensive care patient. The intravenous administration of chlorpromazine in doses of 10 mg to 50 mg every 6 hours may also prove useful in preventing shivering and the associated thermogenesis.

The need for intravascular volume repletion should be individualized and carefully assessed. Dehydration may not be a prominent feature of classic heat stroke syndrome, but is much more common in patients with exertionally related heat injury. Hypotension may be a reflection of either volume depletion, coupled with peripheral vascular vasodilation, or of primary myocardial dysfunction, in which case little volume resuscitation is needed.

MALIGNANT HYPERTHERMIA AND THE NEUROLEPTIC MALIGNANT SYNDROME

Malignant hyperthermia and the neuroleptic malignant syndrome, like environmental heat injury, are disorders of body temperature related to an inequity between heat generation and heat dissipation. Unlike heat stroke, though, endogenous heat production, without the influence of ambient temperatures, is responsible for the elevation in core body temperature. Physiologic mechanisms to dissipate heat, along with the hypothalamic regulation of temperature may also be impaired, particularly in the neuroleptic malignant syndrome. In addition to hyperpyrexia, both of these conditions share profound muscular rigidity as a common feature. Malignant hyperthermia and the neuroleptic malignant syndrome are uniquely characterized by their association with an assortment of drugs. Although other predisposing conditions have been described in these patients, these drugs are usually essential for the development of these syndromes. A complete listing is included in Table 86-3.

TABLE 86-3 DRUGS ASSOCIATED WITH MALIGNANT HYPERTHERMIA AND THE NEUROLEPTIC MALIGNANT SYNDROME

Malignant Hyperthermia
- Volatile anesthetics
  - Halothane
  - Cyclopropane
  - Enflurane
  - Methoxyflurane
  - Isoflurane
  - Sevoflurane
  - Diethylether
- Depolarizing muscle relaxants
  - Succinylcholine
  - Decamethonium

Neuroleptic Malignant Syndrome
- Phenothiazines
  - Fluphenazine
  - Chlorpromazine
  - Levomepromazine

Neuroleptic Malignant Syndrome (cont.)
  - Thioridazine
  - Trimeprazine
  - Trifluoperazine
  - Prochlorperazine
- Butyrophenones
  - Haloperidol
  - Bromoperidol
- Thioxanthenes
  - Thiothixene
- Dibenzoxepines
  - Loxapine
- Dopamine-depleting drugs
  - Alpha-methyltyrosine
  - Tetrabenazine
- Withdrawal of dopamine agonists
  - Levodopa
  - Levodopa/carbidopa
  - Amantadine

CLINICAL PRESENTATION

Malignant hyperthermia is characterized by the development of trismus (seen as the initial event in 50% of patients), followed by whole body rigidity, and a marked increase in core body temperature, as general anesthesia is used. This process may begin at any time during anesthetic induction, or thereafter, and proceed with frightening rapidity. The metabolic consequences of this syndrome include a combined respiratory and metabolic acidosis, along with elevated serum potassium, sodium, and calcium levels. If significant myonecrosis follows, serum potassium concentrations may rise to life-threatening levels, and the serum calcium concentration may fall rapidly as calcium salt deposition occurs in injured muscle. Early findings which suggest a malignant hyperthermic crisis may be imminent include masseter muscle contractions following succinylcholine administration, cyanosis, increasing carbon dioxide production, tachycardia, and hypertension. Strong consideration should be given to aborting anesthesia when these findings appear and malignant hyperthermia is suspected. As the syndrome progresses, the profound increases in core body temperature ususally leave little doubt as to their cause.

The neuroleptic malignant syndrome should be suspected in patients given virtually any neuroleptic drug, but particularly those in Table 86-3, who subsequently develop signs of muscular rigidity, dystonia, or unexplained catatonic behavior. Diaphoresis, tachycardia, hypertension or hypotension, and an increased respiratory rate also accompany its development as markers of the underlying autonomic instability. Temperature elevation usually follows these findings. Laboratory data are variable, with the exception of CK and serum glutamic-oxaloacetic transaminase (SGOT) elevation in those patients who develop rhabdomyolysis.

THERAPY

Successful treatment of either of these two disorders depends on early clinical recognition and prompt withdrawal of the suspected inciting agent. In malignant hyperthermia, discontinuation alone is often adequate therapy, provided the syndrome is not yet well established. Recovery from the neuroleptic malignant syndrome may similarly occur with discontinuation of the drug; however, 5 to 7 days may be needed for the patient to return to baseline.

Sodium dantrolene is the drug of choice in malignant hyperthermia and should be administered to patients in whom hyperpyrexia continues to develop following anesthetic removal. The recommended dose is 2 mg/kg intravenously. This dose may be repeated every 5 minutes, up to a total of 10 mg/kg. This should be accomplished before instituting any other supportive therapeutic measures. Sodium dantrolene acts by inhibiting calcium release from the sarcoplasmic reticulum, thereby decreasing available calcium for ongoing muscle contraction. Muscle weakness may occur following sodium dantrolene administration; however, respiratory muscle function and airway protective measures typically remain intact.

The role of sodium dantrolene in the neuroleptic malignant syndrome is less well defined, although it has been shown to be effective in reducing thermogenesis in multiple case reports. Doses used have been similar to those recommended in malignant hyperthermia. Administration of greater than 10 mg/kg has been associated with hepatic toxicity.

For more information, please see Chapter 59 in Civetta JM, Taylor RW, Kirby RR: Critical Care. *Philadelphia: J. B. Lippincott, 1988*

BIBLIOGRAPHY

Curley FJ, Irwin RS: Disorders of temperature control: Hyperthermia (Part I). *J. Intensive Care Med* 1986; 1:5

Gronert GA: Malignant hyperthermia. *Anesthesiology* 1980; 53:395

Guze BH, Baxter LR: Neuroleptic malignant syndrome. *N Engl J Med* 1985; 313:163

Hart GR, Anderson RJ, Crumpler CP, et al: Epidemic classical heat stroke: Clinical characteristics and course of 28 patients. *Medicine* 1982; 61:189

Jones TS, Liang AP, Kilbourne EM, et al: Morbidity and mortality associated with the July 1980 heat wave in St. Louis and Kansas City, MO. *JAMA* 1982; 247:3327

Kilbourne EM, Choi K, Jones TS, et al: Risk factors for heat-stroke. A case control study. *JAMA* 1982; 247:3332

Martyn JW: Diagnosis and treating hypothermia. *Can Med Assoc J* 1981; 125:1089

Moss J: Accidental severe hypothermia. *Surg Gynecol Obstet* 1986; 162:501

Rueler JB: Hypothermia: Pathophysiology, clinical setting, and management. *Ann Intern Med* 1978; 89:519

87
Electrical Injuries

CLASSIFICATION

Exposure to electrical current can be categorized according to the type of current (alternating or direct) and to the voltage level of the source. Most electrical injuries occur as the result of contact with alternating current whereas injury from direct current is primarily limited to the uncommon lightning injury victim. The electrical source is considered low tension if the voltage potential is less than 1000 volts and high tension when the voltage exceeds this value. Alternating-current injuries are felt to be more dangerous than a direct-current injury of comparable voltage primarily because of the tetanizing effect of alternating current, which often "locks" the victim's grasping hand to the current source and prolongs contact time. This tends to occur less frequently in high-voltage injuries in which the victim is often literally thrown clear from the electrical source. Alternating current also has a definite propensity to induce ventricular fibrillation, an effect not usually seen in victims of direct-current injury.

CLINICAL MANIFESTATIONS AND MANAGEMENT

Because of the complex nature of electrical injury, the clinical manifestations are presented system-by-system and specific management points are addressed therein.

CARDIOPULMONARY

The cardiopulmonary system is particularly sensitive to the acute effects of alternating current. As little as 100 milliamps (ma) of alternating current is sufficient to produce ventricular fibrillation. Relatively low levels of current across the chest also are capable of inducing tetanic contractions of the respiratory muscles leading to respiratory arrest. An effect on the central respiratory center has been postulated but not proven. Institution of cardiopulmonary resuscitation is of critical importance and should be performed even if prolonged arrest has occurred because complete recovery in this situation has been documented. The usual advanced cardiac life support measures should be followed. After resuscitation and transfer to a medical facility, all patients who have sustained loss of consciousness, cardiac arrest, dysrhythmias, EKG changes of acute myocardial infarction, or who have been subjected to a trans-chest current should undergo EKG monitoring.

Nonspecific EKG changes have been seen in up to 50% of electrical injury victims. Housinger and coworkers in a study of electrical injury victims found creatine kinase-MB (CK-MB) isoenzyme elevation in 56% even though ^{99m}Tc pyrophosphate scans and serial EKGs showed no evidence of myocardial infarction. Furthermore, although cases of well-documented myocardial infarction with acute electrical injury exist, review of several large series since 1969 have revealed this to be an uncommon event. It is apparent that cardiac isoenzymes do not reflect actual myocardial damage (the elevation of CK-MB has been rather soundly traced to skeletal muscle origin by the work of McBride). Late cardiac complications, including repetitive or hemodynamically significant dysrhythmias, also appear to be very uncommon. These are important points in that multiple surgical procedures are usually necessary in the electrically injured patient and should not be delayed on the basis of questionable cardiac findings, as these procedures appear well tolerated.

Other cardiac findings include right bundle branch block and transient global hypokinesis.

RENAL

There is little evidence to support direct renal injury from electric current. Instead, renal toxicity in electrical injury victims occurs as a result of volume depletion and shock and most importantly from acute tubular necrosis secondary to pigmenturia. The source of these hemochromogens is primarily necrotic muscle and occasionally hemolysis. Aggressive fluid management is key in preventing this occasionally fatal complication.

NERVOUS SYSTEM

A wide variety of neurologic sequelae have been described in victims of electrical injury and may take the form of cerebral, spinal cord, or peripheral nerve injury. Immediately following electrical exposure, up to 70% of victims experience loss of consciousness or transient paralysis followed by recovery within 5 to 10 minutes. Confusion, agitation, headache, mood disturbance, and retrograde amnesia are common sequelae, while seizures and autonomic disturbances occur less often within the first several days.

Aside from the medical treatment of seizures, these manifestations of electrical injury have limited impact on management. Persistent or late-onset coma is likely to be related to cerebral edema, closed-head trauma or cerebral thrombosis, and generally portends a poor prognosis. A search for potentially reversible conditions with the use of computed tomographic (CT) scanning of the head appears reasonable. An aggressive approach to monitor and control intracranial pressure is advocated by some.

The most commonly injured peripheral neural structures are the ulnar and median nerves. Delayed nerve injury may occur due to scarring.

MUSCULOSKELETAL AND CUTANEOUS INJURIES

Musculoskeletal and cutaneous injuries frequently dominate the clinical picture in these patients and may consist of injuries not directly related to current flow. Examples include trauma as a result of the victim falling or being thrown by the current source, or as a result of the violent tetanic contractions frequently encountered in electrical injury. The end results may include long bone fractures, spinal fracture, joint dislocations, or splenic rupture. The frequency with which these events occur warrants a careful search for underlying traumatic injury by physical and radiographic examination. Unconscious victims should be treated with cervical immobilization until cervical fractures have been ruled out.

The direct tissue damage produced by electric current consists primarily of deep tissue coagulation necrosis. The goals of management are twofold. First, every attempt is made to salvage affected limbs. The second goal is to limit the systemic effects of necrotic muscle. The untoward effects of undebrided tissues include pyomyositis, sepsis, renal injury, and hypotension (several anecdotes attest to the reversal of hypotension following debridement of necrotic muscle—felt to be a result of the elimination of undefined "toxins"). Fortunately, both of these goals are realized simultaneously by the early exploratory surgery of affected limbs. Indications for early fasciotomy include a charred, mummified distal limb, a grossly swollen extremity, or evidence of a compartment syndrome. In other patients, findings are much more subtle and are only apparent on close clinical follow-up. In that setting, marked elevation of serum CK enzyme levels should prompt further search for occult devitalized muscle.

The cutaneous sequelae of electrical injury vary from the focal, full-thickness burns at the entry and exit sites to more extensive flame burns. In general, burns in electrical victims average less than 20% of the total body surface area. At times the extent of cutaneous injury may obscure underlying deep tissue damage. When this possibility exists, exploratory surgery of the involved limbs should be considered. The management of the cutaneous burns should follow standard therapies for thermal injuries.

LIGHTNING INJURY

The direct current of a lightning strike differs from the more common alternating current injury in several ways. It has been often stated that lightning strike results in asystole, unlike the propensity toward ventricular fibrillation seen in alternating-current victims. However, there have been numerous case

TABLE 87-1 MANIFESTATIONS OF LIGHTNING INJURY

Prolonged cardiorespiratory arrest (asystole) followed by complete recovery
Repetitive ventricular dysrhythmias
Myocardial necrosis
Autonomic dsyfunction—labile hypertension, bronchospasm, spontaneous normalization of pulseless, cyanotic limbs
Arborizing, "spiderlike" cutaneous burns
Deep tissue injury uncommon

reports of ventricular fibrillation in lightning victims. This may occur as a result of prolonged respiratory arrest and its attendant hypoxia and acidosis. Repetitive ventricular dysrhythmias may also occur in lightning injury. Myocardial necrosis has been well documented in lightning injury but appears to be uncommon.

A unique occurrence in lightning injury is marked autonomic dysfunction. This includes labile hypertension and bronchospasm and findings of cyanotic, pulseless limbs which spontaneously revert to normal. It is this latter phenomenon which allows for a somewhat expectant approach to the cyanotic limb in lightning victims, with delay of any attempt at fasciotomy for several hours.

Also important are the complete neurologic recoveries reported in lightning victims after prolonged arrest. Some believe that immediate, total cessation of metabolic activity occurs in this setting, delaying degenerative processes and allowing full recovery. It has been suggested that in the setting of multiple victim lightning accidents, triage priority should be given to the apparent "dead" victims rather than the wakeful but confused victims and that advanced resuscitative measures should be continued for several hours.

Deep tissue necrosis and its complications occur distinctly less often in lightning injury victims, but should still be suspected during evaluation. The cutaneous burns often take unusual arborizing or spiderlike configurations. These patterns reflect an external path of the direct current on the victim's skin, resulting in a "flash" burn.

Contrary to population opinion, lightning strike has a generally good prognosis with survival estimated to be 60% to 70% (Table 87-1).

For more information, please see Chapter 63 in Civetta JM, Taylor RW, Kirby RR: Critical Care. *Philadelphia: J. B. Lippincott, 1988*

BIBLIOGRAPHY

Dixon GR: The evaluation and management of electrical injuries. *Crit Care Med* 1983; 11(5):384

Haberal M: Electrical burns: A five-year experience—1985 Evans Lecture. *J Trauma* 1986; 26(2):103

Housinger TA, Green L, Shahangian S, Saffle JR, et al: A prospective study of myocardial damage in electrical injuries. *J Trauma* 1985; 25(2):122
Hunt JL, Sato RM, Baxter CR: Acute electrical burns. *Arch Surg* 1980; 115:434
McBride JW, Labrosse KR, McCoy HG, Ahrenholz DH, et al: Is serum creatinine kinase-MB in electrically injured patients predictive of myocardial injury? *JAMA* 1986; 255(6):764
Parshley PF: Aggressive approach to the extremity damaged by electric current. *Am J Surg* 1985; 150:78
Purdue GF, Hunt JL: Electrocardiographic monitoring after electrical injury: Necessity or luxury. *J Trauma* 1986; 26(2):166
Sances A, Larson SJ, Myklebast J, Cusick JF: Electrical injuries. *Surg Gynecol Obstet* 1979; 149:97

88 Poisoning and Toxic Exposure

Poisoning is a major worldwide health problem causing up to 3% of emergency room attendances and only a slightly smaller percentage of hospital admissions. The incidence of poisoning has been increasing throughout this century and current estimates suggest that between two and ten million events occur annually in the United States.

Five types of poisoning are generally recognized.

1. *Accidental poisoning* is most frequently encountered in children, but also occurs in adults as a result of work and school mishaps (e.g., ingestion of garden poisons previously decanted into beer bottles).
2. *Deliberate self-poisoning* is the most common form in adults and is also referred to as attempted suicide, parasuicide, and pseudocide.
3. *Homicidal poisoning* is uncommon in contemporary society although over the past few years, several such cases have occurred from cyanide-laced analgesic capsules.
4. *Nonaccidental poisoning* is a variant of the battered child syndrome and involves the administration of poison to a child by a parent.
5. *Therapeutic poisoning* results from the over-prescription of pharmacologic agents, herbal medicines, and vitamins by medical or lay practitioners.

EPIDEMIOLOGY

Poisoning occurs most commonly in young women (ages 15–35). The tragedy of poisoning is that most victims are young and potentially salvageable, and do not wish to die. The lonely, isolated, and bereaved are prone to self-poisoning, but the disease knows no social or racial barriers. Drug and alcohol abuse and psychological disorders also predispose to acute poisoning. Although the mortality rate for acute poisoning is low, this rate following an episode of poisoning is many times greater than that of the general population.

The range of potential poisons, both pharmacologic and nonpharmacologic, is enormous. Commonly abused agents include analgesics, sedative hypnotics, antidepressants, and alcohol. Recent trends have seen a declining incidence of barbiturate and benzodiazepine intoxication and a disturbing increase in the incidence of acetaminophen ingestion. Up to 73% of acute poisonings involve more than one agent.

RECOGNITION

In the absence of a reliable history, diagnosis may be difficult because the range of clinical presentations is broad. Only a few poisons (organophosphates, narcotics, anticholinergics, and salicylates) produce classic clinical patterns. Early diagnosis is a high priority since the efficacy of most therapeutic regimens depends on their early administration. Accurate, early diagnosis is also valuable in the avoidance of unnecessary, potentially hazardous, and expensive investigations such as computed cerebral tomography. Accurate diagnosis has important medicolegal significance in nonaccidental poisoning and is invaluable in the management of the convalescent patient who denies attempted suicide. Diagnosis depends on a high index of suspicion in the appropriate clinical situation, a careful history and physical examination, and the judicious use of laboratory facilities. In the absence of a reliable history, evidence of poisoning should be specifically sought where the clinical presentation involves coma, collapse, convulsion, focal cerebral defect, respiratory or cardiac arrest, hyper- or hypothermia, and hypotension.

HISTORY

History is usually available and reliable with children but may not be with adults and adolescents. Relatives, friends, acquaintances, and medical practitioners may be more useful sources of valuable information. A judicious search of the patient and his residence and belongings may provide evidence of poisoning. All medication packets should be assumed to have been full unless certain knowledge to the contrary is available. Previous hospital records may indicate a propensity toward drug abuse and the identity of potential intoxicants.

PHYSICAL EXAMINATION

The initial assessment should address the adequacy of the circulation and ventilation which should be ensured before proceeding. Specific evidence of intoxication may then be sought. Baseline neurologic and cardiorespiratory assessment provides an essential platform for the assessment of therapeutic urgency and subsequent progress. Core temperature must be assessed with a thermometer that can measure subnormal temperatures.

LABORATORY

There are several areas in which both the general and the toxicology laboratory provide useful information. General laboratory tests may suggest other diagnoses (e.g., hypoglycemia as a cause of coma) or provide evidence of poisoning (e.g., hyperosmolar acidosis in methanol intoxication). They are essential to detect and monitor the complications of poisoning. The toxicology laboratory may confirm or exclude specific intoxication and provide a guide to the severity of the poisoning and the need for specific therapy (e.g., acetaminophen levels). However, screening for poisons is a potentially misleading practice because many poisons are not detected by routine drug screens, the severity of poisoning does not (in most instances) correlate with blood concentrations of poison, and both false-positive and false-negative values have been reported. Routine laboratory tests (blood glucose levels, arterial blood gases, electrolytes) are most useful and should always be performed in the comatose patient. Drug screens and assays are beneficial in specific instances and only when the limitations of the available facilities are known.

THERAPY

Most patients with acute poisoning will survive with appropriately administered supportive care. Specific therapeutic maneuvers are effective only if they are instituted early in the course of the poisoning. Antidotes are available for a small minority of poisons only. Other semispecific remedies are indicated in particular instances only when the risk associated with the poisoning is greater than that associated with the therapy.

SUPPORTIVE CARE

The following items are particularly important:

1. Airway protection. Acid aspiration has a higher mortality rate than most poisons.
2. Oxygenation and ventilation.
3. Maintenance of circulation with appropriate fluid and inotropic therapy.
4. Control of cardiac rhythm. Conventional agents may be inappropriate in drug-induced dysrhythmias. Metabolic control may be more effective.
5. Control of temperature and convulsions.
6. Protection of the unconscious patient.

MINIMIZATION OF ABSORPTION

Careful skin washing reduces absorption of agents absorbed transcutaneously. Removal of patients from the source of inhaled toxins is an obvious, important maneuver. Induced gastric emptying with emesis or lavage is potentially dangerous but effective if instituted early. Activated charcoal is generally safe and effective if used early; it also enhances the elimination of agents which are actively or passively secreted into the gastrointestinal tract.

ENHANCED ELIMINATION

This can be achieved for a small number of poisons by the administration of activated charcoal. Hemodialysis and hemoperfusion also have limited applicability for severe intoxication with a similarly small number of drugs. Forced diuresis is now rarely used; it is hazardous and of only limited benefit. Peritoneal dialysis is of only slightly greater efficacy. Fecuresis is dangerous, barely efficacious, and unpleasant for the patient and staff. Most acute poisonings do not require any specific attempt to enhance elimination.

SPECIFIC ANTIDOTES

Alteration of the distribution and metabolism of poisons and the administration of antidotes have a limited overall role, but are life-saving in specific circumstances. These are summarized in Table 88-1.

PSYCHOLOGICAL ASSESSMENT AND INTERVENTION

The subsequent mortality rate of the victims of acute poisoning and the health care costs engendered by repeated parasuicides demand psychological follow-up, although the data indicating its efficacy are conflicting.

TABLE 88-1 AVAILABLE ANTIDOTES

Toxic Agent	Antidote
Acetaminophen	*N*-acetylcysteine
Anticholinergics	Physostigmine
Anticoagulants	Plasma, Vitamin K Protamine sulphate
Beat-blockers	Isoprenaline, glucagon
Cyanide	Nitrites, EDTA, Thiosulphate
Digoxin	Fab fragments
Ethylene glycol	Ethanol
Heavy metals	Dimercaprol
Iron	Deferoxamine
Methanol	Ethanol
Narcotics	Naloxone
Organophosphates	Atropine, pralidoxime
Sympathomimetics	Adrenergic-blockers

SPECIAL CONSIDERATIONS

Right to Die. When suicide is attempted by a patient who has adequately signified his intentions and desire not to be resuscitated, and when it is not possible to alter the physical or psychological factors leading to the suicide, it may not be appropriate to institute therapy.

Poisoning in Hospital. Patients in the hospital may attempt suicide by self-poisoning. In this event, diagnosis may be extremely difficult.

Refusal of Treatment. If patients refuse treatment or aspects of treatment and if such refusal does not have a well-considered, reasonable basis, the physician has a responsibility to provide all requisite life-saving care.

For more information, please see Chapter 60 in Civetta JM, Taylor RW, Kirby RR: Critical Care. *Philadelphia: J. B. Lippincott, 1988*

BIBLIOGRAPHY

Auerbach PS, Osterloh J, Braun O, et al: Efficacy of gastric emptying: Gastric lavage versus emesis induced with impecac. *Ann Emerg Med* 1986; 15:692
Boehnert MT, Lovejoy FH: Value of the QRS duration versus the serum drug level in predicting seizures and ventricular arrhythmias after an acute overdose of tricyclic antidepressants. *N Engl J Med* 1985; 313:474
Cohen MA, Guzzardi LJ: Inhalation of products of combustion. *Ann Emerg Med* 1983; 12:628
Crapo RO: Smoke inhalation injuries. *JAMA* 1981; 246:1694
Done AK: Aspirin overdosage: Incidence, diagnosis and management. *Pediatrics* 1978; 62(suppl):890
Ray JE, Reilly DK, Day RO: Drugs involved in self poisoning: Verification by toxicological analysis. *Med J Aust* 1986; 144:455
Rumack BH, Matthew H: Acetaminophen poisoning and toxicity. *Pediatrics* 1975; 55:871
Rumack BH, Peterson RC, Koch GG, Amara IA: Acetaminophen overdose: 662 cases with evaluation of oral acetylcysteine treatment. *Arch Intern Med* 1981; 141:380
Stern TA, Mulley AG, Thibault GE: Life-threatening overdose: Precipitants and prognosis. *JAMA* 1984; 251:1983
Trunet P, Borda IT, Rouget AV, et al: The role of drug-induced illness in admissions to an intensive care unit. *Int Care Med* 1986; 12:43

89
Snake Envenomation

EPIDEMIOLOGY

Three thousand snake species inhabit the world, of which 300 are dangerous to humans. Twenty poisonous species from a total of 120 residing in the United States are potential human menaces. Close contact with domestic and imported snakes results in 45,000 snake bites per year in this country of which 8,000 are venomous. Approximately 12 deaths occur per year as a result of these envenomations. Equally significant is the suffering, limb loss, loss of function, and loss of economic productivity which result from nonfatal envenomations. Before the advent of antivenin, morbidity in the form of scarring, contractures, or amputations affected 75% of victims and mortality occurred in 10% to 35%.

Venomous reptiles are found in temperate and tropical areas around the world. They include the Colubridae, Elapidae, Hydrophidae, Crotalidae, and Helodermatidae. Ninety percent to 99% of venomous snake bites in the United States are produced by pit vipers (Crotalidae) and most of the remainder are produced by coral snakes (Elapidae).

Precise species identification of a particular snake is difficult for the untrained physician. However, with careful attention to several key morphologic points he should be able to differentiate those snakes which are poisonous from those which are harmless. The identification of poisonous snakes is based on characteristics of dentition, head shields, pupils, and tail and the presence or absence of a heat-sensing pit. All pit vipers (rattlesnakes, cottonmouths, copperheads) have large anterior retractile fangs which are easily recognized and which contain a venom channel. Careful inspection of a pit viper reveals a small depression on the side of its head midway and slightly below a line connecting the eye and nostril. This depression is a heat-sensing pit used by the snake for location of prey. The pupils of pit vipers are elliptical and vertical whereas those of most nonvenomous snakes are round (although venomous coral snakes also have round pupils). The tail of many American pit vipers is modified into several loosely interlocking horny segments which produce a threatening "rattle" when shaken, hence the name "rattlesnake."

The ventral plates caudal to the anus in pit vipers are arranged in a single row while those in the coral snake are arranged in a double row similar to most nonpoisonous snakes.

Coral snakes have shorter, permanently erect anterior fangs which also contain a venom channel or groove. Coral snakes have no loreal shield separating those shields bordering the eyes from those bordering the nostril. The coral snake also has characteristic tricolor bands of black, red, and yellow or white. The red bands are bordered by yellow or white bands and the bands encircle its body. Nonvenomous mimics of the coral snake are enveloped by tricolor bands also but the red borders the black and the bands do not totally encircle the body ("red on black, venom lack; red on yellow, kill a fellow").

The venom glands of poisonous snakes are modifications of salivary glands. The venom of a single snake may contain 5 to 15 enzymes, 3 to 12 nonenzymatic proteins and peptides, and six or more other substances. These substances exert simultaneous toxic or lethal effects on the integumentary, hematologic, nervous, respiratory, and cardiovascular systems. The clinical picture can also be complicated by the effects of other endogenous mediator release, such as histamine, bradykinin, and adenosine. Therefore snake venoms cannot be classified purely as "neurotoxic" or "cardiotoxic." Hyaluronidase is found in all venoms and produces hydrolysis of connective tissue stroma allowing the dispersion of other toxic components. Crotalid venom is rich in proteases, amino acidases, and phospholipases; therefore, it produces clinical changes related to cellular destruction, membrane permeability, and coagulation. Elapid venoms vary widely between species but contain more neurotoxins and cardiotoxins resulting in various expressions of nerve and heart toxicity.

CLINICAL MANIFESTATIONS

The clinical spectrum of abnormalities produced in a single victim by a given snake venom varies with the size and species of snake, the quantity of venom injected, the number and location of bites, the presence of bacteria in the snake's mouth, the age and health of the victim, and any treatment previously rendered. As many as 30% of crotalid bites and 50% of elapid bites may result in no envenomation. The venom channel is recessed above the tip of the fang and the venom injected may be reduced by poor penetration or glancing blows, causing venom to be lost over the skin and clothing surface. The volume of venom available to a particular snake may be reduced by previous feedings.

Most medically significant envenomations are caused by pit vipers. Rattlesnake bites are the most serious, cottonmouth (water moccasin) bites are of intermediate severity, and copperheads usually produce no major systemic injury. The manifestations of snake envenomations can be divided into local and systemic effects. Rattlesnake venom causes local pain, swelling, erythema, ecchymosis, and occasional bleb formation at the puncture site. Later the increased membrane permeability and cellular destruction produced by various proteases result in spreading edema and tissue sloughing. If the bite is on an extremity, a compartment syndrome may result.

Systemic effects of rattlesnake venom involve hematologic abnormalities and effects on the cardiovascular, respiratory, and neurologic systems. The coagulation defects may result in local bleeding, epistaxis, hemoptysis, hematuria, and gastrointestinal bleeding. Also intravascular hemolysis may occur. Neurologic sequelae affecting rattlesnake envenomations include weakness, sweating, numbness, paresthesias, fasciculations, convulsions, and coma. The coma may be secondary to hypovolemia or to a direct effect of the toxin. Other findings include nausea, vomiting, respiratory depression, and pulmonary edema, especially in more severe cases.

Elapids account for the largest number of worldwide deaths but only a small percentage of deaths in the United States. Coral snake bites produce predominantly systemic effects. Local findings are minimal and the puncture site may be missed. The victim may have numbness or weakness in the bitten extremity. Systemic poisoning by coral snake venom produces drowsiness, euphoria, weakness, nausea, vomiting, fasciculations, excessive salivation, extraocular muscle paresis, hypotension, delayed general paresis, and cardiopulmonary failure.

DIAGNOSIS

Proper diagnosis of snake envenomation depends heavily on a description of the snake or examination of the snake itself. The site of envenomation also provides important visual clues. Potentially morbid crotalid bite sites will demonstrate early local swelling and erythema. Therefore, if after a known crotalid bite the victim demonstrates no local changes over several hours of observation he can be released from the hospital. Elapid or coral snake bites are associated with minimal local changes and systemic complications may be delayed. Therefore, specific antivenin therapy may need to be initiated in these victims before any local or clinical signs appear. The diagnosis of any significant envenomation is supported by those clinical manifestations mentioned above. Almost all victims of snake bites can relate some information about the attacker. Immunoassays as well as bioassays have been used experimentally to identify various snake venoms in tissue. Minton, Weinstein, and Wilde prepared an enzyme-linked immunosorbent assay (ELISA) against the venoms of the Western diamondback rattlesnake, the Mojave rattlesnake and the copperhead. They were able to detect venom levels of 0.1 to 0.01 μg/ml in tissue fluid removed from the bite site of several species of rattlesnakes. These assays may be helpful in the future to identify specific venoms in victims from endemic snakebite areas especially if historical information is limited.

TABLE 88-1 TREATMENT OF SNAKE ENVENOMATIONS

First Aid

Tourniquets–mildly occlusive proximal to bite
Cryotherapy–local ice pack for symptom relief
Incision and suction–within 5 min of bite,
–if over 30 min from hospital
–incision through puncture
–30 min of suction

Specific

	*Crotalid
Severity	*Antivenin Crotalidae Polyvalent*
No envenomation	O vials IV
Mild envenomation	1–4 vials IV
Moderate envenomation	4–7 vials IV
Severe envenomation	15 or more vials IV
	*Elapid
Severity	Micruris fulvius *antivenin*
Historical exposure	3–5 vials IV
Onset of symptoms	3–5 vials IV q 4 h prn

Supportive

Debride necrotic tissue
Fasciotomy for compartment syndrome
Immobilize in position of function
Replace consumed coagulation factors
Oxygen, ventilation, hemodialysis prn

*Skin test for allergy to horse serum first.

TREATMENT

The treatment of clinically significant snake envenomations is shrouded in controversy. It can be divided into first aid, specific antivenin therapy, and supportive therapy (Table 88-1).

For more information, please see Chapter 62 in Civetta JM, Taylor RW, Kirby RR: Critical Care. *Philadelphia: J. B. Lippincott, 1988*

BIBLIOGRAPHY

Christopher DG, Rodning CB: Crotalidae envenomation. *South Med J* 1986; 79:159
Curry SC, Kraner JC, Kunkel DB, et al: Noninvasive vascular studies in management of rattlesnake envenomations to extremities. *Ann Emerg Med* 1985; 14:1081
Kunkel DB, Curry, SC, Vance MV, et al: Reptile envenomations. *J Toxicol-Clin Toxicol* 1983–84; 21:503
Lindsey D: Controversy in snake bite—Time for a controlled appraisal. *J Trauma* 1985; 25:462

Minton SA, Weinstein SA, Wilde CE: An enzyme-linked immunoassay for detection of North American pit viper venoms. Clin Toxicol 1985; 22:303

Russell FE, Carlson RW, Wainschel J, et al: Snake venom poisoning in the United States: Experiences with 550 cases. *JAMA* 1975; 233:341

Simon TL, Grace TG: Envenomation coagulopathy in wounds from pit vipers. *N Engl J Med* 1981; 305:443

Stewart ME, Greenland S, Hoffman JR: First aid treatment of poisonous snakebite: Are currently recommended procedures justified? *Ann Emerg Med* 1981; 10:331

Whitesides TE, Haney TC, Morimoto K, et al: Tissue pressure measurements as a determinant for the need of fasciotomy. *Clin Orthopaed Related Res* 1975; 113:43

XV.
Organ Transplantation

90 Vital Organs

Vital organ transplantation has become a treatment modality for end-stage cardiac and liver disease as well as for patients in chronic renal failure. It is no longer considered experimental but is a lifesaving cost-effective measure for many patients. All transplants of nonpaired organs and most kidney transplants come from cadaveric donors. The vast majority of these donors are cared for in intensive care units (ICU) prior to the organ procurement procedure.

ACCEPTABLE DONORS

TRAUMA PATIENTS

Persons who have become brain dead as a result of any type of head injury—including motor vehicle accidents, falls, and gunshot wounds—are acceptable. Homicide and suicide victims are not excluded, although close cooperation with the medical examiner is absolutely essential. Donated organs of child abuse victims with central nervous system (CNS) mortality, although requiring extreme delicacy and medical–legal teamwork, are particularly needed for liver transplantation because of the shortage of comparably sized livers for pediatric recipients with biliary atresia.

CEREBROVASCULAR ACCIDENT (CVA)

Young and middle-aged patients who have become brain dead from CVAs are acceptable as kidney donors in many cases. This is especially true with patients who have had a ruptured Berry aneurysm and are particularly likely to have otherwise normal organs.

PRIMARY BRAIN TUMORS

Because primary brain tumors do not metastasize, being confined by the blood–brain barrier, patients who have become brain dead from brain tumors are acceptable donors.

CEREBRAL ANOXIA

Patients who are brain dead because of anoxia and unsuccessful resuscitative efforts are acceptable donors. Drowning, cardiorespiratory arrest, drug overdose (if not toxic to the organ being considered for transplantation), and crib death victims can all be used if hemodynamic stability is restored after brain death has occurred and other vital organ function is assessed as normal.

UNACCEPTABLE DONORS

PERSONS OVER AGE 65

Renal function deteriorates with age, as does the kidney's ability to recover from the result of preservation. Liver, heart, and pancreas donors need to be even younger than kidney donors. If the patient had a CVA or is very obese, 55 is a better age limit.

CANCER PATIENTS WITH OTHER THAN BRAIN TUMORS

Cancer cells can be transplanted together with the organ and will flourish in the immunosuppressed milieu.

PERSONS WITH ANY TRANSMISSIBLE DISEASE

Septic patients and patients with hepatitis or HIV are examples of unacceptable donors. The risk to an immunosuppressed host is prohibitive.

PATIENTS WITH RENAL COMPROMISE

Diabetics of longer than 5 to 6 years' duration, patients with long-standing hypertension, and patients with systemic lupus erythematosus are examples of unacceptable patients.

CRITERIA FOR BRAIN DEATH

The concept of brain death is simple. There should be no evidence of brain function, and the condition should be irreversible. Laws vary among the states, and protocols vary from hospital to hospital. A call to the transplant center can help, because its personnel can provide the pertinent information. The transplant team cannot pronounce brain death and must avoid a conflict of interest. When brain death has been determined, which requires two physicians in most states, the patient is legally dead and life-support measures must cease. The following guidelines are suggested.

1 Absence of spontaneous movement

2 No response to stimulation

3 Absence of brain-stem reflexes
  a. Pupils
  b. Corneal
  c. Ciliospinal
  d. Doll's eyes
  e. Gag
  f. Calorics

4 Reversibility must be excluded
  a. No evidence of intake of pharmacologic depressants such as barbiturates
  b. No significant hypothermia (95°F)—especially if electroencephalographic (EEG) criteria are to be followed.

5 If 1 through 4 above are met, that may be sufficient. Otherwise a negative cerebral blood flow study or an isoelectric EEG may be sufficient.

MAINTENANCE OF THE POTENTIAL DONOR

The organ donor has had irreversible brain damage. Until brain death has become clear, it is customary to dehydrate the patient in an effort to minimize brain edema. Further, with hypovolemia, hypotension frequently occurs, which in turn is usually treated with vasopressors. These measures impair the function of donated organs and must be reversed. Frequently there is time to do this while waiting for all the necessary consents and proclamations of brain death. This time can be used to improve the physiologic milieu of the donor and to expedite organ procurement. The following measures are recommended.

VIGOROUS HYDRATION

Boluses of appropriate crystalloid solution should be given to reverse dehydration and to maintain a urine output of at least 100 ml/hr. When this level of hydration is instituted, pressors should be weaned to allow good renal perfusion. Dopamine infusions should be 2 to 5 μg/kg/min or less. A systolic blood pressure of over 100 mm Hg should be maintained. If there is bleeding, transfusions may be given. In patients who are heart and liver donors, a good hematocrit (>30) is particularly desirable. Many patients with severe brain damage will have diabetes insipidus. If volume replacement cannot be maintained, a small dose of pitressin may be used. In these cases, avoid exacerbating diuresis with glucosuria, and vigorously correct severe hypernatremia and hypokalemia, which are frequently associated difficulties.

ANTIBIOTICS

A first-generation cephalosporin should be given immediately before the organ retrieval.

DIURETICS

If the urine output is less than 100 ml/hr despite adequate hydration, mannitol and furosemide are used to stimulate urine output.

PULMONARY INFILTRATES

If the patient is to be considered as a cardiopulmonary donor, make a careful check for pulmonary infiltrates.

EYE CARE

Lubrication of the corneas is critical to ensure their usefulness in transplant.

LABORATORY DATA

The following information should be obtained: ABO blood group, blood urea nitrogen (BUN), creatinine, urinalysis, VDRL, HIV, hepatitis surface antigens, blood culture, urine culture, liver function tests in liver donors, electrocardiogram (EKG) in heart donors, and blood gases in heart–lung donors.

A properly maintained organ donor is essential for a good transplant result because all of the tissues will be in the best possible condition as the donor is brought to the operating room. Before proceeding to surgery, the various teams involved are coordinated by the regional transplant center so that the best use of time and tissues can be accomplished.

GENERAL CONSIDERATIONS IN POSTOPERATIVE CARE

Certain postoperative problems relate to technical operative considerations, and therefore details should be known to the ICU team. The transplant kidney is usually placed in the right iliac fossa, close to the bladder, so that only a short segment of donor ureter needs to be used (the standard procedure involves a ureterovesicostomy). An extended inguinal incision is used, and the peritoneal contents are reflected off the iliac vessels after the inferior epigastric vessels and round ligament (or spermatic cord) are ligated (or retracted). The renal vein is anastomosed end-to-side to the iliac vein. The renal artery is anastomosed end-to-side to the external or common iliac artery or end-to-end to the internal iliac artery. If there are multiple arteries, either a patch or multiple implants are used. The ureter is then implanted into the bladder. In pediatric patients, the peritoneum is opened and the right colon displaced to expose the aorta and vena cava. The renal vessels are implanted into these. Often in this age group, a bilateral nephrectomy is performed concomitantly.

During the procedure, fluids are given sparingly until the suturing of blood vessels begins. The anastomosis takes about 30 minutes to complete; in preparation for this time the patient is hydrated vigorously. Studies have shown that this protocol leads to shortening of the postoperative ATN period. Just after the vascular clamps are released and perfusion of the kidney is restored, mannitol and furosemide are administered to promote a brisk diuresis. In many cases an early post-transplant diuresis behaves much like postobstructive diuresis and can be managed similarly. The rate of intravenous infusion is adjusted every 30 minutes to exactly replace urine and insensible and nasogastric losses, and volume is maintained with blood and colloid. It is not unusual to see as much as 500 ml of urine produced every 30 minutes. The intravenous fluids are then administered at a decreasing rate over several days so that more normal urine outputs can be established. The patients are managed "on the wet side" because transplanted kidneys do not tolerate hypovolemia. Neither does the transplanted kidney tolerate hypotension. For this reason the patients are allowed to be mildly hypertensive for the first 48 hours postoperatively. Blood pressures of 160/100 mm Hg in adults are not uncommon. As the patient becomes euvolemic, the blood pressure normalizes; if it does not, antihypertensive medicines are instituted or reinstituted. Oral intake is gauged by bowel activity and ambulation is started early. The Foley catheter typically is left for about 1 week.

EARLY COMPLICATIONS OF KIDNEY TRANSPLANTATION

HYPERACUTE REJECTION

In the rare case when an inaccurate or falsely negative result is obtained on histocompatibility cross matching, hyperacute rejection can be seen. Hyperacute rejection is mediated by preformed cytotoxic donor-specific antibodies. The kidney will turn blue and soft when blood flow is reestablished. Concomitantly active hemorrhage may occur in the wound from platelet consumption. The kidney must be immediately removed and appropriate transfusion instituted. Hyperacute rejection can occasionally be delayed until after the wound is closed, and urine output that may have been reestablished abruptly ceases. However, this is not a usual cause of such findings after a few hours postoperatively.

ACUTE TUBULAR NECROSIS

Delayed function is common in cadaver kidney transplant. Dialysis needs to be used postoperatively in about 20% of patients. It is often seen in kidneys removed from older donors or when recipients have a low-flow state intraoperatively or postoperatively. However, it sometimes occurs capriciously. The kidney will appear normal in the operating room and may produce urine for minutes or even hours, and then function deteriorates. Acute tubular necrosis may persist for weeks and even months after transplant, although usually function returns (*i.e.*, releasing the need for dialysis) within 2 weeks after its onset. Nuclear scanning, showing good flow and impaired function, is helpful but not specifically diagnostic in distinguishing ATN from other complications. With ATN, fluid restriction and dialysis become necessary. However, care must be taken to hydrate these patients adequately when diuresis begins. Serial nuclear scans and occasional renal biopsies are helpful to rule out acute rejection superimposed on ATN.

VASCULAR OCCLUSION

During surgery, vascular occlusion caused by an arterial intimal flap may be seen. Problems from gradual occlusion may also occur with time. Unsuspected trauma in handling the renal artery from the time of organ retrieval or implantation may cause intimal and medial damage leading to vascular occlusion. In exceptional cases the onset of renal failure is subtle, with irreversible changes having occurred by the time a diagnosis is made. Microvascular thrombosis has been reported to occur as an idiosyncratic reaction to cyclosporine A and will be manifested as rapidly rising creatinine. This can be diagnosed by renal biopsy. In these cases the drug needs to be withheld. Such arterial thrombosis may be accompanied by sudden pain in the kidney, fever, and a rising creatinine level. Renal scan will help with the diagnosis. Partial infarction may be compatible with residual renal function if the renal pelvis remains intact. Stenosis of the arterial ostium may occur years after transplant and will present with worsening hypertension and renal function. Captopril exacerbates the increase in creatinine, and a renal scan with captopril may be helpful. Angiography and balloon angioplasty or open repair are indicated.

Venous thrombosis is rarely seen and usually predisposes to graft loss before diagnosis can occur perhaps as a result of inadvertently twisting the renal vein at the time of implantation or by purse-stringing in a pediatric kidney.

ACUTE REJECTION

Usually seen within the first several weeks after transplantation, acute rejection can occasionally occur as early as 5 to 7 days postoperatively. With modern immunosuppression regimens, it is only seen in 33% to 50% of the patients and is accompanied by a rise in creatinine, occasionally fever, graft swelling, and tenderness. The diagnosis is definitively made by biopsy, but usually the clinical setting coupled with a renal scan showing decreased flow and function as compared to baseline may be adequate to institute therapy. Acute rejection is treated with abrupt increase in corticosteroid administration and sometimes by graft irradiation and monoclonal or polyclonal ALG.

CYCLOSPORINE TOXICITY

Drug toxicity is also manifest by rising creatinine with rejection. Cyclosporine serum levels are usually high, and the serum creatinine concentration decreases within 24 to 48 hours as a result of lowering the dose of the drug. However, it is sometimes very difficut to distinguish cyclosporine toxicity from rejection, especially if the two phenomena occur concomitantly, and a renal biopsy may be necessary to make the diagnosis.

URINE LEAKS

In about 2% of patients urine leaks occur. Sometimes the diagnosis can be made by finding urine in the Hemovac drainage catheter, by finding extravasation on the renal scan, or by using ultrasonic techniques. Urinary or local wound symptoms are common and elevation in BUN and creatinine is also frequent, particuarly after the Foley catheter has been removed. Definitive diagnosis frequently can be made with a cystogram. The source of leak can be at the vesicotomy or the ureteral implantation site. Although a few bladder leaks will heal with prolonged catheter drainage, reoperation and closure are strongly urged. More rarely urine leaks occur from slough of the distal ureter or renal pelvis as a result of injury to the blood supply. This serious complication, often accompanied by infection, leads to nephrectomy.

LYMPHOCELE

At any time postoperatively lymphocele may be seen and may be the result of dividing numerous lymphatic channels in the pelvis of the recipient or even in the transplanted kidney. A lymphocele pressing against the pelvis or ureter of the kidney or renal vessels will cause obstruction to urine flow or renal blood flow or even create pressure on the renal parenchyma, causing elevated serum creatinine concentration. Occasionally there is swelling of the ipsilateral leg. Lymphoceles may also be caused by bleeding in the perioperative period associated with an increase in volume in a closed space as tissue fluid enters the liquefying hematoma by osmotic forces. A lucent area may be seen on renal scan, but ultrasonography is the definitive test. These patients may be brought to the operating room for intraperitoneal drainage and marsupialization of the lymphocele.

HEMATURIA

As a result of bleeding from the periureteral vessel, hematuria occurs. Although it is usually self-limited, occasionally cystoscopy and cauterization are necessary. Hematuria can also occur from bladder suture line bleeding or from the transplanted kidney and is usually self-limited.

BLEEDING

Because the uremic state is associated with platelet dysfunction, bleeding into the transplant wound is somewhat more commonly seen than in other types of surgery. There can be a considerable consumptive coagulopathy induced by the allograft even when long-term function will eventually result. These patients need to have blood and blood product replacement and evacuation of the hematoma with hemostasis. Blood pressing on such a kidney is associated with significant transplant dysfunction.

INFECTION

The most common complication seen in transplant patients is infection because of immunosuppression. Infections can range from viruses to bacteria to fungi and opportunistic organisms. Infection is often associated with graft dysfunction and sometimes with rejection. Vigilance is necessary to diagnose infection and institute appropriate therapy early. Usually, decreasing doses of immunosuppressive drugs are necessary.

For more information, please see Chapter 143 in Civetta JM, Taylor RW, Kirby RR: Critical Care. *Philadelphia: J. B. Lippincott, 1988*

BIBLIOGRAPHY

Ad Hoc Committee of the Harvard Medical School: A definition of irreversible coma. *JAMA* 1968; 205, 85
Collins GM, Green RD, Boyer D, et al: *Transplantation* 1977; 23:310
Griffiths AB, Fletcher EW, Morris PJ: Lymphocele after renal transplantation. *Aust NZ J Surg* 1979; 49:626
Hume DM: Progress in clinical renal homotransplantation. *Adv Surg* 1966; 2:419
Korein J (ed): Brain death: Interrelated medical and social issues. *Ann NY Acad Sci;* 1978; 315:1
Lieberman RP, Glass NR, Crummy AB, et al: Nonoperative percutaneous management of urinary fistulas and strictures in renal transplantation. *Surg Gynecol Obstet* 1982; 155:667-672
Marshall VC: Renal preservation. In Morris PJ (ed): *Kidney Transplantation: Principles and Practice,* 2nd ed, pp 129–157. London, Grune & Stratton, 1984
Murray JE, Harrison JH: Surgical management of fifty patients with kidney transplants including eighteen pairs of twins. *Am J Surg* 1963; 105:205
Prout GR, Hume DM, Lee HM, et al: *J Urol* 1967; 97:409
Rankin RS, Crummy AB, Belzer FO: Biplane arteriography for the evaluation of arterial stenosis in renal transplantation. *AJR* 1977; 128:330

Rosenthal JT, Shaw BW, Hardesty RL, et al: Principles of multiple organ procurement from cadaver donors. *Ann Surg* 1983; 198:617
Salvatierra O, Belzer FO: Pediatric cadaver kidneys. *Arch Surg* 1975; 110:181
Starzl TE, Marchioro TL, Dickinson TC, et al: Techniques of renal homotransplantation. *Arch Surg* 1964; 89:87
Starzl TE, Marchioro TL, Morgan WW, et al: A technique for use of adult renal homografts in children. *Surg Gynecol Obstet* 1964; 119:106
Williams GM, Hume DM, Hudson RP, et al: "Hyperacute" renal-homograft rejection in man. *N Engl J Med* 1968; 279:611

91
Intensive Care of Liver Transplant Patients

Patients awaiting liver transplantation are usually chronically ill, as would be expected from the indications for liver transplantation (Fig. 91-1). When portal hypertension is present, gastrointestinal hemorrhage is common. Most adult liver transplant candidates have had at least one episode of acute upper gastrointestinal bleeding. Similarly, most have abnormal coagulation profiles, hypoalbuminemia, and an altered cardiovascular profile that reflects a high output, low peripheral vascular resistance state. It has recently been suggested that end-stage liver failure predisposes to multisystem organ failure (MSOF).

SURGICAL PROCEDURE

DONOR LIVER MANAGEMENT

Once a patient's condition is considered hopeless and brain death is imminent, the focus of care is directed at donor organ maintenance. After brain death certification, all measures are directed at preserving donor organs, not neurologic function. In the operating room during organ procurement, the donor's cardiac output and oxygenation should be maximized. Extensive surgical dissection in the chest and abdomen are performed before cold flushing with the preservation solution. This sequence is used to minimize ischemic injury. Although numerous groups have attempted to prolong the ischemic time limit by altering the preservation solution, none has been shown to be superior to Euro–Collins solution. The primary goal in organ procurement is to minimize organ ischemic time during and after organ harvesting.

VENOVENOUS BYPASS WITHOUT SYSTEMIC ANTICOAGULATION

Extensive dissections are carried out prior to cold flushing with preservative. The primary goal in organ procurement is to minimize organ ischemic time during and after organ harvesting.

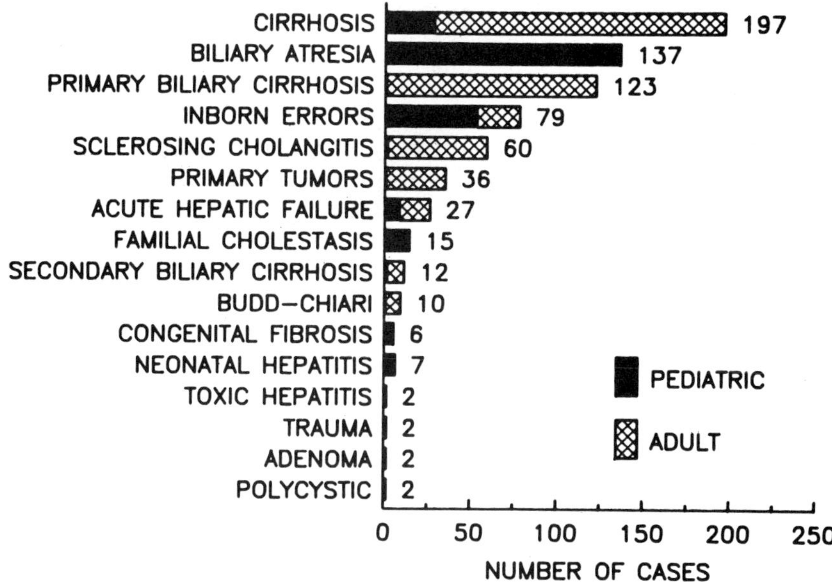

Figure 91-1 Indications for 720 liver transplants performed in Pittsburgh.

Venovenous bypass without systemic anticoagulation has been used to avoid the decrease in cardiac output, deterioration in renal function, and worsening of portal hypertension during the anhepatic phase (from removal of the native liver to return of blood flow to the donor liver). Significantly fewer blood products are required, and the serum creatinine has been lower postoperatively. All biliary tract reconstructions today are performed by either a choledochocholedochostomy with a T-tube stent or a choledochojejunostomy to a Roux-en-Y limb of jejunum. Rapid infusion systems have been developed to deliver diluted, warm blood at rates up to 2 liters per minute.

POSTOPERATIVE INTENSIVE CARE

The postoperative care of the liver transplant patient in the ICU is similar in many ways to the routine postoperative care of any patient who has undergone extensive intra-abdominal surgery. Strict attention is given to intravascular fluid status, electrolyte balance, coagulation, liver and renal function, and cardiovascular performance. Closely monitor filling pressures, arterial blood gases (ABGs), cardiac rhythm, cardiac output, and urine output, as well as the output from all surgical drains. Therapy is directed initially at achieving hemodynamic stability by the titration of routine resuscitative care, which is guided by clinical signs, laboratory data, and the invasive hemodynamic monitoring mentioned above. Beyond this resemblance to the routine postoperative patient care in the ICU, the liver transplant patient has unique problems that stem from the newly transplanted liver and the necessity of immunosuppression.

The routine orders for care of the postoperative liver transplant patient are based on standard principles of surgical management (Table 91-1). Electrocardiogram (EKG) and arterial, central venous, and pulmonary arterial pressures are monitored continuously, as are respiratory variables during mechanical ventilation. Vital signs and fluid balance are recorded frequently because these patients are often unstable in the immediate postoperative period. Many patients have oliguria in the first 24- to 48-hour period because of intraoperative blood loss and its replacement as well as transient hypo-

TABLE 91-1 ORDERS FOR POSTOPERATIVE CARE OF ADULT LIVER TRANSPLANT PATIENTS

Diagnosis: S/P orthotopic liver transplant
Condition: Critical
Vital signs: q15min until stable, then hourly
Hourly CVP, I & O
NPO
Bed rest until tracheal extubation, then up as tolerated
Respiratory care per ICU
Foley catheter to closed gravity drainage
Jackson–Pratt drains to closed bulb suction
T tube to closed drainage
NG tube to low continuous suction—irrigate with 30 ml normal saline q1hr
Riopan 5 ml q2hr per NG tube, clamp for 15 min
Double dose if gastric *p*H < 5
Turn q2hr, endotracheal suctioning q4hr, postural drainage and clamping q4hr
5% dextrose, half-normal saline at 125 ml/hr
Cyclosporine 2 mg/kg IV q12hr at 10 AM and 10 PM daily
Methylprednisolone: 50 mg IV q6hr × 4, then
40 mg IV q6hr × 4, then
30 mg IV q6hr × 4, then
20 mg IV q6hr × 4, then
20 mg IV q12hr × 2, then
20 mg IV qd
Cyclosporine trough level from 9:30 PM blood
Ampicillin 1.0 g IV q6hr × 5d
Cefataxime 1.0 g IV q6hr × 5d
Mycostatin 5 ml swish and swallow qid once NG tube is out (and Mycostatin vaginal suppository tid to women)
CRX now and daily
Stat, then q6hr × 4: CBC, PT, PTT, platelets
q6hr × 4: electrolytes, BUN, creatinine, glucose, amylose
Daily labs: CBC, differential, PT, PTT, platelets, electrolytes, Ca, P, Mg, BUN, creatinine, bilirubin (T/D), SGOT, SGPT, alkaline phosphatase, GTP, total protein, albumin, amylase
Keep 4 U packed RBC on hold

tension or inferior vena caval cross-clamping. Furosemide or colloid therapy is used during this interval. Excessive use of crystalloids, however, can result in pulmonary edema. Therefore, fluids are administered as necessary to maintain CVP at approximately 10 cm H_2O.

HYPERTENSION

Hypertension is a common postoperative problem. Hydralazine and beta-adrenergic blocking agents such as labetalol and propranolol provide initial antihypertensive therapy. These agents are given as intravenous boluses and titrated to effect. In patients who require other antihypertensive therapy because they either cannot receive the above agents or are refractory to them, use minoxidil, clonidine, or captopril. Avoid using alpha-methyldopa because of its hepatotoxic potential. In acute hypertensive emergencies, nifedipine, 10 mg sublingually, is a useful immediate agent in addition to more definitive long-term therapy. In cases of refractory hypertension, labetalol can be given intravenously as 20 mg over 2 minutes, repeated as necessary every 10 minutes to a total dose of 300 mg. Labetalol can also be given as a continuous infusion at an initial dose of 2 mg/min, adjusted according to the arterial pressure.

ANTACIDS

The patient is kept without oral intake until gastrointestinal mobility resumes. A nasogastric (NG) tube, inserted during the operation, is kept to low continuous suction and irrigated hourly with saline. Antacid (Mylanta, 30 ml, or Riopan, 5 ml) is given by the NG tube every 4 hours to keep the gastric *p*H above 5. This dose of antacid is doubled when the gastric *p*H is less than 5. Previous studies have demonstrated significantly less upper gastrointestinal hemorrhage in patients whose gastric *p*H is over 5.

PULMONARY

Pulmonary complications are common and should be treated aggressively. The patient is turned every 2 hours. Pulmonary toilet is achieved by endotracheal suctioning, manual hyperinflations using a self-inflating ventilation bag and instillation of 3 ml saline with repeat suctioning as needed. Sustained (15 sec) manual hyperinflations of the lungs for recruitment are used if arterial hypoxemia develops. The patient is weaned from mechanical ventilation using standard criteria for extubation. If there are no special problems, the patient can be extubated within 12 to 24 hours of surgery.

FLUID THERAPY

Fluid management is very important. Most patients arrive in the ICU in a nonsteady state characterized by a much expanded extracellular fluid volume, increasing vasomotor tone, and hypothermia. Start basal fluid resuscitation with 5% dextrose in half-normal saline, infused at 125 ml/hr. Since excessive administration of crystalloids may precipitate pulmonary edema, use either plasma protein fraction or fresh frozen plasma to provide oncotic pressure and maintain intravascular volume. The goal of this initial therapy is to keep CVP at about 10 cm H_2O and urine output at 0.5 ml/kg/hr. Hypovolemia must be avoided because the combination of hypovolemia and cyclosporine increases the risk of postoperative renal failure.

If hypokalemia occurs during the initial postoperative period, it is best treated with infusion of 20 meq KCl rather than by adding KCl to the maintenance intravenous fluids. Caution must be exercised to avoid hyperkalemia. The patient may be unable to excrete excess potassium because some degree of oliguria is common postoperatively. Further, graft necrosis may occur, with either primary nonfunction or hepatic artery thrombosis, and result in rapid increases in serum potassium.

IMMUNOSUPPRESSION

Immunosuppression is begun preoperatively. Cyclosporine and prednisone are the mainstays of immunosuppression in the liver transplant patient. The first dose of cyclosporine, 17.5 mg/kg, is given orally just before surgery, and the first bolus of steroids, 1 g methylprednisolone, is given intravenously at the time that the donor liver is revascularized. Postoperatively, 2 mg/kg cyclosporine is given intravenously every 12 hours until the patient resumes oral intake. Once the patient is able to take medications orally, 17.5 mg/kg cyclosporine is given in divided doses twice a day, as well as 2 mg/kg intravenously every 12 hours. Methylprednisolone, 200 mg, is given intravenously on the first day in four divided doses and tapered by 40 mg/day until a maintenance dose of 20 mg/day is reached. Once the patient resumes oral intake, switch to prednisone, 20 mg/day, orally. Cyclosporine dosage is monitored by daily cyclosporine trough levels in blood samples drawn 30 minutes before the evening dose. Generally, whole blood trough levels (by radioimmunoassay) of 800 to 1000 ng/ml are considered optimal.

ANTIBIOTICS

Since all patients are immunosuppressed and the procedure requires anastomosis of donor and recipient bile ducts, antibiotics with a spectrum appropriate for biliary tract pathogens such as *Klebsiella, Escherichia coli,* and enterococcus are started preoperatively. Give all patients ampicillin and cefotaxime, 1 g each, intravenously every 6 hours. Other antibiotics are given as guided by culture results. Oral and vaginal candidiasis occur frequently in the liver transplant patient. To suppress these infections, give Mycostatin oral suspension four times a day and, for women, Mycostatin vaginal suppositories three times a day.

If there are no special problems or complications, the patient can usually be transferred to a surgical ward by the second or third postoperative day.

HEPATIC COMPLICATIONS

Primary nonfunction results in total hepatic failure including profound hypoglycemia, uncorrectable coagulopathy, stage IV coma, new onset of renal failure, profound metabolic acidosis, cardiogenic shock, and markedly abnormal liver function test findings. Although prolonged ischemia may lead to primary nonfunction, some hepatic allografts fail to function despite apparently uneventful procurement and transplantation. Improvement rarely occurs after 48 hours of nonfunction. If it persists, the patient should be considered for immediate retransplantation.

Hepatic artery thrombosis is the most common and devastating vascular complication. It may present as acute hepatic gangrene with sepsis and fulminant liver failure, delayed bile leak resulting from ischemic necrosis of the common bile duct, or relapsing bacteremia. The first two entities must be treated by retransplantation, although antibiotic therapy has been successful in some pediatric patients with relapsing bacteremia. Doppler ultrasonography of the liver has been a useful screening device to detect a pulsatile artery. Arteriography may be required to make the definitive diagnosis. Because of the threat of hepatic artery thrombosis, platelet counts as low as 30,000 and prothrombin times (PT) less than 30 seconds are not treated unless patients have active bleeding.

Rejection is the most common cause for hepatic allograft dysfunction. It may present as a swollen and hard liver, a tender abdomen with ascites, deterioration of liver function tests, and decreased quantity and quality of the bile. Prolonged PT is rarely seen. The differentiation of infection from rejection is most important since infection is treated with a decrease in immunosuppression, whereas rejection requires an increase. Liver biopsy may be necessary to differentiate rejection from ischemic injury and various forms of vital hepatitis, especially *Cytomegalovirus* (CMV) infection. Liver rejection may also be assessed by a T-tube cholangiogram. Pruning of the bile ducts within the liver suggests rejection. Ultrasonography can also be used to rule out bile duct obstruction. Computed tomography (CT) of the liver may reveal areas of decreased attenuation consistent with rejection.

Acute rejection is treated with steroid pulse therapy. If liver function continues to deteriorate, the patient should be considered a candidate for antilymphocyte globulin (OKT-3).

Cyclosporine toxicity may be manifest as hypertension, tremulousness, hypertrichosis, gingival hyperplasia, and nephrotoxicity. In fact, cyclosporine toxicity is the most common cause of an increase in blood urea nitrogen (BUN) and creatinine.

RENAL COMPLICATIONS

Hypovolemia and oliguria should be treated by fluid replacement, recognizing that there may be significant third space losses. In patients with preoperative renal dysfunction, postoperative renal failure may occasionally be severe enough to require hemodialysis. If the new liver functions promptly, renal function usually improves rapidly.

BLEEDING AND COAGULATION PROBLEMS

The coagulation defects most commonly seen in the ICU are prolonged PT, partial thromboplastin time (PTT), and thrombocytopenia. With appropriate component therapy, bleeding due to a coagulopathy is a rare problem. Inability to correct a coagulopathy should suggest poor graft function.

INFECTION

The liver transplant patient is not placed in protective isolation. The overwhelming threat to these immunocompromised patients is their own gastrointestinal flora. Evaluation of infections should include CMV, reactivation of tuberculosis, legionella, and hepatitis. Evaluation of fever should be similar to that in other immunocompromised hosts. Herpesvirus and CMV have caused significant infections. Herpesvirus infections can be treated with daily acyclovir, 5 mg/kg in three divided doses for 10 to 14 days. At present there is no specific treatment for CMV infections. The use of bolus injections of steroids during periods of "stress" in the presence of major infection is unwarranted and dangerous. However, maintenance doses must be continued.

For more information, please see Chapter 142 in Civetta JM, Taylor RW, Kirby RR: Critical Care. *Philadelphia: J. B. Lippincott, 1988*

BIBLIOGRAPHY

Bihari, DJ: Acute liver failure—The ultimate cause of multiple organ system failure? *Intensive Crit Care Dig* 1987; 5:39–42

Hastings PR, Skillman JJ, Bushnell LS, et al: Antacid titration in the prevention of acute gastrointestinal bleeding: A controlled randomized trial in 100 critically ill patients. *N Engl J Med* 1978; 208:1041

Matuschak GM, Rinaldo JE, Van Thiel DH, et al: Acute respiratory failure with preexisting end-stage hepatic insufficiency is irreversible. *Am Rev Respir dis* 1985; 131(4, pt 2):A151

Rosenthal JT, Shaw BW Jr, Hardesty RL, et al: *Surg Clin North Am* 1985; 12:5H

Starzl TE, Iwatsuki S, Shaw BW, et al: Evolution of liver transplantation. Hepatology 1984; 4:475

Starzl TE, Fung JJ: OKT-3 in treatment of rejection under cyclosporine steroid therapy. Transplant Proc 1986; 18:'937

Toledo–Pereyra LH, Castellanos J, Chapman M: Failure to preserve liver allographs for 24 hours: Experimental and theoretical considerations. *Transplant Proc* 1987; 19(4):68

XVI. Resuscitation

92
Emergency Resuscitation

AIRWAY MANAGEMENT

TRACHEAL INTUBATION

Orotracheal intubation in the nontrauma patient is best accomplished with the patient's head in the "sniffing" position; a straight or curved blade may be used. The optimal position is ideally established by an assistant. A Yankauer suction catheter should be at the head of the bed for use by the intubating clinician. The laryngoscope blade should be inserted into the right side of the mouth, sweeping the tongue to the left. It should be advanced along the midline, pulling the mandible at a 45° angle in a straight line toward the ceiling. During intubation the stylet should be withdrawn as soon as the tube is past the vocal cords. Adults should ideally be intubated with at least an 8-mm inside diameter (ID) (preferably an 8.5-mm) endotracheal tube.

Nasotracheal intubation can be accomplished as an alternative in the spontaneously breathing patient. If time allows, a topical anesthetic and possibly a topical alpha-adrenergic agent such as neosynephrine should be applied first to anesthetize and shrink the nasal mucosa. The endotracheal tube is lubricated and placed into the naris without a stylet and advanced into the posterior nasopharynx. Breath sounds are auscultated through the proximal end of the tube and when they are heard to be maximal, the tube is quickly but gently advanced forward during inspiration. In the adult, an 8-mm ID tube is optimal for nasotracheal intubation.

If the intubating clinician is experienced and confident that the glottic area can be visualized, he or she may administer succinylcholine (1 mg/kg) to facilitate intubation in the uncooperative patient or in the patient with tense jaw musculature. Bag-valve-mask ventilation must be on standby in either situation in case of unsuspected problems. After intubation, a portable chest radiograph should be obtained to verify tube position.

CIRCULATION

The absence of a pulse mandates chest compressions. In two-person cardiopulmonary resuscitation (CPR) ventilations are delivered after every fifth chest compression, with a compression rate in the adult of 80/min. A carotid pulse implies a systolic pressure of approximately 60 mm Hg; a femoral pulse, a systolic pressure of approximately 70 mm Hg; and a radial pulse, a systolic pressure of approximately 80 mm Hg.

VENOUS ACCESS

A longer catheter inserted centrally provides a lower flow rate than a shorter catheter with the same ID which is inserted peripherally. There is some potential advantage to drugs introduced by the central route, since the peak level may be higher and appear earlier; however these differences are not major considerations. What must be weighed against any potential benefits is the potential disruption of resuscitation, both airway management and chest compressions, during insertion of a central catheter.

RESUSCITATION PHARMACOLOGY

Table 92-1 lists medications routinely used during cardiac arrest.

EPINEPHRINE

Epinephrine is the pressor drug of choice for primary cardiac arrest. It is recommended in patients with ventricular fibrillation and pulseless ventricular tachycardia who are unresponsive to initial defibrillation attempts. Its mechanism of action is not related to its central beta-adrenergic effects, but to its alpha-adrenergic vasoconstrictor effects. In the patient who is converted to a rhythm which generates a pulse, epinephrine may facilitate coronary artery perfusion and cardiac output by raising aortic diastolic pressure.

ATROPINE

Atropine is currently recommended for patients with bradycardiac dysrhythmias and hypotension, asystole, and electromechanical dissociation.

SODIUM BICARBONATE

Sodium bicarbonate should be given only in one or more of the following circumstances:

1 ABG results are available to guide therapy
2 A long "down-time" existed prior to initiation of CPR
3 After failure of standard drug therapy protocol

TABLE 92-1 CRITICAL CARE RESUSCITATION MEDICATIONS

Drug	Preparation (intravenous)	Dosage (intravenous)
Epinephrine	Prefilled syringe: 10 ml (1 mg in 1:10,000 dilution)	0.5–1 mg 5–10 ml (Repeat every 15 min. if dysrhythmia persists.)
Atropine	Prefilled syringe: 10 ml (1 mg)	0.5–1 mg 5–10 ml (If dysrhythmia persists, repeat every 5 min. up to total of 2 mg.)
Lidocaine	Prefilled syringe: 10 ml (100 mg)	1 mg/kg (If dysrhythmia persists, repeat 0.5 mg/kg every 8 min. to total of 3 mg/kg.)
Bretylium	Ampule: 10 ml (500 mg)	5 mg/kg; if necessary, followed every 5 min. by 10 mg/kg (each dose given over 8 min.) to a total of 30 mg/kg
Procanamide	Vial: 10 ml (1000 mg)	Adult: 50 mg/min. to total of 1 g or until dysrhythmia resolves
Verapamil	Ampule: 2 ml (5 mg)	Adult: Bolus up to 10 mg (over 1 min.) may be repeated in 30 min.
Norepinephrine	Ampule: 4 ml (4 mg) (4 mg in 250 ml D_5W) (16 μg/ml)	Initially 2–3 ml min. and titrate upward to desirable blood pressure.
Dopamine	Prefilled syringe: 10 ml (400 mg) (Not for direct injection. Add dopamine (in mg) = patient weight (in kg) × 15 to 250 ml D_5W. Then infusion pump setting will equal dosage in μg/kg/min.	2–20 ug/kg/min
Isoproterenol	Vial: 5 ml (1 mg) (1 mg in 250 ml D_5W) (4 μg/ml)	2–20 μg/min
Sodium bicarbonate	Prefilled syringe: 50 ml (50 meq)	1 meq/kg when indicated. If used in an arrest state, 1/2 meq/kg may be repeated every 10 min. (Potential indications: prolonged down time, unsuccessful resuscitation, per ABG analysis).
Calcium chloride	10 ml (10%) Vial: (100 mg/ml)	5 ml for special resuscitation conditions

ISOPROTERENOL

Isoproterenol should be used only as a secondary drug in patients with sinus bradycardia and atrioventricular blocks with hypotension who do not respond to atropine.

CALCIUM

Calcium is no longer recommended except in: arrest due to calcium channel blockers, documented hypocalcemia, cycloplegic arrest, arrest subsequent to massive stored blood transfusion, or documented hyperkalemia.

DOPAMINE

Dopamine is the drug of choice for hypotension in the successfully resuscitated arrest due to myocardial ischemia.

ANTIARRHYTHMICS

In the hemodynamically unstable patient with life-threatening ventricular dysrhythmia, lidocaine remains the antiarrhythmic of choice. Since procainamide requires excessive time for administration (50 mg/min to a maximum of 1 g) bretylium can be considered a second-line agent.

DEFIBRILLATION

COUNTERSHOCK

Pulseless ventricular tachycardia and ventricular fibrillation are treated identically in the arrested patient. These patients should receive immediate defibrilation with a voltage of 200 joules (J) repeated once and followed by countershock with maximum voltage (360 J). After the initial countershocks, IV access is obtained and intubation performed, if it can be easily accomplished quickly by skilled personnel. If tracheal intubation causes delay in further essential resuscitative measures, bag-valve-mask ventilation is substituted at this point. As soon as tracheal intubation or IV access is established, the patient should receive 1 mg of epinephrine 1:10,000 solution (10 ml), followed by another maximum countershock (360 J). If ventricular tachycardia/fibrillation continues, a lidocaine bolus of 1 mg/kg IV is given and followed by an additional countershock. Subsequent lidocaine boluses (0.5 mg/kg) every 8 minutes to a total of 3 mg/kg (each followed by a countershock) may be given. Alternative drug therapy is bretylium in repetitive doses of 5 mg/kg, 10 mg/kg, and 10 mg/kg, with a countershock after each drug bolus. If the patient transiently converts to a stable rhythm after countershock but the dysrhythmia returns, the same countershock is applied again. Initial infusion dosage for lidocaine should be 2 to 4 mg/min and 2 mg/min for bretylium.

Ventricular Fibrillation and Pulseless Ventricular Tachycardia

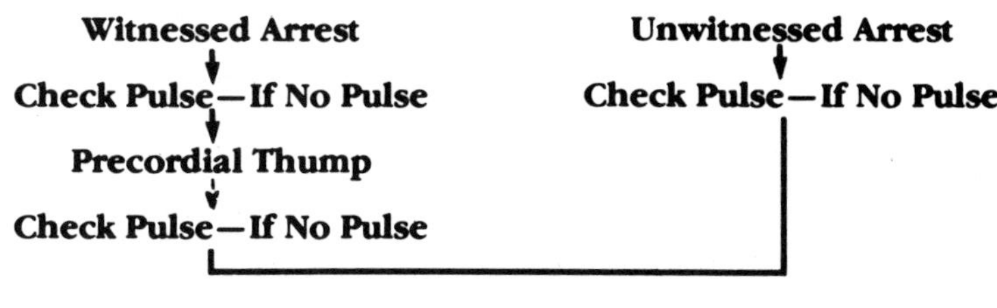

CPR Until a Defibrillator Is Available

↓

Check Monitor for Rhythm—if VF or VT

↓

Defibrillate 200 Joules

↓

Defibrillate 200-300 Joules

↓

Defibrillate With up to 360 Joules

↓

CPR If No Pulse

↓

Establish IV Access

↓

Epinephrine, 1:10,000, 0.5-1.0 mg IV Push

↓

Intubate If Possible

↓

Defibrillate With up to 360 Joules

↓

Lidocaine, 1 mg/kg IV Push

↓

Defibrillate With up to 360 Joules

↓

Bretylium, 5 mg/kg IV Push

↓

(Consider Bicarbonate)

↓

Defibrillate With up to 360 Joules

↓

Bretylium, 10 mg/kg IV Push

↓

Defibrillate With up to 360 Joules

↓

Repeat Lidocaine or Bretylium

↓

Defibrillate With up to 360 Joules

Figure 92-1 Suggested treatment of ventricular fibrillation (*VF*) and pulseless ventricular tachycardia (*VT*) is demonstrated. The flow of the algorithm presumes that VF or pulseless VT is continuing. The algorithm represents suggested management only. Some patients may require care not specified in the figure. (Amerian Heart Association: Standards and guidelines for cardiopulmonary resuscitation and emergency cardiac care. *JAMA* 1986; 255:2841)

In a patient with persistently unresponsive ventricular fibrillation or pulseless ventricular tachycardia, epinephrine should be administered at 5 to 10 minute intervals. Arterial blood gas analysis should be used at the earliest possible time for decisions on bicarbonate therapy.

PRECORDIAL THUMP

The precordial thump is recommended when ventricular fibrillation or ventricular tachycardia are observed while the patient is monitored. Although spontaneous conversion with this technique is low, the minimal risk and insignificant time expenditure make it an acceptable initial maneuver.

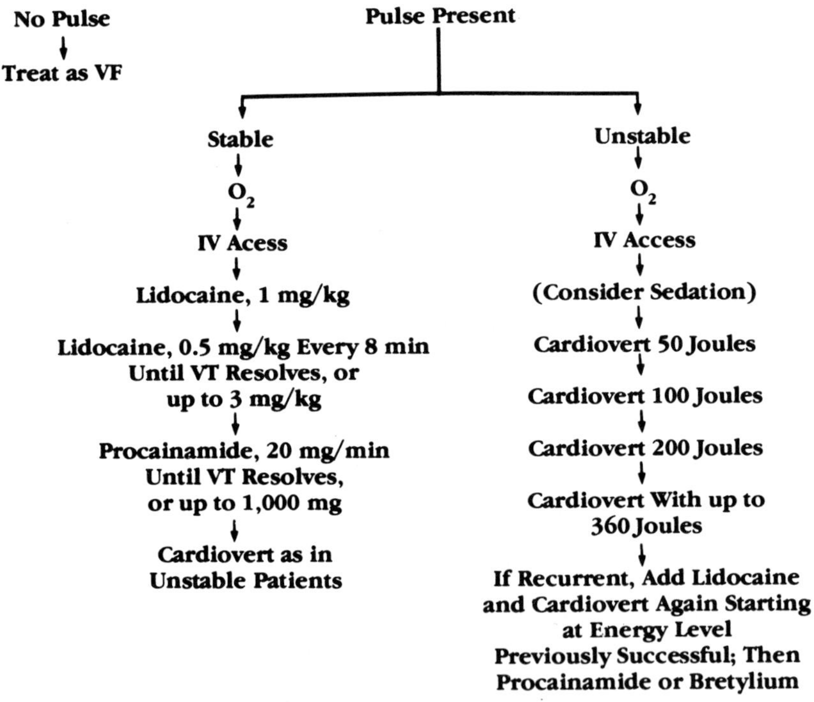

Figure 92-2 Suggested treatment of sustained ventricular tachycardia (VT) is demonstrated. The flow of the algorithm presumes that VT is continuing. Unstable patients include those with chest pain, dyspnea, hypotension (systolic BP < 90 mm Hg), congestive heart failure, ischemia, or myocardial infarction. The algorithm represents suggested management only. Some patients may require care not specified in the figure. (American Heart Association: Standards and guidelines for cardiopulmonary resuscitation and emergency cardiac care. *JAMA* 1986; 255:2841)

Asystole

If Rhythm Is Unclear and Possibly Ventricular Fibrillation, Defibrillate as for VF. If Asystole is Present

↓

Continue CPR

↓

Establish IV Access

↓

Epinephrine, 1:10,000, 0.5-1.0 mg IV Push

↓

Intubate When Possible

↓

Atropine, 1.0 mg IV Push (Repeated in 5 min)

↓

(Consider Bicarbonate)

↓

Consider Pacing

Figure 92-3 Suggested treatment of asystole is demonstrated.The flow of the algorithm presumes that asystole is continuing. The algorithm represents suggested management only. Some patients may require care not specified in the figure. (American Heart Association: Standards and guidelines for cardiopulmonary resuscitation and emergency cardiac care. *JAMA* 1986; 255:2841)

Electromechanical Dissociation

Continued CPR

↓

Establish IV Acess

↓

Epinephrine, 1:10,000, 0.5-1.0 mg IV Push

↓

Intubate When Possible

↓

(Consider Bicarbonate)

↓

Consider Hypovolemia,
Cardiac Tamponade,
Tension Pneumothorax,
Hypoxemia,
Acidosis,
Pulmonary Embolism

Figure 92-4 Suggested treatment of electromechanical dissociation (EMD) is demonstrated. The flow of the algorithm presumes that EMD is continuing. The algorithm represents suggested management only. Some patients may require care not specified in the figure. (American Heart Association: Standards and guidelines for cardiopulmonary resuscitation and emergency cardiac care. *JAMA* 1986; 255:2841)

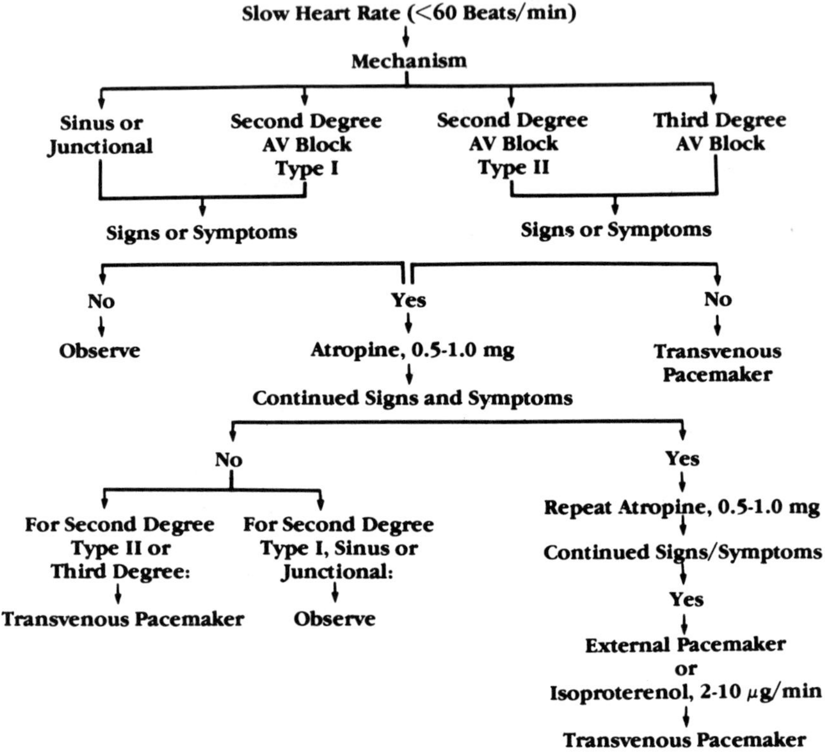

Figure 92-5 Suggested treatment of hemodynamically significant bradycardia is demonstrated. Significant signs and symptoms include hypotension (systolic blood pressure < 90 mm Hg), premature ventricular contractions, altered mental status, chest pain, dyspnea, ischemia, or myocardial infarction. The use of isoproterenol should be considered as temporizing therapy only. The algorithm represents suggested management only. Some patients may require care not specified in the figure. (American Heart Association: Standards and guidelines for cardiopulmonary resuscitation and emergency cardiac care. *JAMA* 1986; 255:2841)

TRACHEAL DRUG ADMINISTRATION

If an endotracheal tube has been inserted but IV access has not yet been obtained, many drugs used in resuscitation can be introduced effectively by the tracheal route. The ideal mechanism is to insert an IV connector tubing catheter into the endotracheal tube and inject the drug into the lower trachea, bypassing the endotracheal tube. Vigorous bag ventilation is then performed

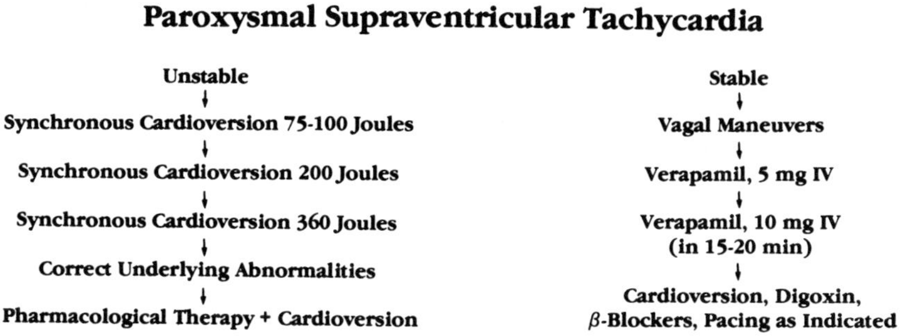

Paroxysmal Supraventricular Tachycardia

Unstable
↓
Synchronous Cardioversion 75-100 Joules
↓
Synchronous Cardioversion 200 Joules
↓
Synchronous Cardioversion 360 Joules
↓
Correct Underlying Abnormalities
↓
Pharmacological Therapy + Cardioversion

Stable
↓
Vagal Maneuvers
↓
Verapamil, 5 mg IV
↓
Verapamil, 10 mg IV (in 15-20 min)
↓
Cardioversion, Digoxin, β-Blockers, Pacing as Indicated

Figure 92-6 Suggested treatment of paroxysmal supraventricular tachycardia (PSVT) is demonstrated. The flow of the algorithm presumes that PSVT is continuing. The algorithm represents suggested management only. Some patients may require care not specified in the figure. (American Heart Association: Standards and guidelines for cardiopulmonary resuscitation and emergency cardiac care. *JAMA* 1986; 255:2841)

to disperse the medication into the lower airway for more rapid absorption. In addition to epinephrine, other drugs that can be introduced by this route include atropine, lidocaine, naloxone, bretylium, and diazepam.

PACEMAKERS

Pacemakers are used in patients with an atrioventricular block or narrow complex sinus bradycardia, and in whom initial therapy with atropine fails. Noninvasive transcutaneous pacers may allow temporary pacing capability with subsequent elective insertion of the transvenous pacer. Emergency temporary transvenous pacer placement may be difficult, particularly in patients with low cardiac output, but may be facilitated by fluoroscopy.

ACQUIRED IMMUNE DEFICIENCY SYNDROME (AIDS)

Patients who may be human immunodeficiency virus positive (HIV+) place the critical care clinician at significant risk. Since it is very difficult to predict which patients are HIV+ the following measures should be strongly considered in the resuscitation of all patients: [1] gloves; [2] eye protection; and [3] extra vigilance to avoid needle sticks.

TREATMENT ALGORITHMS

The American Heart Association advanced cardiac life support algorithm for ventricular fibrillation, ventricular tachycardia, asystole, electromechanical

Ventricular Ectopy

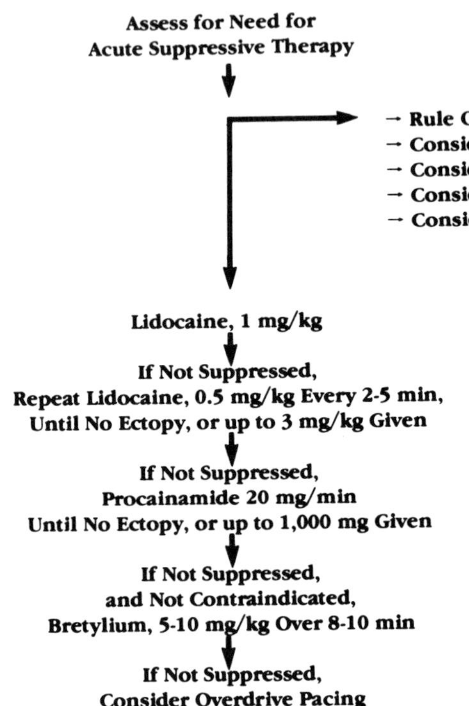

Once Ectopy Resolved, Maintain as Follows:
After Lidocaine, 1 mg/kg...Lidocaine Drip, 2 mg/min
After Lidocaine, 1-2 mg/kg...Lidocaine Drip, 3 mg/min
After Lidocaine, 2-3 mg/kg...Lidocaine Drip, 4 mg/min
After Procainamide...Procainamide Drip, 1-4 mg/min (Check Blood Level)
After Bretylium...Bretylium Drip, 2 mg/min

Figure 92-7 Suggested treatment of ventricular ectopy is demonstrated. The flow of the algorithm presumes that ventricular ectopy is continuing. The algorithm represents suggested management only. Some patients may require care not specified in the figure. (American Heart Association: Standards and guidelines for cardiopulmonary resuscitation and emergency cardiac care. *JAMA* 1986; 255:2841)

dissociation, bradycardia, supraventricular tachycardia, and ventricular ectopy are shown in Figures 92-1 through 92-7.

For more information, please see Chapter 12 in Civetta JM, Taylor RW, Kirby RR: Critical Care. *Philadelphia: J. B. Lippincott, 1988*

BIBLIOGRAPHY

American Heart Association: Standards and guidelines for cardiopulmonary resuscitation and emergency cardiac care. JAMA 1986; 255:2841

Brillman J, Sanders A, Otto CW, et al: Comparison of epinephrine and phenylephrine for resuscitation and neurologic outcome of cardiac arrest in dogs. *Ann Emerg Med* 1987; 16:11

Dalsey WC, Syverud SA, Trott A: Transcutaneous cardiac pacing. *J Emerg Med* 1984; 1:201

Ewy GA: Current status of cardiopulmonary resuscitation. *Mod Concepts Cardiovasc Dis* 1984; 53:43

Feliciano DV, Mattox KL, Grahim JM, et al: Major complications of percutaneous subclavian vein catheters. *Am J Surg* 1979; 138:869

Luce JM, Cary JM, Ross BK, et al: New developments in cardiopulmonary resuscitation. *JAMA* 1980; 244:1366

Majernick TG, Bieniek R, Houston JB: Cervical spine movement during orotracheal intubation. *Ann Emerg Med* 1986; 15:417

Otto CW, Yakaitis RW: The role of epinephrine in CPR: A reappraisal. *Ann Emerg Med* 1984; 13:840

Ralston SH, Tacker WA, Showen L: Endotracheal versus intravenous epinephrine during electromechanical dissociation with CPR in dogs. *Ann Emerg Med* 1985; 14:1044

Sanders AB, Kern KB, Ewy GA, et al: Improved resuscitation from cardiac arrest with open-chest massage. *Ann Emerg Med* 1984; 13:672

Weaver WD, Copass MK, Bufi D, et al: Improved neurologic recovery and survival after early defibrillation. *Therapy and Prevention* 1984; 69:943

93 Whom to Resuscitate

Decisions concerning who should or should not be resuscitated involve multifactorial issues ranging from religious, moral, ethical, legal, humanistic, and medical ones to considerations of patients' rights, the effects on family, and even the availability of medical and financial resources. Decisions not to initiate or to discontinue resuscitation are, at best, based only on *probabilities* of success.

The decision to continue or discontinue resuscitation efforts is best informed by knowledge of published statistics, medical case reports, and, most importantly, the physician's clinical experience and judgment.

RATIONALES AGAINST UNIVERSAL RESUSCITATION

Excepting the perfunctory caveats about hypothermia and certain drug overdoses, the patient's condition is absolutely irreversible when he is found to be cold, stiff with rigor mortis, or with dependent lividity. Equally untreatable conditions are torso transection, complete incineration, decapitation, and decomposition.

It is unrealistic, extraordinarily expensive, and occasionally dangerous to respond to and treat *all* victims of cardiopulmonary arrest. Even when the arrest is witnessed, time estimates are fairly inaccurate. Minutes may have "seemed like hours" to those distraught relatives in the home or to hospital roommates who are anxiously awaiting help. Further, although witnesses report that the patient "went out" at the time of the initial call for help, upon closer questioning it may be revealed that the patient "was still breathing a little" just up to the time of arrival of the rescuers. Perhaps the best indicator of down time is the response to the initial therapy.

If an appropriate electrical depolarization (standard countershock) is delivered immediately to a patient with ventricular fibrillation, the heart should usually be able to return to nearly normal function within seconds (as indicated by return of a normal sinus rate and rhythm, tight QRS complexes, and adequate spontaneous blood pressure). If, however, defibrillation is delayed by 1 or 2 minutes, even with CPR, the heart may be compromised. If the defibrillation is delayed even more (say 5 to 10 minutes), the residual post-defibrillatory state may reflect severe compromise manifested by spontaneous return of only a wide, bizarre ventricular complex on EKG that is not accompanied either by detectable atrial depolarization or by an adequate contractile state (pulseless).

THE TERMINALLY ILL PATIENT

In the hospital setting, a comatose patient with known hypercalcemia and a histologically diagnosed, metastatic terminal cancer who presents to a physician after having made a Living Will is best served by no therapy at all. But the same patient who presents with only a hearsay diagnosis (and little else) should be resuscitated pending further data. It is to be hoped that decisions not to resuscitate should involve consensus and planning before the arrest and not at the time of arrest.

What about "slow code," and "code gray" orders? Some practitioners refer to this process as "going through the motions" to satisfy the family (and the reader of the chart) that aggressive care was provided, when in fact it was not. In most medicolegal opinions, such procedures represent fairly hazardous attempts to equivocate. One should attempt to give full resuscitation efforts or none at all.

NEUROLOGIC CRIPPLES

It has been argued that there is potential for creating a population of neurological cripples. Generally, however, patients either survive awake and neurologically intact or have progressive cerebral edema and systemic deterioration over the next 48 to 72 hours. Most people who die do so within a week of their resuscitation attempt or are declared to be brain dead.

BIBLIOGRAPHY

Bedell SE, Pelle D, Maher PL, et al: Do-not-resuscitate orders for critically ill patients in the hospital. How are they used and what is their impact? *JAMA* 1986; 256:233

Brain Resuscitation Clinical Trial I Study Group: Neurologic recovery after cardiac arrest: The effect of ischemia. *Crit Care Med* 1985; 13:930

Lipton HL: Do-not-resuscitate decisions in a community hospital: Incidence, implications, and outcomes. *JAMA* 1986; 256:1164

McIntyre KM: Medicolegal considerations in cardiopulmonary resuscitation and emergency cardiac care. In Medical Control in Emergency Medical Services Systems. National Research Council, pp 116–119. Washington, DC, National Academy Press, 1981

Weaver WD, Cobb LA, Hallstrom AP, et al: Considerations for improving survival from out-of-hospital cardiac arrest. *Ann Emerg Med* 1986; 15:1181

94 Termination of Resuscitation

ON WHAT SHOULD THE DECISION TO TERMINATE CPR BE BASED?

Cardiopulmonary resuscitation should be terminated if inappropriately initiated. It should not be initiated on those who are obviously dead or when a do-not-resuscitate (DNR) order has been instituted in accordance with appropriate hospital policy, is in effect.

Cardiopulmonary resuscitation should be terminated when it is determined that the cardiovascular system is unresponsive and hence further efforts are futile: [1] 30 minutes of CPR/emergency cardiac care have passed without resumption of intrinsic cardiac output, and [2] bradyasystolic arrest rhythms persist despite attempted myocardial pacing (*i.e.*, external, transvenous, or transthoracic) or intravenous pharmacologic therapy (*i.e.*, atropine or epinephrine), or both. If the decision is made to continue with further resuscitative efforts, it should be based on the consideration that the underlying factors precipitating cardiac arrest (*i.e.*, hypothermia, drug ovedose, or electrolyte disturbance) are treatable; hence, continued resuscitation may be successful. Beyond the two aforesaid conditions, determining when resuscitation is futile becomes more difficult. A consideration of the medical history in addition to the other prearrest and arrest factors that have a negative influence on survival is helpful in formulating this decision (Table 94-1).

SHOULD THE COST OF PATIENT CARE OR THE POSTRESUSCITATION QUALITY OF LIFE BE CONSIDERED IN THE DECISION TO STOP CPR?

In this era of increasing fiscal restraint, cost is a frequently discussed reason for terminating or limiting care. The dramatization of the rising cost of medical care has contributed to the concern that prolonged resuscitation may result in a drawn-out death in the intensive care unit. However, most patients who

TABLE 94-1 PREDICTORS OF MORTALITY FOLLOWING CARDIAC ARREST AND ATTEMPTED CPR

Prearrest
Homebound life-style
Cancer
Cerebrovascular accident with residual neurologic deficit
Renal failure
Sepsis
Left ventricular dysfunction
Hypotension (systolic blood pressure less than 100 mm Hg)
Metabolic acidosis
Recurrent cardiac arrest during the same hospital stay
Arrest
Unwitnessed collapse
CPR delayed more than 4 minutes
Bradyasystolic arrest rhythms (asystole electromechanical dissociation/pulseless idioventricular rhythm)
Fine ventricular fibrillation (ventricular fibrillation amplitude <0.2 mV)
CPR for more than 15 minutes
Dilated pupils despite adequate ventilation and external chest compression
Endotrachel intubation

die do so within 24 hours of the resuscitation effort. Two problems arise when using postresuscitation quality of life in the decision to stop CPR: First, it is impossible to predict which patients will suffer these complications; and second, the termination of treatment based on the quality of life is a special judgment reserved for informed patients. Cost and the postresuscitation quality of life have no bearing on the judgment of when to stop CPR.

WHO SHOULD DECIDE TO TERMINATE CPR?

This decision rests with the physician who has the primary medicolegal responsibility for the patient during the cardiac arrest.

LEGAL IMPLICATIONS OF TERMINATING CPR

There have been surprisingly few litigations involving CPR because of the low expectations and the lack of precedent-setting cases in decisions involving the termination of CPR. Under the principle of proximate cause, it is nearly impossible to demonstrate that terminating CPR resulted in the death of a patient who has already suffered a cardiac arrest. All medical care should be stopped when the patient is determined to be legally dead. A legal pronouncement of death is made when an individual has sustained either [1] irreversible cessation of all functions of the entire brain, including the brain stem, or [2] irreversible cessation of cardiopulmonary functions. During CPR the determination that irreversible cessation of all brain functions has occurred is not possible; hence, the responsiveness of the cardiovascular system is used to determine death. The finding of cardiovascular unresponsiveness (as determined using acceptable medical standards) indicates that the heart has died, and there is not legal purpose to be served in continuing with further procedures or therapeutic intervention.

A prime consideration in withholding or terminating treatment is the competent refusal of such treatment by an individual. In the presence of a Living Will the physician may feel more comfortable in not beginning, restricting, or terminating resuscitation. Do-not-resuscitate orders should be honored when appropriately implemented and documented. Preferably a resuscitation would never begin on such a patient, but, if begun before the DNR orders are discovered and verified, it should be stopped expeditiously once this is realized. The physician will have the least legal risk in terminating a resuscitative effort by practicing high-quality medical care cosistent with the medical community standards. This should be done in a compassionate, caring manner and, when possible, in accordance with the patient's desires and the family's participation.

For more information, please see Chapter 13 in Civetta JM, Taylor RW, Kirby RR: Critical Care. *Philadelphia: J. B. Lippincott, 1988*

BIBLIOGRAPHY

Bedell SE, Delbanco TL, Cook EF, et al: Survival after cardiopulmonary resuscitation in the hospital. *N Engl J Med* 1983; 309:569

Eisenberg MS, Bergner L, Hallstrom A: Cardiac arrest in the community: Importance of rapid provision and implications for program planning. *JAMA* 1979:241:1905

Eisendrath SJ, Jonsen AR: The living will: Help or hindrance? *JAMA* 1983; 249:2054

Eliastam M: When to stop CPR. In Auerbach PS, Budossi SA (eds): *Cardiac Arrest and CPR,* pp 215–219. Rockville, MD, Aspen Publishing Co, 1983

Goldberg AH: Cardiopulmonary arrest. *N Engl J Med* 1974; 290:381

Guidelines for the determination of death. *JAMA* 1981; 246:2184

Herskovits v. Group Health, 99 Wn. 2d 609, 664 P.2d 474 (1983)

Hollingsworth JH: The results of cardiopulmonary resuscitation: A three year university hospital experience. *Ann Intern Med* 1969; 71:459

McIntyre KM: Medicolegal aspects of decision-making in resuscitation and life support. *Cardiovasc Rev Rep* 1983; 4:46

Mackintosh AF, Crabb ME, Grainer R, et al: The Brighton resuscitation ambulances: Review of 40 consecutive survivors of out-of-hospital cardiac arrest. *Br Med J* 1978; 1:1115

Miles SH, Cranford R, Schultz AL: The do-not-resuscitate order in a teaching hospital: Considerations and a suggested policy. *Ann Intern Med* 1982; 96:660

Nachlas MM, Miller DI: Closed-chest cardiac resuscitation in patients with acute myocardial infarction. *Am Heart J* 1965; 69:448

Peatfield RC, Sillet RW, Taylor D, et al: Survival after cardiac arrest in hospital. *Lancet* 1977; 2:1223

Smith JP, Bodai BI: Guidelines for discontinuing prehospital CPR in the emergency department—A review. *Ann Emerg Med* 1985; 14:1093

Standards and guidelines for cardiopulmonary resuscitation and emergency cardiac care. *JAMA* 1986; 255:2980

Stemmler EJ: Cardiac resuscitation: A 1-year study of patients resuscitated within a university hospital. *Ann Intern Med* 1965; 63:613

Weaver WD, Cobb LA, Dennis D, et al: Amplitude of ventricular fibrillation waveform and outcome after cardiac arrest. *Ann Intern Med* 1985; 102:53

Index

Page numbers followed by *f* indicate illustrations; those followed by *t* indicate tabular material.

ISBN 0-397-51030-6